Essential Interventional Cardiology

Essential Interventional Cardiology

Second Edition

MICHAEL S. NORELL, MD, FRCP
Consultant Interventional Cardiologist & PCI Programme Director
The Heart & Lung Center
Wolverhampton
UK

JOHN PERRINS, MD, BSc, FRCP, FACC
Consultant Cardiologist
Leeds Nuffield Hospital
Leeds, UK

BERNHARD MEIER, MD, FACC, FESC
Professor and Chairman of Cardiology
Swiss Cardiovascular Center Bern
University Hospital
Bern, Switzerland

A. MICHAEL LINCOFF, MD
Professor of Medicine
Cleveland Clinic Lerner College of Medicine of Case Western
    Reserve University
Department of Cardiovascular Medicine
The Cleveland Clinic Foundation
Cleveland, OH

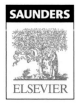

SAUNDERS

ELSEVIER

SAUNDERS
ELSEVIER

1600 John F. Kennedy Blvd.
Ste 1800
Philadelphia, PA 19103-2899

ESSENTIAL INTERVENTIONAL CARDIOLOGY   978-0-7020-2981-3
Copyright © 2008, 2001 by Saunders an imprint of Elsevier Ltd.

Notice

Knowledge and best practice in this field are constantly changing. As new research and
experience broaden our knowledge, changes in practice, treatment, and drug therapy
may become necessary or appropriate. Readers are advised to check the most current
information provided (i) on procedures featured or (ii) by the manufacturer of each product
to be administered, to verify the recommended dose or formula, the method and duration of
administration, and contraindications. It is the responsibility of the practitioner, relying on
his or her experience and knowledge of the patient, to make diagnoses, to determine
dosages and the best treatment for each individual patient, and to take all appropriate safety
precautions. To the fullest extent of the law, neither the Publisher nor the Editors assume
any liability for any injury and/or damage to persons or property arising out of or related to
any use of the material contained in this book.

Library of Congress Cataloging-in-Publication Data

Essential interventional cardiology / Michael S. Norell ... [et al.]. -- 2nd ed.
    p. ; cm.
    Includes bibliographical references.
    ISBN 978-0-7020-2981-3
    1. Heart--Diseases--Treatment. 2. Coronary heart disease--Treatment.
3. Cardiology. I. Norell, Michael S.
    [DNLM: 1. Cardiovascular Diseases--therapy. 2.
Catheterization--methods. WG 166 E7785 2008]

RC683.8.E77 2008
616.1'2--dc22

                                                                    2007039758

Acquisitions Editor: Natasha Andjelkovic
Developmental Editor: Isabel Trudeau
Project Manager: Bryan Hayward
Design Direction: Gene Harris

Working together to grow
libraries in developing countries

www.elsevier.com | www.bookaid.org | www.sabre.org

ELSEVIER   BOOK AID International   Sabre Foundation

Printed in United States of America

Last digit is the print number: 9   8   7   6   5   4   3   2   1

Contributors

Sorin Brener, MD, FACC
Director, Angiography
  Core Laboratory
Interventional Cardiology
The Cleveland Clinic
  Foundation
Cleveland, OH
*Chapter 20: Percutaneous
Coronary Intervention in Acute
Myocardial Infarction*

John Caplin
Consultant Cardiologist
and Clinical Governance
Lead Castle Hill Hospital
Cottingham East Yorkshire
*Chapter 36: Balloon
pericardiotomy*

Ryan D. Christofferson, MD
Interventional Fellow
  Cardiology
Cleveland Clinic
Cleveland, OH
*Chapter 22: Percutaneous
Coronary Intervention for
Chronic Total Occlusions*

Antonio Columbo, MD
Director Cardiac Cath Lab
and Interventional
  Cardiology Unit
San Raffaele University
  Hospital and EMO
  Centro Cuore Columbus
Milano, Italy
*Chapter 23: Percutaneous
Coronary Intervention for
Bifurcation Lesions*

**James Cotton, MBBS,
MD, MRCP**
Honorary Senior Lecturer
University of Birmingham
Consultant Cardiologist
Heart and Lung Centre
Wolverhampton, UK
*Chapter 11: Arterial Puncture
Site Closure and Aftercare*

Alain Cribier
Professor of Medicine
Cardiology, University
  Hospital
University of Rouen
Chief of the Department of
  Cardiology
University Hospital Charles
  Nicolle
Rouen, France
*Chapter 32: Aortic Valve
intervention*

Michael Cusack
Consultant
Cardiologist Heart
  & Lung Centre
New Cross Hospital
Wolverhampton
*Chapter 10: Pressure Wire
and Related Technologies*

**Adam de Belder, BSc, MD,
MRCP**
Consultant
Cardiologist Brighton and
  Sussex University Hospital
Brighton, UK
*Chapter 19: Circulatory
Support in Percutaneous
Coronary Intervention*

**Mark Andrew de Belder,
MA, MD, FRCP**
Consultant Cardiologist
The James Cook
  University Hospital
Middlesbrough, UK
*Chapter 14: Directional and
Rotational Atherectomy*

**Brendan Duffy, MB,
MRCPI**
Interventional Cardiology
  Fellow
Cleveland Clinic
Cleveland, OH
*Chapter 22: Percutaneous
Coronary Intervention for
Chronic Total Occlusions*

**Duncan Ettles, MD, FRCP
(Ed), FRCR**
Consultant
Cardiovascular and
  Interventional
  Radiologist
Department of Radiology
  Hull Royal Infirmary
Kingston upon Hull
East Yorkshire
*Chapter 30: Percutaneous
Vascular Intervention in the
Venous System*

Nezar M. Falluji, MD, MPH
*Chapter 13: Restenosis and
In-Stent Restenosis*

John M. Galla, MD
Fellow
Cardiovascular Medicine
  Cleveland Clinic
Cleveland, OH
*Chapter 6: Adjunctive
Pharmacotherapy During
Percutaneous Coronary
Intervention*

Anthony Gershlick
Consultant
  Cardiologist/Honorary
  Senior Lecturer
Cardiology
Glenfield Hospital
  Leicester
*Chapter 40: Current Major
Trials in Interventional
Cardiology*

**Ever Grech, MB BS, MD,
FRCP, FACC**
Consultant Cardiologist
Honorary Clininical
  Lecturer
*Chapter 37: Foreign body
retrieval*

v

Contributors

Roger V. Hall, MD
Professor of Clinical
  Cardiology
University of East Anglia
Norwich
*Chapter 31: Percutaneous
Mitral Valvuloplasty and Repair*

Jagath Herath, MD
Consultant Cardiologist
Provincial General
  Hospital, Badulla
Badulla
Sri Lanka
*Chapter 25: Percutaneous
Coronary Intervention in
Saphenous Vein Graft Disease*

**Richard R Heuser, MD,
FACC, FACP, FESC**
Clinical Professor of
  Medicine Director of
  Interventional Fellowship
  Program
University of Arizona
College of Medicine
Director of Cardiology
Chief of Cardiac
  Catherization Laboratory
St. Luke's Hospital and
  Medical Center
Phoenix, Arizona
*Chapter 28: Percutaneous
Management of Aortic and
Peripheral Vascular Disease*

David Hildick-Smith
Consultant
Cardiologist
Cardiology Department
  Royal Devon & Exeter
  Hospital
Exeter, UK
*Chapter 32: Aortic Valve
intervention*

David R. Holmes, Jr., MD
Consultant, Cardiovascular
  Disease Professor of
  Medicine
Mayo Clinic,
Mayo Medical School
Rochester, MN
*Chapter 24: Percutaneous
Coronary Intervention in Small
Vessels*

Ioannis Iakovou, MD
Attending Physician
Army Hospital of
  Thessaloniki
Thessaloniki, Greece
*Chapter 23: Percutaneous
Coronary Intervention for
Bifurcation Lesions*

**Samir R. Kapadia, MD,
FACC**
Staff and Director,
  Interventional Cardiology
  Fellowship
Cleveland Clinic
  Foundation
Cleveland, OH
*Chapter 35: Septal ablation for
HCM*

Juhana Karha, MD
Fellow in Cardiovascular
  Medicine
Cleveland Clinic
Cleveland, OH
*Chapter 20: Percutaneous
Coronary Intervention in Acute
Myocardial Infarction*

**Sadia Khan, MBBS
(Karachi); FCPS Medicine,
FCPS Cardiology
(Pakistan).**
Consultant Cardiologist
Assistant Professor
Department of Medicine
Aga Khan University
  Hospital, Karachi
Cardiology Section
Aga Khan University
  Hospital
Karachi
Pakistan
*Chapter 18: Laser Use in
Percutaneous Coronary
Intervention*

**Saib Khogali, MB.ChB.,
MD, FRCP**
Consultant Interventional
  Cardiologist
The Heart and Lung Center
New Cross Hospital
Wolverhampton
UK
*Chapter 2: Pathology of
Balloon Dilatation*

Young-Hak Kim, MD, PhD
Division of Cardiology,
  Asan Medical Center,
Seoul, Korea
*Chapter 21: Percutaneous
Coronary Intervention in Left
Main Stem Disease*

Pramod Kuchulakanti, MD
*Chapter 17: Intracoronary
Brachytherapy*

**Babu Kunadian, MBBS,
MRCP**
Specialist Registrar in
  Cardiology
Mersey deanery Liverpool,
  United Kingdom
*Chapter 14: Directional
and Rotational Atherectomy*

Harry M. Lever, MD
Staff Cardiologist and
  HCM Specialist
Cleveland Clinic
  Foundation
Cleveland, OH
*Chapter 35: Septal ablation for
HCM*

A. Michael Lincoff, MD
Vice Chairman,
  Department of
  Cardiovascular Medicine
Cleveland Clinic
Cleveland, OH
*Chapter 6: Adjunctive
Pharmacotherapy During
Percutaneous Coronary
Intervention*

Ted Lo
Consultant Cardiologist
  Cardiothoracic Center
North Staffordshire
  Hospital Stoke on Trent
Staffordshire
*Chapter 5: Vascular Access for
Percutaneous Coronary
Intervention*

Matthew Lovell
PhD Student with
  Dr. Mathur
*Chapter 38: Gene therapy and
stem cell technology*

Iqbal Malik
Honorary Senior Lecturer
Department of Cardiology
Imperial College
Consultant Cardiologist
Imperial College Healthcare
  NHS Trust
London, UK
*Chapter 26: Carotid Artery
  Stenting*

**Anthony Mathur, MA, MB,
Bchir, MRCP, PhD**
Senior Lecturer and
  Consultant Cardiologist
*Chapter 38: Gene therapy and
  stem cell technology*

**Bernhard Meier, MD,
FACC, FESC**
Professor and Head
  of Cardiology
Department of Cardiology
Swiss Cardiovascular Center
Bern University Hospital
Bern
Switzerland
*Chapter 34: ASD, PFO and left
  atrial appendage closure*

David J. Moliterno, MD
Chief, Cardiovascular
  Medicine Professor and
  Vice Chair
Internal Medicine
  University of Kentucky
Lexington, KY
*Chapter 13: Restenosis and
  In-Stent Restenosis*

Roger KG Moore, MD
Consultant Interventional
  Cardiologist
Royal Preston Hospital
Preston Lancashire
United Kingdom
*Chapter 16: Cutting Balloon
  Angioplasty*

**Tony Nicholson, BSc,
MSc, MB ChB, FRCR**
Consultant
Vascular Radiologist
Radiology, Jubillee Wing
  Leeds Teaching Hospitals
Leeds, Yorkshire UK
*Chapter 29: Coarctation of the
  Aorta*

James Nolan
Consultant Cardiologist
  Cardiothoracic Center
North Staffordshire
  Hospital Stoke on Trent
Staffordshire
*Chapter 5: Vascular Access for
  Percutaneous Coronary
  Intervention*

**Michael S. Norell, MD,
FRCP**
Consultant Interventional
  Cardiologist & Programme
  Director
The Heart and Lung Center
Wolverhampton
UK
*Chapter 1: History,
  Development and Current
  Advances in Coronary
  Intervention*

**Andrew T. L. Ong, MBBS,
PhD, FRACP, FCSANZ,
FESC, FACC**
Clinical Senior Lecturer
  University of Sydney
Sydney, NSW
Consultant Interventional
  Cardiologist
Westmead Hospital
Westmead, NSW
Australia
Chapter 8: Drug-Eluting Stents

Seung-Jung Park, MD, PhD
Division of Cardiology,
  Asan Medical Center,
  Seoul, Korea
*Chapter 21: Percutaneous
  Coronary Intervention in Left
  Main Stern Disease*

**John Perrins, MD BSc
FRCP FACC**
Consultant Cardiologist
Leeds Nuffield Hospital
Leeds
UK
*Chapter 7: Intracoronary
  Stenting*

Raphael A. Perry
Clinical Lecturer
Liverpool University
  Medical School
Consultant
Cardiologist & Associate
  Medical Director
  Cardiothoracic Centre
Liverpool NHS Trust
  Liverpool, UK
*Chapter 16: Cutting Balloon
  Angioplasty*

Srinivasa P. Potluri
*Chapter 27: Percutaneous
  Management of Renal Arterial
  Disease*

**Bernard Prendergast,
B Med Sci, BM, BS, DM,
FRCP**
Consultant
Cardiologist
Wythenshawe Hospital
Manchester, UK
*Chapter 31: Percutaneous
  Mitral Valvuloplasty and Repair*

**Shakeel Ahmed Qureshi,
MS ChB, FRCP**
Consultant
Paediatric Cardiologist
Department of Congenital
  Heart Disease
Evelina Children's Hospital
Guy's & St Thomas
  Hospital NHS Tru
London, UK
*Chapter 33: Pulmonary
  valvuloplasty*

Contributors

Stephen Ramee, MD
Section Head,
  Interventional Cardiology
Director, Cardiac
  Catheterization
  Laboratory
*Chapter 27: Percutaneous
  Management of Renal Arterial
  Disease*

**David R. Ramsdale, MD,
FRCP**
Consultant Cardiologist
Cardiothoracic Center
Liverpool
*Chapter 37: Foreign
  body retrieval*

**Peter Schofield, MBChB,
FRCP, MD, FACC, FESC**
Lecturer
Department of Medicine
Cambridge University
  Consultant Cardiologist
Papworth Hospital
Cambridge, England
*Chapter 18: Laser Use in
  Percutaneous Coronary
  Intervention*

**Arun Sebastian, MRCP,
FRCR**
Radiologist
Department of Radiology
Hull Royal Infirmary
Kingston upon Hull
East Yorkshire
*Chapter 30: Percutaneous
  Vascular Intervention in the
  Venous System*

Amy L. Seidel, MD
Fellow, Interventional
  Cardiology Emory
  University Hospital
Atlanta, GA
*Chapter 35: Septal ablation for
  HCM*

**Patrick W. Serruys,
MD, PhD**
Professor of Interventional
  Cardiology
Thoraxcenter Erasmus
  Medical Center
The Netherlands
Chapter 8: Drug-Eluting Stents

Norman Shaia, MD
Cardiologist
*Chapter 28: Percutaneous
  Management of Aortic and
  Peripheral Vascular Disease*

Man Fai Shiu, MD, FRCP
Honorary Associate
  Professor
Warwick University
Consultant Cardiologist
University Hospital
Coventry and
  Warwickshire
Coventry, England
*Chapter 15: PCI in the
  Presence of Significant
  Intraluminal Thrombus*

David Smith
Consultant Cardiologist
Cardiology Department
Royal Devon & Exeter
  Hospital
Barrack Road, Exeter
*Chapter 12: Complications
  of Percutaneous Coronary
  Intervention*

Paul Sorajja
Director, Cardiac Cath Lab
  and Interventional
Cardiology EMO Centro
  Cuore Columbus and
  San Raffaele Hospital
Milan
Italy
*Chapter 24: Percutaneous
  Coronary Intervention in Small
  Vessels*

**Rod Stables, MA, DM,
BM BCh, FRCP**
Consultant Cardiologist
Cardiothoracic Centre
Liverpool
Liverpool, UK
*Chapter 3: Patient Selection
  for Percutaneous Coronary
  Intervention*

**Ian R. Starkey, MBChB,
FRCP**
Consultant Cardiologist
  Western General Hospital
Edinburgh
Scotland
*Chapter 4: Investigation,
  Work-Up and Patient
  Preparation before PCI*

**Martyn Thomas, MD,
FRCP**
Interventional Cardiologist
BCIS President
Kings College Hospital
  Denmark Hill
London UK
*Chapter 39: Training and
  Practice Guidelines for
  Percutaneous Coronary
  Intervention*

**John Thomson, BM, BS,
Bmed Sci**
Consultant
Paediatric Cardiologist,
  Congenital Heart Disease,
  Leeds general Infirmary
University of Leed Leeds,
  Yorkshire, UK
*Chapter 33: Pulmonary
  valvuloplasty*

Murat Tuzcuu, MD
Vice Chairman
Department of
  Cardiovascular Medicine
Cleveland Clinic
  Cleveland, OH
*Chapter 35: Septal ablation for
  HCM*

Neal Uren
Consultant Cardiologist
Department of Cardiology
New Royal Infirmary of
  Edinburgh
Edinburgh
*Chapter 9: Intravascular
  Ultrasound in Coronary Artery
  Disease*

Contributors

Alec Vahanian
Head of Cardiology
  Department
Bichat Hospital
Professor of Cardiology
Department of Cardiology
  Paris Universite
VII Paris, France
*Chapter 31: Percutaneous
  Mitral Valvuloplasty and Repair*

Sophia Vaina, PhD, FESC
Consultant Interventional
  Cardiologist
1st Department of
  Cardiology
Athens Medical School
Hippokration Hospital
Athens, Greece
Chapter 8: Drug-Eluting Stents

Ron Waksman, MD
Associate Chief of
  Cardiology
Director of Experiental
  Angioplasty & New
  Technologies
Washington Hospital
  Center
Professor of Medicine
Cardiology
Georgetown University
Washington, DC
*Chapter 17: Intracoronary
  Brachytherapy*

Patrick L. Whitlow
Director, Interventional
  Cardiology
Cleveland Clinic
Cleveland, Ohio
*Chapter 22: Percutaneous
  Coronary Intervention for
  Chronic Total Occlusions*

Stephan Windecker, MD
Director, Invasive
  Cardiology
Department of Cardiology
University Hospital Bern
  Bern, Switzerland
*Chapter 34: ASD, PFO and left
  atrial appendage closure*

**Azfar G. Zaman, BSc,
MBChB, MD, FRCP**
Honorary Senior Lecturer
  Cardiology
Newcastle University
Consultant Cardiologist
Freeman Hospital
  Newcastle-upon-Tyne,
  UK
*Chapter 25: Percutaneous
  Coronary Intervention in
  Saphenous Vein Graft Disease*

Preface

The first edition of Essential Interventional Cardiology, published in 2001, described percutaneous coronary intervention (PCI) as it was practiced at the time. As anyone working in the field of cardiovascular intervention can attest, this is a rapidly advancing area of practice. Some techniques have forged ahead while others have fallen by the wayside. Coronary stenting with drug-eluting devices has become commonplace but their use has been tempered by issues of cost-effectiveness and late thrombosis. While a few procedures such as directional coronary atherectomy, intramyocardial laser and brachytherapy may have seen their day, they have been supplanted by percutaneous aortic valve replacement, gene therapy and carotid intervention.

In the age of the Internet a book such as this cannot necessarily keep at the cutting edge of the latest advances in a medical field as dynamic as cardiovascular intervention. Nevertheless, as with the first edition, we trust that its contents will lay the foundations upon which further knowledge and experience can be built. This second edition is aimed at the more experienced practitioner as well as the PCI trainee, and has been significantly updated and enlarged in order to include the many advances that this speciality has seen.

We have expanded its authorship to reflect the international impact that intervention has seen in the 30 years since Andreas Gruntzig made the first steps on this fascinating journey. Authors from across the world have been asked to contribute to this edition because of their knowledge and skill in particular aspects of PCI. In addition to updating previous chapters, others – such as that on primary PCI in AMI – have been enlarged in keeping with their increasing importance. Techniques such as carotid, renal, aortic and peripheral vascular intervention have also been incorporated as we recognise that the skill and expertise perfected by the coronary practitioner can equally well be put to good use in other vascular territories.

The first section of the new edition describes the fundamental principles of PCI in terms of its techniques and devices. A section on adjunctive technology is followed by an enlarged section devoted to PCI in particular lesion subsets or clinical scenarios. Similarly a section on non-coronary intervention has been expanded to include both peripheral vascular intervention as well as the treatment of cardiac conditions remote from the coronary vascular tree. As in the first edition, we have included a chapter devoted to guidelines that support best practice and training, whilst a comprehensive final chapter describes the major trials upon which much of our current PCI activity is founded.

We recognize that all our contributing authors are very busy in their daily practice of interventional cardiology and yet took the time to write a chapter on their particular area of expertise. For all their effort, time and enthusiasm, we are sincerely grateful.

Michael S. Norell
E. John Perrins
Bernhard Meier
A. Michael Lincoff

Contents

Contents

Contents

Section One

Fundamental
Techniques and
Devices for
Percutaneous
Coronary
Intervention

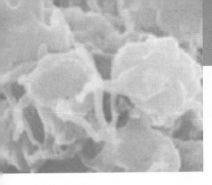

1

History, development and current activity in coronary intervention

MICHAEL S. NORELL

KEY POINTS

- Following the first percutaneous coronary angioplasty in 1977, growth in the procedure has been exponential.

- It is estimated that in 2000, approximately one million angioplasty procedures were undertaken worldwide.

- In the USA the number of percutaneous transluminal coronary angioplasties (PTCAs) performed annually exceeds that of coronary artery bypass graft (CABG) procedures.

- Despite major technological advances in equipment, and the increasing applicability of PTCA to a variety of patient subsets, the basic principles of the technique remain unchanged.

- UK rates for PTCA remain below those in the USA and Western Europe as a result of restricted resources and limited access to cardiological investigation.

HISTORICAL PERSPECTIVE

Cardiac catheterisation and coronary angiography

More than two decades have passed since Andreas Grüntzig (Fig. 1.1) first attempted the percutaneous relief of a coronary stenosis. This single event, representing the culmination of many years of experimentation, has now passed into legend. Percutaneous coronary revascularisation has emerged as a routine cardiac procedure, but the trials and tribulations of workers in the field of invasive cardiology, whose efforts led stepwise to that day in September 1977, are nevertheless worthy of review.

The era of invasive cardiac investigation and intervention began with the pioneering efforts of Forssman in 1929. The latter half of the previous century had seen Claude Bernard and later, Chaveau and Marey, develop the concept of 'cardiac catheterisation' in animal subjects employing intra-arterial or intravenous intubation in horses or dogs, but it was Forssman who demonstrated its feasibility and safety in humans. Taking advantage of his friendship with a nurse, Gerda Ditzen, he was able to cut down on his own cephalic vein and advance a rubber urethral catheter to his right atrium, documenting its progress with X-ray fluoroscopy. Right heart catheterisation was further developed with the work of Cournand and Ranges (1941), while investigation of the left heart proceeded via parasternal, subxiphoid, apical, suprasternal, transbronchial, papravertebral and transseptal approaches; until Zimmerman reported the results of retrograde left heart catheterisation in 1949.

Other developments also allowed cardiac catheterisation to progress to a stage recognisable in the present day. In 1953, Seldinger introduced his technique of entering arteries percutaneously. Serious peri-procedural cardiac arrhythmias could be addressed with closed chest cardiac compression (1960) and the

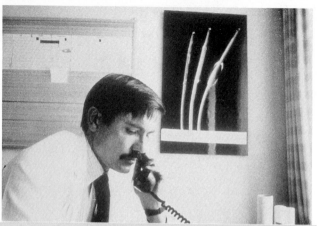

Figure 1.1:
Andreas Grüntzig.

introduction of direct current (DC) defibrillation by Lown in 1962. X-ray documentation had been limited to single plate exposures until the image intensifier coupled to film exposure at rapid frame rates resulted in the emergence of true cineangiography. Cardiac events could thereby be visualised in 'real time' incorporating less contrast volume and less radiation exposure to both patient and operator.

By the mid-1950s, visualisation of the coronary circulation had been achieved only by flush injection into the aortic root. A number of modifications to this technique were in use, including power injection into the sinus of Valsalva. It was during one such procedure in 1958, that an National Institute of Health (NIH) catheter inadvertently migrated into the right coronary artery and the subsequent injection of contrast opacified the vessel without the patient experiencing ill effects; Mason Sones had thereby demonstrated that selective coronary arteriography was possible. During the next few years, the first 1000 coronary angiograms were performed with only 2 deaths and a 2% incidence of ventricular fibrillation. Pre-formed polyethylene catheters were introduced in 1962 and were further modified by Judkins heralding the modern era of comprehensive percutaneous cardiac investigation.

Coronary angioplasty

Initial non-surgical attempts to address arterial obstruction focused on the peripheral circulation. Charles Dotter, together with Judkins in 1964, first reported a successful approach in leg arteries using co-axial sheaths to allow sequential dilatations. In an initial series of nine patients with severe perpheral ischaemia; six improved and four amputations were avoided. However, it was recognised that a better mechanical method of dilatation was required which exerted radial, rather than longitudinal force, on the vessel wall. A latex balloon was initially tried, but it was then appreciated that a non-elastic dilator was preferable. In 1974 Andreas Grüntzig developed a sausage-shaped polyvinyl chloride (PVC) balloon, mounted at the end of a catheter, which could be inflated to a predetermined diameter to exert a radial force of 3 to 5 atmospheres. This was initially used in the iliac and femoropopliteal system with satisfactory results, and was then extended to address disease in renal, basilar, coeliac and subclavian arteries.

Miniaturisation of this balloon system allowed it to be considered for coronary stenoses. Initial experiments in relieving mechanically produced strictures in canine coronaries, were reported in 1976. In May 1977, after careful planning, Grüntzig together with Richard Myler, decided to attempt balloon dilatation in a patient undergoing bypass surgery in San Francisco. During the operation, a balloon tipped catheter was passed retrogradely up the left anterior descending (LAD) artery from a distal arteriotomy. Following balloon expansion, no debris was produced downstream, and reinvestigation after surgery showed that vessel dilatation had been successful. A further 15 peri-operative cases were undertaken in San Francisco and Zurich before true percutaneous transluminal coronary angioplasty (PTCA) was attempted in the human subject.

Gruntzig's description of the first PTCA, performed in Zurich on 16 September 1977, was later quoted in an article by Hurst:

After working seven years to develop peripheral arterial dilatation, using animal experiments, post-mortem examinations and intraoperative dilatations, we were ready to use the technique for coronary artery dilatation in man .... It happened in September 1977 that we did coronary angiography on a 37-year-old insurance salesman with severe and exercise induced angina pectoris. The coronary angiography revealed single vessel disease with a proximal stenosis in the left anterior descending artery located immediately before the take-off of a large diagonal branch .... The guiding catheter was placed in the left coronary orifice and the dilatation catheter was inserted ... a roller pump (was in place to start coronary perfusion) through the main lumen of the dilatation catheter (if this became necessary). The stenosis was severe but the catheter slipped through it without resistance. (The balloon was inflated.) To the surprise of all of us, no ST elevation, ventricular fibrillation or even extrasystole occurred and the patient had no chest pain. At this moment, I decided not to start the coronary perfusion with the roller pump. After the first balloon deflation, the distal coronary pressure rose nicely. Encouraged by this positive response, I inflated the balloon a second time to relieve the residual gradient .... Everyone was surprised about the ease of the procedure and I started to realise that my dreams had come true.

This first case was reported in a letter to *The Lancet* in 1978. In it, Grüntzig prophetically stated:

This technique, if it proves successful in long-term follow-up studies, may widen the indications for coronary angiography and provide another treatment for patients with angina pectoris.

A report of the first 50 cases was published in *The New England Journal of Medicine* in 1979, indicating success in 32 patients. Stenosis severity fell from 84% to 34%, with a reduction in the translesional pressure gradient from 58 to 19 mmHg. Seven patients required emergency coronary artery bypass graft

(CABG); there was a 5% incidence of myocardial infarction, but no procedural deaths. In a book prepared before his untimely death in 1985, Grüntzig wrote:

> Whatever becomes of the method I have left one mark on medicine. Forssman demonstrated that man could place a catheter into his heart successfully. Mason Sones studied the coronary arteries selectively by angiography without significant mortality. I have shown that man can work therapeutically within the coronary arteries themselves in the face of an alert, comfortable patient.

In September 1977, coronary revascularisation had entered a new era of rapidly advancing technology. The subsequent 20 years have seen the subspecialty of interventional cardiology become one of the most exciting and rewarding fields in modern medicine.

TECHNOLOGICAL DEVELOPMENTS

The procedure of coronary angioplasty, although modified over the last 20 years by enhanced technology, still conforms to the original descriptions of the technique (Figs. 1.2 and 1.3). Under radiographic control and local anaesthesia, the coronary arterial ostium is engaged with a guiding catheter and the target lesion traversed with an atraumatic guidewire. A balloon-tipped catheter is then advanced over the guidewire until it reaches the site of atheromatous obstruction, at which point the balloon is inflated with diluted contrast medium. The size of balloon, inflation pressure and the number and duration of inflations, varies according to the lesion characteristics. When the angiographic appearances suggest adequate lesion dilatation, all the equipment is removed and the patient is returned to the ward.

The original Grüntzig balloon material was PVC and of low compliance. It would rupture rather than exceed its designed maximal outer diameter. The catheter shaft incorporated a double lumen which allowed the balloon to be expanded and voided, and for pressure to be monitored at the catheter tip. Other than for a short-fixed guidewire, steerability was not possible. Balloon material limited inflation pressures to 5 atmospheres, the catheter shaft diameter was almost 5 French (F) (1.7 mm) and crossing profiles were high. The subsequent 15 years witnessed a rapid growth in technology resulting in marked improvements in guiding catheters and guidewires, as well as in balloon design.

Guiding catheters

Although coronary angioplasty represented an extension of diagnostic angiography, the construction of guiding catheters needed modification as these would need to support the passage of high profile and inflexible balloon catheters through tortuous vessels and across high-grade obstructions, rather than simply allow contrast injection. Initial examples had large outer diameters with poor memory and torque control. In the early 1980s, bonded, multilayer guiding catheters were developed comprising an inner surface of Teflon (to decrease friction), a middle layer of woven mesh (for torque control) and an outer layer of polyurethane (to maintain form). The variety of preformed shapes available for diagnostic work (Judkins, Amplatz), were reflected in the design of guides for

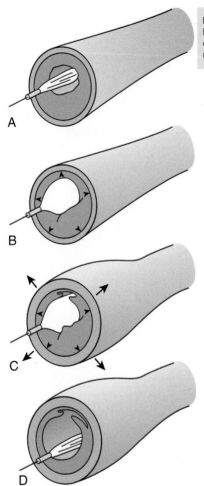

Figure 1.2:
Diagrammatic transverse cross section of coronary dilatation. Note the development of intimal fissuring as a result of balloon barotrauma.

interventional use, with many additional configurations to deal with atypical anatomy (e.g. Voda, Multipurpose, El Gamal, Hockey Stick).

Soft-tipped guides meant a reduced likelihood of catheter induced trauma to the coronary ostium, while thinner walls allowed increased internal lumens to incorporate other non-balloon devices. In the early 1980s, 9 or 10 F (3 or 3.3 mm diameter) guides were routinely used, but with advancing technology, notably in reducing the profiles of balloons and other devices, guiding catheter diameters came down in size. While in the early 1990s 8 F (2.7 mm) guides were commonplace; 7 and 6 F (2.3 or 2.0 mm) catheters are now increasingly employed. This results in less femoral arterial trauma and more rapid patient ambulation after the procedure, as well as allowing PTCA to be undertaken from alternative sites of vascular access, particularly the radial artery.

Guidewires

A short wire was fixed to the distal tip of the balloon catheter in 1979, but a major advance was made in 1982 when Simpson developed a long moveable and

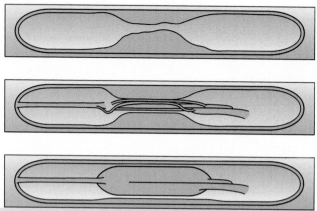

Figure 1.3:
Diagrammatic representation of the principles of balloon coronary angioplasty. The deflated balloon catheter is positioned across a coronary stenosis and inflated (middle). It is then deflated leaving the atheromatous lesion compressed and the stenosis relieved (bottom).

independent guidewire that was inserted through the central lumen. This allowed better tip control and steerability enabling access to distal coronary lesions. The initial 0.018 wires were later to be reduced in diameter and incorporate a variety of lubricious coatings to reduce friction and enhance passage through severe stenoses. Another modification was the introduction of a low profile balloon able to be moved only over a limited segment of reduced diameter wire (Hartzler 'Micro').

Guidewire control could be restricted by its passage through the balloon catheter lumen and contrast injection was also limited. Furthermore, the exchange of balloons was problematical involving wire extension to avoid having to rewire the target lesion. This was overcome by Kaltenbach's introduction of the long (300 cm) wire technique in 1984. Currently used wires measure 0.014 inches in diameter. The radiopaque distal few centimetres varies in flexbility, as does the shaft, providing increased support when addressing tortuous anatomy with relatively inflexible devices.

Balloon catheters

The balloon catheter itself has sustained a number of major modifications since its original design in 1977. A large variety of balloon lengths and expanded diameters became available, increasing the scope of possible lesions. Balloon material was also developed which could withstand far higher pressures (currently in excess of 20 atmospheres) and yet expand in a predictable fashion. Operators could choose from balloon materials with a range of compliance characteristics to suit particular lesion types. As balloon and shaft design improved, so did trackability and steerability, and as the crossing profile of the balloon reduced it became axiomatic that if a wire could cross the stenosis then so would the balloon catheter.

Balloon preparation was often problematical as the material did not collapse easily with aspiration and thus de-airing was frequently incomplete. Until the development of superior materials, this was overcome with a specific air venting tube which was integral in the Simpson–Roberts balloon catheter system.

The original fixed wire design re-emerged in the mid-1980s with the 'balloon on a wire' concept. This was particularly valuable for distal lesions, or cases when preservation of wire position or balloon exchange was considered not to be a priority. Erbel and Stack produced continuous perfusion balloons that allowed the anterograde flow of blood beyond the inflated balloon and could thereby limit ischaemia during long balloon inflations.

A milestone in balloon catheter development occurred in the 1986 with the introduction of the 'monorail' system by Bonzel. By only requiring a relatively short segment of guidewire to run through the distal catheter tip and shaft, lesions could be independently wired before selection of the balloon catheter, and balloon exchange was simplified. 'Over the wire' systems remained in limited use as they provided easier wire exchange (when occasionally required) and the ability to measure distal pressure. However, the emergence of superior fluoroscopy and digital X-ray systems with online quantitative coronary angiography (QCA), meant that operators could assess the results of angioplasty visually without having to rely on abolition of the translesional pressure gradient. Thus, in Europe, monorail systems represent the majority of activity while in the USA such 'rapid exchange' devices are more restricted by regulatory issues.

As the technique of PTCA necessarily incorporates the temporary occlusion of an epicardial coronary artery, it is not surprising that much research activity capitalised on this model of controlled myocardial ischaemia. A multitude of publications have emerged in the literature as a result of harnessing this therapeutic modality and thereby studying the effects of transient coronary occlusion in man. Examination of these effects has involved action potential changes, coronary sinus blood sampling, electrocardiographic and haemodynamic alteration, and analysis of ventricular contraction during balloon inflation employing echocardiography or contrast left ventriculography.

Such research has clarified the sequence of abnormalities occurring in left ventricular myocardium rendered ischaemic as a result of transient coronary occlusion. Initially diastolic dysfunction (abnormal relaxation and reduced compliance), is followed by systolic contractile changes indicated by hypokinesis, akinesis or dyskinesis of myocardial segments subtended by the treated artery. Electrocardiogram (ECG) abnormalities then develop, manifest as ST segment changes in leads overlying the ischaemic territories. Cardiac chest pain is a final and unpredictable occurrence in this cascade of ischaemic events all of which totally resolve in the reverse sequence when ischaemia is relieved. These ischaemic effects may be mitigated by collateral flow to the index artery, and there is now much interest surrounding the role of preconditioning in this setting.

These, and other technological advances steadily increased the scope of PTCA allowing a larger variety of lesions to be treated more successfully and with greater safety. Angioplasty had grown from a pioneering and unpredictable experiment to become a routine therapy for patients with coronary disease. A further breakthrough was to occur in 1987 which, in significance, was second only to Grüntzig's pioneering efforts; this was the first implantation in man of an intracoronary stent (see Chapter 6).

WORLDWIDE ACTIVITY

Initial enthusiasm for PTCA resulted in an understandable rush to learn the technique. This prompted leaders in the field to convene a workshop in June 1979, in Bethesda, USA, under the auspices of the National Heart, Lung, and Blood Institute (NHLBI). Here it was decided to limit the availability of PTCA to centres with clearly defined and agreed protocols. Even the commercial provider of the equipment agreed to abide by these guidelines such that operators could not obtain balloon catheters without having undergone approved instruction in the technique. Results of procedures were pooled in a unified and systematic fashion so that many of the first insights into PTCA and its outcomes derived from this NHLBI registry.

Between 1977 and 1982 data on 3079 patients were entered into the registry from 106 institutions. Of these patients, 77% were male with a mean age of 54 years, two-thirds having Canadian Heart Class III or IV symptoms. Almost three-quarters had single vessel disease, the LAD artery being the most commonly addressed. Left main stem disease was attempted in 1% and bypass graft dilatation performed in 4%.

At this early stage several drawbacks were apparent when PTCA was compared with coronary artery surgery. First, the initial and long-term results were unpredicatable and the definition of a successful procedure was uncertain; a 20% reduction in stenosis severity was achieved in 67% of the original registry. Secondly, the risks of PTCA were not clearly superior to surgery (myocardial infarction: 5.5%, emergency CABG: 6.6%, death: 0.9%) acknowledging that the majority had single vessel disease. Thirdly, it became apparent that a relatively small volume of procedures was being undertaken by an increasingly large number of operators thus potentially diluting an initially small experience. Finally, technical factors like vessel angulation or tortuosity, distal disease and lesion calcification, eccentricity or chronic occlusion, were anticipated to limit PTCA to perhaps 10 or 15% of patients considered for surgical revascularisation.

The technical advances in PTCA described in this chapter resulted in greater applicability of the procedure and thereby an exponential increase in activity. Emory University in Atlanta, where Grüntzig had undertaken much of his later work, was in the vanguard of interventional research. Their experience, reported in 1985, indicated a learning curve for the technique and improving results associated with increasing experience and the new emerging technology. For example, the circumflex artery became more accessible with steerable systems rising from 7% to 16% of all procedures and enjoying similar success rates as with the other main arteries. Their experience in 3500 consecutive cases set a standard to which other interventional units could aspire with success in 89%, myocardial infarction in 2.6%, emergency CABG in 2.7% and death in 0.1% of patients.

The growth in activity has been seen worldwide, with the USA particularly generating large volumes. It is interesting to note that ten years after the first report of coronary artery bypass grafting in 1968, 100,000 operations had been performed in the USA. However this figure had been overtaken by the number of PTCA procedures (106000) undertaken within only seven years of its first reported series in 1978. Recent UK data suggest that CABG rates may now be on the decline as PTCA activity continues to increase (Fig. 1.4).

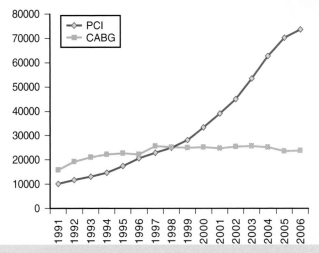

Figure 1.4:
Comparison of rates of PCI and CABG in the UK. Source: BCIS Audit Returns (2006) (www.bcis.org.uk)

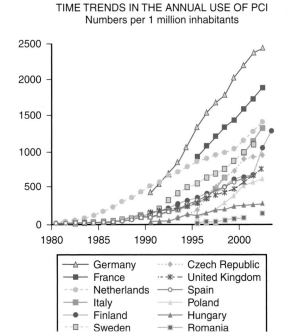

Figure 1.5:
Comparison of time trends in European PCI activity. Source: Euroheart Survey, 3rd Report
(www.escardio.org)

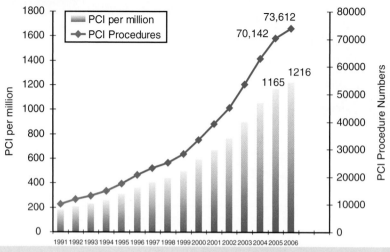

Figure 1.6:
Annual PCI activity in the UK. Source: BCIS audit returns, 2006 (www.bcis.org.uk)

In 1995, there were an estimated 350 000 PTCA cases performed in the USA, with almost 500 000 undertaken worldwide. In Europe, activity has been similarly increasing from approximately 250 000 in 1995, to almost 300 000 in 1997. Individual European countries differ in interventional activity and thus in the PTCA rates per million of the population (Fig. 1.5). Growth in activity in the UK, although substantial, nevertheless lags behind that of other European countries like France, Germany and Belgium. This discrepancy in the UK compared with other Western European nations is primarily a funding issue within the National Health Service (NHS). A lack of resources limits the number of patients coming forward for angiographic investigation, and thereby the number available for revascularisation with CABG as well as PTCA.

In the UK, data on PTCA activity is collected by the British Cardiovascular Intervention Society (BCIS) on an annual basis. Input from participating centres has been voluntary, but nevertheless the volumes recorded have always been in concordance with those suggested by industry sources when equipment sales have been examined. Thus in 1991, 52 centres in the UK undertook 9933 PTCA procedures representing 174 cases per million population. The annual growth in activity has varied between approximately 12% and 19%, the average since 1991 being 15% per year. In 2006, a total of 91 centres reported almost 74 000 procedures, giving a rate per million of 1216 (Fig. 1.6).

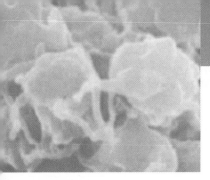

2

Pathology of balloon dilatation in a coronary artery

SAIB S. KHOGALI, MD FRCP

KEY POINTS

▥ Morphological changes of coronary arteries can result after a balloon dilation injury.

▥ Quantitative and qualitative assessments of the immediate effect of balloon injury on atherosclerotic plaque can be provided by a combination of coronary angiography and intravascular ultrasound.

▥ Balloon size relative to vessel diameter is an important consideration prior to balloon angioplasty to avoid intra and post procedural complications.

▥ The healing and repair process start at the site of angioplasty with re-modelling of the atherosclerotic plaque.

▥ The histological changes associated with the healing process begin with cellular infiltration of monocytes (becoming macrophages) and lymphocytes, with subsequent neointimal smooth muscle cell proliferation.

INTRODUCTION

Balloon dilatation injury in human coronary arteries results in morphological changes. These are largely dependent on: atherosclerotic plaque composition, eccentrictity of treated segment, and balloon barotraumas. The reactive healing response to balloon injury leads to intimal hyperplasia – the major mechanism responsible for restenosis.

MECHANISMS OF BALLOON INJURY

The morphological and histological changes after balloon dilatation are observed in two time periods:
(i) early (<30 days) changes post coronary angioplasty (POBA); or
(ii) late (>30 days) post POBA – healing, repair and re-modelling at the angioplasty site

EARLY CHANGES POST CORONARY BALLOON ANGIOPLASTY

The effect of balloon dilatation is dependent on plaque composition and eccentricity. Atherosclerotic plaque in human coronary arteries is mostly composed of fibrous tissue with variable amounts of calcific deposits (hard plaque). Rarely, a patient may have 'soft plaque' – without dense collagen or calcific deposits.

Quantitative and qualitative assessments of the immediate effect of balloon injury on atherosclerotic plaque can be provided by a combination of coronary angiography and intravascular ultrasound. These observations and data from animal model studies[1] have provided consistent evidence for the mechanisms of balloon injury down at tissue and cellular levels.

Inflation of a balloon results in six main mechanisms of balloon injury (Figs. 2.1a and 2.b) as observed angiographically and by IVUS[2]:

1. compression of plaque;
2. vessel stretch – seen in eccentric lesions;
3. superficial tear;
4. deep tear or dissection/subintimal – reaching the media;
5. submedial dissection; and
6. extensive deep dissection.

In the context of balloon angioplasty alone, balloon size relative to vessel diameter is an important consideration prior to balloon angioplasty. Under-sizing results in under-dilatation and is associated with restenosis and over-sizing increases the risk of acute complications such as coronary dissections, perforations and the need for coronary bypass surgery.

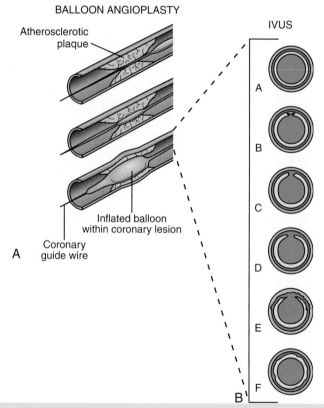

Figure 2.1:
Mechanism of balloon angioplasty injury and cross-sectional IVUS appearance.
Cross-sectional schema of coronary artery and mechanisms of balloon injury:
A = plaque compression; **B** = superficial tear/fissure (intimal); **C** = deeper sub-intimal tear; **D** = sub-intimal tear with localized dissection; **E** = deep subintimal tear with extensive dissection reaching media and **F** = circular sub-intimal dissection. In eccentric lesions, stretching of vessel wall (without plaque) and sub-medial dissection can occur.

Optimal balloon-to-artery ratios achieve the best expansion with minimal residual stenosis at a lower risk of acute dissection. A ratio of 0.9–1.0 and inflation at a lower pressure is advocated rather than under-sizing and a higher inflation pressure with a higher risk of acute complications.[3,4]

The early angiographic appearances after POBA injury can vary between no change angiographically, in a heavily calcified lesion, to an excellent stent-like result in a soft plaque lesion. Between these two ends of a spectrum other angiographic appearances that may be seen include:

- haziness within the treated segment – due to disruption of intima and/or inherent thrombus;
- dissection/intimal flaps – which can be extensive or localized; and
- contrast 'hang-up' in treated segment where POBA has caused dissection into adventitial layer.

Angiographic and IVUS imaging before and after POBA
Angiography post POBA is useful in demonstrating the impact of balloon angioplasty on coronary stenosis as shown in Fig. 2.2a and b. IVUS images of this same stenosis before and after POBA demonstrates the morphology of the lesion and the effect of balloon inflation on the intima with increase in lumen caliber (Figs. 2.2c and d).

Tissue cross-sectional views of coronary stenosis pre- and post- POBA
Schematic representation of cross-sectional views of coronary stenoses – typically lipid rich atheromatous plaque after angioplasty, reveal the early changes of balloon inflation including intimal tears, dissections and deep medial tears (Fig. 2.3a). The different histological patterns of the intima, media and adventitia are outlined (Fig. 2.3b). Optical coherence tomography (OCT) is a new research tool which provides enhanced images of the intimal region allowing closer examination of the effects of balloon injury (Fig. 2.3c).

Late changes of balloon angioplasty injury After successful POBA there is a healing and repair process at the site of angioplasty, with re-modelling of the atherosclerotic plaque. These late changes at >30 days, can result in either maintained lumen caliber with little change (angiographically) since POBA or a decrease in lumen size because of restenosis.

Coronary restenosis This tends to occur to variable degrees at three to six months post POBA. Clinically, restenosis is manifest by a recurrence of anginal symptoms and angiographically with a reduced vessel diameter. Angiographic restenosis and its quantitation will be the subject of a later chapter. In general terms, a diameter stenosis of >50% constitutes angiographic restenosis. The latter, however, often poorly correlates with the patient's symptoms.

Late histological and morphological changes after POBA The pathophysiological process is complex and involves early, intermediate and late changes (three months post POBA). The histological changes associated with the healing process begins

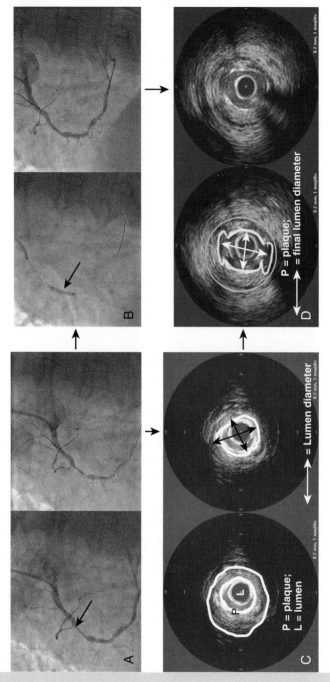

Figure 2.2:
Angiographic and IVUS appearance after balloon angioplasty
A Mid-RCA lesion (black arrow);
B Balloon inflation (black arrow) POBA angiographic result; **C** IVUS pre POBA. IVUS images of mid-RCA final POBA result before stenting.

CORONARY BALLOON ANGIOPLASTY EFFECTS AT THE TISSUE LEVEL

Tissue cross-sectional view of lipid rich coronary stenosis with reduced lumen (black arrow) before POBA

Increase in lumen size (black arrow) post POBA with evidence of intimal tears (white arrow in enhanced IVUS below)

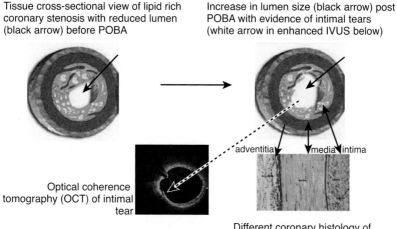

Optical coherence tomography (OCT) of intimal tear

adventitia media intima

Different coronary histology of intima, media and adventitia

Figure 2.3:
Balloon angioplasty effects at the tissue level
A Tissue cross-sectional view of lipid rich coronary stenosis with reduced lumen (black arrow) before POBA. Increase in lumen size (black arrow) post POBA with evidence of intimal tears (broken arrow in enhanced IVUS below). B different coronary histology of intima, media and adventitia; C OCT of intimal tear (*courtesy of Lightlab imaging*).

with cellular infiltration of monocytes (becoming macrophages) and lymphocytes, with subsequent neointimal smooth muscle cell proliferation. These cells in time produce an extracellular matrix which is the main restenotic tissue. In some cases no intimal proliferation is found and only atherosclerotic plaque (usually eccentric lesions) in which elastic recoil must have taken place at the time of POBA[5].

REFERENCES

1. Takagi, M., *et al.*, The Watanabe heritable hyperlipidemic rabbit is a suitable experimental model to study differences in tissue response between intimal and medical injury after balloon angioplasty, Arterioscler Thromb Vasc Biol, 1997, 17(12): p. 3611–19.

2. Honye, J., *et al.*, Morphological effects of coronary balloon angioplasty in vivo assessed by intravascular ultrasound imaging, Circulation, 1992, 85(3): p. 1012–25.

3. Roubin, G.S., *et al.*, Influence of balloon size on initial success, acute complications, and restenosis after percutaneous transluminal coronary angioplasty. A prospective randomized study, Circulation, 1988, 78(3): p. 557–65.

4. Azuma, A., *et al.*, Quantitative measurements of balloon-to-artery ratios in coronary angioplasty, J Cardiol, 1991. 21(4): p. 879–88.

5. Waller, B.F., *et al.*, Morphological observations late (greater than 30 days) after clinically successful coronary balloon angioplasty, Circulation, 1991, 83(2 Suppl): p. I28–41.

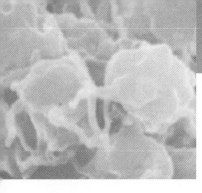

3

Patient selection for percutaneous coronary intervention

ROD STABLES

KEY POINTS

▨ Case selection is an essential element in the practice of percutaneous coronary intervention (PCI) and has a direct and immediate bearing on outcome.

▨ The enthusiasm for PCI must be tempered with the realisation that:
 – the potential for clinical gain is real but can be modest;
 – performance is associated with morbidity and mortality; and
 – alternative therapeutic strategies exist.

▨ The process involves the interaction of a number of factors:
 – the training and experience of the interventionist;
 – access to equipment and facilities;
 – the availability of surgical or other support;
 – characteristics of the patient;
 – nature of the clinical presentation; and
 – the details of the epicardial coronary anatomy to be addressed.

▨ Assessment of appropriateness can be complex and involves a consideration of symptoms and functional testing.

INTRODUCTION

In the practice of PCI the aim is to deliver maximum clinical gain at the lowest possible levels of risk. Case selection is an essential element in this process and is one of the few factors in the control of the cardiologist that has a direct and immediate bearing on outcome. The development of the skill (or art!) of case selection should be a central component of training but is often neglected, with increasing emphasis on procedural issues.

Careful review will identify cases that would be best managed by alternative treatments but can also provide important information to guide the conduct of a proposed intervention. The need for specialised equipment or adjunctive medication can be identified and provision assured. Appropriate scheduling of catheter laboratory, ward and other clinical areas can be performed. Unusual or high-risk cases may demand the collaboration of other interventionists or surgical and anaesthetic colleagues. Furthermore, the process of informed consent is improved if patients can be appraised of a case specific assessment of likely gains and potential risks.

GENERAL CONSIDERATIONS

Most interventionists will accept that PCI has established limitations. The enthusiasm to recommend this form of therapy should be tempered in the light of this reality.

The potential for clinical gain is real but can be modest

No study has been able to demonstrate that, in patients with stable angina, management with PCI confers prognostic advantage. In this setting, randomised controlled trials against medical therapy have shown that an interventional strategy does result in better resolution of symptoms but the gains are modest and attenuate over medium term follow-up.[1-3] The role of early angiography and revascularisation in the acute coronary syndromes is, to some extent still the subject of debate[4,5] but there is now general agreement that an invasive strategy will benefit a selected proportion of patients.[6-9] As in the management of acute ST segment elevation myocardial infarction, prompt access to facilities and appropriately trained staff may be required at a specific point in the natural history if benefits are to be realised.[10]

Performance is associated with some level of morbidity and mortality

All trials comparing PCI with medical therapy have shown an increased rate of major adverse cardiac events in the intervention group, mostly related to complications at the time of revascularisation.[2,3] All interventionists will be familiar with the potential for other forms of procedure-related morbidity. Although these events may not be reported as formal outcome measures in the trial literature, they have important implications for the patient's perception of outcome and for the consumption of health-care resources.

Alternative therapeutic options exist and are effective

Advances in medical therapy options for symptom management, support of impaired left ventricular function and secondary prevention (particularly lipid lowering[11]) have revolutionised the so-called conservative approach. A major, multicentre trial (COURAGE) has been initiated in the United States and Canada to reassess the value of PCI over continued modern medical therapy.

In the management of more advanced disease, CABG remains an effective and widely applicable treatment option. A meta-analysis of the first generation trials comparing PTCA and CABG has been published.[12] Rihal and Yusuf[13] extended these observations to include the bypass angioplasty revascularisation investigation (BARI) trial producing a combined sample size of 5200 patients. The overall mortality rate was 7.8% and 6.6% in the PTCA and CABG groups respectively (odds ratio 1.20, 95% CI 0.97–1.48). This represents a trend to increased mortality in the PTCA group that approaches conventional levels of statistical significance. The PTCA strategy was also limited by a greater need for repeat revascularisation procedures (34% PTCA vs 3.3% CABG in the first year of follow-up), and less effective relief of angina symptoms.

The results of similar trials from the stent era have now been reported[14,15] and show that the routine use of coronary stents has improved the rate of repeat revascularisation with PCI, but that this remains around four times higher than that observed in patients managed with bypass grafting. Five-year follow up from the ARTS study also seems to support the BARI trial, in reporting a reduced mortality for diabetic patients managed with surgery (8.3% v 13.4%, p = 0.27).[16]

The potential for drug eluting stent technology to further erode the surgical advantage is the subject of ongoing randomized trials.[17]

CASE SELECTION – ASSESSING APPROPRIATENESS

The process of case selection is complex and multifactorial. Many aspects are difficult to characterise and hence describe. The appropriateness of any given procedure will be influenced by the skills and experience of the interventionist, the availability of other therapeutic options and the attitude of the patient to the potential for benefit and risk. The management of specific clinical syndromes will evolve over time and be influenced by the development of (and access to) new techniques, equipment and adjunctive medications.

These difficulties are perhaps best exemplified by retrospective studies designed to rate the appropriateness of interventional procedures. Most have used the opinions of 'Expert Panels' using a methodology designed by the RAND Corporation and the University of California.[18–21] Raw data from these panels consists of tables of thousands of situation-specific rankings that can be difficult to apply to routine clinical practice. Furthermore the data becomes obsolete over time, can be influenced by the composition of the panel[22,23] and do not necessarily translate from one nation to another.[24]

Other investigators have adopted a more simplified approach. The University of Maryland revascularisation appropriateness scoring system (RAS) combines information on symptoms, clinical presentation, coronary anatomy, non-invasive tests of functional significance, left ventricular function and co-morbidity to derive a simple index of suitability (Fig. 3.1).[25] A German group has developed a computer program to predict the outcome of coronary interventions. Initial weightings for predictive factors were derived from retrospective data and tested on new prospective cases.[26] The potential for artificial intelligence computer systems to 'learn' from cases as they are added to the registry means that this type of tool may be able to remain current with practice evolution, though routine clinical application is still several years away.

The leading professional societies issue guidelines for the practice of coronary intervention and for the management of common clinical presentations.[27,28] These seek to establish Class 1, 2 and 3 indications for the performance of PCI and are updated on a regular basis. They should also be read in conjunction with more recent guidelines examining the management of specific clinical scenarios.[6,29] These documents are available from the professional society websites (http://www.escardio.org), (http://www.acc.org).

CASE SELECTION – A PRACTICAL APPROACH

A structured approach to case selection or risk stratification might consider three elements:

- Factors related to the nature of the clinical presentation.
- Factors related to the clinical characteristics of the patient.
- Factors related to the proposed target lesion(s).

The established clinical indications for PCI are subject to continued expansion and refinement. Its role in the management of many presentations (for example – acute

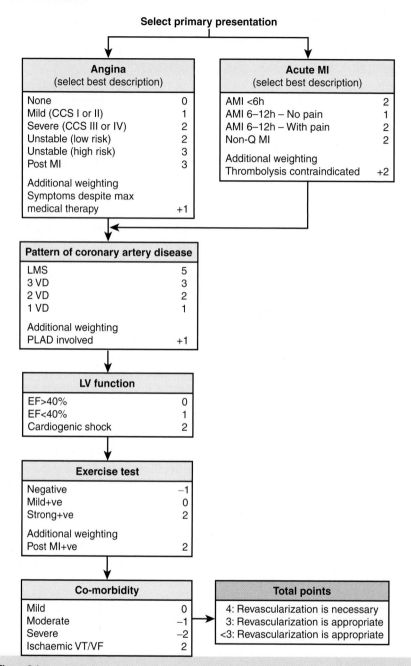

Figure 3.1:
Calculation of the University of Maryland revascularization appropriateness scoring (RAS). (Adapted from Ziskind et al.[25])

myocardial infarction, acute coronary syndromes, cardiogenic shock, multivessel disease and small vessel disease) are still the subject of continuing evaluation. A detailed review of this area is beyond the scope of this text and the role of PCI in a number of key clinical presentations is explored in other chapters.

Assessment of the status and clinical characteristics of the patient can be considered in the following terms.

General cardiac status

The state of the circulation has an immediate and significant impact on the performance of any PCI procedure. Cardiogenic shock precipitated by acute ischaemia represents a clear but very high-risk indication. Less florid left ventricular failure is another negative prognostic factor and may compromise the ability of the patient to lie supine on the examination table. The need for elective ventilation or circulatory support (for example, intra-aortic balloon pumping) is a marker of adverse outcome. Post procedural reduced perfusion or hypotension can precipitate subacute vessel closure. In this respect a vaso-vagal response or disturbance of cardiac rhythm with brady or tachycardia can have important implications.

Details of the coronary anatomy

The operator must contemplate the likely impact of transient balloon occlusion or an abrupt closure event at each proposed target lesion. This analysis demands a thorough review of current angiographic findings, including bypass graft conduits, if present. Flow limiting lesions or occlusive disease in non-target vessels increase procedural risk. Procedures to a 'last remaining conduit' represent one extreme in this continuum. In certain clinical situations (for example, thrombus laden lesions, saphenous vein graft disease or rotational atherectomy) the sequelae of embolisation of material to the distal vascular bed should be considered.

The left main stem (or right ostium) and proximal portions of the principal vessels may be subjected to mechanical trauma by the guide catheter and other equipment. Plaque or other atherosclerotic disease in these territories increases the risk of vessel dissection or abrupt closure.

Suitability for CABG

Angiographic review should also involve a consideration of the options for surgical therapy, either as an elective alternative to PCI or in a bailout setting. There is merit in involving surgical colleagues in this process. Suitability for CABG will be influenced by co-morbid factors beyond the coronary vasculature, particularly respiratory, renal and hepatic function. Lack of a surgical 'rescue' option increase the risk of any proposed procedure but may, of course, represent an appropriate procedure for patients in need of revascularisation.

Peripheral and great vessels

Adequate stability of the guiding catheter is an essential pre-requisite for successful PCI. Atherosclerotic or other disease of the peripheral vessels may deny access for the catheter of choice and for additional equipment, for example, an intra-aortic balloon pump (IABP). Unfolding or excessive tortuosity of the aorta can further compromise guide catheter positioning.

Procedural morbidity will be increased in cases with widespread vascular disease. The risk of catheter-related embolic release to the head and neck or peripheral vessels is real. Complications at the vascular access site can result in embolisation, occlusion or bleeding. Co-existing hypertension, obesity or systemic anticoagulation can confound these problems.

Renal function

Chronic renal failure (CRF) is an established risk factor for coronary artery disease. Nevertheless emerging data suggests that the results of PCI at any individual lesion may be less favourable in patients with established CRF.[30,31] For patients with any degree of renal impairment the nephrotoxicity of radiographic contrast can precipitate acute renal failure. Even with precautionary measures such as fluid administration or elective filtration, the scope and duration of any PCI procedure will be limited by the need to minimise exposure to contrast agent.

Diabetes mellitus

Diabetes mellitus (DM) is often a marker of more widespread and diffuse coronary artery disease. This pattern of disease is difficult to manage with PCI and CABG may provide a better revascularisation strategy. In the BARI and ARTS trials, comparing multivessel PTCA with conventional CABG, the advantages of the surgical approach were most marked in patients with DM.[16,32]

The reasons for this are not fully established and may extend beyond the simple presence of more extensive disease. At individual lesions, the restenosis rate seems to be higher in diabetic patients. Recent studies suggest that use of a GPIIb/IIIa receptor blocking antiplatelet agent (abciximab) seems to confer particular advantage in diabetic patients.[33] This may suggest that other mechanisms, some platelet mediated, may be involved.

REFERENCES

1. Hueb W, Bellotti G, Almeida de Oliveira S *et al*. The medicine, angioplasty or surgery study (MASS): a prospective randomised trial of medical therapy, balloon angioplasty or bypass surgery for single proximal left anterior descending artery stenoses. J Am Coll Cardiol 1995; 25:1600–5.

2. Parisi AF, Folland ED, Hartigan P, on behalf of the Veterans Affairs ACME Investigators. A comparison of angioplasty with medical therapy in the treatment of single-vessel coronary artery disease. N Engl J Med 1992; 326:10–16.

3. RITA-2 trial participants. Coronary angioplasty versus medical therapy for angina: the second Randomised Intervention Treatment of Angina (RITA-2). Lancet 1997; 350: 461–8.

4. Van de WF, Gore JM, Avezum A, Gulba DC, Goodman SG, Budaj A *et al*. Access to catheterisation facilities in patients admitted with acute coronary syndrome: multinational registry study. BMJ 2005 Feb 26; 330(7489):441.

5. Clayton TC, Pocock SJ, Henderson RA, Poole-Wilson PA, Shaw TR, Knight R, *et al.* Do men benefit more than women from an interventional strategy in patients with unstable angina or non-ST-elevation myocardial infarction? The impact of gender in the RITA 3 trial. [see comment]. European Heart Journal 2004 Sep; 25(18):1641–50.

6. Bertrand ME, Simoons ML, Fox KA, Wallentin LC, Hamm CW, McFadden E, *et al.* Management of acute coronary syndromes in patients presenting without persistent ST-segment elevation. [erratum appears in Eur Heart J. 2003 Jun;24(12):1174–5]. European Heart Journal 2002 Dec; 23(23):1809–40.

7. Lagerqvist B, Husted S, Kontny F, Naslund U, Stahle E, Swahn E, *et al.* A long-term perspective on the protective effects of an early invasive strategy in unstable coronary artery disease: two-year follow-up of the FRISC-II invasive study. [see comment]. Journal of the American College of Cardiology 2002 Dec 4; 40(11):1902–14.

8. Diderholm E, Andren B, Frostfeldt G, Genberg M, Jernberg T, Lagerqvist B, *et al.* The prognostic and therapeutic implications of increased troponin T levels and ST depression in unstable coronary artery disease: the FRISC II invasive troponin T electrocardiogram substudy. American Heart Journal 2002 May; 143(5):760–7.

9. Fox KA, Poole-Wilson PA, Henderson RA, Clayton TC, Chamberlain DA, Shaw TR, *et al.* Interventional versus conservative treatment for patients with unstable angina or non-ST-elevation myocardial infarction: the British Heart Foundation RITA 3 randomised trial. Randomized Intervention Trial of unstable Angina. [see comment]. Lancet 2002 Sep 7; 360(9335):743–51.

10. Keeley EC, Boura JA, Grines CL. Primary angioplasty versus intravenous thrombolytic therapy for acute myocardial infarction: a quantitative review of 23 randomised trials. [see comment]. [Review] [41 refs]. Lancet 2003 Jan 4; 361(9351):13–20.

11. Pitt B, Waters D, Brown WV *et al.* Aggressive lipid-lowering compared with angioplasty in stable coronary artery disease. N Engl J Med 1999; 341:70–76.

12. Pocock SJ, Henderson RA, Rickards AF *et al.* Meta-analysis of randomised trials comparing coronary angioplasty with bypass surgery. Lancet 1995; 346:1184–9.

13. Rihal CS, Yusuf S. Chronic coronary artery disease: drugs, angioplasty or surgery. BMJ 1996; 312:265–6.

14. Serruys PW, Unger F, Sousa JE, Jatene A, Bonnier HJ, Schonberger JP, *et al.* Comparison of coronary-artery bypass surgery and stenting for the treatment of multivessel disease. N Engl J Med 2001 Apr 12; 344(15):1117–24.

15. Coronary artery bypass surgery versus percutaneous coronary intervention with stent implantation in patients with multivessel coronary artery disease (the Stent or Surgery trial): a randomised controlled trial. Lancet 2002 Sep 28; 360(9338):965–70.

16. Serruys PW, Ong AT, van Herwerden LA, Sousa JE, Jatene A, Bonnier JJ, *et al.* Five-year outcomes after coronary stenting versus bypass surgery for the treatment of multivessel disease: the final analysis of the Arterial Revascularization Therapies Study (ARTS) randomized trial. J Am Coll Cardiol 2005 Aug 16; 46(4):575–81.

17. Serruys PW, Lemos PA, van Hout BA. Sirolimus eluting stent implantation for patients with multivessel disease: rationale for the Arterial Revascularisation Therapies Study part II (ARTS II). Heart 2004 Sep; 90(9):995–8.

18. Hilborne LH, Leape LL, Bernstein SJ et al. The appropriateness of use of percutaneous transluminal coronary angioplasty in New York State. JAMA. 1993; 269:761–5.

19. Hilborne LH, Leape LL, Kahan JP, Park RE, Kamberg CJ, Brook RH. Percutaneous transluminal coronary angioplasty: a literature review and ratings of appropriateness and necessity. Santa Monica, CA, USA: The RAND Corporation. JRA–01, 1991.

20. Meijler AP, Rigter H, Bernstein SJ et al. The appropriateness of intention to treat decisions for invasive therapy in coronary artery disease in the Netherlands. Heart 1997; 77:219–24.

21. Bernstein SJ, Brorsson B, Abert T et al. Appropriateness of referral of coronary angiography patients in Sweden. Heart 1999; 81:470–77.

22. Shekelle PG, Kahan JP, Bernstein SJ, Leape LL, Kamberg CJ, Park RE. The reproducibility of a method to identify the overuse and underuse of medical procedures [see comments]. N Engl J Med. 1998; 338:1888–95.

23. Ayanian JZ, Landrum MB, Normal SL, Guadagnoli E, McNeil BJ. Rating the appropriateness of coronary angiography – do practicing physicians agree with an expert panel and with each other? [see comments]. N Engl J Med. 1988; 338:1896–1904.

24. Brook RH, Kosecoff JB, Park RE, Chassin MR, Winslow CM, Hampton JR. Diagnosis and treatment of coronary disease: comparison of doctor's attitudes in the USA and the UK. Lancet 1988; 1:750–53.

25. Ziskind AA, Lauer MA, Bishop G, Vogel RA. Assessing the appropriateness of coronary revascularisation: The Universtiy of Maryland Revascularization Appropriateness Score (RAS) and its comparison to RAND expert panel ratings and ACC/AHA guidelines with regard to assigned appropriateness rating and ability to predict outcome. Clin Cardiol 1999; 22:67–76.

26. Budde T, Haude M, Hopp HW et al. A prognostic computer model to individually predict post-procedural complications in interventional cardiology: the INTERVENT Project [see comments]. Eur Heart J. 1999; 20:354–63.

27. Silber S, Albertsson P, Aviles FF, Camici PG, Colombo A, Hamm C et al. Guidelines for percutaneous coronary interventions. The Task Force for Percutaneous Coronary Interventions of the European Society of Cardiology. Eur Heart J. 2005 Apr; 26(8):804–47.

28. Smith SC, Jr., Dove JT, Jacobs AK, Kennedy JW, Kereiakes D, Kern MJ et al. ACC/AHA guidelines of percutaneous coronary interventions (revision of the 1993 PTCA guidelines)— executive summary. A report of the American College of Cardiology/American Heart Association Task Force on Practice Guidelines (committee to revise the 1993 guidelines for percutaneous transluminal coronary angioplasty). J Am Coll Cardiol 2001 Jun 15; 37(8):2215–39.

29. Antman EM, Anbe DT, Armstrong PW, Bates ER, Green LA, Hand M et al. ACC/AHA guidelines for the management of patients with ST-elevation myocardial infarction; A report of the American College of Cardiology/American Heart Association Task Force on Practice Guidelines (Committee to Revise the 1999 Guidelines for the Management of patients with acute myocardial infarction). J Am Coll Cardiol. 2004 Aug 4; 44(3):E1–E211.

30. Schoebel FC, Gradaus F, Ivens K et al. Restenosis after elective coronary balloon angioplasty in patients with end stage renal disease: a case–control study using quantitative coronary angiography. Heart. 1997; 78:337–42.

31. Ix JH, Mercado N, Shlipak MG, Lemos PA, Boersma E, Lindeboom W *et al*. Association of chronic kidney disease with clinical outcomes after coronary revascularization: the Arterial Revascularization Therapies Study (ARTS). Am Heart J. 2005 Mar; 149(3):512–19.

32. BARI Investigators. Comparison of coronary bypass surgery with angioplasty in patients with multivessel disease. N Engl J Med. 1996; 335:217–25.

33. Lincoff AM, Califf RM, Moliterno DJ *et al*. Complementary clinical benefits of coronary-artery stenting and blockade of platelet glycoprotein IIb/IIIa receptors. Evaluation of platelet IIb/IIIa inhibition in stenting investigators. N Engl J Med. 1999; 341:319–27.

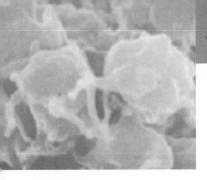

4

Investigation, workup and patient preparation before PCI

IAN R. STARKEY

KEY POINTS

■ No matter how urgent the clinical situation, it is essential that certain preliminaries be observed prior to performing a PCI procedure.

■ Basic essentials can be summarised under the general headings of:
Oreliminary investigations;
Therapeutic alterations;
Consent; and
Anticipation (and possible prevention) of problems (PTCA).

INTRODUCTION

In 2006, nearly 74,000 PCI procedures were performed in 91 centres in the UK, a rate of just over 1200 per million population (British Cardiovascular Intervention Society [BCIS] annual survey – unpublished data). PCI has now overtaken CABG as the commonest form of myocardial revascularisation procedure performed on patients with obstructive coronary artery disease. It is important to remember that such procedures, while 'routine' for some operators and exciting for others, may be frightening, painful and dangerous for the patients on whom they are performed, even though statistically the success rate is high. Before such a procedure begins, much can be done to diminish the patient's fear and pain, minimise the danger and increase further the likelihood of procedural and clinical success. The essential components of this preparation are:

P   preliminary investigations;
T   therapeutics;
C   consent; and
A   anticipation (of possible complications).

There is inevitably some overlap between these elements, all of which require consideration in all patients. The emergency nature of some procedures (e.g. primary PCI for a patient with an acute ST-elevation myocardial infarction) may curtail the time available for preparation of the patient, but should never result in omission of the basic essentials.

PRELIMINARY INVESTIGATIONS

These are needed to allow three questions to be answered:

1. Is percutaneous coronary intervention (PCI) appropriate for this patient?
    With few exceptions, PCI should only be considered in a patient with symptoms of coronary artery disease, objective evidence of myocardial

ischaemia/infarction and an anatomically suitable lesion(s), as demonstrated by coronary angiography. As a preliminary to such a procedure, therefore, the interventional cardiologist should review the patient's history and the results of any non-invasive and invasive investigations. While all this information should be available in advance of procedures performed electively, it is now increasingly common that patients, especially those with acute coronary syndromes (ACS: unstable angina or acute myocardial infarction), have combined diagnostic (i.e. coronary angiography) and therapeutic (i.e. PCI) procedures performed. In this situation, it is especially important for the interventional cardiologist to retain a capacity for objective judgement, so that, for instance, a patient who might best be treated surgically does not receive sub-optimal treatment simply because it is 'convenient' and it has been scheduled.

2. If PCI is appropriate, is the patient fit for the procedure?

Before arrival in the cardiac catheterisation laboratory, *every* patient should have a clinical history documented and a physical examination performed (Fig. 4.1). These should be supplemented by some basic investigations, although the number of these will be kept to a minimum in emergency situations (Table 4.1).

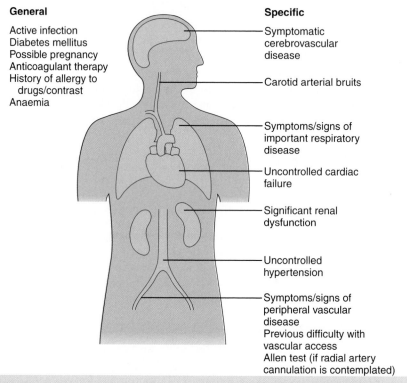

General

Active infection
Diabetes mellitus
Possible pregnancy
Anticoagulant therapy
History of allergy to
   drugs/contrast
Anaemia

Specific

Symptomatic
cerebrovascular
disease

Carotid arterial bruits

Symptoms/signs of
important respiratory
disease

Uncontrolled cardiac
failure

Significant renal
dysfunction

Uncontrolled
hypertension

Symptoms/signs of
peripheral vascular
disease
Previous difficulty with
vascular access
Allen test (if radial artery
cannulation is contemplated)

Figure 4.1:
History and examination of patient prior to PCI.

TABLE 4.1 - INVESTIGATIONS PRIOR TO PCI
ALL PATIENTS
Full blood count Blood urea, creatinine and electrolytes 12-lead ECG Blood group and save
SOME PATIENTS
INR (patients on warfarin) Chest X-ray (if clinically indicated) Others (respiratory function tests, plasma glucose, etc. according to clinical indication)

It is of particular importance to discover conditions that might increase the technical difficulty or risk of an invasive cardiac procedure. Some such factors can be corrected but awareness of others may lead to changes in peri-procedural drug therapy (see Therapeutics below), the information provided to the patient (see Consent below) or an ability to predict, and hopefully prevent, possible complications (see Anticipation below).

3. Can anything be done to improve his/her fitness?

This is mostly discussed in the ensuing sections of this chapter. The discovery of some intercurrent medical conditions might appropriately result in the postponement of an elective procedure. Examples would include severe anaemia (especially if this may be related to active or recent bleeding), active or suspected infection, uncontrolled hypertension and possible/definite pregnancy. On rare occasions, the discovery of serious non-cardiac disease (e.g. advanced malignancy) might lead to cancellation of a planned PCI procedure.

THERAPEUTICS (TABLE 4.2)

Anti-anginal drugs

Most patients with symptomatic coronary artery disease are taking regular anti-anginal medication, which can be continued until, and indeed, after the interventional procedure. Treatment with a long-acting nitrate and/or a calcium-channel blocker may actually be of benefit in the prevention of coronary artery spasm during/after the procedure. Although there is no convincing evidence that cholesterol-lowering therapy (e.g. statin drugs) specifically affects the short-term outcome of coronary interventional procedures, such treatment is an important part of the long-term management of patients with coronary artery disease and should, likewise, be continued.

Oral anti-platelet therapy

Most patients with coronary artery disease are taking Aspirin, which inhibits the platelet cyclo-oxygenase pathway, thus reducing the formation of thromboxane A_2, prostaglandin E_2 and prostacyclin. In the unusual circumstance of a patient not taking regular Aspirin presenting for PCI, this drug (300 mg) should be given,

TABLE 4.2 - DRUG THERAPY PRIOR TO PCI

DRUG CLASS	ACTION REQUIRED
Oral anti-anginal drugs	Continue
Cholesterol-lowering therapy	Continue
Oral anti-platelet therapy	Ensure that aspirin has been taken
	ADMINISTER LOADING DOSE OF CLOPIDOGREL (IF NOT ALREADY PRESCRIBED)
Warfarin	Discontinue if possible
	Measure INR and correct excessive anticoagulation
	TAKE APPROPRIATE MEASURES TO AVOID HAEMORRHAGE AT VASCULAR ACCESS SITE
IV Heparin	Continue
	Measure ACT and consider reduced bolus dose
SC Low molecular-weight heparin	Administer last injection >12 hours prior to PCI (if possible)
GP IIb/IIIa receptor antagonists	Continue but consider the use of a reduced, weight-adjusted heparin regime
Pre-medication	If necessary, use diazepam 5–20 mg orally
Antidiabetic medication	See text
Other drug therapy	Continue unchanged

preferably at least two hours before the start of the procedure. Aspirin (75–300 mg daily) should be continued long term thereafter.

As the overwhelming majority of PCI procedures now involve the placement of one or more coronary stents, combined anti-platelet therapy, using Aspirin and Clopidogrel (a thienopyridine derivative that inhibits adenosine diphosphate (ADP)-induced platelet aggregation[1]), has become normal practice even though Clopidogrel is not currently licensed for this indication. Many patients undergoing urgent PCI procedures for the treatment of ACS may already be taking Clopidogrel but patients undergoing elective or emergency procedures should receive a loading dose of Clopidogrel before the procedure. Available evidence suggests that maximal platelet inhibition is not achieved until at least six hours after a loading dose of 300mg; this time can be reduced to around two hours by administering a loading dose of 600mg.[2]

Anticoagulant therapy

Some patients may be anticoagulated with Warfarin, usually for reasons other than the presence of coronary artery disease (e.g. prosthetic heart valve, atrial fibrillation, venous thrombo-embolic disease). It may be impossible or undesirable to discontinue such treatment, but it is imperative that its effect is measured (by international normalised ratio (INR)), preferably before the start of the procedure and certainly prior to the removal of the arterial access sheath. Excessive anticoagulation should be corrected, but even therapeutic anticoagulation increases the risk of haemorrhage, especially at the vascular access site – anticipation of such a problem should lead to the use of appropriate prophylactic measures (see below).

Most patients with acute coronary syndromes are treated with Heparin. Intravenous unfractionated Heparin can be continued until the patient's arrival in the catheterisation laboratory. Measurement of the activated clotting time (ACT) will then allow the administration of an appropriate bolus of intravenous

Heparin, which may not actually be substantially different from that given to a patient not pre-treated with Heparin.[3] If a twice-daily regime of subcutaneous low molecular-weight Heparin is being used, the last injection should be given at least 12 hours before any planned coronary interventional procedure.[4] At the start of the procedure, an intravenous bolus of unfractionated Heparin can then be given in the usual way. In 'emergency' procedures, performed less than 12 hours after the last dose of low molecular-weight Heparin, it is normal practice to use a reduced dose of IV Heparin (<70 U/kg).

Platelet glycoprotein IIb/IIIa receptor antagonists

The results of randomised placebo-controlled clinical trials of several agents of this type demonstrate a clear benefit in patients with acute coronary syndromes, those undergoing percutaneous coronary interventional treatment or both. A detailed discussion of the use of such drug treatment is outwith the scope of this chapter – suffice it to say that it is clear that PCI can be performed safely after/during administration of such agents provided that a reduced, weight-adjusted heparin regime is used, in order to reduce the risk of major bleeding.[5]

Pre-medication

Despite explanation and reassurance, many patients remain anxious about undergoing PCI. If anxiety is overt and/or the patient expresses a desire for a sedative, a benzodiazepine such as Diazepam 5–20 mg orally may be given $1–1\frac{1}{2}$ hours before the start of the procedure. Benzodiazepines are also effectively absorbed when administered sublingually, but this method conveys no great advantage, as the onset of action is unlikely to be any more rapid. Some patients undergoing PCI will have had many previous invasive procedures, so that femoral arterial access may be difficult and painful. Prior administration of an opiate drug (Pethidine or Morphine), combined with generous quantities of local anaesthetic (Lignocaine) will be much appreciated by such patients.

Diabetes mellitus[6]

Since patients are usually fasted for several hours before PCI procedures, special precautions may be required to prevent hypoglycaemia in patients with diabetes mellitus. If possible, an elective procedure in a diabetic should be scheduled at the beginning of the list, to avoid the patient having to fast for an unpredictable and excessive length of time.

Treatment with sulphonylureas should be omitted on the morning of the day of the procedure. The administration of significant quantities of glucose-containing IV fluids should be avoided if possible. Insulin treatment is unlikely to be required. Drug treatment can be restarted at the time of the patient's first meal after the procedure.

Although lactic acidosis associated with treatment with Metformin occurs only rarely, it is more common in diabetics with impaired renal function. There have been a number of reports of cases of Metformin-associated lactic acidosis in patients with acute renal failure precipitated by iodinated contrast material, as is used during diagnostic and therapeutic cardiac procedures. This has led to the manufacturer's current recommendation that Metformin should be discontinued at the time of, or prior to, any such procedure and withheld for 48 hours after the procedure. Treatment should be re-instituted only after renal function has been re-evaluated and found to be normal. In all but emergency cases, renal function should be checked in all patients taking Metformin *before* the procedure. As Metformin is contraindicated in the presence of abnormal renal function, such patients should have their drug therapy reviewed, although PCI can be performed provided that special precautions are taken[7,8] (see Anticipation below).

Patients controlled with Insulin should receive no subcutaneous Insulin on the day of the procedure. An IV infusion of GKI (e.g. 500 ml 10% glucose with 10 mmol potassium chloride and 15 U Insulin at 100ml/hour) should be commenced before the procedure and continued until a normal diet and subcutaneous Insulin can be restarted safely. The blood glucose level should be checked at least every two hours using one of the commercially available bedside test strips. Depending on the result, the amount of Insulin may require adjustment (if plasma glucose >11 mmol/l, increase Insulin to 20 U; if <6.5 mmol/l, decrease to 10 U).

Other drug therapy

In general terms, there is no need for other drug therapy to be discontinued or changed. Even long-term steroid therapy is unlikely to need enhancement, although the need for this should be reviewed in the event of a major complication, especially significant myocardial infarction (MI) and/or emergency CABG.

CONSENT[9]

In an emergency, if consent cannot be obtained, medical treatment may be provided to anyone who needs it, provided that the treatment is limited to what is immediately necessary to save life or avoid significant deterioration in the patient's health. With this exception, an interventional cardiological procedure should not be performed without the patient giving his/her informed consent. This implies a two-stage process, involving the provision of information to the patient, who then decides voluntarily whether or not to consent to undergo the proposed procedure.

The information that a patient wants or ought to know, before deciding whether to consent to an interventional cardiological procedure, should include:

- Details of the diagnosis and prognosis, including the likely prognosis if the proposed treatment is not carried out.
- Other options for treatment of his/her condition, including the option not to treat.
- The purpose of the proposed procedure and details of exactly what is involved (including the likely duration of the procedure and the hospital stay).
- Details of what he/she might experience during or after the procedure (e.g. 'will it hurt?'), including a discussion of the risks and the probability of success.
- Advice about whether any part of the proposed procedure is experimental.
- The name of the doctor who will have overall responsibility for the treatment.
- Whether doctors in training will be involved.

● A reminder that a patient can change his/her mind about a decision at any time and has a right to seek a second opinion.

It is important to ensure that this information is provided in such a way that the patient has sufficient time to consider it carefully and ask questions before giving consent. In practical terms, it may well be the case that information is given in stages, sometimes by different people working in different institutions. For instance, a patient may be given information about his/her cardiac condition (and a possible need for an invasive procedure) after coronary angiography performed by a physician/cardiologist working in a district general hospital (DGH). Staff at the Regional Cardiac Centre might then provide further information about the proposed procedure, both before and at the time of the patient's admission for that procedure. It is important that any information given is both consistent and accurate. Medical staff performing interventional procedures should provide their audited results to colleagues in their referring DGHs.[10] It is also important that the facts provided are relevant to the patient's particular clinical situation. For example, it would be misleading to cite an average risk of death during coronary angioplasty as <1% when talking to a patient (or his/her relatives) about performing coronary angioplasty as treatment for cardiogenic shock following acute myocardial infarction – in this fortunately rare clinical situation, the likelihood of survival is considerably less than 99%!

Provided that the patient agrees, especially in high-risk clinical situations, it may well be appropriate to provide information about the proposed procedure to the next of kin (and/or other relatives/friends). In the worst-case scenario, it will not be the patient who will be asking what went wrong and why!

Ideally the doctor undertaking the procedure should discuss it with the patient and obtain consent, but if this is not practicable, the task can be delegated to another person, provided that he/she is suitably trained and qualified and has sufficient knowledge of the proposed procedure and its risks.

Although in an emergency a patient can indicate their informed consent orally, it is good clinical practice to make a routine of obtaining written consent for a cardiac interventional procedure. Following appropriate discussion, the patient should be asked to give consent for the treatment of any complications that may arise (e.g. emergency CABG). It is also important to ascertain whether there are any procedures to which the patient would object and which, therefore, should *not* be performed: the consent form should be worded appropriately. Most institutions have special consent forms for Jehovah's witnesses, whose religious beliefs preclude the transfusion of blood or blood products.

ANTICIPATION

Before and during a cardiac laboratory procedure, it is imperative for the interventional cardiologist to maintain an air of calm and cheerful optimism, as uncertainty will quickly be detected by other members of staff and the patient, with potentially unfortunate consequences. In reality it is important to be thinking at least one step ahead as anticipation of possible problems is a vital step towards preventing them or at least dealing with them swiftly and efficiently if or when they occur. While almost anything can happen to any patient, some are especially vulnerable to particular problems, and appropriate prophylactic measures should be undertaken.

All patients

The 'easy procedure' can only be defined in retrospect and one should never assume that an apparently straightforward procedure will necessarily be so. An interventional procedure should only be undertaken by, or under the direct supervision of, a trained operator, with ancillary staff (nurses, technicians and radiographers) who experience a sufficient number of cases in their centre to ensure personal and institutional competence. It is also vital that the procedure is carried out in a fully equipped cardiac catheter laboratory, with an adequate range of equipment and drugs available at all times. This must include full facilities for cardiopulmonary resuscitation, including an intra-aortic balloon pump. There can be no place for a 'quick angioplasty' performed by an inexperienced operator in an ill-equipped location.[10]

Most patients

Although emergency CABG is now required in less than 0.1% of all reported PTCA procedures performed in the UK, the possibility of surgical intervention should be anticipated in all but a very small subgroup of patients in whom a decision is made before the procedure that emergency CABG would be inappropriate. In practical terms this means that coronary interventional procedures should be carried out on patients who have given informed consent for CABG if it should be deemed necessary and have donated a blood sample for blood grouping + formal cross-matching. In other than emergency situations, patients should undergo a three-hour liquid fast and a six-hour solid fast before the procedure. The arrangements for surgical cover for such procedures will vary according to local conditions, but the generally accepted national guideline is that it must be possible to establish cardiopulmonary bypass within 90 minutes of the referral being made to the cardiac surgical service.[10]

Some patients

It can be anticipated that patients with significant impairment of left ventricular (LV) systolic function may experience considerable haemodynamic deterioration during a cardiac interventional procedure, especially if this is prolonged or complex. If such a procedure is to be performed, systemic circulatory support, most often with intra-aortic balloon pump (IABP) counter-pulsation should be used or at least on standby.

Although no patient is immune from the development of 'contrast nephropathy', patients with pre-existing renal dysfunction are especially vulnerable. In such patients, measures that may help prevent the development of this condition[7] include:

- Minimising the volume of contrast medium used.
- Avoiding concomitant use of other nephrotoxic drugs (especially non-steroidal anti-inflammatory drugs).
- Ensuring adequate hydration. This usually implies the administration of IV fluid to a fasting patient – as a general rule at 300–500ml of IV hydration

(normal or half-normal saline) should be given before the contrast medium is administered, whilst post-procedure hydration should be adjusted to achieve a diuresis of at least 150ml/hour.

- The use of low-osmolar non-ionic contrast media, especially iodixanol (Visipaque®).

- N-acetylcysteine (NAC): although this product is used increasingly commonly in this situation, there are considerable uncertainties surrounding its effectiveness. The commonest regimen employed is 600mg orally twice daily for two days, starting the day before the procedure, although clearly this may be impractical for urgent and (especially) emergency cases.[10]

A history of 'allergy' to contrast media is often unconfirmed on checking. Serious reactions are unusual following arterial administration, but should be anticipated in patients with a confirmed history of anaphylactic reactions during previous procedures. Pre-treatment with Prednisolone 40–60 mg daily, preferably for 3–4 days, may be helpful. In an emergency, hydrocortisone 200 mg IV immediately before the procedure, repeated 4-hourly, is a reasonable alternative. Although Chlorpheniramine is often given in addition, there is no convincing evidence that it is of value.

Finally, as has already been stated, patients taking oral anticoagulant therapy are at increased risk of haemorrhage, especially from the vascular access site. A number of measures may lessen this risk, including the use of small-calibre sheaths, conservative heparin dosing, selective or routine use of arterial closure devices and/or pneumatic compression systems and obtaining arterial access via the radial artery.

REFERENCES

1. Brookes CIO, Sigwart U. Taming platelets in coronary stenting: ticlopidine out, clopidogrel in? Heart 1999; 82:651–53.

2. Longstreth K L, Wertz J R. High-dose clopidogrel loading in percutaneous coronary intervention. Ann Pharmacother. 2005; 39:918–22.

3. Blumenthal RS, Wolff MR, Resar JR *et al*. Preprocedural anticoagulation does not reduce angioplasty heparin requirements. Am Heart J. 1993; 125:1221–5.

4. FRISC II Investigators. Invasive compared with non-invasive treatment in unstable coronary-artery disease: FRISC II prospective randomised multicentre study. Lancet 1999; 354: 708–15.

5. Topol EJ, Byzova TV, Plow EF. Platelet GPIIb–IIIa blockers. Lancet 1999; 353:227–31.

   Gill GV, Albert KGMM. The care of the diabetic patient during surgery. In: Alberti KGMM, Zimmet P, DeFronzo RA *et al*. (eds) International textbook of diabetes mellitus, 2nd edn. Chichester: John Wiley, 1997, pp. 1243–53.

6. Ansell G. Complications of intravascular iodinated contrast media. In: Ansell G, Bettman MA, Kaufman JA *et al*. (eds) Complications in diagnostic imaging and interventional radiology, 3rd edn. Cambridge, MA: Blackwell Science, 1996, pp. 245–300.

7. Heupler FA. Guidelines for performing angiography in patients taking Metformin. Cathet Cardiovasc Diag. 1998; 43:121–3.

8. General Medical Council. Seeking patients' consent: the ethical considerations. London: General Medical Council, 1998.

9. Joint working group on coronary angioplasty of the British Cardiac Society and British Cardiovascular Intervention Society. Coronary angioplasty: guidelines for good practice and training. Heart. 2000; 83:224–35.

10. Shalansky SJ, Pate GE, Levin A *et al.* N-acetylcysteine for prevention of radiocontrast induced nephrotoxicity: the importance of dose and route of administration. Heart. 2005; 91:997–9.

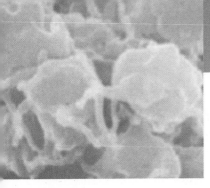

5

Vascular access for percutaneous coronary intervention

TED S. N. LO AND JAMES NOLAN

KEY POINTS

■ Percutaneous transfemoral intervention is still employed by many cardiologists although this is associated with a significant risk of access site neurovascular complication.

■ The percutaneous transradial approach is the safest route available for percutaneous coronary intervention even in the setting of multiple potent antiplatelet agents.

■ Cost benefit, improved short-term quality of life and patient preference all favour the transradial approach.

■ A learning curve exists for the transradial technique but the long-term gain outweighs this short-term disadvantage.

■ For experienced transradial operators, radiation exposure, total procedure times and PCI success rates are comparable to those obtained with transfemoral access.

INTRODUCTION

The arterial access site chosen for PCI can have an important influence on procedural costs and procedural related morbidity and mortality.[1] Access site complications can cause major disability and death. With the exponential rise in PCI procedures and the use of multiple potent antiplatelet agents as standard practice, containing access site complications is an important clinical challenge. Until the late 1980s, most cardiologists utilised the femoral or brachial artery as their access site of choice. The femoral artery has been the preferred route of access ever since the percutaneous Seldinger technique superseded the more technically challenging brachial cut-down approach. There are, however, well documented vascular access complications with the femoral approach especially with concurrent use of glycoprotein (GP) IIb/IIIa inhibitors.[2] It has, therefore, become increasingly apparent that a safer route of arterial access would be highly desirable.[1]

The radial artery has been widely used for many years for haemodynamic monitoring with a low risk of significant neurovascular complications. Two important anatomical features contribute to reducing the risk profile of this access site. First, the vessel is superficial and, in the majority of patients, is not an end artery. Radial artery occlusion does not, therefore, result in major ischaemic complications. Haemostasis is easily achieved by pressure over the point of arterial puncture, while any bleeding is easily recognised allowing prompt action. Second, no major veins or nerves lie close to the radial artery, limiting the risk of neurological damage or arterio-venous fistula formation. The development of small calibre diagnostic catheters facilitated the use of the radial artery for coronary angiography, first described by Campeau in 1989.[3] The success of these diagnostic cardiac procedures has led other cardiologists to explore the use of the radial artery as an access site for PCI.[4]

A COMPARISON OF ARTERIAL ACCESS SITES FOR CORONARY INTERVENTION

When a surgical cut down approach to the brachial artery is employed for cardiac procedures, operator skill and experience are important factors in limiting the rate of complications associated with this technically demanding approach. Skilled high volume operators can achieve low complication rates even in the setting of intensive antithrombotic therapy.[5] For less skilled or infrequent operators, most series consistently reported a 5–10% incidence of major complications [1,6–11] (Fig. 5.1). Major neurovascular complications resulting in acute arm ischaemia or median nerve palsy occur in around 5% of patients (Fig. 5.2). An alternative method to this approach employs a percutaneous Seldinger technique to position a sheath in the brachial artery. This technique is technically much simpler than a surgical cut down, but is associated with a similar risk of important neurovascular complications.[11] Because of these issues brachial access is now rarely employed.

Following the introduction of the Seldinger technique, the percutaneous femoral approach revolutionized the practice of invasive cardiology and remains the access of choice in many institutions.[12] The femoral approach facilitates rapid

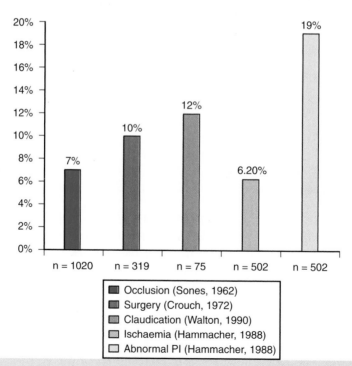

Figure 5.1:
Neurovascular complications after Brachial cut-down procedures.

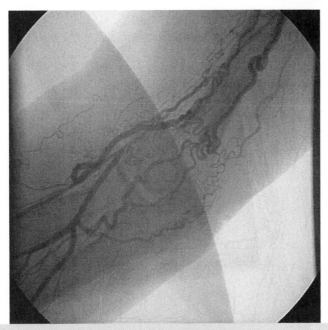

Figure 5.2:
Arteriogram in a patient with arm claudication following a PTCA performed via a surgical cut down approach to the brachial artery. There is total occlusion of the brachial artery at the level of the antecubital fossa with collateral formation limiting forearm ischaemia at rest.

and simple access to the left side of the heart and usually facilitates good catheter support as well as access to large-diameter devices. Such advantages are partially offset by bleeding complications, often mandating prolonged bed rest and further treatment (including compression or thrombin injection for a pseudoaneurysm, blood transfusion or surgical intervention) (Figs. 5.3 and 5.4). These can lead to further discomfort and a longer hospital stay, consuming additional institutional resources. In a minority of patients femoral vascular complications can be severe and lead to death. The incidence of significant neurovascular complications ranges from 1% following a simple diagnostic procedure to 17% when large bore catheters are employed in association with aggressive antithrombotic therapy in PCI (Fig. 5.5).[1,13–17] Concealed retroperitoneal bleeding, although uncommon, is an ominous complication that has a reported mortality rate of 15%.[18] One-third of patients who sustain an iatrogenic femoral nerve injury related to a cardiac procedure have a permanent neurological deficit.[19] These problems have not been resolved with the use of vascular closure device. A meta-analysis of 30 randomised trials (with a total sample size of 4000 patients) indicated that vascular closure device increases the risk of femoral access site complications compared to manual compression.[20] In addition to these complications, access via a brachial or femoral access site is impossible in 5–10% of patients, due to anatomical variation, peripheral vascular disease or obesity, and the radial access site may allow such patients to be investigated and treated.[21]

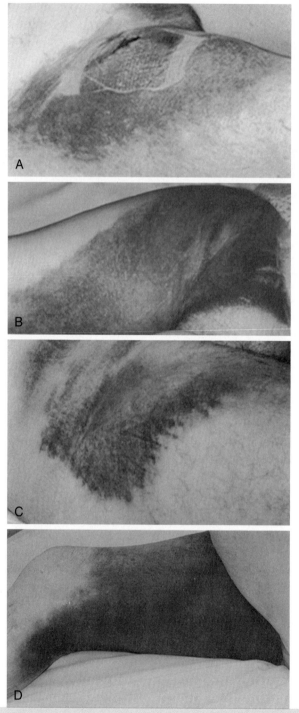

Figure 5.3:
A-B-C-D Large femoral haematoma.

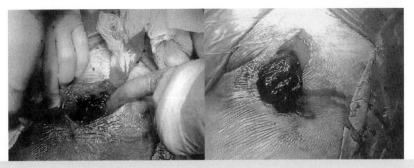

Figure 5.4:
Surgical repair of femoral pseudoaneurysm with large haematoma.

Multiple studies have compared the radial approach with femoral or brachial access. The best know study, The Access Trial[22] examined the relative merits of the percutaneous brachial, femoral and radial access sites in 900 patients undergoing elective PCI. It demonstrates that the radial approach is the safest, with no significant vascular complications occurring, compared to rates of 2% in the femoral group and 2.3% in the brachial group. There was no increase in total procedure duration or radiation exposure when transradial procedures were compared with percutaneous femoral procedures. A recent meta-analysis of

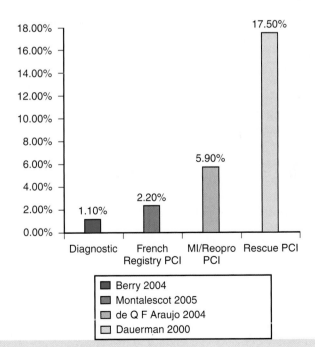

Figure 5.5:
Femoral access site complications in current practice.

12 randomized control trials further confirmed that the transradial approach is a highly safe technique with comparable procedural duration, radiation exposure and clinical results to that of the transfemoral approach.[23] More importantly, vascular access site complications are virtually abolished (0.3%) by the transradial approach.

Given the demonstrated reduction in the risk of vascular complications, the radial artery is a particularly attractive option in the setting of anticoagulation, post thrombolysis or aggressive antiplatelet therapy. Hildick-Smith *et al* reported low rate of radial access complications in fully anticoagulated patients with INR >2 who had a transradial coronary angiography.[24] In a comparison of vascular access site complications in patients undergoing PCI with adjunctive intravenous GP IIbIIIa inhibitor therapy, 7.4% of the transfemoral patients had a major vascular access site complication (despite the use of weight adjusted heparin, small calibre guiding catheters and femoral artery closure devices in the majority of these patients), compared to none of the similarly treated radial patients.[25] In the setting of rescue PCI with adjunct GP IIbIIIa inhibitor, the reported rate of major femoral vascular complications ranges from 20–39%[2,26–28] and around 10% even if vascular closure device is employed.[29] Emerging data assessing the efficacy of transradial PCI in such a setting have all reported near complete elimination of vascular complications and with comparable procedural success rate as transfemoral approach.[30]

Patient comfort and preference are also important considerations in the comparison of these access sites. Delayed mobilisation after transfemoral procedures is common, due to inguinal pain, while bed rest itself has been shown to have an adverse effect on outcome.[31,32] Patients undergoing elective transradial PCI can be mobilised immediately after the completion of these procedures with no adverse effects or risks, which allows PCI to be performed on a day case basis.[33,34] Coronary angiography via the radial artery as opposed to the femoral artery is associated with short-term improvements in quality of life, whilst at the same time reducing hospital costs.[1,35,36] The radial approach for intervention was preferred by 73% of patients in whom preceding diagnostic films were performed by the femoral route.[4] As a result of the shorter hospital stay and reduced complication rates associated with transradial procedures, hospital costs of coronary stent deployment can be reduced by 15% when compared with the femoral route.[36] The transradial technique, therefore, fulfils the requirements for a safer access site for interventional procedures with the added advantages of cost savings and improved quality of life.

THE TRANSRADIAL APPROACH

Case selection

The radial artery is a superficial vessel palpable in the forearm proximal to the flexor retinaculum of the wrist. Any patient with good radial pulsation and a favourable Allen test may be considered to be suitable for a transradial approach.[37] The Allen test is performed by completely occluding the radial and ulnar arterial supply to the hand using digital pressure. The patient is then asked to repeatedly flex and extend their fingers, producing a blanched palmar surface when the hand is opened. With the hand in the open position, the occlusive pressure applied to the ulnar artery is released. If palmar flushing appears within ten seconds the Allen test is regarded as favourable. A favourable Allen test (present in over 90% of the population) confirms that an adequate collateral supply to the hand by the ulnar artery is present, and that occlusion of the radial artery after cannulation will not result in major distal ischaemia. In patients with an unfavourable Allen test, further evaluation with pulse oximetry should be carried out.[38] A pulse oximeter is placed on the thumb, demonstrating a normal high saturation phasic pattern. The radial artery is then occluded by manual compression for two minutes. If a normal high saturation phasic pattern persists, a patent ulnar palmer arch is present. If pulsatile flow is initially abolished but returns within two minutes, an adequate recruitable collateral circulation is present. Radial catheterization is safe in both of these situations should radial occlusion occur. If pulsatile flow is abolished by radial compression and does not reappear, there is a risk of thumb ischaemia if radial occlusion occurs. An alternative access should be employed for these patients. Asymptomatic occlusion of the radial artery has been reported to occur in 2–9% of patients following a transradial procedure, with spontaneous recanalisation in half of these cases.[39–43] Performing a transradial procedure does not preclude the use of the radial artery as a surgical conduit since the contralateral artery can be utilised

RADIAL ARTERY CANNULATION

The patient's right arm is prepared by removing all hand and wrist jewellery before shaving and disinfecting the wrist. The design of most catheterisation laboratories and operator preference favours the use of the right arm, but the left radial artery can be utilised if required or preferred. Any intravenous lines should be placed in the opposite arm. The right arm is supported on an arm board and a small volume of local anaesthetic (1 ml of 1–2% lignocaine) infiltrated over the radial artery 1–2 cm proximal to the styloid process. Care should be taken at this stage not to obliterate the pulse by injecting a large volume of anaesthetic, or to puncture the artery (which may induce spasm).

Radial artery puncture can be performed using either a dedicated transradial introducer system (ARROW International Inc., Reading, PA) or an open needle radial kit (TERUMO Medical Corp, Somerset, NJ; COOK, Bloomington, IN; VYGON UK Ltd, Gloucestershire) using the Seldinger technique. The ARROW system consists of an outer plastic cannula mounted over a small calibre puncture needle. The puncture needle is co-axial with an integrated guidewire housed within a clear observation barrel. When the anterior wall of the radial artery is punctured, arterial blood flows back into the observation barrel, and the integrated guidewire advanced into the radial artery followed by the integral soft plastic outer cannula. The needle, wire and delivery tube are then removed leaving the cannula insitu in the radial artery. A 'cocktail' of anti-spasmolytic drugs such as verapamil and nitrates are then given through the cannula (after warning the patient to expect a short-lived burning sensation in their forearm and hand), and a long guidewire advanced. The cannula is then removed and a radial sheath inserted over the guide wire. Although this system has the advantage of administrating vasodilator cocktail before sheath insertion and may reduce the risk of inducing radial artery spasm, it does have a learning curve of its own.

The open needle Seldinger based technique for radial artery cannulation, which most femoral trained operators are familiar with, appears to be easier to master. A specific radial puncture kit which consists of a short, small caliber needle with a flat-sided hub should be used. The guide wire supplied has a soft tip to aid atraumatic entry into the radial artery whilst the shaft is considerably stiffer to facilitate tracking the sheath into the artery. The puncture site and proximal artery are palpated by the non-dominant hand, and the needle is introduced at a 30 degree angle to the skin directly above the planned puncture site. The radial artery usually lies only a few millimetres below the skin surface, and arterial blood will flow back from the needle hub when the anterior wall of the artery is punctured. Because the puncture needle is small caliber, a low volume, less pulsatile bleed back (compared to vigorous pulsatile flow with puncture of femoral artery) is evidence of satisfactory puncture. The needle position is then fixed with the non-dominant hand, and the guide wire is introduced. If the wire will not easily exit from the tip of the needle, it is important not to attempt to forcefully advance it against resistance. The wire should be removed and the needle position adjusted before further attempts at wire introduction. Usually, this difficulty occurs because the needle bevel is partially embedded in the posterior wall of the artery, and slightly withdrawing the needle will facilitate easy guide wire entry. If the wire enters the artery with no difficulty but resistance is encountered in the mid or upper forearm, the wire has usually entered a small side branch. Withdrawal (for 1–2 cm) and rotation of the wire will usually allow satisfactory wire advancement. A scalpel is then used to make a small incision in the skin at the wire entry point. This is to facilitate sheath introduction, and is particularly important when 6 F or larger sheaths are required. Following this the sheath is usually easily inserted over the wire.

Specific radial access sheaths should also be used in all cases as they have design features optimised to facilitate sheaths introduction into a small caliber radial artery. These include very tapered dilators and hydrophilic coating on the sheaths. The choice of sheath length is between short (7 or 11 cm) or long (23 cm). Long sheaths are best suited for operators during learning curve as they minimize the risk of inducing radial artery spasm related to excessive catheter torquing manoeuvres, but may occasionally be difficult to remove. For experienced radial operators short sheaths are usually satisfactory as catheter manipulation is reduced and spasm less likely. Short sheaths have the advantage of being easier to remove and causing fewer traumas to the artery. When a short sheath is used, it should be secured with a cannula dressing to prevent accidental sheath removal during catheter exchange.

GUILDING CATHETER SELECTION AND MANIPULATION

The majority of patients will have an adequate radial lumen to accommodate a 6 F sheath, which is compatible with kissing balloon techniques or the use of adjunctive devices such as intravascular ultrasound and rotablation. The reduction in size of guide catheters from 8 to 6 F can cause problems with the well established techniques of acquiring adequate guiding catheter back-up. The selection of an optimal catheter configuration is, therefore, vitally important when using the transradial technique. The guiding catheter must provide support

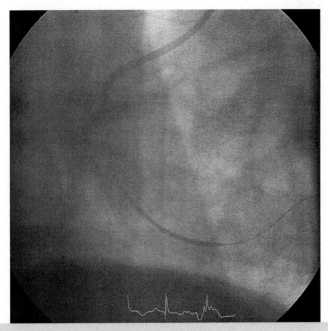

Figure 5.6:
Deep intubation of a 6 F guiding catheter in the right coronary artery, facilitating distal delivery of a stent despite tortuous proximal anatomy and a proximal stent.

from the opposite aortic wall, whilst being co-axial with the coronary ostium. Deep intubation of the catheter may be necessary (Fig. 5.6), in which case the guide catheter must have a soft, atraumatic tip and be flexible enough to be inserted into the vessel. The use of coronary stents requires the guide catheter to have gentle, flexible curves to allow the passage of the stent system with a minimum of friction. The guide catheters available include those designed for the femoral approach and dedicated radial catheters.[39] The left coronary artery may be engaged with the left Judkins, Extra backup (EBU), left Amplatz (AL) and Multipurpose catheters, the Kimny Radial or MUTA radial left. The right coronary is similarly approached with the right Judkins (JR), Multipurpose, right (or left) Amplatz, the Kimny Radial or MUTA radial right. We normally use an EBU or an AL for PCI to the left coronary system and a JR4 or an AL1 for PCI to the right coronary artery. We only use dedicated radial catheters when these fail.

Some complex PCI procedures require the use of large calibre devices or adjunctive supportive therapy such as balloon pumping and coronary pacing. Published data suggests that many individuals have a radial artery capable of accommodating large calibre sheaths, and 7 F or 8 F sheaths can be used in many patients.[44] Where necessary, an antecubital vein can be percutaneously punctured to allow access to the right side of the heart for pacing or pressure measurement. Simultaneous positioning of a radial and femoral sheath will allow PCI to be performed with balloon pump support, without the necessity for bilateral groin punctures.

THE LEARNING CURVE

Performing percutaneous transradial procedures provides new technical challenges and are associated with an important learning curve. During the learning phase, the operator must reliably puncture the relatively small calibre radial artery, successfully manipulate catheters from a distal access site in the right arm, and perform interventions utilising a different range of guiding catheter configurations, calibres and operating techniques. Initial failure rates for radial artery cannulation of 3.8% improving to 1.2% have been reported during a 650 patient series.[45]

A common problem during the initial part of the learning curve is radial artery spasm (Fig. 5.7) which occurs in up to 10% of cases in an initial series making successful cannulation less likely and catheter manipulation more difficult, as well as causing pain during the procedure and making sheath removal unpleasant.[46] The occurrence of spasm is predominantly related to operator experience and to the degree of patient anxiety, such that a successful, painless first pass will be least likely to provoke spasm. The following points may help reduce the occurrence of spasm:

- adequate patient sedation if necessary;
- effective local anaesthetic;
- successful first pass cannulation (avoiding haematoma formation and the initiation of spasm before cannulation);

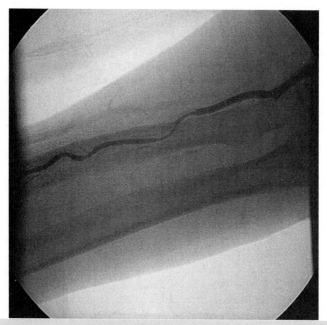

Figure 5.7:
Radial artery spasm prior to introduction of a guidewire.

- use of an anti-spasmolytic, either via the cannula or after insertion of a short length of the sheath. Verapamil and nitrates are commonly used;
- use of a long sheath to protect the vessel wall during catheter movement;
- use of an exchange length guidewire to minimise vessel trauma; and
- operator experience is important (more frequent successful first punctures and shorter procedure times).

If spasm occurs, the patient should be warned that sheath removal will be painful. Extreme spasm (and pain) may make immediate withdrawal impossible, in which case patient sedation and analgesia is required, and sublingual nitrate should be administered. Intra-arterial nitrates and verapamil can be re-administered, whilst warm compresses applied to the arm may reduce the spasm. If the problem persists, increased analgesia and an hour's wait may be sufficient, but if this is unsuccessful, an axillary block will rapidly remove radial spasm. Ongoing research to quantify radial artery spasm and allow comparisons of sheath length and coating and the use and composition of anti-spasmolytic cocktails are currently underway.

CONCLUSION

Coronary intervention performed via a brachial or femoral access site is associated with a significant risk of important neurovascular complications. The use of aggressive antithrombotic regimes in association with acute unstable patients will increase this risk, which cannot be eliminated by the use of vascular access closure devices. Transradial PCI almost eliminates the risk of arterial access site complications. In addition, patients prefer transradial procedures, and hospital costs can be significantly reduced compared with procedures performed via the femoral or brachial artery. The major limitation to widespread clinical use of this access site is the learning curve associated with reliably puncturing the radial artery, and performing PCI from a distal upper limb access site. With improvements in technique and equipment the learning curve has been considerably shortened, and a committed interventionist should have no difficulty in developing a transradial service.[47]

REFERENCES

1. Eccleshall S, Muthusamy T, Nolan J. The transradial access site for cardiac procedures: A clinical perspective. Stent 1999; 2(3):74–9.

2. Sundlof D, Rerkpattanapitat P, Wongpraparut N *et al*. Incidence of bleeding complications associated with abciximab use in conjunction with thrombolytic therapy in patients requiring percutaneous transluminal angioplasty. Am J Cardiol 1999; 83:1569–71.

3. Campeau L. Percutaneous radial artery approach for coronary angiography. Cathet Cardiovasc Diagn 1989; 16(1):3–7.

4. Kiemeneij F. Transradial artery coronary angioplasty and stenting: History and single centre experience. J Invas Cardiol 1996; 8 (Suppl. D):3D–8D.

5. Nolan J, Batin P, Welsh C *et al*. Feasibility and applicability of coronary stent implantation with the direct brachial approach: Results of a single-centre study. Am Heart J 1997; 134(939–44).

6. McCollum CH, Mavor E. Brachial artery injury after cardiac catheterization. J Vasc Surg. 1986; (4):355–9.

7. Hammacher ER, Eikelboom BC, van Lier HJ, Skotnicki SH, Wijn PF. Brachial artery lesions after cardiac catheterisation. Eur J Vasc Surg. 1988; (3):145–9.

8. Adams DF, Fraser DB, Abrams HL. The complications of coronary arteriography. Circulation. 1973; 48(3):609–18.

9. Walton J, Greenhalgh RM. Brachial artery damage following cardiac catheterisation. When to re-explore. Eur J Vasc Surg. 1990; 4(3):219–22.

10. Sones FM Jr. Complications of coronary arteriography and left heart catheterization. Cleve Clin Q. 1978; 45(1):21–3.

11. Hildick-Smith DJ, Khan ZI, Shapiro LM, Petch MC. Occasional-operator percutaneous brachial coronary angiography: first, do no arm. Catheter Cardiovasc Interv. 2002; 57(2):161–5.

12. Noto TJ Jr, Johnson LW, Krone R, Weaver WF, Clark DA, Kramer JR Jr, Vetrovec GW. Cardiac catheterization 1990: a report of the Registry of the Society for Cardiac Angiography and Interventions. Cathet Cardiovasc Diagn. 1991; 24(2):75–83.

13. Oweida SW, Roubin GS, Smith RB 3rd, Salam AA. Postcatheterization vascular complications associated with percutaneous transluminal coronary angioplasty. J Vasc Surg. 1990; 12(3):310–15.

14. Berry C, Kelly J, Cobbe SM, Eteiba H. Comparison of femoral bleeding complications after coronary angiography versus percutaneous coronary intervention. Am J Cardiol. 2004; 94(3):361–3.

15. Montalescot G, Chevalier B, Dalby MC, Steg PG, Morice M-C, Cribier A, Meyer P, Alor F. Description of modern practices of percutaneous coronary intervention and identification of risk factors for adverse outcome in the French nationwide OPEN registry. Heart 2005; 91:89–90.

16. Dauerman HL, Prpic R, Andreou C, Vu MA, Popma JJ. Angiographic and clinical outcomes after rescue coronary stenting. Catheter Cardiovasc Interv. 2000; 50(3):269–75.

17. de Queiroz Fernandes Araujo JO, Veloso HH, Braga De Paiva JM, Filho MW, Vincenzo De Paola AA. Efficacy and safety of abciximab on acute myocardial infarction treated with percutaneous coronary interventions: a meta-analysis of randomized, controlled trials. Am Heart J. 2004; 148(6):937–43.

18. Sreeram S, Lumsden AB, Miller JS, Salam AA, Dodson TF, Smith RB. Retroperitoneal hematoma following femoral arterial catheterization: a serious and often fatal complication. Am Surg. 1993; 59(2):94–8.

19. Kent KC, Moscucci M, Gallagher SG, DiMattia ST, Skillman JJ. Neuropathy after cardiac catheterization: incidence, clinical patterns, and long-term outcome. J Vasc Surg 1994; 19(6):1008–13.

20. Koreny M, Riedmuller E, Nikfardjam M, Siostrzonek P, Mullner M. Arterial puncture closing devices compared with standard manual compression after cardiac catheterization: systematic review and meta-analysis. JAMA. 2004; 291(3):350–7.

21. Al-Allaf K, Eccleshall S, Muthusamy T, Nolan J. Selection of arterial access sites for cardiac procedures. Br J Cardiol. 2000; 7:422–5.

22. Kiemeneij F, Laarman GJ, Odekerken D, Slagboom T, van der Wieken R. A randomized comparison of percutaneous transluminal coronary angioplasty by the radial, brachial and femoral approaches: the Access study. J Am Coll Cardiol. 1997; 29(6):1269–75.

23. Agostoni P, Biondi-Zoccai GG, de Benedictis ML, Rigattieri S, Turri M, Anselmi M, Vassanelli C, Zardini P, Louvard Y, Hamon M. Radial versus femoral approach for percutaneous coronary diagnostic and interventional procedures; Systematic overview and meta-analysis of randomized trials. J Am Coll Cardiol. 2004; 44(2):349–56.

24. Hildick-Smith DJR, Walsh JT, Lowe MD, Petch MC. Coronary angiography in the fully anticoagulated patient: the transradial route is successful and safe. Catheter Cardiovasc Interv. 2003; 58(1):8–10.

25. Choussat R, Black A, Bossi I, Fajadet J, Marco J. Vascular complications and clinical outcome after coronary angioplasty with platelet IIb/IIIa receptor blockade. Eur Heart J 2000; 21:662–7.

26. Ellis SG, Da Silva ER, Spaulding CM, Nobuyoshi M, Weiner B, Talley JD. Review of immediate angioplasty after fibrinolytic therapy for acute myocardial infarction: insights from the RESCUE I, RESCUE II, and other contemporary clinical experiences. Am Heart J. 2000; 139(6):1046–53.

27. Sutton AG, Campbell PG, Graham R, Price DJ, Gray JC, Grech ED, Hall JA, Harcombe AA, Wright RA, Smith RH, Murphy JJ, Shyam-Sundar A, Stewart MJ, Davies A, Linker NJ, de Belder MA. A randomized trial of rescue angioplasty versus a conservative approach for failed fibrinolysis in ST-segment elevation myocardial infarction: the Middlesbrough Early Revascularization to Limit INfarction (MERLIN) trial. J Am Coll Cardiol. 2004; 44(2):287–96.

28. O'Neill WW, Weintraub R, Grines CL, Meany TB, Brodie BR, Friedman HZ, Ramos RG, Gangadharan V, Levin RN, Choksi N. A prospective, placebo-controlled, randomized trial of intravenous streptokinase and angioplasty versus lone angioplasty therapy of acute myocardial infarction. Circulation, 1992. 86(6): p. 1710–17.

29. Boccalandro F, Assali A, Fujise K, Smalling RW, Sdringola S. Vascular access site complications with the use of closure devices in patients treated with platelet glycoprotein IIb/IIIa inhibitors during rescue angioplasty. Catheter Cardiovasc Interv. 2004; 63(3):284–9.

30. Kassam S, Cantor WJ, Patel D, Gilchrist IC, Winegard LD, Rea ME, Bowman KA, Chisholm RJ, Strauss BH. Radial versus femoral access for rescue percutaneous coronary intervention with adjuvant glycoprotein IIb/IIIa inhibitor use. Can J Cardiol. 2004 Dec; 20(14):1439–42.

31. Allen C, Glasziou P, Del Mar C. Bed rest: a potentially harmful treatment needing more careful evaluation. Lancet. 1999; 354:1299–33.

32. Foulger V. Patients' views of day-case cardiac catheterisation. Prof Nurse. 1997; 12:478–80.

33. Laarman GJ, Kiemeneij F, van der Wieken LR, Tijssen JG, Suwarganda JS, Slagboom T. A pilot study of coronary angioplasty in outpatients. Br Heart J. 1994; 72(1):12–15.

34. Kumar S, Anantharaman R, Das P, Hobbs J, Densem C, Ansell J, Roberts DH. Radial approach to day case intervention in coronary artery lesions (RADICAL): a single centre safety and feasibility study. Heart. 2004; 90(11):1340–1.

35. Mann JT 3rd, Cubeddu MG, Schneider JE, Arrowood M. Right Radial Access for PTCA: A Prospective Study Demonstrates Reduced Complications and Hospital Charges. J Invasive Cardiol. 1996; 8 Suppl D:40D–44D.

36. Cooper CJ, El-Shiekh RA, Cohen DJ, Blaesing L, Burket MW, Basu A, Moore JA. Effect of transradial access on quality of life and cost of cardiac catheterization: A randomized comparison. Am Heart J. 1999; 138(3 Pt 1):430–6.

37. AlAllaf K, Eccleshall S, Kaba R, Nolan J. Arterial access for cardiac procedures utilising the percutaneous transradial approach. Br J Cardiol 2000; 7:548–52.

38. Barbeau GR, Arsenault F, Dugas L, Simard S, Lariviere MM. Evaluation of the ulnopalmar arterial arches with pulse oximetry and plethysmography: comparison with the Allen's test in 1010 patients. Am Heart J. 2004; 147(3):489–93.

39. Kiemeneij F. Transradial approach for coronary angioplasty and stenting. Stent 1998; 1:83–88.

40. Stella PR, Kiemeneij F, Laarman GJ, Oderkerken D, Slagboom T, van der Wieken R. Incidence and outcome of radial artery occlusion following transradial artery coronary angioplasty. Cathet Cardiovasc Diagn. 1997; 40(2):156–8.

41. Bertrand B, Sene Y, Huygue O, Monségu J. Doppler ultrasound imaging of the radial artery after catheterization. Ann Cardiol Angeiol (Paris), 2003; 52(3):135–8.

42. Lotan C, Hasin Y, Mosseri M, Rozenman Y, Admon D, Nassar H, Gotsman MS. Transradial approach for coronary angiography and angioplasty. Am J Cardiol. 1995; 76(3):164–7.

43. Nagai S. Ultrasonic assessment of vascular complications in coronary angiography and angioplasty after transradial approach. Am J Cardiol. 1999; 83(2):180–6.

44. Saito S, Ikei H, Hosokawa G, Tanaka S. Influence of the ratio between radial artery inner diameter and sheath outer diameter on radial artery flow after transradial coronary intervention. Cathet Cardiovasc Intervent. 1999; 46:173–8.

45. Louvard Y, Harvey R, Pezzano M, Bradai R, Benaim R, Morice M. Transradial complex coronary angioplasty: The influence of a single operator's experience. J Invas Cardiol. 1997; 9 (Suppl. C):647–9.

46. Barbeau G, Carrier G, Ferland S, Létourneau L, Gleeton O, Larivière M. Right transradial approach for coronary procedures: Preliminary results. J Invas Cardiol. 1996; 8 (Suppl. D):19D–21D.

47. Eccleshall SC, Banks M, Carroll R, Jaumdally R, Fraser D, Nolan J. Implementation of a diagnostic and interventional transradial programme: resource and organisational implications. Heart. 2003; 89(5):561–2.

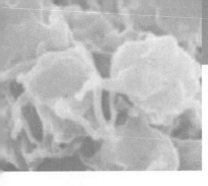

6

Adjunctive pharmacotherapy during PCI

JOHN M. GALLA, MD AND A. MICHAEL LINCOFF, MD

KEY POINTS

■ Given the inherent risk of thrombosis following percutaneous coronary intervention, anticoagulant pharmacotherapy is crucial to both the short- and long-term success of these procedures (Table 6.1).

■ All patients without documented allergy who undergo PCI should maintain or initiate aspirin therapy with daily doses between 75 and 150 mg.

■ Patients who receive intracoronary stents should receive clopidogrel as a loading dose of 300–600 mg followed by 75 mg daily.

■ Therapy should be continued for at least one month following deployment of bare metal stents; three months for sirolimus eluting stents and six months for paclitaxel eluting stents with consideration for longer duration therapy if affordable and well-tolerated.

■ The body of clinical evidence suggests that aside from the lowest risk patients, optimal outcomes with PCI are associated with an advanced anticoagulation regimen including either bivalirudin or a heparin plus GP IIb/IIIa antagonist.

■ GP IIb/IIIa inhibition plus a heparin is currently the preferred approach in patients with acute MI and severe ACS although results of ongoing trials with bivalirudin may demonstrate similar efficacy.

■ For non-emergent interventions, a bivalirudin regimen may be preferred due to reductions in bleeding risk and cost considerations.

INTRODUCTION

The release of thrombogenic subendothelial components is an unavoidable consequence of the deployment of percutaneous coronary devices. The subsequent activation of platelets and the clotting cascade is responsible for the formation of intracoronary thrombus, the major acute complication of percutaneous intervention. Pharmacotherapy directed at inhibition of these pathways is critical to the successful completion and durability of any intracoronary procedure.

ANTIPLATELET THERAPY

Aspirin

The primary antiplatelet mechanism of aspirin is achieved through the irreversible inactivation of cyclooxygenase through acetylation. This inhibition blocks the production of thromboxane A_2, a potent platelet aggregator, which is released by platelets in response to numerous activating factors. Aspirin has been extensively evaluated in the setting of myocardial ischemia. For patients undergoing PTCA, a retrospective analysis showed aspirin to produce a robust reduction in the rate of recurrent occlusive intracoronary thrombosis. Prospective data have shown that patients receiving antiplatelet therapy, including aspirin, experience

TABLE 6.1 - DOSING SUMMARY OF ADJUNCTIVE MEDICATIONS DURING PCI

SUMMARY OF ADJUNCTIVE MEDICATIONS

Drug	Dose
Antithrombin agents	
Unfractionated Heparin (UFH)	With GP IIb/IIIa – 60–70 U/kg IV to target ACT >200–225 sec
	Without GP IIb/IIIa – 100U/kg IV to target ACT >300 sec
LMWH (enoxaparin)	0.75 mg/kg IV
Bivalirudin (Angiomax®)	0.75 mg/kg bolus, 1.75 mg/kg·hr infusion
Antiplatelet agents	
Aspirin	75–162 mg po qd
clopidogrel (Plavix®)	300–600 mg loading dose
	75 mg po qd
	Minimum of one month for BMS, 3–6 mo for DES
ticlopidine (Ticlid®)	250 mg po bid × 2–4 weeks, optional 500 mg po loading dose
abciximab (ReoPro®)	0.25 mg/kg bolus 0.125 mcg/kg·min (max 10 mcg/min) × 12 hrs post PCI
eptifibatide (Integrilin®)	180 mcg/kg bolus, 2.0 mcg/kg·min infusion for 72–96 hrs
	For PCI, second 180 mcg/kg bolus administered ten minutes after first bolus
tirofiban (Aggrastat®)	0.4 mcg/kg load × 30 minutes, then 0.1 mcg/kg·min × 48–96 hrs

GPIIb/IIIa – glycoprotein IIb/IIIa inhibitor

U – units

IV – intravenous

ACT – activated clotting time

BMS – bare metal stent

DES – drug-eluting stent

mcg – microgram

kg – kilogram

PCI – percutaneous coronary intervention

min – minute

max – maximum

significantly fewer periprocedural ischemic events.[1] Based on these and other data, aspirin has become the foundation of interventional antiplatelet therapy.

Patients undergoing percutaneous interventions are likely to be either stabilized on chronic aspirin therapy for secondary prevention in chronic coronary arterial disease or have been recently initiated through the primary treatment of an acute coronary syndrome. The typical dose of 325 mg is likely more than sufficient to completely inhibit platelet thromboxane synthesis. Research has suggested that a dose between 75 and 150 mg is as effective for chronic therapy as higher doses in reducing ischemic events with a lower risk for bleeding events.[2]

THIENOPYRIDINES

The thienopyridine class includes ticlopidine (Ticlid®) and clopidogrel (Plavix®) which both exert antiplatelet activity through irreversible blockade of the P2Y12 ADP receptor. Initial trials [3–7] establishing the additive value of thienopyridines to aspirin were conducted with ticlopidine and demonstrated a reduction in relevant clinical endpoints when compared to warfarin-based therapy. Following its success in the CAPRIE trial,[8] clopidogrel was compared to ticlopidine in a head-to-head trial of patients undergoing PCI. This CLASSICS trial[9] demonstrated equivalent efficacy in the reduction of cardiac endpoints but that clopidogrel had a significantly superior safety profile with little gastrointestinal intolerance or bone marrow suppression.

Once established as the preferred thienopyridine, investigators pursued the application of clopidogrel in the acute coronary syndromes (ACS), specifically non-ST-segment elevation (NSTE) ACS in the CURE trial.[10] As a substudy of CURE, PCI-CURE [11] detailed the outcomes of the 2638 patients who underwent PCI following pretreatment with clopidogrel or placebo for a median treatment duration of six days. Patients in the active arm experienced a durable reduction in major adverse cardiac events from the initial 30 days through 12 months of follow-up suggesting that pretreatment with clopidogrel was responsible for the observed difference. As the management of ACS included an increasing number of patients undergoing early PCI, concerns arose about the effect of the duration and dosage of clopidogrel pre-treatment. Compared to the median clopidogrel pre-treatment of six days in PCI-CURE, the CREDO trial[12] evaluated the efficacy of pre-treatment 3–24 hours prior to elective PCI. A loading dose of 300mg more than six hours before stent deployment demonstrated a trend toward lower cardiac endpoints. The loading dose of clopidogrel in PCI has been further investigated given the frequency of early intervention in the NSTE-ACS population. The ARMYDA-2 trial[13] recruited 255 patients who were treated with a loading dose of 600 mg (vs. 300 mg) administered 4–8 hours before PCI and demonstrated reduced periprocedural myocardial infarctions without an increased risk of bleeding. The ISAR-REACT[14] trial also evaluated the increased 600mg clopidogrel loading dose (given as late as two hours prior to PCI) and found no benefit of added IIb/IIIa receptor blockade in the setting of low-risk PCI.

With the introduction of drug eluting stents, there was a concomitant shift in the recommended minimum duration of therapy following stent deployment. Patients who received bare metal stents typically were continued on thienopyridine therapy for a minimum of 30 days – a duration which reflected the time necessary to re-endothelialize the stented arterial segment. In addition to reducing the incidence of neointimal hyperplasia, both sirolimus and paclitaxel eluting stents delay luminal re-endothelialization to varying degrees. There is currently a Class I (Level of Evidence B) recommendation from the ACC/AHA to continue clopidogrel therapy for three months following sirolimus eluting and six months following paclitaxel eluting stents.[15] Following the durable benefit seen in CURE and CREDO (Fig. 6.1), many operators advise continuation of dual antiplatelet therapy with aspirin and clopidogrel for 9–12 months or more after stent placement.

GLYCOPROTEIN IIb/IIIa INHIBITORS

The platelet surface receptor for glycoprotein IIb/IIIa binds either fibrinogen or von Willebrand factor and is the final common pathway to platelet aggregation. There are three approved parenteral inhibitors of GPIIb/IIIa: a chimeric monoclonal antibody fragment abciximab (ReoPro®); a disulfide-linked

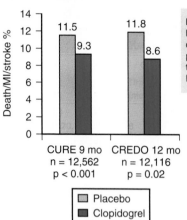

Figure 6.1:
Reduction in ischemic events with long-term (9–12 months) clopidogrel use in addition to aspirin in the CURE trial of patients with unstable ischemic syndromes and the CREDO trial of patients undergoing percutaneous revascularization. MI=myocardial infarction.

heptapeptide eptifibatide (Integrilin®); and, a non-peptide derivative of tyrosine tirofiban (Aggrastat®). For patients undergoing PCI, the blockade of GPIIb/IIIa receptors has demonstrated clear benefit with a consistent reduction in acute ischemic events by as much as 50–60% (Fig. 6.2).

The periprocedural use of abciximab was associated with significant reductions in the 30–day rate of death, myocardial infarction or urgent target vessel revascularization for patients undergoing elective percutaneous interventions.[16–18] Benefit was seen in these trials across numerous interventional

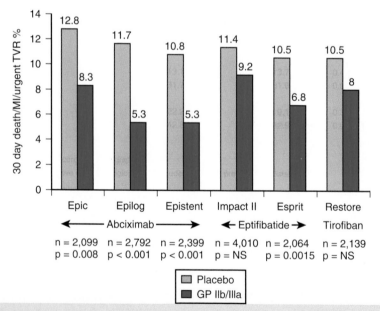

Figure 6.2:
Reduction in 30-day major adverse cardiac events with glycoprotein IIb/IIIa receptor inhibitor (GP IIb/IIIa) use in patients with unstable ischemic syndromes undergoing percutaneous revascularization. MI = myocardial infarction, TVR = target vessel revascularization, NS = non-significant.

techniques including balloon angioplasty, directional atherectomy and coronary stenting. From a pooled analysis, 30-day mortality trended lower by 29% and was significantly lower at six and twelve months by a similar magnitude.[19] Abciximab has been broadly evaluated in the setting of percutaneous revascularization for the primary treatment for ST-segment elevation myocardial infarction (STEMI).[20–24] A meta-analysis which included these 3666 patients confirmed the significant reductions in both short and long-term hard ischemic outcomes without increases in major bleeding events for patients.[25] However, pretreatment with abciximab was of no benefit for patients receiving medical management of NSTE-ACS.[26] The benefits of abciximab have been particularly powerful in high-risk subgroups including patients with diabetes mellitus and unstable angina. Thus, abciximab is efficacious in a variety of clinical settings for patients undergoing percutaneous intervention and confers a durable and robust reduction in important ischemic clinical endpoints including mortality.

For patients undergoing elective percutaneous revascularization, tirofiban and eptifibatide have been evaluated and at lower doses found to be ineffective at reducing ischemic outcomes[27,28]; only eptifibatide at higher doses was found to produce significant reductions relative to placebo, although it is not clear that the magnitude of benefit was the same as that with abciximab in a similar setting.[29] As an adjunct in the management of NSTE-ACS, eptifibatide and tirofiban have been studied in three randomized trials which included over 15 000 patients.[30–32] Relative risk reductions in death or myocardial infarction from these trials ranged from 8–27% and were greatest in patients who underwent early PCI. Benefits were seen in both preprocedural stabilization and reduction of ischemic events following stenting. In the low-risk patient population undergoing PCI (absence of recent MI, unstable angina, angiographic thrombus, LV ejection fraction <30%, hemodynamic instability or insulin-dependent diabetes mellitus), glycoprotein IIb/IIIa inhibition with abciximab failed to demonstrate additional benefit for patients treated with 600mg of clopidogrel at least two hours prior to stent deployment.[14]

Complications of GPIIb/IIIa inhibition include bleeding and idiopathic thrombocytopenia. Bleeding complications most commonly occur at the site of vascular access and have been reduced in frequency by appropriate weight-based algorithms for both GPIIb/IIIa and antithrombin therapy during PCI. Early removal of vascular sheaths and appropriate care of cannulation sites are important measures which help reduce bleeding complications of these drugs. Life-threatening bleeding can be controlled by discontinuing drug administration and in the case of abciximab, platelet transfusion. Concern exists over the possible increased risks for patients needing to undergo CABG shortly after abciximab infusion. Analysis of trial data[17,18] suggests that there was not an increase in perioperative blood loss; however, re-exploration for bleeding was more common but was balanced by a lower frequency of ischemic events. Thrombocytopenia occurs rarely with the GPIIb/IIIa inhibitors but is more frequent with abciximab than tirofiban or eptifibatide and can be extreme in both onset and magnitude

Antithrombin therapy

In addition to platelet activation, rupture of intracoronary plaque during percutaneous intervention is a potent activator of the clotting cascade and the administration of antithrombin therapy is critical to the prevention of periprocedural thrombotic complications. Compounds directed against this pathway include unfractionated heparin (UFH), low-molecular-weight heparins (LMWH) and direct thrombin inhibitors (DTI).

Heparin

Heparin exerts its antithrombotic effect by complexing with anti-thrombin and catalyzing its activity against thrombin and factor Xa. It was widely utilized to prevent abrupt vessel thrombosis during PTCA and has continued to be a mainstay of therapy during PCI. Dosing of heparin is typically monitored through the use of the activated clotting time (ACT) and through early retrospective analyses, patients undergoing PCI with an ACT above 300 seconds appeared to be associated with lower rates of ischemic complications. With the advent of more advanced pharmacologic and mechanical therapies in the catheterization lab additional analyses, have suggested that heparin dosing and ACT targets can be reduced during PCI. When used with glycoprotein IIb/IIIa receptor inhibitors, ACT has been shown to have no impact on efficacy outcomes.[33] A more updated analysis confirmed the absence of effect of ACT on efficacy, but did find increases in bleeding complications with increased ACT.[34] Heparin has continued as standard antithrombin therapy throughout the increasingly complex pharmacologic environment of the cardiac catheterization lab and operators in the current environment typically aim for lower range heparinization: 70–100U/kg, ACT>250 without GP IIb/IIIa blockade, 50–70 U/kg, ACT > 200 sec with GP IIb/IIIa blockade.

Low molecular weight heparins (LMWH)

Low molecular weight heparins (LMWH) are formed by the chemical or enzymatic depolymerization of UFH and have been evaluated for use in the setting of PCI. Their antithrombotic activity is mediated through a specific pentasaccharide sequence which is more specifically directed to inhibition of factor X than thrombin. Compared with UFH, LMWH are less protein bound, yielding better bioavailability, longer half-life and a more predictable anticoagulant response.[35] In most settings, these benefits preclude the need for routine monitoring. Dosing of enoxaparin (Lovenox®), the most widely studied LMWH approved for use in the United States, is typically weight-based and given subcutaneously every 12 hours. In patients undergoing PCI, dosing strategy of enoxaparin was prospectively evaluated and showed that patients can safely undergo intracoronary stenting within eight hours of last enoxaparin without additional antithrombin therapy.[36] For patients who undergo PCI between 8 and 12 hours after last dose, a single intravenous bolus of 0.3 mg/kg is sufficient to prevent major thrombotic events.[37]

The largest experience with LMWH in the setting of PCI comes from four randomized trials comparing LMWH to UFH in NSTE-ACS.[38-41] These large trials complimented small registry data[42] which suggested LMWH was as effective as UFH in the setting of PCI. PCI rates in these prospective trials ranged from 15–47% and the total population included over 20 000 patients. The largest trial to be reported was SYNERGY representing almost half the total population

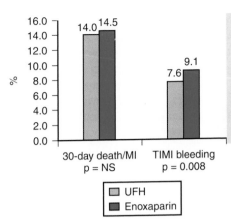

Figure 6.3:
Statistical equivalence in ischemic outcomes and increase in major bleeding between low-molecular-weight heparin (enoxaparin) and unfractionated heparin in patients with unstable ischemic syndromes undergoing percutaneous revascularization from SYNERGY (n = 10,027). MI = myocardial infarction, TIMI = Thrombolysis In Myocardial Infarction and UFH = unfractionated heparin, NS = non-significant.

and recruited high-risk patients with NSTE-ACS who were to be managed with an early invasive strategy. There was no significant difference in the incidence of 30-day death or MI between the groups treated with enoxaparin or UFH. Enoxaparin did meet criteria for non-inferiority to UFH, but was associated with a significant excess risk of major bleeding (Fig. 6.3). Additional analyses from this trial of a modern ACS paradigm suggest patients who undergo a change in antithrombin therapy choice have worse outcomes compared to those who remain on consistent therapy.

Direct thrombin inhibitors (DTIs)

Thrombin (factor II) plays an integral role in the formation of clot within the damaged vessel. In comparison to the heparins, DTIs are active on both free and clot-bound thrombin, are less protein bound and are less susceptible to circulating inhibitors.[43] The direct thrombin inhibitors hirudin (Lepirudin®), a peptide derived from the saliva of the medicinal leech, and bivalirudin (Angiomax®), a peptide analog of hirudin, have been developed and tested for the prevention of thrombosis in several settings including PCI. Following early lessons from investigations of the use of DTIs in ACS[44], bivalirudin was approved as a substitute for UFH during PCI. Regulatory approval of this agent was based on trial data from patients undergoing balloon angioplasty for unstable angina[45], where bivalirudin was shown to provide somewhat better protection against ischemic events and markedly reduce bleeding complications compared with UFH.

With the advent of newer pharmacologic and percutaneous therapies, bivalirudin was re-evaluated in an updated treatment strategy to include the use of thienopyridines, GPIIb/IIIa inhibitors and intracoronary stents.[46] The trial tested the hypothesis that bivalirudin as alternate antithrombin therapy would preclude the need for routine GPIIb/IIIa blockade typically employed with UFH. Patients were randomized to receive a weight-based strategy of bivalirudin and provisional GPIIb/IIIa inhibitor or heparin with planned GPIIb/IIIa inhibitor. The bivalirudin regimen, with only 7.2% of patients requiring provisional GP IIb/IIIa blockade, was associated with similarly low rates of ischemic complications as

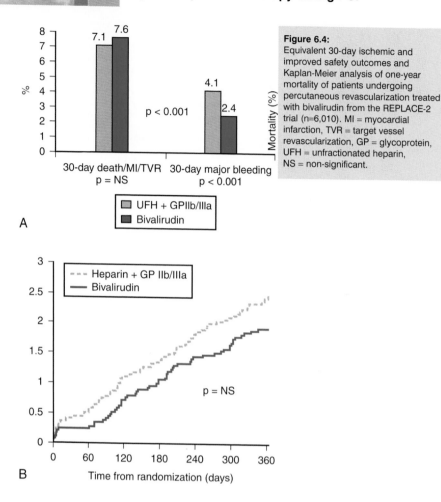

Figure 6.4:
Equivalent 30-day ischemic and improved safety outcomes and Kaplan-Meier analysis of one-year mortality of patients undergoing percutaneous revascularization treated with bivalirudin from the REPLACE-2 trial (n=6,010). MI = myocardial infarction, TVR = target vessel revascularization, GP = glycoprotein, UFH = unfractionated heparin, NS = non-significant.

was heparin with routine use of a GP IIb/IIIa inhibitor. Major bleeding rates were significantly reduced by 41% in patients randomized to bivalirudin when compared to the heparin group. No differences in mortality were observed by 1-year; however, there was a trend that favored bivalirudin therapy (Fig. 6.4A and B). These data confirmed the effectiveness and safety of bivalirudin with discrete use of GPIIb/IIIa blockade as an effective strategy for reducing thrombotic complications of PCI. Patients with high-risk ACS or acute MI were not tested in REPLACE-2, and are under evaluation in other dedicated trials.

REFERENCES

1. Schwartz L, Bourassa MG, Lesperance J, *et al.* Aspirin and dipyridamole in the prevention of restenosis after percutaneous transluminal coronary angioplasty. N Engl J Med 1988; 318:1714–19.

2. Collaborative meta-analysis of randomised trials of antiplatelet therapy for prevention of death, myocardial infarction, and stroke in high risk patients. Br Med J 2002; 324:71–86.

3. Leon MB, Baim DS, Popma JJ, *et al.* A clinical trial comparing three antithrombotic-drug regimens after coronary-artery stenting. Stent Anticoagulation Restenosis Study Investigators. N Engl J Med 1998; 339:1665–71.

4. Urban P, Macaya C, Rupprecht HJ, *et al.* Randomized evaluation of anticoagulation versus antiplatelet therapy after coronary stent implantation in high-risk patients: the multicenter aspirin and ticlopidine trial after intracoronary stenting (MATTIS). Circulation 1998; 98: 2126–32.

5. Schuhlen H, Hadamitzky M, Walter H, Ulm K, Schomig A. Major benefit from antiplatelet therapy for patients at high risk for adverse cardiac events after coronary Palmaz-Schatz stent placement: analysis of a prospective risk stratification protocol in the Intracoronary Stenting and Antithrombotic Regimen (ISAR) trial. Circulation 1997; 95:2015–21.

6. Schomig A, Neumann FJ, Kastrati A, *et al.* A randomized comparison of antiplatelet and anticoagulant therapy after the placement of coronary-artery stents. N Engl J Med 1996; 334:1084–9.

7. Bertrand ME, Legrand V, Boland J, *et al.* Randomized multicenter comparison of conventional anticoagulation versus antiplatelet therapy in unplanned and elective coronary stenting. The full anticoagulation versus aspirin and ticlopidine (fantastic) study. Circulation 1998; 98:1597–603.

8. A randomised, blinded, trial of clopidogrel versus aspirin in patients at risk of ischaemic events (CAPRIE). CAPRIE Steering Committee. Lancet 1996; 348:1329–39.

9. Bertrand ME, Rupprecht HJ, Urban P, Gershlick AH, Investigators FT. Double-blind study of the safety of clopidogrel with and without a loading dose in combination with aspirin compared with ticlopidine in combination with aspirin after coronary stenting: the clopidogrel aspirin stent international cooperative study (CLASSICS). Circulation 2000; 102:624–9.

10. Yusuf S, Zhao F, Mehta SR, Chrolavicius S, Tognoni G, Fox KK. Effects of clopidogrel in addition to aspirin in patients with acute coronary syndromes without ST-segment elevation. N Engl J Med 2001; 345:494–502.

11. Berger PB, Steinhubl S. Clinical implications of percutaneous coronary intervention-clopidogrel in unstable angina to prevent recurrent events (PCI-CURE) study: a US perspective. Circulation 2002; 106:2284–7.

12. Steinhubl SR, Berger PB, Mann JT, 3rd, *et al.* Early and sustained dual oral antiplatelet therapy following percutaneous coronary intervention: a randomized controlled trial. JAMA 2002; 288:2411–20.

13. Patti G, Colonna G, Pasceri V, Pepe LL, Montinaro A, Di Sciascio G. Randomized trial of high loading dose of clopidogrel for reduction of periprocedural myocardial infarction in patients undergoing coronary intervention: results from the ARMYDA-2 (Antiplatelet therapy for Reduction of Myocardial Damage during Angioplasty) study. Circulation 2005; 111:2099–106.

14. Kastrati A, Mehilli J, Schuhlen H, *et al.* A clinical trial of abciximab in elective percutaneous coronary intervention after pretreatment with clopidogrel. N Engl J Med 2004; 350:232–8.

15. Antman EM, Anbe DT, Armstrong PW, *et al.* ACC/AHA guidelines for the management of patients with ST-elevation myocardial infarction—executive summary. A report of the American College of Cardiology/American Heart Association Task Force on Practice Guidelines (Writing Committee to revise the 1999 guidelines for the management of patients with acute myocardial infarction). J Am Coll Cardiol 2004; 44:671–719.

16. Use of a monoclonal antibody directed against the platelet glycoprotein IIb/IIIa receptor in high-risk coronary angioplasty. The EPIC Investigation. N Engl J Med 1994; 330:956–61.

17. Platelet glycoprotein IIb/IIIa receptor blockade and low-dose heparin during percutaneous coronary revascularization. The EPILOG Investigators. N Engl J Med 1997; 336:1689–96.

18. Randomised placebo-controlled and balloon-angioplasty-controlled trial to assess safety of coronary stenting with use of platelet glycoprotein-IIb/IIIa blockade. The EPISTENT Investigators. Evaluation of Platelet IIb/IIIa Inhibitor for Stenting. Lancet 1998; 352:87–92.

19. Kereiakes DJ, Lincoff AM, Anderson KM, et al. Abciximab survival advantage following percutaneous coronary intervention is predicted by clinical risk profile. Am J Cardiol 2002; 90:628–30.

20. Brener SJ, Barr LA, Burchenal JE, et al. Randomized, placebo-controlled trial of platelet glycoprotein IIb/IIIa blockade with primary angioplasty for acute myocardial infarction. ReoPro and Primary PTCA Organization and Randomized Trial (RAPPORT) Investigators. Circulation 1998; 98:734–41.

21. Montalescot G, Barragan P, Wittenberg O, et al. Platelet glycoprotein IIb/IIIa inhibition with coronary stenting for acute myocardial infarction. N Engl J Med 2001; 344:1895–903.

22. Neumann FJ, Kastrati A, Schmitt C, et al. Effect of glycoprotein IIb/IIIa receptor blockade with abciximab on clinical and angiographic restenosis rate after the placement of coronary stents following acute myocardial infarction. J Am Coll Cardiol 2000; 35:915–21.

23. Antoniucci D, Rodriguez A, Hempel A, et al. A randomized trial comparing primary infarct artery stenting with or without abciximab in acute myocardial infarction. J Am Coll Cardiol 2003; 42:1879–85.

24. Stone GW, Grines CL, Cox DA, et al. Comparison of angioplasty with stenting, with or without abciximab, in acute myocardial infarction. N Engl J Med 2002; 346:957–66.

25. De Luca G, Suryapranata, H, Stone, GW, et al. Abciximab as adjunctive therapy to reperfusion in acute ST-segment elevation myocardial infarction. JAMA 2005; 293:1759–65.

26. Simoons ML. Effect of glycoprotein IIb/IIIa receptor blocker abciximab on outcome in patients with acute coronary syndromes without early coronary revascularisation: the GUSTO IV-ACS randomised trial. Lancet 2001; 357:1915–24.

27. Randomised placebo-controlled trial of effect of eptifibatide on complications of percutaneous coronary intervention: IMPACT-II. Integrilin to Minimise Platelet Aggregation and Coronary Thrombosis-II. Lancet 1997; 349:1422–8.

28. Effects of platelet glycoprotein IIb/IIIa blockade with tirofiban on adverse cardiac events in patients with unstable angina or acute myocardial infarction undergoing coronary angioplasty. The RESTORE Investigators. Randomized Efficacy Study of Tirofiban for Outcomes and REstenosis. Circulation 1997; 96:1445–53.

29. Novel dosing regimen of eptifibatide in planned coronary stent implantation (ESPRIT): a randomised, placebo-controlled trial. Lancet 2000; 356:2037–44.

30. Inhibition of platelet glycoprotein IIb/IIIa with eptifibatide in patients with acute coronary syndromes. The PURSUIT Trial Investigators. Platelet Glycoprotein IIb/IIIa in Unstable Angina: Receptor Suppression Using Integrilin Therapy. N Engl J Med 1998; 339:436–43.

31. A comparison of aspirin plus tirofiban with aspirin plus heparin for unstable angina. Platelet Receptor Inhibition in Ischemic Syndrome Management (PRISM) Study Investigators. N Engl J Med 1998; 338:1498–505.

32. Inhibition of the platelet glycoprotein IIb/IIIa receptor with tirofiban in unstable angina and non-Q-wave myocardial infarction. Platelet Receptor Inhibition in Ischemic Syndrome Management in Patients Limited by Unstable Signs and Symptoms (PRISM-PLUS) Study Investigators. N Engl J Med 1998; 338:1488–97.

33. Chew DP, Bhatt DL, Lincoff AM, et al. Defining the optimal activated clotting time during percutaneous coronary intervention: aggregate results from 6 randomized, controlled trials. Circulation 2001; 103:961–6.

34. Brener SJ, Moliterno DJ, Lincoff AM, Steinhubl SR, Wolski KE, Topol EJ. Relationship between activated clotting time and ischemic or hemorrhagic complications: analysis of 4 recent randomized clinical trials of percutaneous coronary intervention. Circulation 2004; 110:994–8.

35. Weitz JI. Low-molecular-weight heparins. N Engl J Med 1997; 337:688–98.

36. Martin JL, Fry ET, Sanderink GJ, et al. Reliable anticoagulation with enoxaparin in patients undergoing percutaneous coronary intervention: The pharmacokinetics of enoxaparin in PCI (PEPCI) study. Catheter Cardiovasc Interv 2004; 61:163–70.

37. Collet JP, Montalescot G, Lison L, et al. Percutaneous coronary intervention after subcutaneous enoxaparin pretreatment in patients with unstable angina pectoris. Circulation 2001; 103:658–63.

38. Cohen M, Demers C, Gurfinkel EP, et al. A comparison of low-molecular-weight heparin with unfractionated heparin for unstable coronary artery disease. Efficacy and Safety of Subcutaneous Enoxaparin in Non-Q-Wave Coronary Events Study Group. N Engl J Med 1997; 337:447–52.

39. Antman EM, McCabe CH, Gurfinkel EP, et al. Enoxaparin prevents death and cardiac ischemic events in unstable angina/non-Q-wave myocardial infarction. Results of the thrombolysis in myocardial infarction (TIMI) 11B trial. Circulation 1999; 100:1593–601.

40. Ferguson JJ, Califf RM, Antman EM, et al. Enoxaparin vs unfractionated heparin in high-risk patients with non-ST-segment elevation acute coronary syndromes managed with an intended early invasive strategy: primary results of the SYNERGY randomized trial. JAMA 2004; 292:45–54.

41. Blazing MA, de Lemos JA, White HD, et al. Safety and efficacy of enoxaparin vs unfractionated heparin in patients with non-ST-segment elevation acute coronary syndromes who receive tirofiban and aspirin: a randomized controlled trial. JAMA 2004; 292:55–64.

42. Kereiakes DJ, Grines C, Fry E, et al. Enoxaparin and abciximab adjunctive pharmacotherapy during percutaneous coronary intervention. J Invasive Cardiol 2001; 13:272–8.

43. Lefkovits J, Topol EJ. Direct thrombin inhibitors in cardiovascular medicine. Circulation 1994; 90:1522–36.

44. Direct thrombin inhibitors in acute coronary syndromes: principal results of a meta-analysis based on individual patients' data. Lancet 2002; 359:294–302.

45. Bittl JA, Chaitman BR, Feit F, Kimball W, Topol EJ. Bivalirudin versus heparin during coronary angioplasty for unstable or postinfarction angina: Final report reanalysis of the Bivalirudin Angioplasty Study. Am Heart J 2001; 142:952–9.

46. Lincoff AM, Bittl JA, Harrington RA, *et al*. Bivalirudin and provisional glycoprotein IIb/IIIa blockade compared with heparin and planned glycoprotein IIb/IIIa blockade during percutaneous coronary intervention: REPLACE-2 randomized trial. JAMA 2003; 289:853–63.

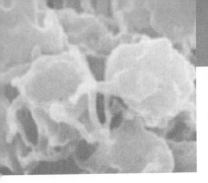

7

Intra coronary stenting

DR E. JOHN PERRINS, MD BSC FRCP FACC

KEY POINTS

▪ Stents are a landmark technology and are used in the majority of PCI.

▪ Modern stents are both radially strong and conformable.

▪ Balloon expandable slotted tube stents predominate.

▪ Stents are available pre-mounted on balloons with a wide variety of diameters and lengths.

▪ Stents reduce restenosis and reintervention in PCI.

▪ Stents reduce acute complications of conventional balloon angioplasty and reduce the need for emergency bypass surgery.

▪ Bifurcations, long diffuse lesions and small vessels have higher restenosis rates.

▪ In-stent restenosis is difficult to treat.

INTRODUCTION

The development and widespread use of coronary stents has probably been the single most significant advance in the field of interventional cardiology over the last 20 years. So much so that the use of a stent at the time of coronary artery dilatation is now carried out in more than 98% of all intra coronary angioplasty procedures and so, in many ways, coronary angioplasty has become coronary stenting. Despite this coronary stenting is still perceived as a relatively immature technology, there is still very significant and important debate concerning its exact role and there is a proliferation of stent designs, stent technologies and stent coatings which continue to challenge the interventional cardiologist to try and utilise them to their best ability. The increased cost of stenting represents financial challenges that have been taken up to a greater or lesser extent in different health care systems and countries. The United Kingdom, as in so many other things, tends to lag behind other developed countries in this regard (Fig. 7.2).

The fundamental principle of coronary stenting is that a mechanical scaffold will be placed at the site of the treated segment of the coronary artery. The scaffold increases the radial strength of the vessel wall thereby preventing elastic recoil. In addition by pressing the intima firmly against the media of the arterial wall, it will tend to prevent disruption of the plaque or dissected flaps from proliferating or expanding and may cause more rapid healing at the site of the intervention. Equally the stent itself will introduce new properties into the treated segment of artery. It will alter the fundamental elasticity of that vessel and the stent itself may induce subsequent biological changes, for example, intimal hyperplasia, which may to some extent undo the initial advantages of placing the stent in the first place (restenosis).

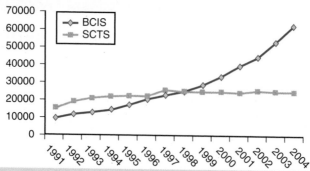

Figure 7.1:
Rapid annual growth of UK PCI procedures with static numbers for CABG. 95% of all UK PCI procedures in 2004 used one or more stents. (From BCIS audit returns 2004.) (www.bcis.org.uk)

Fundamental challenges in stenting

- The actual mechanical design of the stent itself.
- The problem of physically delivering the stent to the coronary artery in question.
- Expanding the stent to its proper dimensions.
- Ensuring that the stent is evenly and properly applied to the intimal surface of the vessel.
- The ensuing biological response to the stent itself.

The rapid and continued growth of stenting in the UK is illustrated by Fig. 7.1.

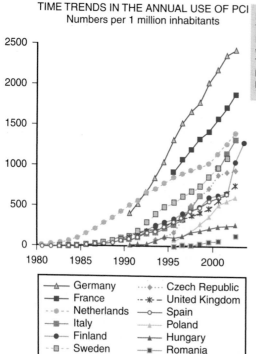

TIME TRENDS IN THE ANNUAL USE OF PCI
Numbers per 1 million inhabitants

Figure 7.2:
Time trends in annual PCI rates from Euro Heart Survey 3rd report. www.escardio.org/knowledge/ehs/slides/ The UK has increased its rates steadily but has made no progress in closing the gap between its main European partners.

HISTORICAL OVERVIEW

Although the widespread use of stents is a relatively recent phenomenon in the world of PCI the concept of using a device to maintain the lumen goes right back to the originators of angioplasty itself. Charles Dotter who originally described the use of progressive dilating devices to push through and create an opening in occluded peripheral vessels, in 1964 also, proposed that a silastic supporting device might be placed in an artery following such a procedure to maintain patency.[1] Dotter and Judkins were also, first to coin the term 'stent' to describe an intra-vascular implant in a peripheral artery in 1969. The origin of the word stent itself is obscure but may be related to the work of a dentist, Charles Thomas Stent, who developed a material for taking dental impressions. In 1977, of course, Grunzig made his first description of balloon coronary angioplasty and the subsequent very rapid interest and growth of that technique, for a while at least caused the concept of stenting to be put somewhat into the background. In 1983, Dotter and his colleagues described the use of trans-catheter placement of nitinol coil stents into canine arteries.[2] Shortly after, Maass and his colleagues described the use of steel springs as a stenting device.[3] In 1985, Palmaz and his team hit upon the idea of using an angioplasty balloon to assist in the deployment of a stent in the peripheral arteries. They came up with the entirely novel concept of using a balloon to expand the stent within the coronary arteries. The technique that has now become more or less the de facto technique for intra-coronary stenting today. In 1987, Palmaz and Schatz described the implantation of balloon expandable stents in the canine coronary circulation.[4] Between 1986 and 1988 a number of initial implantations of both balloon expandable and self-expanding (wall stent) were reported in humans. All of the early stent experience was plagued by the problems of thrombosis of the stent after placement and the difficulty of manipulating relatively rigid and bulky stent devices into the appropriate part of the coronary circulation.

Whilst these early attempts at developing coronary stent devices were taking place, it was becoming apparent from the wider application of simple balloon angioplasty that this technique was not without its problems. In particular the problems of vessel dissection, acute closure and restenosis were starting to become a major limitation in the application of angioplasty. It was apparent to many of the pioneering investigators at that time that stenting might well provide a partial solution to all of these problems. In the early 1990s, when the balloon expandable Palmaz Schatz stent was really the most practical and proven of the available devices, two seminal studies were commenced, the Benenstent in Europe and the Stress Study in North America.[5,6] These two randomized controlled studies focused on the use of coronary stenting in the single discrete lesion and looked specifically at restenosis rates compared to simple balloon angioplasty. Both studies showed a very important reduction in restenosis (Benenstent: 22% stent, 32% balloon. Stress: 32% stent, 42% balloon). These trials although they have been extensively analyzed and criticized triggered an explosion in stenting which had continued unabated.

There have, of course, been numerous highly significant developments since Benestent and Stress were published. Antonio Colombo[7] is widely regarded as having realised that one of the fundamental problems with stent placement (particularly with the Palmaz Schatz stent) was failure to completely expand all of the stent when placed in the coronary vessel. He proposed the technique of high pressure stent deployment, initially with the thought of over expanding the stent but subsequently realising, particularly with ultrasound, that the stents simply required a high pressure to completely expand them. Although many stents are now manufactured claiming to require lower deployment pressures most operators will still deploy stents with pressures in the region of 10–16 atmospheres in the deploying balloon. The recognition that anti-platelet agents reduce sub acute stent thrombosis, in particular the early use of Ticlopidine further opened the way to widespread stent usage. Controlled trials[8] showing that Warfarin actually added nothing and possibly increased complications in elective stenting allowed the abandonment of Warfarin with marked reduction in femoral arterial closure complications and, of course, the subsequent development of closure devices has largely eliminated these problems. The introduction of Clopidogrel into routine PCI practice has largely eliminated stent thrombosis and intravascular ultrasound has allowed us to fully appreciate the difficulties of actually estimating the proper diameter of the intra-coronary vessel, the adequacy of deployed stent expansion and the importance of covering all of the at risk lesion. Most of all, of course, it has been the tremendous amount of technological development carried out by the stent manufacturers themselves, in producing balloon expandable stents, that have a low profile, high flexibility and are easy to use.

Drug eluting and other coatings have in some countries almost completely replaced the bare metal stent. They will be fully discussed in another chapter.

STENT DESIGN

Most articles on coronary stenting tend to describe the various stent designs available at the time of writing the book or chapter. In my view, all this does is uniquely date the text as stent design and development is progressing so rapidly that even in the relatively short time it has taken to produce this book any such information would be out of date. However, it is fair to say that the balloon expandable stent currently reigns supreme and as nearly all of the balloon expandable stents share common design features I will concentrate on those. Julio Palmaz had the brilliant idea that if one took a very thin stainless steel tube and cut small longitudinal slots in that tube using a laser cutter; if the tube was then expanded by a balloon the expanded slotted tube would become a mesh. Clearly the shape and properties of that mesh would depend entirely upon the way the tube was cut, the material from which the tube was made and the way in which the tube was expanded with the balloon. Like so many good ideas he initially found it difficult to interest a manufacturer to produce it. Johnson & Johnson Inc. (who had had very little prior involvement with cardiac intervention) eventually listened to his suggestions and the balloon expandable stent was born. Figure 7.3 shows the appearances of a balloon mounted slotted tube stent in expanded and unexpanded forms.

Desirable design features for stents
- biologically inert;
- good radio-opacity;

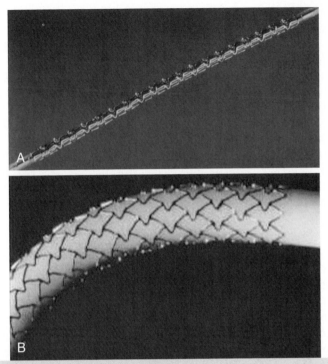

Figure 7.3:
A, An unexpanded NIR stent (Boston Scientific Inc). The complex slots in the steel tube are evident.
B, The same stent expanded on the balloon. The slotted tube becomes a tubular mesh which is both radially strong and conformable.

- flexible when mounted on delivery balloon;
- radial strength and conformable when expanded;
- smooth surface and/or coating;
- good side branch access through stent cells;
- availability of wide range of diameters and lengths;
- reduced metal or cell design for smaller vessels, increased for larger diameter vessels; and
- low cost.

The design of any stent is always a trade off between a number of desirable characteristics. The stent requires radial strength in order to prevent the collapse of the stent and to hold the wall of the stented segment of artery, firmly in place. However, at the same time the stent needs to be conformable and flexible, both when it is compressed upon the delivery balloon and when it is expanded within the coronary vessel, as coronary vessels, of course, have highly complex 3D shapes. The material of the stent requires to be biologically inert. It is a highly desirable characteristic that the stent can be seen during its placement, by utilizing x-ray screening equipment. The radio opaqueness of the stent is, therefore, a vital factor when actually implanting it. The surface of the stent needs to be as smooth as possible in order to attract as little platelet interest as possible. In early stent designs because of the problems of the rigidity of the slotted tube small segments of slotted tube were linked together by articulations, this allowed the stent to bend in certain places but obviously meant that the coverage of the wall of the vessel would be incomplete at the point of articulation. Numerous clever geometric designs in the method of cutting the stainless steel tube have now resulted in stents that are both flexible, but have radial strength. The size of the associated cells in the expanded mesh is, therefore, not too large. Many manufacturers now produce different stents for different sizes of vessel particularly different diameters as obviously if one stent is used for all coronary diameters then the larger the stent is expanded the less amount of vessel wall will be covered. The stent may, therefore, have too much metal coverage in small vessels and too little in large vessels. Most stents are made from some form of stainless steel, although other metals have been used particularly nitinol and tantalum. In addition changing the metal composition of the stainless steel particularly in varying the chromium content (e.g. Guidant Vision and Medtronic driver) has improved the surface properties of the metal itself.

Stents have also been coated in a range of various materials, most of which have had a fairly neutral effect, although there has been some suspicion curiously that coating the stent with gold may actually produce adverse consequences. More recently a lot of attention has focused on other methods of coating a stent, for example, the PC coating process (Biocompatibles Inc.) and the Carmeda coating process – bonding Heparin to the surface of the stent (Cordis Inc.). These designs have been largely replaced with drug eluting coatings although other approaches such as antibody binding may yet be effective. Obviously modifying the surface properties of the stent may eventually allow lower platelet activation and reduce the amount of intimal hyperplasia but there is no real clinical evidence to support this yet.

In the early days of stenting, the stent was supplied on its own and had to be crimped, usually by hand, on to an angioplasty balloon. Modern stents, however, almost invariably consist of a stent pre-mounted on the balloon and in fact balloons are now designed specifically to accept stents and many stents are heat sealed on to the balloon so that it is almost impossible to detach the stent whilst the balloon is deflated.

There are many other stent designs (Fig. 7.4). Some have used coiled or twisted wire to produce expandable cells which can then be welded together to form longer stents (e.g. AVE Micro stent and GFX stents). Some are made entirely from complex coils which when expanded are similar to mesh stents (Cordis Crossflex). Others have used a steel backbone to which are attached segments which can be expanded. Finally there was the Wallstent, a lattice work of stainless steel wires which when unconstrained expand to form a tube. The device is held in its collapsed state by a sheath which when withdrawn allows the stent to self expand. Although still used in larger peripheral vessels the wallstent is rarely used in the coronary circulation today.

The paper by Lau and Sigwart[9] examines in detail the relationships between different stent technologies and possible clinical impact. The need for manufacturers to produce distinguishable and patentable designs has caused a

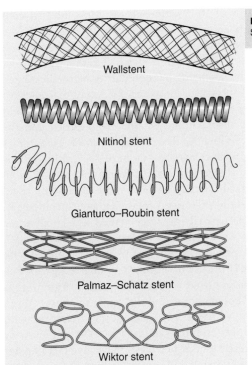

Figure 7.4:
Some different early stent designs.

Wallstent

Nitinol stent

Gianturco–Roubin stent

Palmaz–Schatz stent

Wiktor stent

number of poor designs to be tested in man, and similar problems will plague drug-eluting stent technologies for many years to come.

Covered stents
All the stents discussed so far are various kinds of meshes which have holes in them. Covered stents aim to totally cover the intimal surface of the treated vessel in a manner similar to a tube graft. Most designs have a polymer tube sandwiched between two stents or covering the outside of one. As the stent is expanded the polymer stretches and forms a tube graft. So far long term results with restenosis have been very poor, they do have a unique place, however, in the treatment of coronary perforation and in the exclusion of coronary aneurysms.

TECHNIQUE OF STENT DEPLOYMENT
The technique of stent deployment is relatively simple in theory! Following conventional arterial access ordinary guiding catheters are used and a guide wire usually 0.14 is used to cross the target lesion. Until relatively recently pre dilatation of the target lesion was always required as the stent was too bulky to pass directly across the narrow vessel. However, in the last two to three years balloon mounted stents have become significantly lower in profile and have increased flexibility to allow direct crossing of the undilated lesion in a high proportion of cases, so called primary or direct stenting. Once the stent is positioned satisfactorily the balloon is inflated and generally the stent deployed

at a pressure somewhere in the region of 10–16 atmospheres. Most modern stent deployment balloons allow a high enough pressure to be used so that the deploying balloon can carry out the final deployment of the stent. In addition stents are now mounted on balloons whose length is matched to that of the stent removing the risk of either end of the deploying balloon damaging the unstented vessel wall when expanded to high pressure. However, for many reasons post inflation of the stent may sometimes be required, often with a shorter balloon at even higher pressures. The wire is then withdrawn, the groin closed and the patient generally discharged the following day. Periprocedural Heparin is generally considered to be essential, most centres will monitor KCT although this is not always universal and with the use of or increasing use of GP2a/3b inhibitors such as Reo-Pro, weight adjusted Heparin is more commonly used. Clopidogrel and Aspirin are universally prescribed following stent deployment. Some centres will only use Aspirin particularly in larger stented segments but the majority of centres, particularly in the UK, will use Aspirin and Clopidogrel. There is no absolute agreement either on the duration of treatment required with anti-platelet drugs or on the doses but the use of 75 mg Clopidogrel and 300 mg Aspirin for at least two weeks and often four weeks following the procedure is common and most patients will be maintained on Aspirin at lower doses indefinitely unless they are hyper-sensitive to it. Adequate pre-treatment with clopidogrel is now recognized to be essential and up to 600 mg may be administered if the patient is not already established on it. In elective PCI I favour at least one week's treatment with clopidogrel and aspirin prior to the procedure. Warfarin is generally not used in the context of coronary stenting nowadays. In patients who have a pre existing high risk requirement for warfarin (e.g. prosthetic heart valve) aspirin and clopidogrel may be combined with the warfarin but formal safety of this approach is unknown.

GENERAL INDICATIONS FOR STENTING

The clinical selection of patients for intervention is covered elsewhere in this book. Stents are placed in the following situations:

- bail out;
- elective with pre dilatation;
- elective without pre dilatation;
- following a preceding device therapy (e.g. after rotablator);
- urgent – ACS; and
- urgent – STEMI.

In the early days of stenting stent placement for bailout indications after unsatisfactory or unsuccessful balloon angioplasty or other device intervention was the primary indication. However, following the realisation that elective stenting reduced restenosis, bail-out stenting is now uncommon (Fig. 7.5). Provisional stenting has also largely disappeared from UK practice. Primary stenting (see below) is unquestionably quicker and cheaper to perform electively than provisional stenting (i.e. balloon angioplasty first and only stent if angiographic result is unsatisfactory) (Fig. 7.6).

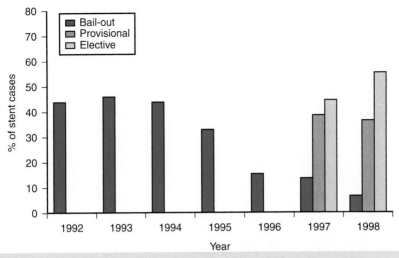

Figure 7.5:
Use of bail-out stenting in the UK 1992–2004. Bail-out and provisional stenting have largely disappeared. (www.bcis.org.uk)

PERI PROCEDURAL COMPLICATIONS OF STENTING

Procedural complications primarily relate to whether it is possible to deliver a stent to the intended site in the coronary artery. As operators started to use stenting in more and more complex coronary arteries the limitations of the mechanical properties of the stent – balloon combination not infrequently led to the situation whereby the unexpanded stent could not be taken forward to the desired place. Thereby inevitably requiring an attempt at withdrawing the stent balloon or deploying the stent in an unwanted area. Withdrawal of the undeployed stent on the balloon used to represent a considerable risk of the stent being pulled off the balloon and being left unexpanded, but left within the coronary circulation. This is now a very rare complication as most stents if they have been applied to the balloon by the manufacturer are very resistant to being loosened in this way but there are many operator errors which can still allow this to occur, for example, if the balloon has been inflated at all at any time during the procedure the stent may have been loosened. If the balloon is left on negative pressure during deployment (the routine for balloon angioplasty) the balloon may loosen from the stent enough to allow it to come off the balloon. Sometimes when withdrawing a stent back into a guiding catheter the edge of the guiding catheter will lift up the back of the stent and then strip it off the balloon as the balloon is withdrawn. It cannot be emphasised enough the importance of screening the balloon and stent whenever the balloon and stent are moved together but particularly during withdrawal. It is vital to ensure that the tip of the guide catheter and the stent are as coaxial as possible during withdrawal. Even when the stent balloon is not being intentionally withdrawn it may move between the time at which the stent was in the right position and the time at which the balloon is actually inflated. It is very important to continue to screen at the time of the inflation.

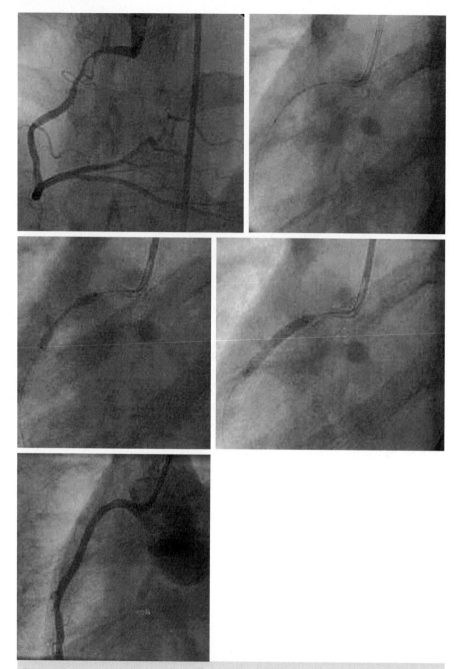

Figure 7.6:
These five angio frames show a primary stent procedure to the right coronary vessel in a patient with unstable angina. The lesion is crossed with a 014 wire and a Cordis Velocity 3.5mm × 23mm stent. The final result is excellent. Procedure time 8.5 minutes.

UNDER EXPANSION OF THE STENT

The second major group of procedural complications relate to inability or failure to deploy the stent adequately even though it may be in the right place. Routine use of relatively high pressure balloon expansion together with more compliant balloon designs have made this complication less common but adequate expansion of the stent is fundamentally predicated by having selected a stent of the correct diameter for the lumen of the vessel and the routine use of QCA is still to be highly recommended to ensure proper selection of stent size so long as, of course, QCA is carried out properly and calibrated properly. Strict attention to the appearance of the stent following deployment in more than once projection remains vital to assessing whether the stent is actually deployed both completely and at the right diameter. As mentioned earlier in this chapter under deployment of the stent is one of the fundamental causes of sub-acute stent thrombosis and unquestionably contributes to a higher restenosis rate. Some X-ray screening manufacturers are developing digital technolgies to image the expanded stent without contrast to examine it more closely. Drug eluting stents are definitely less forgiving of inadequate deployment or undersizing and IVUS remains important particularly in key positions such as the left main stem.

EDGE DISSECTIONS

Stenting, of course, fundamentally reduces the risk of dissection at the point at which the stent is placed. However, sometimes a dissection will propagate from the end of the stent. Most commonly this is a distal edge dissection. If there is just a very small shelf or irregularity at the end of the stent then it may not be necessary to do anything further but it is very important to observe the lesion for a minute or two if nothing else is done. However, in the author's experience one commonly ends up having to place another stent at the outflow of the first one. Although intravascular ultrasound is well described as a way of helping to manage these kinds of complications the fact that it is not used routinely generally leads operators to place another stent. Anterograde dissection is much less common but potentially very serious, as if a dissection propagates proximally towards the ostium of the stented vessel there is the risk of involvement of the main stem or another major proximal side branch. It is easy for the operator to miss proximal problems related to the stent. It should also be remembered that it is possible to dissect the proximal vessel during the passage of a stent particularly if that stent passage has been difficult. Prompt stenting of the affected proximal segment of the vessel is essential and may be life saving. Proximal dissections can sometimes involve the wall of the aorta itself.

SIDE BRANCHES

Obviously whenever a stent is placed over the ostium of a side branch unpredictable consequences may occur. If the side branches are relatively small and there is clearly good angiographic flow down the side branch then experience has shown that no further attention to that side branch is required. However, often a side branch may appear nipped or may even disappear when a stent is expanded across it. Most modern stents will allow the passage of a wire through the mesh into a side branch which can then generally be dilated and even stented itself.

As soon as the operator moves into that realm he has to face up to the techniques and limitations of bifurcation stenting which will be discussed in a later section.

Vessel rupture

Vessel rupture during stenting itself is relatively rare although obviously may occur particularly during pre dilatation. Occasionally if a lesion is very resistant to dilatation and very high pressure is required a balloon rupture may still cause a vessel perforation despite a stent having been placed. Stenting may, of course, be a life saving maneouvre when vessel rupture has occurred for other reasons and the covered stent particularly is very useful in that rare but very dramatic situation. Inflation of a standard angioplasty balloon in the vessel proximal to the perforation will often prevent major bleeding into the pericardium. Pre dilatation of occlusions with very small diameter balloons initially may reduce the risk of rupture when the guide wire has entered a small branch leading from the occlusion. Never give Reo-Pro before you have opened an occlusion successfully.

DISTAL EMBOLISATION

Significant embolisation of material following a stent expansion in a stable chronic atheromatous plaque is very rare. However, as stenting is used more and more both in acute unstable syndromes and in myocardial infarction, stents are increasingly used in situations where embolisation may occur. It is the author's personal experience that in this situation primary or direct stenting comes into its own as the balloon and stent can be placed directly across a soft friable lesion and the stent expanded and deployed with a single balloon dilatation. Embolisation often occurs if post dilatation of such a stent is then attempted and it is the author's opinion that post dilatation should not be carried out on stents in these acute and friable lesions. This is particularly important in the context of acute myocardial infarction or where stents are being placed in bulky friable vein grafts. The management of embolisation is difficult, Reo-Pro would generally be considered to be mandatory unless there were some fundamental contra-indication to its use. Intra-coronary nitrates and particularly intra-coronary Verapamil may help to combat the no reflow situation that occurs. More recently devices are becoming available which may catch embolic material in particular high risk situations (e.g. Cordis Angioguard) and a whole new technology of clot removal and dispersal devices has arrived and will be discussed in another chapter.

POST PROCEDURAL COMPLICATIONS

By far away the most important complication in the early days of stenting was sub acute stent thrombosis with abrupt closure of the vessel, usually within the first 7–14 days of stent placement. Modern anti-platelet treatment, high pressure ballooning and adequate stent to vessel sizing have largely eliminated this problem, however, and in modern practice sub acute stent thrombosis rates are well below 1%. Paradoxically it is now so rare that it may be missed altogether if a patient represents. Curiously if a sub acute stent thrombosis does occur simple ballooning of the stent together with Heparin or Reo-Pro generally results in an excellent angiographic appearance and repeated sub acute thrombosis seems to be virtually non-existent and presumably it all relates to the mechanics of the initial stent dilatation.

RESTENOSIS

Restenosis remains a fundamental complication of any percutaneous intervention and although stenting fundamentally reduces restenosis it does not by any stretch of the imagination eliminate it. It is difficult to get a true perspective as to what the clinical impact of restenosis is. It is well known that angiographic restenosis rates are higher than clinical restenosis rates a consistent feature in nearly all interventional trials. Clearly there is a fundamental difference between a restenosis and re-presentation following interventional procedure. Within the UK at least restenosis appears to be being treated in between 7–10% of patients. The treatment of restenosis is a complex topic and in my view fundamentally relates to the context in which the original intervention was done and in particular whether additional moderate or perhaps more severe disease is still present in other vessels. Coronary artery by-pass grafting is an excellent treatment for restenosis and it is essential that patients are offered surgical revascularisation if it is clearly the most appropriate option. All known methods of treating restenosis themselves result in a higher rate of further restenosis. In the author's view diffuse disease in long stents should always been treated by surgery unless there is a contraindication. Focal restenosis may well be susceptible either to balloon inflation, cutting balloon inflation or re-stenting. Because the material within the stent in a restenotic lesion is smooth and rubbery it is often the case that if a balloon is inflated within a restenosed stent the balloon prolapses either antro-gradely or distally and does not expand the material. Repeated attempts to expand the stent in this situation can lead to catastrophic damage to the vessel and if migration of the balloon is occurring prompt re-stenting is the treatment of choice as the stent is able to engage the intimable hyperplasia and can then be deployed without migration of the balloon. Similarly the blades in the cutting balloon will cut into the intimal hyperplasia, generally allowing dilatation of the segment without balloon migration. Unfortunately it may be difficult to place the cutting balloon in the stented segment due to its rigidity and it may be difficult to get a good match of length of cutting balloon to length of restenotic segment. There has been a lot of focus on the use of radiation both for the treatment of restenosis and for its prevention and this is covered elsewhere in this book.

STENTING IN LESIONS SUBSETS

Small vessels

All of the randomised trials of stenting v balloon angioplasty have shown a fundamental relationship between vessel size and restenosis. As vessel size gets smaller restenosis becomes more common. This data relates to stents which have not specifically been designed for small vessels. Newer designs allowing less wall coverage and with improved surface coatings may allow small vessel stenting with similar results to larger vessels but clinical trial results are not yet available. Small vessel stenting probably relates to the use of stents in vessels between 2.25 and 2.75 mm internal diameter. Whether any intervention at all it is justified in vessels smaller than 2 mm is probably not known.

At the moment it is hard to justify the use of stents in an elective scenario for small vessels. However, because small vessels are frequently involved in interventional procedures and are certainly no less likely to suffer complications of dissection than larger vessels it is often necessary to stent smaller vessels. It is important to attain the largest possible lumen size in these situations and the availability of quarter-sized balloons particularly 2.75 mm balloons is important but not always generally recognised or available. Results with drug eluting stents may be disappointing in very small vessels.

LEFT MAIN STEM

The left main stem used to be an absolute contraindication to angioplasty or stenting and although in general terms surgery should always be offered there are many circumstances where surgery may be at particularly high risk or impossible. There have been a number of studies recently presented of elective stenting in the left main stem and this will be fully covered in a later chapter. Stenting of the left main in poor surgical candidates is now accepted and trials are now ongoing to assess elective left main stenting with drug-eluting stents compared to CABG.

SAPHENOUS BY-PASS GRAFTS

The management of the diseased by-pass graft is a difficult problem for everybody treating patients who have been revascularised. The graft is frequently diffusely diseased, often has fiable material within it and often is of large diameter which may stretch the mechanical properties of stents to their limits. It should be remembered that nearly all of the longitudinal studies of stenting and angioplasty in vein grafts show a consistently higher restenosis rate and perhaps much more importantly a very significant chronic occlusion rate in the graft within two years of the procedure. With current technologies stenting of a by-pass graft cannot really be considered to be a definitive treatment. Careful attention should always be paid to the native vessels as if it is possible to revascularise the native vessel to which the graft is attached that is generally a better procedure to carry out and is likely to have a better long term outcome. There is no convincing evidence that the use of Reo-Pro reduces the risk of complications from graft angioplasty other than where thrombus is clearly present. The newer thrombus collecting devices are generally accepted to improve long-term outcomes but they are still not routinely used in all graft PCI in the UK. I believe primary stenting offers a fundamental advantage in the treatment of the by-pass graft as by avoiding pre dilatation and then placing the stent with one inflation the risk of embolisation seems to be reduced and primary stenting should be employed wherever possible in the saphenous vein graft.

OSTIAL LESIONS

Treatment of ostial lesions either of grafts or the right coronary artery is made simpler by stenting but the restenosis rates are significantly higher than in the body of the vessel. It can be very difficult to accurately size the ostium without intravascular ultrasound. Placement of the stent right up to the ostium can be difficult and careful guide catheter selection and positioning is required. It is very easy to miss the first 2–3 mm of the vessel with subsequent restenosis. The use of a longer stent (18mm or greater) even in short discrete ostial lesions may be helpful as it allows easier positioning and decreases the chance of the stent moving during deployment. High pressures are required in the ostium but dissection of the main aortic wall is possible.

BIFURCATION LESIONS

The treatment of coronary bifurcations remains the most technically challenging and contentious area of intervention. All current routine treatments have higher restenosis and adverse event rates than for lesions in the body of the vessel. This applies as much to stenting as to other device technologies discussed elsewhere in this book. Coronary bifurcations are a heterogeneous collection of anatomical variations and different strategies are employed according to whether both limbs are involved, the angulation, the proximal segment, etc. The presence of significant bifurcation disease, particularly at the LAD/Diagonal position mandates a careful consideration of the benefits of CABG. If other adverse factors such as diabetes are present then surgery has to be the strategy of first choice. A detailed discussion of bifurcation stenting is beyond the scope of this chapter.

Bifurcation stenting – key points

- There is a steep learning curve.
- The use of two guidewires and simultaneous inflation of both predilating and post deployment balloons is associated with improved results.
- Primary stenting is currently not possible.
- Larger lumen guide catheters are helpful.
- Stent the most important (generally larger) vessel first.
- Culotte stenting (where both stents are in the proximal segment as well as in each limb) is widely advocated but early clinical results are uncertain.
- Wrapping of the two guide wires either in the guide catheter or in the proximal vessel can produce catastrophic "jamming" of the two balloons or stents.
- A bifurcation restenosis is even more difficult to treat than the original lesion.

LONG LESIONS

Stents are now generally available in a variety of lengths up to 40 mm. Longer lesions may require more aggressive predilatation and the use of support wires may facilitate stent passage. Longer stented segments are probably associated with higher rates of in-stent restenosis. Very careful attention needs to be paid to adequate stent expansion. Post dilatation to high pressure is more commonly needed and it is vital to taper the stent if the reference diameter at the start of the lesion is more than 0.5mm of the distal lesion. Calcified long lesions are particularly likely to have some areas of poor stent expansion. Ideally intravascular ultrasound should be used in this situation to optimise deployment.

Urgent PCI for ACS and STEMI

These topics will be covered at length in other sections of this book but it is clear that emergency or acute intervention will become the dominant mode of treatment as a number of trials have clearly shown benefit to early interventional treatment, the RITA3 trial being typical.[10] This requires fundamental reconsideration of the method of service delivery and the relationships between small and large centres. In 2004 in the UK 50% of PCI procedures were acute and this will rise sharply as primary PCI is rolled out.

CONCLUSIONS AND FUTURE DIRECTIONS

Stenting will continue to dominate PCI for some years to come. Primary PCI for acute STEMI is now established but roll out throughout the UK will take time. The management of ACSs will dominate emergency PCI for some time to come and it is likely that cold elective PCI will reduce in numbers as will elective CABG. Drug-eluting stents have sufficient unsolved problems to ensure technological growth for many years to come and the totally absorbable stent either a polymer or a soluble metal remains a tantalising proposition. Data is emerging suggesting linkages between procedural volumes and outcomes particularly in the treatment of STEMI and ACS. Coronary care units are already outmoded and need to be replaced by acute revascularisation centres (ARC).

REFERENCES

1. Dotter CT, Judkins MP. Transluminal treatment of arteriosclerotic obstruction. Circulation 1964; 30:654–70.

2. Dotter CT, Buschman PAC, McKinney MK, Rosch J. Transluminal expandable nitinol coil stent grafting. Radiology 1983; 147:259–60.

3. Maas D, Zollikofer CL, Largiader F, Senning A. Radiological follow-up of transluminally inserted vascular endoprostheses: an experimental study using expanding spirals. Radiology 1984; 152:659–63.

4. Schatz RA, Palmaz JC, Tio FO, Garcia F, Garcia O, Reuter SR. Balloon expandable intra-coronary stents in the adult dog. Circulation 1987; 76:450–7.

5. Serruys PW, De Jaegre P, Kiemeneij F et al, for the Benestent study group. A comparison of balloon-expandable stent implantation with balloon angioplasty in patients with coronary artery disease. New Engl J Med 1994; 331:489–95.

6. Fischman DL, Leon MB, Baim DS et al, for the stent restenosis study investigators. A randomised comparison of coronary stent placement and balloon angioplasty in the treatment of coronary artery disease. New Engl J Med 1994; 331:496–501.

7. Colombo A, Hall P, Nakamura S et al. Intracoronary stenting without anticoagulation accomplished with intravascular ultrasound guidance. Circulation 1995; 91:1676–88.

8. Schomig A, Neuman FJ, Kastrati A et al. A randomised comparison of antiplatelet and anticoagulant therapy after placement of Intracoronary stents. N Engl J Med 1996; 334: 1084–9.

9. Lau KW, Mak K, Hung J, Sigwart U. Clinical impact of stent construction and design in percutaneous coronary intervention. Am Heart J 2004; 147:764–73.

10. Fox KAA *et al*. Interventional versus conservative treatment for patients with unstable angina or non-ST-elevation myocardial infarction: the British Heart Foundation RITA 3 randomised trial. Randomized Intervention Trial of unstable Angina Lancet. 2002 Sep 7; 360 (9335):743–51.

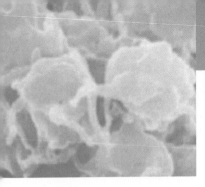

8

Drug-eluting stents

SOPHIA VAINA MD, ANDREW T. L. ONG MBBS, FRACP,
PATRICK W. SERRUYS MD, PHD

KEY POINTS

- Stent implantation was developed to overcome the acute recoil of balloon angioplasty, but resulted in the development of chronic in-stent restenosis related to specific factors regarding patient, lesion and procedural characteristics.

- Drug-eluting stents are a novel approach in stent technology and design with local drug delivery to inhibit intimal thickening by interfering with different pathways.

- Both the drug and the delivery vehicle must fulfill pharmacological, pharmacokinetic and mechanical requirements.

- Current successful drug eluting stents require a polymer coating for drug delivery.

- Clinical trials examining several pharmaceutical agents, particularly sirolimus and paclitaxel, have demonstrated marked reduction in restenosis following stenting.

- Treatment of coronary stenosis with sirolimus or paclitaxel-eluting stents has been associated with a sustained clinical benefit with low rates of target vessel revascularization and major adverse cardiac events.

INTRODUCTION

Coronary artery disease is one of the major causes of morbidity and mortality in developed countries. In addition to medical treatment, percutaneous coronary stent implantation is for many patients, the method of choice for the management of coronary atherosclerosis. This is because stents prevent acute vessel closure and early vessel recoil, and improve the long-term patency of vessels. However, restenosis still remains a problem. The pathogenesis of restenosis can be divided into four phases, which can take place from hours to weeks and months: early elastic recoil, mural thrombus formation, neointimal proliferation with extracellular matrix formation, and chronic geometric arterial changes (months).[1] Some risk factors such as long, complex lesions, small vessels and diabetes have been clearly identified, and others are at present discussed.[2] Local delivery of immunosuppressive agents using drug-eluting stents, targets the inhibition of excessive cell growth, inflammation, migration, proliferation and/or secretion of the extracellular matrix. Several different compounds, which interfere in various sites of this vicious process, have been proposed. Currently, in clinical practice rapamycin and paclitaxel eluting stents are widely used, whereas extended research is ongoing for the evaluation of new agents and novel stent designs.

PATHOGENESIS OF RESTENOSIS

Restenosis is a local vascular manifestation of the general biological response to injury. The response to balloon inflation and stent implantation is initially determined by the extent of the arterial injury, which is associated with endothelial cell loss exposing the underlying vessel wall.[3] This leads to immediate accumulation of platelets, macrophages and polymorphonuclear neutrophils, aiming to cover the location of the injury.[4] Platelets and leukocytes contain chemotactic factors and mitogens, which are released in the injured vessel wall. Chemokines increase the amount of matrix metalloproteinase, which induces remodeling of the extracellular matrix and smooth muscle cell migration.[5,6] Furthermore, injury also causes stretching and lysis of some of the cells, mainly vascular smooth muscle cells of the underlying layers, which are thus activated. As a result, these cells shift from a contractile to a synthetic phenotype, leading to proliferation, migration and synthesis of extra-cellular matrix responsible for intimal thickening.[3] Smooth muscle cells are also stimulated to increase the expression of genes involved in cell division[7]. Compared to restenosis after balloon angioplasty, the pathophysiology of in-stent restenosis may be different, with more profound cellular and proliferative response and less thrombogenic potential.

DRUG-ELUTING STENTS

The concept of delivering immunosuppressive agents locally to prevent in stent restenosis arose from similarities observed between tumor cell growth and tissue proliferation that characterises intimal hyperplasia following stenting. Drug release at the site of vascular injury achieves an effective local concentration of the drug for a certain period of time, while simultaneously avoiding systemic toxicity. The safety and efficacy of drug-eluting stents depend on the combination of drug, delivery system, and kinetics of release.[8] Two different delivery systems have been explored, with and without additional coatings. Uncoated metal stents that have a drug attached to their surface or embedded within macroscopic fenestrations or microscopic nanopores, enabling rapid drug delivery are under investigation and are not yet commercially available. Metal stents coated with an outer layer of polymer (bioabsorbable or non-bioabsorbable) can be drug-loaded, thus providing more controlled and sustained drug delivery, which might allow more optimal drug–tissue interactions.[9] Polymer coatings have been proven to be durable, and deliver drug in a uniform and controlled way.

Sirolimus eluting stents

The Johnson and Johnson "Cypher" stent consists of a BX Velocity™ stent (Cordis/J&J, Miami Lakes, FL, USA), and a polymer coating. The incorporation of an additional drug-free polymer matrix prolongs drug release to more than 28 days in the slow release formulation.[10]

Sirolimus is natural macrocyclic lactone that binds to specific cytosolic proteins called FK506 binding protein which blocks G1 to S cell cycle progression by inhibiting the activation of a protein known as mTOR (mammalian target of rapamycin) (Fig. 8.1)[11]. This also suppresses cytokine driven T cell proliferation. The first in man (FIM) implantation study of the sirolimus-eluting stent was performed in Rotterdam and Sao Paolo. Since then, four randomized trials have been conducted, and are summarized in Tables 8.1, 8.2 and 8.3. The first randomized trial of sirolimus eluting stent was the RAVEL study (RAndomized study with the

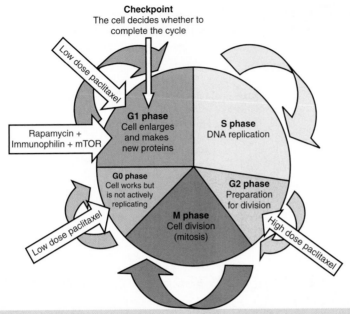

Figure 8.1:
Sirolimus and paclitaxel site of action on cell cycle. The sirolimus immunophilin complex blocks G1 to S cell cycle progression by interacting with a specific target protein (mTOR) and inhibiting its activation. High doses (>12nM) of paclitaxel cause G2/M arrest, whereas low doses (3–6nM) arrest primarily G0 to G1 and G1 to G2 phases.

sirolimus-coated bx VELocity™ balloon expandable stent in the treatment of patients with de novo native coronary artery lesions). At six months, the degree of neointimal proliferation, manifested as the mean late luminal loss, was significantly lower in the sirolimus-stent group than the standard stent group. At one year follow-up, the overall rate of major cardiac events was 5.8% in the sirolimus eluting stent group and 28.8% in the bare metal stent group (p<0.001)(12). The early RAVEL results appear to be maintained out to three years.[13]

The US based SIRIUS trial (Multicenter, randomized, double blind study of the SIRolImUS-eluting Bx-Velocity™ balloon expandable stent in the treatment of patients with de novo coronary artery lesions) randomized 1058 patients in to treatment with rapamycin-coated or bare metal Bx Velocity™ balloon expandable stents.[14] At 12 months, target-lesion revascularization (TLR) was 4.9% in the sirolimus arm versus 20% in the bare metal arm (p<0.001).[15] SIRIUS was the only trial in which edge restenosis, predominantly located at the proximal margin of the stent was observed and was attributed to balloon injury occurring outside the stent.[14]

The C-SIRIUS (The Canadian Study of the Sirolimus-Eluting Stent in the Treatment of Patients With Long De Novo Lesions in Small Native Coronary Arteries)[16] and the E-SIRIUS (the European study)[17] confirmed the effectiveness of the sirolimus-eluting stent in smaller populations (Tables 8.1, 8.2 and 8.3).

TABLE 8.1 - RANDOMIZED TRIALS COMPARING BARE METAL STENTS WITH POLYMER-COATED DRUG-ELUTING STENTS

	STUDY CHARACTERISTICS		
	Design	Inclusion Criteria	Study Groups
SIROLIMUS			
RAVEL (12, 67)*	randomized double-blind	de novo lesion native vessel single lesion lesion length <18 mm vessel diameter 3 – 3.5mm	Polymer-coated sirolimus-eluting stent (n = 120 pts) Bare stent (n = 118 pts)
SIRIUS (14)[†]	randomized double-blind	de novo lesion native vessel single lesion lesion length 15 – 30 mm vessel diameter 2.5 – 3.5mm	Polymer-coated sirolimus-eluting stent (n = 533 pts) Bare stent (n = 525 pts)
E-SIRIUS (17)*	randomized double-blind	de novo lesion native vessel single lesion lesion length 15 – 32 mm vessel diameter 2.5 – 3.0mm	Polymer-coated sirolimus-eluting stent (n = 175 pts) Bare stent (n = 177)
C-SIRIUS(16)*	randomized double-blind	single de novo coronary lesion Stable or unstable angina or documented silent ischemia Lesion length 15 – 32 mm Vessel diameter 2.5 – 3.0 mm	Polymer-coated sirolimus-eluting stent (n = 50 pts) Bare stent (n = 50 pts)
PACLITAXEL (polymer-coated)			
TAXUS I (61)[‡]	randomized double-blind	single lesion, single stent restenotic or de novo lesions lesion length ≤12 mm vessel diameter 3.0 – 3.5mm	Polymer-coated slow-release paclitaxel-eluting stent (n = 31 pts) Bare stent (n = 30 pts)
TAXUS II (68)[§]	randomized double-blind	single lesion, single stent native vessel de novo lesions lesion length ≤12 mm vessel diameter 3.0 – 3.5mm	Polymer-coated slow-release paclitaxel-eluting stent (n = 131 pts) Bare stent control for SR-paclitaxel (n = 136 pts) Polymer-coated moderate-release paclitaxel-eluting stent (n = 135 pts) Bare stent control for MR-paclitaxel (n = 137 pts)
TAXUS IV(69)[||]	randomized double-blind	single de novo lesions length 10 – 28 mm vessel diameter 2.5 –3.75mm	Polymer-coated moderate-release paclitaxel-eluting stent (n = 662 pts) Bare stent control for MR-paclitaxel (n = 652 pts)
TAXUS V(24)[¶] ∂	randomized double-blind	single de novo lesions lesion length 10 – 46 mm vessel diameter 2.25 – 4.0mm	Polymer-coated SR paclitaxel-eluting stent (n = 586 pts) Bare stent (n = 586 pts)

TABLE 8.1 - RANDOMIZED TRIALS COMPARING BARE METAL STENTS WITH POLYMER-COATED DRUG-ELUTING STENTS—cont'd

	STUDY CHARACTERISTICS		
	Design	Inclusion Criteria	Study Groups
TAXUS VI(25)	randomized double-blind	lesion length 20.6 mm	Polymer-coated moderate-release paclitaxel-eluting stent (n = 219) Bare stent (n = 227 pts)

* Aspirin lifelong, clopidogrel for two months
† Aspirin lifelong, clopidogrel for three months
‡ Aspirin for at least twelve months, clopidogrel for six months
§ Aspirin lifelong, clopidogrel for at least six months
|| Aspirin lifelong, clopidogrel for six months
¶ Aspirin for nine months, clopidogrel for six months

Paclitaxel-eluting stents

Paclitaxel promotes polymerization of tubulin and inhibits the disassembly of microtubules, which stabilizes microtubules and results in inhibition of cell division. Cell replication is inhibited in the G_0/G_1 and G_2/M phases (Fig. 8.1).[18] Additionally, paclitaxel affects cell motility, shape, and transport between organelles.

Two delivery methods have been used in clinical trials, either with or without a polymer carrier. In the pivotal US trial DELIVER 1, paclitaxel was loaded without a polymer. No significant benefit was seen in the treated group and the stent was not commercialized.[19]

Boston Scientific Corporation pursued the development of paclitaxel stents eluted from a polymeric carrier. The randomized TAXUS I trial evaluated the safety of the TAXUS™ – NIRx™ stent system[20] and was followed by TAXUS II[21] and TAXUS IV. In the TAXUS IV trial, compared with the bare-metal stent the paclitaxel-eluting stent [paclitaxel-coated Express2™ stent (Boston Scientific Co., USA)] reduced the 12-month rates of TLR by 73%, the target-vessel revascularization (TVR) by 62%, and composite major adverse cardiac events (MACE) by 49%. Additionally, between 9 and 12 months, there were significantly fewer myocardial infarctions, TVR, and MACE in the paclitaxel-eluting stent than in the control stent group.[22] Among patients with diabetes, compared to the bare-metal stent the TAXUS™ stent reduced the rate of 9-month binary angiographic restenosis by 81%, and reduced the 12-month rates of TLR by 65%, TVR by 53%, and composite MACE by 44%.[23] The TAXUS V trial assessed the efficacy of the slow release stent compared with the bare metal stents in long lesions and small vessels. At nine-months follow-up, overall MACE rate in the TAXUS group was 15% compared with 21.2% in the control group (p=0.0084).[24] The TAXUS VI trial tested the moderate release formulation stent (not commercially available) and included complex and long lesions, treated with multiple stents. Two-year clinical results reported a TVR rate of 13.9% in the TAXUS MR group and 21.9% in the control group (p = 0.0335).[25] Clinical studies utilizing polymer-coated paclitaxel-eluting stents are summarized in Tables 8.1, 8.2 and 8.3.

TABLE 8.2 - RANDOMIZED TRIALS COMPARING BARE METAL STENTS WITH POLYMER-COATED SIROLIMUS- OR PACLITAXEL-ELUTING STENTS – QUANTITATIVE CORONARY ANGIOGRAPHY FOLLOW-UP

Study	Time (months)	QUANTITATIVE CORONARY ANGIOGRAPHY FOLLOW-UP Diameter Stenosis (% ± SD)	Restenosis (%)	Late Loss (mm ± SD)
SIROLIMUS				
RAVEL (67, 70, 71)[†]	6			
Sirolimus		14.7±7.0*	0*	–0.01±0.33*
Bare stent		36.7±18.1	26.6	0.80±0.53
SIRIUS (14)[‡]	8			
Sirolimus		23.6±16.4*	8.9*	0.24±0.47*
Bare stent		43.2±22.4	36.3	0.81±0.67
E-SIRIUS (17)[‡]	8			
Sirolimus		24.7±14.7*	5.9*	0.19±0.39*
Bare stent		48.3±23.4	42.3	0.80±0.57
C-SIRIUS(16)[†]	8			
Sirolimus		20.5±10.3	2.3*	0.09±0.31*
Bare stent		47.8±24.5	52.3	0.79±0.74
PACLITAXEL (polymer-coated)				
TAXUS I (61)[†]	6			
Paclitaxel		13.56±11.77*	0	0.36±0.48*
Bare stent		27.23±16.69	10	0.71±0.47
TAXUS II (68)[‡]	6			
Paclitaxel-SR		26.8±12.8*	5.5*	0.31±0.38*
Bare stent-SR		35.1±15.1	20.1	0.79±0.45
Paclitaxel-MR		26.8±13.1*	8.6*	0.30±0.39*
Bare stent-MR		37.1±17.8	23.8	0.77±0.50
TAXUS IV(22, 69)[‡]	9			
Paclitaxel		26.3±15.5*	7.9*	0.23±0.44*
Bare stent		39.8±18.5	26.6	0.61±0.57
TAXUS V(24)[†]	9			
Paclitaxel-SR		13.15±11.97*	13.7*	0.49±0.61*
Bare stent		31.78±15.14	31.9	0.90±0.62*
TAXUS VI(25)[†]	9			
Paclitaxel-MR		22.2±19.15*	9.1*	0.39±0.56*
Bare stent		42.8±20.90	32.9	0.99±0.5

* p<0.05 vs. control
[†] In-stent quantitative coronary angiography
[‡] In-segment quantitative coronary angiography (includes the 5-mm proximal and distal edges)

Comparisons between sirolimus and paclitaxel

The 1,386 patient REALITY trial compared SES versus PES. At eight-month follow-up, there were no differences in in-stent or in-lesion binary restenosis (primary end-point) rates and in TLR rates, although the late loss was significantly less with SES.[26] The SIRTAX study was also designed to compare the safety and efficacy of the SES versus the PES. Patients treated with SES stents had significantly better clinical and angiographic outcomes.[27] The ISAR-DIABETES study randomized 250 patients with diabetes to SES or PES. At nine-month follow-up, there was no significant difference between the two groups with

TABLE 8.3 - RANDOMIZED TRIALS COMPARING BARE METAL STENTS WITH POLYMER-COATED SIROLIMUS- OR PACLITAXEL-ELUTING STENTS – CLINICAL FOLLOW-UP

			CLINICAL FOLLOW-UP			
Study	Time (months)	Death (%)	Myocardial infarction (%)	Repeat revascularization (%)	Any event (%)	Stent thrombosis (%)
SIROLIMUS						
RAVEL (67, 70, 71)	12					
Sirolimus		1.7	3.3	0*	5.8*	0
Bare stent		1.7	4.2	22.9	28.8	0
SIRIUS (14)	9					
Sirolimus		0.9	2.8	3.8*	7.1*	0.4
Bare stent		0.6	3.2	15.8	18.9	0.8
E-SIRIUS (17)	9					
Sirolimus		1.1	4.6	4.0*	8.0*	1.1
Bare stent		0.6	2.3	20.9	22.6	0
C-SIRIUS(16)	9					
Sirolimus		0	2	4	4	2
Bare stent		0	4	18	18	2
PACLITAXEL (polymer-coated)						
TAXUS I (61)	24					
Paclitaxel		0	0	3	3	0
Bare stent		0	0	10	10	0
TAXUS II (68)	12					
Paclitaxel-SR		0	2.3	10.1*	10.9*	0.7
Bare stent-SR		1.5	5.1	15.9	22.0	0
Paclitaxel-MR		0	3.7	6.9*	9.9*	0
Bare stent-MR		0	5.2	19.1	21.4	0
TAXUS IV(22, 69)	12					
Paclitaxel		1.4	3.5	6.8*	10.6*	0.6
Bare stent		1.2	4.6	16.7	19.8	0.8
TAXUS V(24)	9					
Paclitaxel-SR		0.5	5.3	12.1*	15*	0.7
Bare stent		0.9	4.6	17.3	21.2	0.7
TAXUS VI(25)	24					
Paclitaxel-MR		0.5	8.8	13.9*	21.3	0.5
Bare stent		1.4	6.8	21.9	25.1	0.9

* p<0.05 vs. control

respect to the incidence of death or myocardial infarction. However, the primary endpoint of the study, late lumen loss, was significantly greater with PES, both in-segment and in-stent as were angiographic restenosis rates. No significant difference between the two groups with regard to the incidence of target lesion revascularization or angiographic restenosis was noted, but the study was underpowered.[28] Finally, the ISAR-DESIRE trial (The Intracoronary Stenting or Angioplasty for Restenosis Reduction – Drug-Eluting Stents for In-Stent REstenosis) was designed to investigate the effectiveness of SES and PES compared with balloon angioplasty in patients with in-stent restenosis. Late lumen loss was significantly lower in the SES group with no difference in restenosis rates although TVR was lower in the SES group.[29]

DRUG-ELUTING STENTS IN THE "REAL WORLD"

Rapamycin and paclitaxel registries

In the RESEARCH registry the one-year clinical outcomes of the first 508 consecutive patients treated exclusively with SES were compared to 450 patients who received bare stents in the period immediately prior to the introduction of SES; and demonstrated an overall reduction of 38% in the composite risk of death, myocardial infarction, or re-interventions.[30] Following on, the T-SEARCH registry compared the first 576 patients exclusively treated with PES against the 508 patients treated with SES from the RESEARCH registry. At one year, the unadjusted MACE rate was 13.9% in the PES group and 10.5% in the SES group (p = 0.1) and following multivariate adjustment had a hazard ratio of 1.16 (95% CI 0.81 to 1.64, p = 0.4). The one-year incidence of clinically driven TVR was 5.4% vs. 3.7%, respectively (p = 0.3).[31] These results suggest a similar efficacy between the two devices.

Complex lesions

Angiographic restenosis after drug-eluting stent implantation in complex patients is an infrequent event, occurring mainly in association with lesion-based characteristics and diabetes mellitus.[32] The effectiveness of drug-eluting stent implantation for left main stenoses has been investigated. Despite the higher-risk patients and lesion profiles in the DES compared to the BMS group, the incidence of MACE at a six-month clinical follow-up was lower.[33] The short- and long-term clinical outcome of left main percutaneous coronary intervention in 181 patients was recently reported. With a median follow-up of 503 days, the cumulative incidence of MACE was lower in the DES than in the BMS cohort with significantly lower rates of both myocardial infarction and TVR in the drug-eluting stent group.[34]

Percutaneous treatment of coronary bifurcation lesions is considered a technical challenge. Follow-up data demonstrates a high technical success rate. However, with conventional stents restenosis rates higher than 30% have been reported in most studies. Introduction of DES has resulted in a lower event rate and reduction of main vessel restenosis in comparison with historical controls.[35,36]

Chronic total occlusion is limited by high rates of subacute reocclusion and late restenosis. Preliminary results from two studies investigating SES implantation in patients with chronic total occlusion demonstrated less restenosis rates and TLR after six months compared with BMS.[37,38] Similar promising results were observed after PES implantation in a non-randomized study assessing the efficacy of PES in chronic total coronary occlusions.[39]

Treatment of saphenous vein graft disease is an emerging problem, due to the increasing number of patients undergoing bypass surgery. Stent implantation has better long-term outcome compared to balloon angioplasty.[40] In a preliminary study, SES were implanted in 19 patients with saphenous vein graft lesions and reported an in-hospital MACE of 11%, whereas over a mean 12.5+/-2.6 month follow-up, TLR was 5% and event-free survival 84%.[41] Improved mid-term and long-term efficacy of DES implantation compared to BMS implantation in saphenous vein graft lesions was confirmed in two studies, which included 61 and 40 patients, respectively.[42,43]

The treatment of in-stent restenosis remains a therapeutic dilemma, since many pharmacological and mechanical approaches have shown disappointing results. In a recent study 16 patients with severe, recurrent in-stent restenosis were treated with sirolimus-eluting stents.[44] Four months follow-up demonstrated that in-stent late lumen loss averaged 0.21 mm and the volume obstruction of the stent was 1.1%. At nine months clinical follow-up, three patients had experienced four MACE.[44] Similar results were reported in Sao Paulo, Brazil, where no patient had in-stent or stent margin restenosis at four months, and only one patient developed in-stent restenosis at one-year follow-up.[45] In a subgroup of 44 patients in RESEARCH with complex in-stent restenosis, the data showed at one year that the incidence of repeat intervention due to re-restenosis was 11.6%, with no stent thromboses or deaths.[46] The TROPICAL study, a prospective multicenter registry, assessed the effectiveness and safety of SES in the treatment 162 patients with in-stent restenosis. The nine-month rate of death was 1.2% and that of nonfatal myocardial infarction was 1.2%.[47] These findings confirm the efficacy of SES in the treatment of in-stent restenosis.[47] The TAXUS III trial investigated the feasibility and safety of PES for the treatment of in-stent restenosis. No subacute stent thrombosis occurred up to 12 months and MACE rate at was 29%.[48] The ISAR DESIRE randomized trial showed that DES are superior to balloon angioplasty.[29] However, the results were less remarkable than those for de novo lesions. The TAXUS V ISR pivotal trial, designed to compare PES with intra-coronary brachytherapy for in-stent restenosis, has completed enrolment and the results are pending.

Stent thrombosis

There is concern that DES implantation results in subsequent thrombosis. Early stent thrombosis is a complication observed within the first 30 days post procedurally, and is due to the arterial injury caused by the stent struts[49], while delayed endothelialization associated with DES implantation may result in late stent thrombosis (>30 days).

In sequential consecutive cohorts of 506 patients with BMS, 1,017 with SES, and 989 with PES, the incidence of angiographically proven early stent thrombosis was 1.2%, 1.0%, and 1.0% respectively.[50] Including possible stent thrombosis, the respective incidences were 1.4%, 1.5% and 1.6%, indicating a similar risk profile in all three groups. Early stent thrombosis was associated with bifurcation stenting and was more prominent in the acute myocardial infarction setting. Additionally, a meta-analysis of eight trials in 3,817 patients with coronary artery disease who were randomised to either PES or BMS suggested that standard dose paclitaxel-eluting stents do not increase the hazard of stent thrombosis compared to bare metal stents.[51] Similar results were reported in a pooled analysis including ten randomized studies, where 2,602 were allocated to drug-eluting stents and 2,428 patients to bare metal stents.[52] In "real world" patients increased late thrombosis after drug-eluting stent implantation has been observed and has been associated with premature antiplatelet therapy discontinuation, renal failure, bifurcation lesions, diabetes, and low ejection fraction.[53,54] Late angiographic stent thrombosis has been reported with an incidence of 0.35% with a mean follow-up of 1.5 years[55], and using a broader definition to include sudden death, between 0.5 – 0.8% with 9-month follow-up.[53] Importantly, patients with DES should remain on antiplatelet therapy lifelong following DES implantation unless an absolute contraindication supervenes.

Drug-eluting stents versus CABG

ARTS II compared SES in multivessel disease with the outcomes in ARTS I. The results clearly showed that use of drug-eluting stents in this study was better than the bare metal stent arm results in ARTS 1, and although overall events were similar to the CABG arm of ARTS I, the need for repeat revascularization remained lower with surgery.[56] The SYNTAX randomized, multi-center clinical trial is designed to compare 12-month event free survival of PCI using the PES with CABG for three vessel disease or left main disease.[57] In the trial, 1,500 patients are being randomized to either PES implantation or CABG at up to 90 sites in Europe and the United States, with nested registries of CABG and PCI. The FREEDOM multi-center trial (future revascularization evaluation in patients with diabetes mellitus: optimal management of multivessel disease) will randomize 2,400 DM patients with multi-vessel coronary disease to PCI with DES or CABG; with the primary outcome of five-year mortality.

NEW GENERATION DRUG-ELUTING STENTS

As we extend the use of DES to treat more indications, more efficacious agents and improved stent platforms may be required.

The Endeavor drug-eluting stent system

The Endeavor drug-eluting stent system (Medtronic, Minneapolis, Minnesota) consists of a Medtronic's Driver™ coronary stent, a phosphorylcholine polymer coating and an anti-proliferative drug agent, the ABT-578. The ABT-578 is a tetrazole-containing macrocyclic immunosuppressant and potent antiproliferative agent. The pilot safety ENDEAVOR I trial[58] has been followed by the randomized ENDEAVOR II (Endeavor drug-eluting stent vs. the Driver™ bare metal stent) trial, which demonstrated a significantly higher TLR-free survival in the Endeavor drug-eluting stent system (95.4% vs. 87.8%, p <0.001).[59] Based on these results, the Endeavor ABT-578-eluting stent received CE approval for sale in Europe. The results of ENDEAVOR III (Endeavor drug-eluting stent vs. the Cypher™ Sirolimus-eluting stent) are expected in October 2005, while ENDEAVOR IV will compare against PES.

ZoMaxx drug-eluting coronary stent

The ZoMaxx™ drug-eluting stent consists of the TriMaxx™ stent (Abbott Laboratories, Illinois, U.S.A), a polymer carrier and the immunosuppressant drug ABT-578. The TriMaxx™ stent has a unique tri-layer sandwiching stainless steel and tantalum. ZOMAXX I conducted in Europe, Australia and New Zealand and ZOMAXX II in North America are prospective and randomized clinical trials designed to evaluate the safety and efficacy of ZoMaxx™ drug-eluting stent system in comparison to PES.

Everolimus-eluting stent

Everolimus is a sirolimus analogue, arresting the cell cycle at the G1 to S phase. The FUTURE I and II trials evaluated both safety and feasibility of the everolimus-eluting stent.[60,61] The SPIRIT I trial investigated the safety and effectiveness of the everolimus-eluting VISION™ stent (Guidant Corporation, Indianapolis, Indiana).[62] The SPIRIT III in USA will compare the XIENCE™ V system an everolimus-eluting MULTI-LINK VISION® Coronary Stent (Guidant Corporation, Indianapolis, Indiana) with the TAXUS™ Express 2™ stent. The SPIRIT II clinical trial will initiate in Europe in the very near future.

Biolimus A9™-eluting stent

Biolimus A9™ is also a sirolimus derivative that inhibits growth factor-driven cell proliferation, such as T-cells and vascular smooth muscle cells. The STEALTH trial (Stent Eluting A9 BioLimus Trial in Humans) was the FIM study to investigate the safety and efficacy of a biolimus A9-eluting stent, the BioMATRIX™ stent (Biosensors International, Singapore).[63] Recently, a second trial with a biolimus A9™-eluting stent has begun enrollment. The NOBORI 1 clinical trial will compare the Nobori™ biolimus A9™-eluting coronary stent system (TERUMO Europe NV, Belgium) with the Taxus™ stent and plans to prospectively randomize approximately 400 patients in up to 30 centers in Europe, Australia and Asia.

The Conor™ stent

The Conor™ Medstent (Conor Medsystems, USA) has a unique stent design that allows laser cut wells to be filled with a combination of polymer and drug by using a piezoelectric dispenser that injects multiple drops of polymer/drug solution directly into each hole, and does not place drug nor polymer on the strut surface. The current generation is made of cobalt-chrome alloy and offers lower profiles and greater flexibility, while maintaining excellent radiopacity. Additionally, the current Conor™ systems use erodable polymer, which release drug by a combination of diffusion and erosion. The DepoStent trial was the first evaluation of the Conor stent in humans. The PISCES study was a multi-center dose optimization registry[64] as was the SCEPTER trial. Quantitative coronary angiography results were favorable in the groups with long elution times. The COSTAR trial is designed to evaluate several doses, in order to define the dose response curve for Paclitaxel. Finally, the EUROSTAR trial is looking at 10 and 30μg, long release formulations with six-month follow-up.

Tacrolimus-eluting stent

Tacrolimus (FK506) is a water-insoluble macrolide immunosuppressant. It has been widely used to reduce the incidence and severity of allograft rejection after organ transplantation and to treat other inflammatory conditions such as atopic dermatitis. The JUPITER II trial investigated the safety and the efficacy of the Janus™ tacrolimus-eluting carbostent (Sorin Group) compared to the bare metal Tecnic™ carbostent (Sorin Group). Early clinical outcomes demonstrated low MACE rate in both groups. These results were sustained up to six months follow-up.[65]

The Genous™ Bio-engineered R stent™

Endothelial progenitor cells have been identified as a key factor for re-endothelialization. The Genous™ Bio-engineered R stent™ (OrbusNeich, Fort Lauderdale, Florida) was developed to enhance accumulation of endothelial progenitor cells at the site of arterial injury after stent implantation, in order to rapidly create a functional endothelial layer and thus reduce potential thrombosis and restenosis. Endothelial progenitor cell recruitment is achieved through surface immobilized antibodies directed toward endothelial progenitor cell – surface antigens. The HEALING-FIM (Healthy Endothelial Accelerated Lining Inhibits Neointimal Growth-First In Man) registry was the first clinical investigation and nine-month composite major adverse cardiac and cerebrovascular events rate was 6.3%.[66] This preliminary study demonstrated the safety and feasibility of the Genous™ Bio-engineered R stent™. The HEALING II, 60 patient, multi-center, prospective, non-randomized trial, assesses the safety and efficacy, of the Genous™ Bio-engineered R stent™.

CONCLUSIONS

Drug eluting stents have undoubtedly improved the outcomes following stenting. Sirolimus and paclitaxel eluting stents have lived up to early promise with consistent results in increasingly complex trial lesions and in worldwide registries. New drugs and stent designs are being tested in clinical trials and if successful, will add to the current generation of devices available.

REFERENCES

1. Dangas G, Fuster V. Management of restenosis after coronary intervention. Am Heart J 1996; 132(2 Pt 1):428–36.

2. Kastrati A, Mehilli J, Dirschinger J, Pache J, Ulm K, Schuhlen H, et al. Restenosis after coronary placement of various stent types. Am J Cardiol 2001; 87(1):34–9.

3. Van Belle E, Bauters C, Asahara T, Isner JM. Endothelial regrowth after arterial injury: from vascular repair to therapeutics. Cardiovasc Res 1998; 38(1):54–68.

4. Liu MW, Roubin GS, King SB, 3rd. Restenosis after coronary angioplasty. Potential biologic determinants and role of intimal hyperplasia. Circulation 1989; 79(6):1374–87.

5. Filippatos G, Parissis JT, Adamopoulos S, Kardaras F. Chemokines in cardiovascular remodeling: clinical and therapeutic implications. Curr Mol Med 2003; 3(2):139–47.

6. Galis ZS, Khatri JJ. Matrix metalloproteinases in vascular remodeling and atherogenesis: the good, the bad, and the ugly. Circ Res 2002; 90(3):251–62.

7. Winslow RD, Sharma SK, Kim MC. Restenosis and drug-eluting stents. Mt Sinai J Med 2005; 72(2):81–9.

8. Regar E, Sianos G, Serruys PW. Stent development and local drug delivery. Br Med Bull 2001; 59:227–48.

9. Rogers CD. Optimal stent design for drug delivery. Rev Cardiovasc Med 2004; 5 Suppl 2:S9–S15.

10. Serruys PW, Regar E, Carter AJ. Rapamycin eluting stent: the onset of a new era in interventional cardiology. Heart 2002; 87(4):305–7.

11. Gingras AC, Raught B, Sonenberg N. mTOR signaling to translation. Curr Top Microbiol Immunol 2004; 279:169–97.

12. Morice MC, Serruys PW, Sousa JE, Fajadet J, Ban Hayashi E, Perin M, et al. A randomized comparison of a sirolimus-eluting stent with a standard stent for coronary revascularization. N Engl J Med 2002; 346(23):1773–80.

13. Fajadet J, Morice MC, Bode C, Barragan P, Serruys PW, Wijns W, et al. Maintenance of long-term clinical benefit with sirolimus-eluting coronary stents: three-year results of the RAVEL trial. Circulation 2005; 111(8):1040–4.

14. Moses JW, Leon MB, Popma JJ, Fitzgerald PJ, Holmes DR, O'Shaughnessy C, et al. Sirolimus-eluting stents versus standard stents in patients with stenosis in a native coronary artery. N Engl J Med 2003; 349(14):1315–23.

15. Holmes DR, Jr., Leon MB, Moses JW, Popma JJ, Cutlip D, Fitzgerald PJ, et al. Analysis of 1-year clinical outcomes in the SIRIUS trial: a randomized trial of a sirolimus-eluting stent versus a standard stent in patients at high risk for coronary restenosis. Circulation 2004; 109(5):634–40.

16. Schampaert E, Cohen EA, Schluter M, Reeves F, Traboulsi M, Title LM, et al. The Canadian study of the sirolimus-eluting stent in the treatment of patients with long de novo lesions in small native coronary arteries (C-SIRIUS). J Am Coll Cardiol 2004; 43(6):1110–15.

17. Schofer J, Schluter M, Gershlick AH, Wijns W, Garcia E, Schampaert E, et al. Sirolimus-eluting stents for treatment of patients with long atherosclerotic lesions in small coronary arteries: double-blind, randomised controlled trial (E-SIRIUS). Lancet 2003; 362(9390):1093–9.

18. Giannakakou P, Robey R, Fojo T, M.V. B. Low concentrations of paclitaxel induce cell type-dependent p53, p21 and G1/G2 arrest instead of mitotic arrest: molecular determinants of paclitaxel-induced cytotoxicity. Oncogene 2001; 20(29):3806–13.

19. Lansky AJ, Costa RA, Mintz GS, Tsuchiya Y, Midei M, Cox DA, et al. Non-polymer-based paclitaxel-coated coronary stents for the treatment of patients with de novo coronary lesions: angiographic follow-up of the DELIVER clinical trial. Circulation 2004; 109(16):1948–54.

20. Grube E, Silber S, Hauptmann KE, Mueller R, Buellesfeld L, Gerckens U, et al. TAXUS I: six- and twelve-month results from a randomized, double-blind trial on a slow-release paclitaxel-eluting stent for de novo coronary lesions. Circulation 2003; 107(1):38–42.

21. Serruys PW, Degertekin M, Tanabe K, Russell ME, Guagliumi G, Webb J, et al. Vascular responses at proximal and distal edges of paclitaxel-eluting stents: serial intravascular ultrasound analysis from the TAXUS II trial. Circulation 2004; 109(5):627–33.

22. Stone GW, Ellis SG, Cox DA, Hermiller J, O'Shaughnessy C, Mann JT, *et al*. One-year clinical results with the slow-release, polymer-based, paclitaxel-eluting TAXUS stent: the TAXUS-IV trial. Circulation 2004; 109(16):1942–7.

23. Hermiller JB, Raizner A, Cannon L, Gurbel PA, Kutcher MA, Wong SC, *et al*. Outcomes with the polymer-based paclitaxel-eluting TAXUS stent in patients with diabetes mellitus: the TAXUS-IV trial. J Am Coll Cardiol 2005; 45(8):1172–9.

24. Stone GW, Ellis SG, Cannon L, Greenberg JD, Tift Mann JT, Spriggs D, *et al*. Outcomes of the Polymer-Based, Paclitaxel-Eluting Taxus Stent In Complex Lesions: Principal Clinical and Angiographic Results From the Taxus-V Pivotal Randomized Trial. 54th Annual Scientific Session 2005.

25. Grube E. Randomized Trial of Moderate-Rate Release Polymer-Based Paclitaxel-Eluting TAXUS stent for the Treatment of Longer Lesions. EUROPCR 2005, Paris, France 2005.

26. Morice MC, Serruys PW, Colombo A, Meier B, Tamburino C, Guagliumi G, *et al*. Prospective Randomized Multi-Center Head-to-Head Comparison of the Sirolimus-Eluting Stent (Cypher) and the Paclitaxel-Eluting Stent (Taxus) (REALITY). Sunday, Mar 06, 2005 2005; 54th ACC Annual Scientific Session, Orlando, USA.

27. Windecker S. SIRTAX: Randomized Comparison of a Sirolimus- vs a Paclitaxel-Eluting Stent for Coronary Revascularization. In: 54 th ACC Annual Scientific Session; 2005; Orlando, USA; 2005.

28. Kastrati A, Dibra A, Mehilli J, Pache J, Schuhlen H, von Beckerath N, *et al*. ISAR-DIABETES: Paclitaxel-Eluting Stent Versus Sirolimus-Eluting Stent for the Prevention of Restenosis in Diabetic Patients With Coronary Artery Disease. In: 54th ACC Annual Scientific Session; 2005; Orlando, USA; 2005.

29. Kastrati A, Mehilli J, von Beckerath N, Dibra A, Pache J, Schühlen H, *et al*. ISAR-DESIRE: Drug-Eluting Stents for In-Stent Restenosis. In: European Society of Cardiology Congress 2004; 2004; Munich, Germany; 2004.

30. Lemos PA, Serruys PW, van Domburg RT, Saia F, Arampatzis CA, Hoye A, *et al*. Unrestricted utilization of sirolimus-eluting stents compared with conventional bare stent implantation in the "real world": the Rapamycin-Eluting Stent Evaluated At Rotterdam Cardiology Hospital (RESEARCH) registry. Circulation 2004; 109(2):190–5.

31. Ong AT, Serruys PW, Aoki J, Hoye A, van Mieghem CA, Rodriguez-Granillo GA, *et al*. The unrestricted use of paclitaxel- versus sirolimus-eluting stents for coronary artery disease in an unselected population: one-year results of the Taxus-Stent Evaluated at Rotterdam Cardiology Hospital (T-SEARCH) registry. J Am Coll Cardiol 2005; 45(7):1135–41.

32. Lemos PA, Hoye A, Goedhart D, Arampatzis CA, Saia F, van der Giessen WJ, *et al*. Clinical, angiographic, and procedural predictors of angiographic restenosis after sirolimus-eluting stent implantation in complex patients: an evaluation from the Rapamycin-Eluting Stent Evaluated At Rotterdam Cardiology Hospital (RESEARCH) study. Circulation 2004; 109(11):1366–70.

33. Chieffo A, Stankovic G, Bonizzoni E, Tsagalou E, Iakovou I, Montorfano M, *et al*. Early and mid-term results of drug-eluting stent implantation in unprotected left main. Circulation 2005; 111(6):791–5.

34. Valgimigli M, van Mieghem CA, Ong AT, Aoki J, Granillo GA, McFadden EP, *et al*. Short- and long-term clinical outcome after drug-eluting stent implantation for the

percutaneous treatment of left main coronary artery disease: insights from the Rapamycin-Eluting and Taxus Stent Evaluated At Rotterdam Cardiology Hospital registries (RESEARCH and T-SEARCH). Circulation 2005; 111(11):1383–9.

35. Colombo A, Moses JW, Morice MC, Ludwig J, Holmes DR, Jr., Spanos V, *et al.* Randomized study to evaluate sirolimus-eluting stents implanted at coronary bifurcation lesions. Circulation 2004; 109(10):1244–9.

36. Sharma SK. Simultaneous kissing drug-eluting stent technique for percutaneous treatment of bifurcation lesions in large-size vessels. Catheter Cardiovasc Interv 2005; 65(1):10–6.

37. Nakamura S, Muthusamy TS, Bae JH, Cahyadi YH, Udayachalerm W, Tresukosol D. Impact of sirolimus-eluting stent on the outcome of patients with chronic total occlusions. Am J Cardiol 2005; 95(2):161–6.

38. Ge L, Iakovou I, Cosgrave J, Chieffo A, Montorfano M, Michev I, *et al.* Immediate and mid-term outcomes of sirolimus-eluting stent implantation for chronic total occlusions. Eur Heart J 2005; 26(11):1056–62.

39. Werner GS, Krack A, Schwarz G, Prochnau D, Betge S, Figulla HR. Prevention of lesion recurrence in chronic total coronary occlusions by paclitaxel-eluting stents. J Am Coll Cardiol 2004; 44(12):2301–6.

40. Hanekamp CE, Koolen JJ, Den Heijer P, Schalij MJ, Piek JJ, Bar FW, *et al.* Randomized study to compare balloon angioplasty and elective stent implantation in venous bypass grafts: the Venestent study. Catheter Cardiovasc Interv 2003; 60(4):452–7.

41. Hoye A, Lemos PA, Arampatzis CA, Saia F, Tanabe K, Degertekin M, *et al.* Effectiveness of the sirolimus-eluting stent in the treatment of saphenous vein graft disease. J Invasive Cardiol 2004; 16(5):230–3.

42. Ge L, Iakovou I, Sangiorgi GM, Chieffo A, Melzi G, Cosgrave J, *et al.* Treatment of saphenous vein graft lesions with drug-eluting stents: immediate and midterm outcome. J Am Coll Cardiol 2005; 45(7):989–94.

43. Tsuchida K, Ong AT, Aoki J, van Mieghem CAG, Rodriguez-Granillo GA, Valgimigli M, *et al.* Immediate and one-year outcome of percutaneous intervention of saphenous vein graft disease with paclitaxel-eluting stents. Am J Cardiol 2005; in press.

44. Degertekin M, Regar E, Tanabe K, Smits PC, van der Giessen WJ, Carlier SG, *et al.* Sirolimus-eluting stent for treatment of complex in-stent restenosis: the first clinical experience. J Am Coll Cardiol 2003; 41(2):184–9.

45. Sousa JE, Costa MA, Abizaid A, Sousa AG, Feres F, Mattos LA, *et al.* Sirolimus-eluting stent for the treatment of in-stent restenosis: a quantitative coronary angiography and three-dimensional intravascular ultrasound study. Circulation 2003; 107(1):24–7.

46. Saia F, Lemos PA, Arampatzis CA, Hoye A, Degertekin M, Tanabe K, *et al.* Routine sirolimus eluting stent implantation for unselected in-stent restenosis: insights from the rapamycin eluting stent evaluated at Rotterdam Cardiology Hospital (RESEARCH) registry. Heart 2004; 90(10):1183–8.

47. Neumann FJ, Desmet W, Grube E, Brachmann J, Presbitero P, Rubartelli P, *et al.* Effectiveness and safety of sirolimus-eluting stents in the treatment of restenosis after coronary stent placement. Circulation 2005; 111(16):2107–11.

48. Tanabe K, Serruys PW, Grube E, Smits PC, Selbach G, van der Giessen WJ, *et al.* TAXUS III Trial: in-stent restenosis treated with stent-based delivery of paclitaxel incorporated in a slow-release polymer formulation. Circulation 2003; 107(4):559–64.

49. Komatsu R, Ueda M, Naruko T, Kojima A, Becker AE. Neointimal tissue response at sites of coronary stenting in humans: macroscopic, histological, and immunohistochemical analyses. Circulation 1998; 98(3):224–33.

50. Ong AT, Hoye A, Aoki J, van Mieghem CA, Rodriguez Granillo GA, Sonnenschein K, *et al.* Thirty-day incidence and six-month clinical outcome of thrombotic stent occlusion after bare-metal, sirolimus, or paclitaxel stent implantation. J Am Coll Cardiol 2005; 45(6):947–53.

51. Bavry AA, Kumbhani DJ, Helton TJ, Bhatt DL. What is the risk of stent thrombosis associated with the use of paclitaxel-eluting stents for percutaneous coronary intervention?: a meta-analysis. J Am Coll Cardiol 2005; 45(6):941–6.

52. Moreno R, Fernandez C, Hernandez R, Alfonso F, Angiolillo DJ, Sabate M, *et al.* Drug-eluting stent thrombosis: results from a pooled analysis including 10 randomized studies. J Am Coll Cardiol 2005; 45(6):954–9.

53. Iakovou I, Schmidt T, Bonizzoni E, Ge L, Sangiorgi GM, Stankovic G, *et al.* Incidence, predictors, and outcome of thrombosis after successful implantation of drug-eluting stents. Jama 2005; 293(17):2126–30.

54. McFadden EP, Stabile E, Regar E, Cheneau E, Ong AT, Kinnaird T, *et al.* Late thrombosis in drug-eluting coronary stents after discontinuation of antiplatelet therapy. Lancet 2004; 364(9444):1519–21.

55. Ong AT, McFadden EP, Regar E, de Jaegere PP, van Domburg RT, Serruys PW. Late angiographic stent thrombosis (LAST) events with drug-eluting stents. J Am Coll Cardiol 2005; 45(12):2088–92.

56. Serruys PW, Ong AT, Colombo A, Dawkins K, de Bruyne B, Fajadet J, *et al.* Arterial Revascularization Therapies Study Part II: Sirolimus-Eluting Stents for the Treatment of Patients With Multivessel De Novo Coronary Artery Lesions. 54th ACC Annual Scientific Session, Orlando, USA 2005; Sunday, Mar 06, 2005.

57. Ong AT, Serruys PW, Mohr FW, Morice MC, Kappetein AP, Holmes DR, *et al.* The SYNergy between Percutaneous Coronary Intervention with TAXus™ and Cardiac Surgery (SYNTAX) Study: Design, Rationale and Run-In Phase. Am Heart J 2005; in press.

58. Meredith I. ENDEAVOR I clinical trial. One year follow-up. In: EUROPCR; 2004; Paris, France; 2004.

59. Wijns W, Fajadet J, Kuntz RE. A randomized comparison of the endeavor ABT-578 drug Eluting Stent With a Bare Metal Stent for Coronary Revascularization: Results of the Endeavor II Trial. In: 54th ACC Annual Scientific Session; 2005; Orlando, USA; 2005.

60. Grube E, Sonoda S, Ikeno F, Honda Y, Kar S, Chan C, *et al.* Six- and twelve-month results from first human experience using everolimus-eluting stents with bioabsorbable polymer. Circulation 2004; 109(18):2168–71.

61. Grube E. FUTURE II: Multicenter evaluation of the bioabsorbable polymer-based everolimus-eluting stent. In: TCT; 2003; Washington, USA; 2003.

62. Serruys PW, Ong ATL, Piek JJ, Neumann FJ, van der Giessen WJ, Wiemer M, *et al.* A randomized comparison of a durable polymer Everolimus-eluting stent with a bare metal coronary stent: The SPIRIT first trial. EuroIntervention 2005; 1(1):58–69.

63. Grube E, Hauptmann KE, Buellesfeld L, Lim V, Abizaid A. Six-month results of a randomized study to evaluate safety and efficacy of a Biolimus A9™ eluting stent with a biodegradable polymer coating. EuroIntervention 2005; 1:53–7.

64. Serruys PW, Sianos G, Abizaid A, Aoki J, den Heijer P, Bonnier H, *et al.* The effect of variable dose and release kinetics on neointimal hyperplasia using a novel paclitaxel-eluting stent platform: the Paclitaxel In-Stent Controlled Elution Study (PISCES). J Am Coll Cardiol 2005; 46(2):253–60.

65. Morice MC. JUPITER II Trial. Six-month interim clinical data. In: EuroPCR 2005; 2005; Paris, France; 2005.

66. Aoki J, Serruys PW, van Beusekom H, Ong AT, McFadden EP, Sianos G, *et al.* Endothelial progenitor cell capture by stents coated with antibody against CD34: the HEALING-FIM (Healthy Endothelial Accelerated Lining Inhibits Neointimal Growth-First In Man) Registry. J Am Coll Cardiol 2005; 45(10):1574–9.

67. Regar E, Serruys PW, Bode C, Holubarsch C, Guermonprez JL, Wijns W, *et al.* Angiographic findings of the multicenter Randomized Study With the Sirolimus-Eluting Bx Velocity Balloon-Expandable Stent (RAVEL): sirolimus-eluting stents inhibit restenosis irrespective of the vessel size. Circulation 2002; 106(15):1949–56.

68. Colombo A, Drzewiecki J, Banning A, Grube E, Hauptmann K, Silber S, *et al.* Randomized study to assess the effectiveness of slow- and moderate-release polymer-based paclitaxel-eluting stents for coronary artery lesions. Circulation 2003; 108(7):788–94.

69. Stone GW, Ellis SG, Cox DA, Hermiller J, O'Shaughnessy C, Mann JT, *et al.* A polymer-based, paclitaxel-eluting stent in patients with coronary artery disease. N Engl J Med 2004; 350(3):221–31.

70. Morice MC, Serruys PW, Costantini C, Wuelfert E, Wijns W, Fajadet J, *et al.* Two-Year Follow-Up of the RAVEL Study: A Randomized Study With the Sirolimus-Eluting Bx VELOCITY™ Stent in the Treatment of Patients With De-Novo Native Coronary Artery Lesions. J Am Coll Cardiol 2003; 41(6 (suppl A)):32A [abstract].

71. Morice MC, Serruys PW, Sousa JE, Fajadet J, Ban Hayashi E, Perin M, *et al.* A randomized comparison of a sirolimus-eluting stent with a standard stent for coronary revascularization. N Engl J Med 2002; 346(23):1773–80.

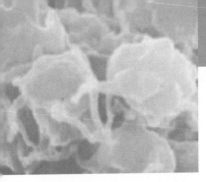

9

Intravascular ultrasound in coronary artery disease

NEAL G. UREN

KEY POINTS

- The observation of the three-layered appearance by intravascular ultrasound occurs due to the acoustic impedance between adjacent structures.

- The earliest accumulations of atherosclerotic plaque consist of crescentic intimal thickening of an intermediate echointensity.

- With a greater accumulation of plaque, there is a greater complexity to the plaque which may be differentiated by broad ultrasound criteria relating to echoreflectivity.

- Intravascular ultrasound provides accurate online quantitative information regarding lumen size and residual plaque load before and after interventional procedures.

- Intravascular ultrasound has confirmed that with increasing plaque accumulation, there is a remodelling process whereby the vessel initially expands to accommodate the plaque load up to around 40% of vessel area.

- During balloon angioplasty, localised calcium has a direct role in promoting dissection by increasing shear stress within the plaque at the junction between tissue types with differing elastic properties.

- A strong argument for the use of IVUS in balloon angioplasty is that it may allow a 'stent-like' result to be achieved by optimising the acute lumen gain from balloon dilatation alone.

- In the MUSIC trial of additional IVUS guidance in optimal stent deployment, criteria for stent expansion were defined and even with only 80% of patients achieving these criteria, a six-month angiographic restenosis rate of 8.3% was reported.

- In the CRUISE study comparing IVUS and angiographic guidance of stenting, the former group demonstrated superior stent expansion and at nine-month follow-up, a 44% reduction in target vessel revascularisation was demonstrated.

- In the OPTICUS trial comparing IVUS and angiographic guidance of stenting with angiographic follow-up, clinical and angiographic outcome was no different comparing both groups.

INTRODUCTION

The development of intravascular ultrasound (IVUS) has been a major development in the invasive imaging of coronary arteries. Clinical studies in intravascular ultrasound began in 1989 with the development of catheters initially in the 5–6 French gauge (F) range with the most recent catheter size miniaturised to 2.6 F.[1] Intravascular ultrasound has permitted not only a greater understanding of plaque morphology and its response to interventional procedures but has provided accurate online quantitative information regarding lumen size and residual plaque load, an important predictor of restenosis. The presence of disease not only at the site of focal stenosis but also in reference segments believed by angiography to be free of disease has modified interventional practice significantly. With continued improvement in image quality through increasing ultrasound frequency from 30 MHz through 40 MHz currently available and ultimately 50 MHz, the morphology of plaque and the offline ability to characterise plaque will provide additional information in the management of atherosclerotic disease. It is likely that continued technical developments will enhance and define the role of intravascular ultrasound in coronary interventional practice.

BASIC INTERPRETATION

An appreciation of the coronary anatomy and its relationship to structures around it is important to the accurate interpretation of intravascular ultrasound images. These spatial relations are best appreciated at the time of slow catheter pull-back from distal to proximal vessel done using an automated pull-back device. Advances in image quality and improved tissue penetration has allowed the use of epivascular structures in addition to side branches as reference points for tomographic and axial orientation (Fig. 9.1).

There are three concentric layers in the epicardial coronary arterial wall demonstrable at histology and seen by intravascular ultrasound imaging. The intima is the innermost layer and consists of endothelial cells and the subendothelial layer of smooth muscle cells and fibroblasts in a connective tissue matrix. The overall thickness of this layer can be just a few cells thick in childhood expanding to 150–200 *gmm in the adult. Beneath this, there is the internal elastic lamina which is intact in the normal state, consisting of fenestrated elastic fibres with a thickness less than 25 *gmm.

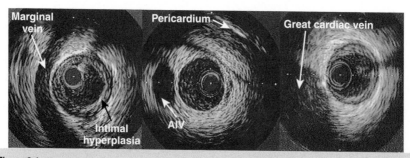

Figure 9.1:
The left panel is an image in the left coronary artery. Marginal veins cross around the artery in the horseshoe pattern, often associated with and opposite to the branch points of the right ventricular marginal arteries. Recurrent atrial branches generally emerge on the opposite side of the artery to the marginal branches.

The middle panel is an image of the proximal LAD artery. The anterior interventricular vein (AIV) lies to the left of the proximal artery in the majority of people (85%), with the first two diagonal branches on the same side. In one third of the people, the interventricular vein branches into two after second diagonal to lie either side of the LAD more distally. Pericardium may be seen as a bright reflection on the anterior side of the artery. Diagonal branches emerge on the same side as the AIV. Septal branches emerge from the LAD in a perpendicular fashion to myocardium, on the opposite side of the pericardium.

The right image is of the proximal left circumflex artery. Distally, the CFX is accompanied by the posterior left ventricular vein whereas in its proximal section, it is crossed and shadowed superiorly by the great cardiac vein. Recurrent atrial branches emerge from the circumflex artery towards the great cardiac vein in the opposite direction to obtuse marginal branches.

The media consists of multiple layers of smooth muscle cells arranged helically and circumferentially around the lumen of the artery, woven through a matrix of elastic fibers and collagen. The coronary arteries are less elastic than other similar sized arteries and thus resemble a transition towards more muscular peripheral arteries. The normal medial thickness ranges from 125–350 *gmm (mean 200 *gmm) although in the presence of plaque, the medial thickness may be considerably thinner, approximately 100 *gmm,[2] or completely involuted and replaced by plaque in severe disease. The external elastic lamina encircles the medial layer. It is composed of elastin but is thinner and more fenestrated than the internal lamina, and is not more than 20 *gmm in thickness.

The adventitia is essentially fibrous tissue, i.e. collagen (type III) and elastin, with the collagen orientated longitudinally in general, and to a lesser tissue density than media. It is a layer that is surrounded by the vaso vasorum, nerves and lymphatic vessels. The adventitia can extend from 300 to 500 *gmm in diameter beyond which it is considered perivascular stroma and epicardial fat.

The appearance of the three-layered appearance by intravascular ultrasound occurs due to the acoustic impedance between adjacent structures. For example, the lumen and intima are usually well-delineated due to the large acoustic impedance between fluid and tissue. The three-layered appearance of the vessel wall is dependent on the intima being of sufficient size to be identified with the resolution of the current generation of ultrasound transducers and in the presence of a sufficient acoustic interface between media and adventitia.[3] At a frequency of 30 MHz, the threshold of intimal thickening required to resolve a definite intimal layer is approximately 160 *gmm. Previous work has shown that there is a progressive increase in the thickness of the intimal layer with increasing age.[4] In an autopsy study done to evaluate the relationship between ultrasound images and tissue histology in 16 intact hearts from subjects ranging in age from 13 to 55 years with no history of coronary artery disease, segments with a three-layered appearance had a significantly greater intimal thickness (243 *b+ 105 *gmm) than non-layered segments (112 *b+ 55 *gmm) with a threshold between the two of 178 *gmm.[4] As this threshold is crossed in males over the age of 30 years, it is apparent that histologically normal arteries will only have a two-layered appearance in the rare patients younger than this undergoing ultrasound examination.

The media appears as a thin middle layer by intravascular ultrasound and is often referred to as the sonolucent zone as it is less echodense than the intima or adventitia due to a lesser collagen content. Intravascular ultrasound imaging was performed in vitro on 6 histologically normal and 104 minimally diseased arteries in patients aged 13 to 83 years to test the hypothesis that normal coronary arteries produce a three-layer image that corresponds to the histologic layers of intima, media and adventitia.[5] The results showed a very strong correlation between area of the echolucent ultrasound layer with the media and the inner echogenic layer with intimal area. In addition, a three-layered appearance was consistently seen when the internal elastic membrane was present with or without intimal hyperplasia. If the internal elastic membrane was absent, a three-layer appearance was still seen if the collagen content of the media was low. However, a two-layer appearance was observed when there was absence of the internal elastic membrane as well as a high collagen content of the media.[5] In addition, the relative composition of the intimal layer also determined the ability to discriminate the three vessel wall layers. Thus, over a given coronary artery segment, the three-layered appearance may alternate with a two-layered appearance due to the relative content of elastin and collagen. However, for the purposes of quantitation, the acoustic impedance between the combination of adventitia and external elastic lamina with the intima permits accurate measurement of plaque and vessel area. In the left main stem and at the proximal part of the right coronary artery, the three-layered appearance may be lost due to the increase in elastin content in transition from the highly elastic aortic root.

ATHEROSCLEROTIC DISEASE

Intravascular ultrasound is the current imaging technology of choice for studying the morphology of atherosclerotic plaque in vivo and continues to have an important diagnostic role (Table 9.1). Early studies used a large 8 F catheter to correlate ultrasound appearances with histological findings in arteries collected at the time of autopsy.[6] The arteries studied were a combination of elastic, transitional (musculo-elastic) and muscular types with respect to media/adventitia appearance. The results confirmed that a highly accurate measurement of luminal area was achieved comparing ultrasound to direct measurement of perfused isolated arteries. A distinct interface between media and adventitia was obtained only where there was a significant difference in the acoustic qualities of the two layers (namely, loose collagen in the adventitia of elastic arteries or where there was a minimal smooth muscle cell component in the adventitia of transitional/ muscular arteries). The interface between plaque and media was only apparent where there was a dense internal elastic lamina or a significant amount of necrotic material in the plaque.

The earliest accumulations of atherosclerotic plaque consist of crescentic intimal thickening of an intermediate echointensity. A common site for initial and increased plaque accumulation occurs at branch points and bifurcations due to the shear stress effect of blood flow. Transplant vasculopathy is a good model for the early development of coronary artery disease as these patients undergo ultrasound studies at angiographic follow-up early after transplantation. In one study, intravascular ultrasound was used to study epicardial arteries in 25 recently transplanted hearts from young donors (mean age 28 years).[7] In this unique study group, all donors aged under 25 years had a homogeneous non-layered vessel wall. Another group of donors of mean age 32 years manifested a three-layered

TABLE 9.1 - DIAGNOSTIC ROLE OF IVUS
Detection of angiographically silent disease
– ostial lesions
– syndrome X
– transplant vasculopathy
Assessment of an ambiguous angiographic appearance
Estimation of functional stenosis severity

appearance. In five hearts, significant eccentric intimal thickening >500 *gmm was shown in donors with risk factors for coronary disease, implying early coronary disease in the presence of angiographically normal arteries. Subsequent work by the same group in a larger group of transplant recipients over a period of long-term follow-up has shown that all 60 hearts had variable degree of concentric intimal thickening after one year, 42 of whom had normal coronary arteries at angiography.[8]

Occasionally, image interpretation can be obscured in abnormal vessels due to incorrect assumptions of the borders of the vessel layers traced manually. This can occur because the internal elastic lamina may not be a separate layer in the presence of plaque. Media may also appear unusually thick due to attenuation of the ultrasound beam passing through intimal plaque. By contrast, the media layer may also be thinner than expected due to the spread of the signal from an area of high reflectivity (plaque) to a low one (media). For these reasons, the outer border of the plaque is usually defined as at the media/adventitia border (the external elastic lamina) which is believed to be a fair assumption given the relative contribution of media to the plaque area. It is implicit in image interpretation that frames are selected with the best image quality and done so by an experienced operator.

With a greater accumulation of plaque, there is a greater complexity to the plaque which may be differentiated by broad ultrasound criteria. A fibrous plaque has an echodensity intermediate between less echodense media or lipid and more echodense calcification. Thus by comparing the brightness of the tissue in question to that of the adventitia, a relative grading of the plaque may be obtained. Such fibrous plaques with similar brightness to adventitia may then be described as hard or soft (with respect to the grey scale) depending on the presence or absence of shadowing behind the plaque (Fig. 9.2). Fatty plaques are significantly more echolucent and when large may be appreciated as lipid pools. However, because shadowing in relation to a fibrous plaque may be

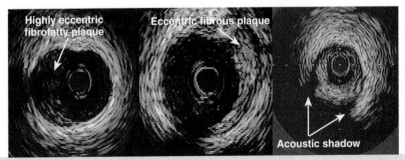

Figure 9.2:
These three panels demonstrate different plaque morphologies. The left panel shows a concentric mild fatty plaque which is less echodense then adventitia. The middle panel shows an extensive fibrofatty plaque with echodensity similar to adventitia. The right panel is a more echodense eccentric plaque with an area of acoustic shadowing between 5 and 8 o'clock due to the presence of dense fibrous plaque.

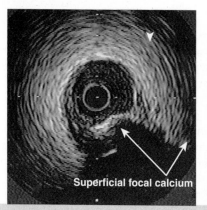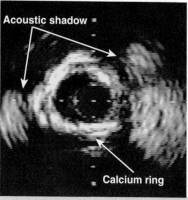

Figure 9.3:
These two images demonstrate the ultrasound fingerprint of (left) a superficial fibrocalcific plaque with an acoustic shadow immediately behind the calcific rim and an acoustic reverberation in this area at 5 o'clock, and (right) a dense cicatrix of calcium in all four quadrants of the image with an extensive acoustic shadowing.

misinterpreted as a lipid collection, there is a tendency to broadly classify plaques containing lipid as fibrofatty in nature.

Calcification is commonly seen by intravascular ultrasound as a bright echo with shadowing behind often associated with reverberation artifact in the area of the shadow due to oscillation of the ultrasound beam between calcium and transducer (Fig. 9.3). Calcium may be seen in relatively small plaque accumulations indicating the age of the plaque or the site of previous plaque rupture and repair. In one series of patients undergoing balloon angioplasty, 82% of arterial segments exhibited small areas of calcium which were visible in only 8% of angiograms at the lesion site or in 155 of more proximal segments by fluoroscopy.[9] In the GUIDE (Guidance by Ultrasound Imaging for Decision Endpoints) trial (Phase I), 70% of target lesions had areas of calcium by ultrasound, compared to 40% of angiograms.[10] Calcification may be graded from absent (0) to severe (3+) by the extent of the arc subtended by a fibrocalcific matrix.[11] In general, at least 180 degrees of calcium is required to achieve a mass of calcium identifiable by angiography (74% identification by fluoroscopy) increasing to 86% of cases identified if more than two quadrants or calcium length *vm 6 mm is present.[12]

By definition, plaque calcification results in shadowing of deeper structures, obscuring evaluation of underlying arterial wall components. Furthermore, shadowing may occur without any obvious calcification as the calcium may be out of plane and not visualised unless hit by the ultrasound beam in a perpendicular fashion. The calcium may be distributed in the plaque in several ways: as a deep deposit in an arc at the intima-media border, in a superficial rim at the luminal surface, or as a concretion within a fibrous plaque (Fig. 9.4). In one study of 110 patients, superficial calcium was present in 50%, deep calcium in 15% and both in 35%.[12] On occasion, the fibrous cap may be intensely echoreflective with shadowing extending to and around the periphery of

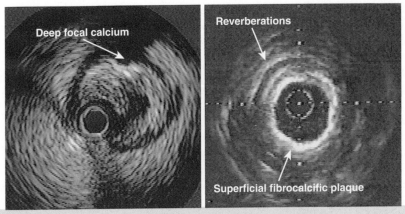

Figure 9.4:
These images demonstrate different distributions of calcium. The left panel demonstrates an area of echodensity between 12 and 1 o'clock posterior to the intimal plaque indicative of deep wall calcium. The right panel represents a superficial ring of calcium with reverberations readily visible (arrows).

the artery suggesting a more uniform distribution of calcium throughout the wall. Dense fibrotic plaques may be sufficiently underpenetrated by the ultrasound beam to cause significant shadowing, and such plaques are usually referred to as fibrocalcific.

The presence of thrombus is often more difficult to establish as it is frequently mistaken for soft plaque.[13] Thrombus often appears as a scintillating mass with a lobular edge and classically moves in an undulating manner separate from the movement of the artery. Incomplete microchannels are sometimes identified but many intra-coronary thrombi may be very difficult to differentiate as they may be relatively small and not very separate from the arterial wall. Luminal blood is characterised by a continually mobile speckled pattern. In contrast to conventional echocardiography, the gain of the intravascular ultrasound console should be set to allow its identification separate from possible thrombus. Where the flow of blood is significantly impaired, the backscatter may be sufficiently intense to mimic thrombus or soft plaque. It may be differentiated from the latter by injection of saline converting the lumen briefly to greater echolucency. Advanced signal analysis of the radiofrequency pattern may help to provide a rational and objective criteria to differentiate thrombus from fibrofatty plaque.[14]

Intravascular ultrasound has confirmed the observations first made by Glagov *et al.* that with increasing plaque accumulation, there is a remodelling process whereby the vessel expands to accommodate the plaque load.[15] The extent of remodelling in a given artery may be highly variable with segments of positive remodelling, no change, and negative remodelling (shrinkage). Even in angiographically normal segments, the average plaque burden in the normal reference segment may comprise 40% of the total vessel cross-sectional area. The inability of angiography to detect this occult disease is due to the presence of positive arterial remodelling and the diffuse nature of disease throughout the entire vessel length in many patients. It has been suggested that discrete coronary artery lesions only become apparent angiographically when the accumulation of plaque above a threshold of 40% of vessel area, for example, overcomes the ability of the vessel to expand any further.[16–18]

CORONARY INTERVENTION

Intravascular ultrasound has provided an invaluable insight into the characteristics of atherosclerotic plaque with an accurate online means for measuring the dimensions of the index artery prior to and after intervention. Furthermore, the reduction in the diameter of ultrasound catheters (to less than 1 mm in diameter) has allowed an assessment to be made prior to intervention as well as describing vessel morphology after the procedure. Additionally, it may provide additional prognostic information regarding the likelihood of acute and subacute vessel closure and longer-term restenosis. In the context of stenting, an improved clinical outcome may be achieved with ultrasound guidance (Table 9.2).

Pre-intervention imaging

With the development of catheters as small as 2.6 F, intravascular ultrasound may be used to assess lesions prior to intervention and direct appropriate therapy. In general, there are two major determinants of device selection – plaque load or burden, and the extent and severity of calcification. With an extensive plaque load, a debulking strategy has become common in interventional practice. Directional coronary atherectomy has been used to debulk lesions although it is only generally successful when the lesion is free of superficial calcium. In the latter case, high speed rotational atherectomy may be used to ablate superficial calcium in lesions with a large plaque load, either as a stand alone procedure or in preparation for further treatment.[19]

In one study of pre-intervention imaging, 313 target lesions underwent intravascular ultrasound resulting in a change of therapy in 40% of cases.[20] This comprised 6% of patients who underwent therapy where none had been planned due to a significant disparity in the assessment of lesion severity between ultrasound and angiography; 7% had revascularisation deferred for the same reason, and a further 13% had a change in revascularisation strategy or selection including referral for bypass surgery in 1% due to demonstration of unsuspected significant unprotected left main involvement.[20]

TABLE 9.2 - INTERVENTIONAL ROLE OF IVUS
PRE INTERVENTION
Accurate quantitation and balloon sizing
Assessment of reference segment disease
Device selection strategy with respect to plaque load and calcification
POST INTERVENTION
Recognition of dissection and thrombus
Prognostic assessment
Optimal stent deployment

Accurate balloon sizing is central to achieving the largest acute lumen gain after balloon angioplasty and with ultrasound, it is possible to demonstrate arterial remodelling and vessel expansion adjacent to diseased segments and balloon size accordingly. A strong argument for the use of intravascular ultrasound (IVUS) in balloon angioplasty is that it may allow a 'stent-like' result to be achieved by optimising the acute lumen gain from balloon dilatation alone. To investigate the safety of such an approach in selected cases, the CLOUT (Clinical Outcomes with Ultrasound Trial) pilot trial has been reported.[21] This is a multicentre investigation of the use of IVUS in balloon 'over-sizing' to achieve an improved acute outcome. The authors hypothesised that adaptive remodelling at the lesion site and in adjacent segments would accommodate this approach. Angiographically guided balloon angioplasty was performed in 104 lesions in 102 patients (types B1 and B2 lesions). IVUS was then performed to measure the proximal and distal reference segments, and if remodelling was present, a larger balloon size was calculated from whichever of the proximal or distal reference segments was smallest from the formula: balloon size = (mean lumen diameter + mean vessel diameter)/2. Quarter-size balloons were then used to achieve this with increased balloon sizes ranging from 0.25 to 1.25 mm. The mean reference segment plaque area was 51 ± 15%. A total of 73% of patients had balloon up-sizing, increasing the balloon:artery ratio from 1.12 ± 0.15 to 1.30 ± 0.17. As a result, minimum lumen diameter increased from 1.95 ± 0.49 to 2.21 ± 0.47 mm (percent diameter stenosis decreased from 28 ± 15% to 18 ± 14%). Despite this more aggressive balloon sizing strategy, the angiographic dissection rate was unchanged (37% vs 40%) with no increase in major complication rate (1.9%). Whether or not this more aggressive approach impacts on clinical outcome is awaited.

One study performed to see whether IVUS guidance of balloon angioplasty leads to better outcome is the SIPS (Strategy of IVUS-guided PTCA and Stenting) trial.[22] Patients enrolled in the study were randomised to either IVUS-guidance using the ORACLE FOCUS™ balloon – a combined balloon catheter and ultrasound transducer – or angiographic guidance of standard practice of balloon dilatation. The aim of the study was to achieve >65% reference minimal lumen area. A total of 355 lesions in 269 patients were enrolled with a 50% stent rate in both arms of the study. IVUS-guided angioplasty resulted in an increased MLD with a reduction in percent diameter stenosis (Table 9.3). A similar acute gain was also seen in patients receiving stents with IVUS-guidance, perhaps reflecting smaller vessels in the IVUS-guided stent group. Procedural success was higher in the IVUS-guided group. No significant difference in duration, contrast use, maximum inflation pressure or equipment used was seen although there was a trend towards a lower number of balloon catheters used in the IVUS-guided arm, 1.22 ± 0.94 vs 1.39 ± 1.03. With respect to acute outcome, there were no deaths and no difference in myocardial infarction (MI), but there was an increase in target vessel revascularisation in the standard angioplasty group, 4.6% vs 0.8%, resulting in a major adverse cardiac event rate (MACE) of 6.1% vs 0.8% (p < 0.05), compared with the IVUS-guided group. Of interest, those undergoing IVUS-guided PTCA had the lowest target segment revascularisation over the follow-up period of almost two years. This reflected the fact that stenting was

TABLE 9.3 - THE SIPS TRIAL			
	ANGIO-GUIDED	IVUS-GUIDED	P VALUE
Follow up (days)	594 ± 280	623 ± 294	
Acute gain (mm)			
– All	2.36 ± 0.6	2.54 ± 0.6	0.02
– PTCA	1.94 ± 0.5	2.16 ± 0.5	<0.0001
– Stent	2.75 ± 0.5	2.88 ± 0.5	NS
Acute success	87.7%	94.5%	0.03
TLR (total)	29%	18%	NS
TLR in vessels <3 mm	28%	15%	0.04

conditional and many patients received a stent because of a complication at the time of intervention. Furthermore, with IVUS-guidance, larger balloons were used due to the recognition of remodelling in diseased segments, accounting for stenting in smaller vessels in this group. Once stented, no difference was seen with respect to major events however. The long-term clinical results of this trial are awaited.

Post intervention imaging

One of the common indications for an intravascular ultrasound study is to assess the appearance of a coronary artery following an interventional procedure. This is performed for several reasons – to examine the resulting morphologic appearance from the intervention, to judge success, to complement angiographic assessment, to quantitate lumen enlargement and plaque reduction, and to consider whether or not to proceed to further intervention including stent implantation. Once stenting is undertaken, ultrasound may used to guide optimal expansion which has been investigated in several trials completed or nearing completion.

Balloon angioplasty Initial *in vitro* validation studies were done to correlate the appearance of diseased arteries at ultrasound post balloon dilatation with histology.[23] The consistent finding following balloon dilatation was tearing of the plaque with separation of the ends of the tear and an increase in lumen cross-sectional area, with some stretching of the less diseased wall. In this study, the lumen area by ultrasound and at section were similar ($R = 0.88$).[23] Dissection of the plaque (separation of intima from media) was a common finding which appeared as an increase in the sonolucent area corresponding to media. One feature described was the presence of arterial flaps with protrusion of plaque into the lumen, less frequently seen *in vivo* due to blood flow.

The presence of calcium in a coronary lesion determines the response of the artery to balloon dilatation. In one study of patients after balloon angioplasty of peripheral and coronary vessels, intralesional calcium and the relative size of dissection for each lesion was determined.[24] A total of 76% of patients had significant dissection/plaque fracture after angioplasty. In 71% of these patients, significant localised calcium deposits were identified within the plaque, and the vast majority of dissections (87%) were adjacent to the calcific portion of the wall. Comparing the relative size of dissections with respect to the neoluminal area, dissections in calcified areas were larger than those in lesions without calcium, 28% vs 11%, respectively. It was concluded that localised calcium had a direct role in promoting dissection by increasing shear stress within the plaque at the junction between tissue types with differing elastic properties.[25] Given these findings, it may be that deep calcium deposits protect against deep medial injury despite a large plaque fracture by deflecting the pressure axially. Further characterisation of lesion morphology with newer ultrasound catheters is required to address these issues in a clinical context.

An important use for intravascular ultrasound in interventional procedures is that it can accurately measure lumen and vessel area both at the lesion site and at the reference segment allowing the operator to size angioplasty balloons more exactly. In a key study of 223 coronary vessels treated by a Palmaz–Schatz stent, directional atherectomy or laser balloon angioplasty, 83% of patients underwent follow-up angiography six months after treatment.[25] The traditional dichotomous definition of restenosis (*vm 50% diameter stenosis) was used along with a cumulative graphical method. Although the restenosis rates were 19%, 31% and 50% for stents, directional atherectomy, and laser balloon angioplasty respectively, the late lumen loss was equivalent across the groups. This indicated that the major procedural determinant on restenosis was the acute lumen gain (2.6, 2.2, and 2.0 mm in the three groups) leading to the 'Bigger is Better' hypothesis.[25]

Stent deployment The MUSIC (Multicentre Ultrasound guidance of Stents In Coronaries) trial was designed to examine the additional value of IVUS in determining optimal stent deployment with Aspirin alone in vessels >3.0 mm (Fig. 9.5). Using the initial criteria of complete apposition (symmetry >0.7) and complete expansion (minimum stent area [MSA] >90% average of proximal/distal segments or MSA >100% of lowest reference segment or MSA >90% proximal segment, and subsequently revised to 80%, 90%, 80% respectively if MSA >9 mm²), a subacute thrombosis rate of 1.3% was reported at follow-up of mean 198 days.[26] The need for bypass surgery was 0.6% and repeat angioplasty was 4.5%. Of interest, even using the revised IVUS criteria, only 80% of patients achieved this. A six-month angiographic restenosis rate of 8.3% was reported (9.3% if the stent thrombosis cases were included) which is a remarkable result suggesting a major clinical benefit form IVUS-guided stent deployment and this data largely led to the design of the OPTICUS trial.

In OPTICUS (OPTimal Intra-Coronary Ultrasound in Stenting), a multicentre, *randomised* trial of 550 patients with angiographic follow-up has been recently reported.[27] The primary endpoints were defined as binary restenosis and angiographic MLD at six months follow-up. The secondary endpoints were 6- and 12-month clinical follow-up and the economics of ultrasound-guided stenting. Again, patients were randomised to angiography- or IVUS-guided stent deployment of either Palmaz–Schatz or NIR stents (thus giving OPTICUS the angiography arm for comparison that MUSIC didn't have). Lesions were more

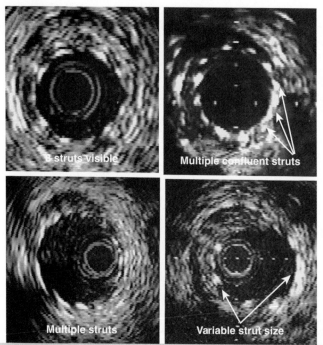

Figure 9.5:
A series of fully deployed intra-coronary stents. A The MicroStents, which has a basic design of continuous wire segments in a zig-zig design with eight axial struts connected by eight radiused crowns. On ultrasound imaging, this stent is identifiable by the presence of eight equally spaced struts/frame when fully expended. B The Wallstent, which is a self-expanding mesh design and made of a cobalt-based alloy with a platinum core. The ultrasound appearance is characterised by a multiple struts closely apposed around the lumen interface. C The MultiLink™ Stent, a slotted tube stent with multiple visible struts by ultrasound. D The Crossflex stent, which is a coil design with the stainless steel wire describing a sinusoidal pattern giving an appearance of unequal arcs by ultrasound.

challenging than described in the Benestent or Stress trials with 62% AHA/ACC type B2 and 15% type C lesions. The MUSIC expansion criteria were achieved in 64% of patients. Initial reports from the study have confirmed a reduction in the need for repeat in-hospital angioplasty although at follow-up despite an improved minimal luminal diameter (MLD) post-stent (and an impressive increase in angiography-guided post-stent MLD), clinical and angiographic outcome was no different comparing both groups.[27]

To evaluate objectively whether ultrasound-guided stent deployment results in an additional clinical benefit over angiography alone, the CRUISE (Can Routine Ultrasound Influence Stent Expansion?) substudy of STARS (STent Anti-thrombotic Regimen Study) has now been reported.[28] Patients undergoing ultrasound-guided stent deployment in nine centres were compared with seven centres in which stenting was guided by angiography alone followed by blinded IVUS assessment (IVUS-documentary). A total of 499 patients were followed up from an initial 525 patients with larger balloon sizing (3.88 *b+ 0.51 vs 3.69 *b+ 0.59 mm, p <0.001) and greater dilatation pressure (18.0 *b+ 2.6 vs 16.6 *b+ 3.0 atmospheres,

TABLE 9.4 - THE CRUISE TRIAL			
	ANGIO-GUIDED	IVUS-GUIDED	p VALUE
Number of patients	229	270	–
Death	2	0	NS
MI	14	19	NS
TVR	35 (15.3%)	23 (8.5%)	0.02

p <0.001) used in the IVUS-guided and IVUS-documentary groups, respectively. A total of 36% of patients in the IVUS-guided group had a change in deployment strategy based on the ultrasound images. This was associated with superior stent expansion (MSA) in the IVUS-guided group, 7.78 *b+ 1.72 mm2 vs 7.06 *b+ 2.13 mm2 (p < 0.001). At nine-month follow-up, a 44% reduction in the clinical end-point of target vessel revascularisation (TVR) was demonstrated (8.5% vs 15.3%, p < 0.05) (Table 9.4).[28] This was an encouraging clinical outcome although the apparent benefits of IVUS guidance could have been accentuated by other differences in treatment between the different centres, given the operators' individual discretion regarding optimisation of final stent deployment. Also, a clinical restenosis rate (TVR) rather than angiographic restenosis rate was selected as a primary endpoint in CRUISE and yet a significantly greater number of multivessel disease patients were in the IVUS-documentary group (44%) compared with the IVUS-guided group (27%), although this was not an independent predictor of TVR by multivariate analysis.[28]

The AVID (Angiography Versus Intravascular ultrasounD) trial is a multicentre comparison of IVUS-guided stenting with angiography-guided stenting, similar in concept to the CRUISE study. The initial results were reported in 1999.[29] A total of 759 patients undergoing elective single or multiple stent placement in native vessels >2.5 mm or saphenous vein grafts in 24 centres were included. Patients were randomised after optimal angiography-guided stent deployment (<10% residual stenosis). In the angiography-guided group, documentary IVUS was performed (with un-blinding only if significant dissection was noted [2.6%]). In the IVUS-guided group, larger balloons or additional stents were required in 43% of cases to achieve the criteria of full stent apposition and MSA >90% of the distal reference area. As a result, the final MSA was greater in the IVUS-guided group (7.54 *b+ 2.86 mm2 vs 6.94 *b+ 2.46 mm2, p< 0.01). After 12 months follow-up, the primary clinical endpoint of target lesion revascularisation (TLR) was 8.4% in the IVUS-guided group versus 12.4% in the angiography-guided group (p = 0.08). When protocol violations such as the inclusion of vessels smaller than 2.5 mm were excluded, the difference achieved statistical significance, 4.9% vs 10.8% (p = 0.02). The benefit of IVUS-guidance was particularly evident in three subgroups – saphenous vein grafts (TLR 5.7% vs 20.4%, p = 0.05), vessels with a diameter stenosis greater than 70% (TLR 3.5% vs 14.9%, p = 0.003), and vessels with a distal reference diameter less than 3.25 mm (TLR 7.9% vs 14.6%, p = 0.04).

Although the availability of recent generation balloon expandable stents has diminished the practice of high pressure (>14 atmospheres) dilatation, the OSTI

TABLE 9.5 - THE OSTI TRIAL	12 ATM	15 ATM	18 ATM	p VALUE
Balloon diameter (mm)	3.30	3.38	3.48	0.0001
Balloon: artery ratio	1.06	1.08	1.13	0.0001
MLD by QCA (mm)	2.78	2.84	2.86	NS
MLD by IVUS (mm)	2.72	2.91	3.04	0.0001
% Diameter stenosis (QCA)	10.6%	9.1%	8.5%	NS
% Diameter stenosis (IVUS)	6.2%	−0.4%	−4.7%	0.0001
Lumen area by IVUS	7.1	8.0	8.6	0.0001

(Optimal StenT Implantation) trial was completed in North America. This trial was designed to study the relationship between balloon pressure and stent deployment by IVUS. To date, 89 Palmaz–Schatz stents have been implanted in 79 lesions in 76 patients, post-dilating at 12, 15 and 18 atmospheres.[30] Palmaz–Schatz stent dimensions increase with increasing post-dilatation pressure which was described by IVUS but not quantitative angiography. Of interest, routinely used criteria for stent expansion, e.g. MUSIC criteria (37% at 12 bar, 61% at 15 bar, 74% at 18 bar) may still not be met despite 18 atmospheres pressure and a balloon: artery ration >1.1 (Table 9.5). In the second OSTI study, focal balloons achieved maximal stent expansion within 0.2 mm of the external elastic lamina resulting in a clinical restenosis rate (target lesion revascularisation) of 8.3%.[31]

High-speed rotational atherectomy Rotational atherectomy uses a rotating diamond-coated burr to abrade atherosclerotic plaque at speeds as high as 180 000 rpm. The technique works through the method of differential cutting whereby the burr selectively abrades harder tissue and is deflected away from normal vessel wall thus removing superficial calcium and dense fibrous plaque through micro-embolisation, pushing softer plaque away from the cutting path of the device. The appearance of vessels undergoing rotational atherectomy as a debulking strategy has been described.[32] In this study, 28 patients (22 calcified plaques, a third of which were circumferential) underwent ultrasound imaging after the procedure (with 71% having adjunct balloon angioplasty). Following rotablation, a distinct, circular intima-lumen interface was achieved with the lumen size 20% larger than the largest burr used. Deviations from a circular geometry occurred only in areas of soft plaque or superficial tissue disruption of calcified plaque. This study confirmed that there was no significant damage to the media and no dissections were caused by the procedure. A residual plaque load of 54% was reported indicating that athero-ablation using a burr strategy of 70–80% of the reference vessel lumen by angiography still resulted in a significant residual plaque even with adjunctive balloon dilatation in the majority of patients.[32]

A subsequent study of sequential ultrasound imaging before and after rotational atherectomy did confirm dissection planes in 26% of cases following rotablation increasing to 76% of cases after adjunct balloon dilatation with spread of the dissection plane to areas not only with the calcified plaque but also adjacent to the plaque, in part contributing to the expansion of the lumen area.[33] There was a reduction in plaque area from 15.7 *b+ 4.1 to 13.0 *b+ 4.7 mm^2 after initial rotablation, but still a residual percent cross-sectional narrowing of 74% indicating the need for adjunct balloon angioplasty to achieve an adequate final lumen area. In this study, the arc of calcium decreased significantly with full thickness calcium removal in some patients. Even without a measurable decrease in calcium arc, significant calcium ablation still occurred as evidenced by an increase in lumen area, uncovering of deeper calcium deposits, and the uncovering of deeper adventitial structures not seen pre-rotational atherectomy. In everyday practice, pre-interventional ultrasound scanning can direct athero-ablation appropriately. Superficial calcium not apparent by angiography is amenable to successful rotablation if the calcium arc is >180 degrees and extends to more than half of the lesion length. This preliminary debulking may then be supplemented by balloon angioplasty or intra-coronary stenting.

One particular complementary role of IVUS and rotablation may be in the treatment of in-stent restenosis. Although several small studies exist, it is only within the last two years that a randomised controlled trial has been conceived – ARTIST (Angioplasty versus Rotablation for Treatment of Intra-STent Stenosis/Occlusion).[34] This is a multicentre trial randomising patients with intra-stent restenosis or occlusion to balloon angioplasty or rotablation in restenosed or occluded stents in native vessels. Important exclusion criteria are coil stents, stents deployed distal to or at bend points >45 degrees, and stents not fully expanded by angiography or pre-procedure ultrasound. The primary endpoints of the study are acute success with quantitative angiographic assessment after the procedure (diameter stenosis <30% visually without additional stenting is defined a procedural success) and at six months follow-up. Preliminary data has reported an angiographic restenosis rate of 42% with a clinical restenosis rate of 36%.[34] The acute and long-term outcome in 100 patients was recently reported and confirmed slow-flow in only 3% with only 2% sustaining an enzyme rise of >3 *bx creatine-kinase.[35] With quantitative IVUS, 77% of acute gain occurred through rotablation and 23% through adjunctive balloon dilatation. At a mean of 13 months follow-up, repeat in-stent restenosis occurred in 28% with a target vessel revascularisation (TVR) of 26%.

REFERENCES

1. Yock PG, Fitzgerald PJ, Popp RL. Intravascular ultrasound. Sci Am 1995; 2:68–77.

2. Waller BF. The eccentric coronary atherosclerotic plaque: morphologic observations and clinical relevance. Clin Cardiol 1989; 12:14.

3. Picano E, Landini L, Lattanzi F et al. Time domain echo pattern evaluations from normal and atherosclerotic arterial walls: a study in vitro. Circulation 1988; 3:654.

4. Fitzgerald PJ, St. Goar FG, Connolly RJ et al. Intravascular ultrasound imaging of coronary arteries. Is three layers the norm? Circulation 1992; 86:154–8.

5. Maheswaran B, Leung CY, Gutfinger DE *et al.* Intravascular ultrasound appearance of normal and mildly diseased coronary arteries – correlation with histologic specimens. Am Heart J 1995; 130:976–86.

6. Nishimura RA, Edwards WD, Warnes CA *et al.* Intravascular ultrasound imaging: in vitro validation and pathologic correlation. J Am Coll Cardiol 1990; 16:145–54.

7. St. Goar FG, Pinto FJ, Alderman EL *et al.* Intra-coronary ultrasound in cardiac transplant recipients: *in vivo* evidence of 'angiographically silent' intimal thickening. Circulation 1992; 85:979–87.

8. St. Goar FG, Pinto FJ, Alderman EL *et al.* Detection of coronary atherosclerosis in young adult hearts using intravascular ultrasound. Circulation 1992; 86:756–63.

9. Tobis JM, Mallery J, Mahon D *et al.* Intravascular ultrasound imaging of human coronary arteries in vivo: analysis of tissue characterization with comparison to in vitro histological specimens. Circulation 1991; 83:319–26.

10. GUIDE trial investigators. IVUS-determined predictors of restenosis in PTCA and DCA: final report from the GUIDE trial, Phase II. J Am Coll Cardiol 1996; 27:156A (Abstract).

11. Farb A, Virmani R, Atkinson JB, Kolodgie FD. Plaque morphology and pathologic changes in arteries from patients dying after coronary balloon angioplasty. J Am Coll Cardiol 1990; 16:1421–9.

12. Mintz GS, Douek P, Pichard A *et al.* Target lesion calcification in coronary artery disease: an intravascular ultrasound study. J Am Coll Cardiol 1992; 20:1149–55.

13. Siegel RJ, Ariani M, Fishbein MC *et al.* Histopathologic validation of angioscopy and intravascular ultrasound. Circulation 1991; 84:109–17.

14. Metz JA, Preuss P, Komiyama N *et al.* Discrimination of soft plaque and thrombus based on radiofrequency analysis of intravascular ultrasound. J Am Coll Cardiol 1996; 27(Suppl. A);200A (Abstract).

15. Glagov S, Weisenberg E, Zarins CK, Stankunavicius R, Kolettis GJ. Compensatory enlargement of human atherosclerotic arteries. N Engl J Med 1987; 316:1371–5.

16. Kakuta T, Currier JW, Haudenschild CC, Ryan TJ, Faxon DP. Differences in compensatory vessel enlargement, not intimal formation, account for restenosis after angioplasty in the hypercholesterolemic rabbit model. Circulation 1994; 89:2809–15.

17. Post MJ, Borst C, Kuntz RE. The relative importance of arterial remodeling compared with intimal hyperplasia in lumen renarrowing after balloon angioplasty. Circulation 1994; 89:2816–21.

18. Currier JW, Faxon DP. Restenosis after percutaneous transluminal coronary angioplasty: have we been aiming at the wrong target? J Am Coll Cardiol 1995; 25:516–20.

19. Ellis SG, Popma JJ, Buchbinder M *et al.* relation of clinical presentation, stenosis morphology, and operator technique to the procedural results of rotational atherectomy-facilitated angioplasty. Circulation 1994; 89:882–92.

20. Mintz GS, Pichard AD, Kovach JA *et al.* Impact of pre-intervention intravascular ultrasound imaging on transcatheter treatment strategies in coronary artery disease. Am J Cardiol 1994; 73:423–30.

21. Stone GW, Linnemeier T, St. Goar FG, Mudra H, Sheehan H, Hodgson JMcB. Improved outcome of balloon angioplasty with intra-coronary ultrasound guidance – core lab angiographic and ultrasound results from the CLOUT study. J Am Coll Cardiol 1996; 27 (Suppl. A):155A (Abstract).

22. Frey AW, Dörfer K, Lange W, Hodgson JB. The impact of vessel size on long-term outcome after intra-coronary ultrasound guidance on provisional stenting. Circulation 1998; 98(Suppl. I):1494 (Abstract).

23. Tobis JM, Mallery JA, Gessert J *et al*. Intravascular ultrasound cross-sectional arterial imaging before and after balloon angioplasty in vitro. Circulation 1989; 80:873–82.

24. Fitzgerald PJ, Ports TA, Yock PG. Contribution of localized calcium deposits to dissection after angioplasty: an observational study using intravascular ultrasound. Circulation 1992; 86:64–70.

25. Kuntz RE, Safian RD, Levine MJ, Reis GJ, Diver DJ, Baim DS. Novel approach to the analysis of restenosis after the use of three new coronary devices. J Am Coll Cardiol 1992; 19:1493–9.

26. de Jaegere P, Mudra H, Figulla H *et al*. for the MUSIC Study Investigators. Intravascular ultrasound-guided optimized stent deployment. Immediate and 6 months clinical and angiographic results from the Multicenter Ultrasound Stenting in Coronaries Study (MUSIC study) Eur Heart J 1998; 19:1214–23.

27. Mudra H, Macaya C, Zahn R *et al*. Interim analysis of the Optimization with ICUS to reduce stent restenosis. Circulation 1998:98(Suppl. I):1908 (Abstract).

28. Fitzgerald PJ, Oshima A, Hayase M *et al*. Final results of the Can Routine Ultrasound Influence Stent Expansion (CRUISE) study? Circulation 2000; 102:523–30.

29. Russo RJ, Attubato MS, Davidson CJ, DeFranco AC, Fitzgerald PJ, Iaffaldano RA *et al*. Angiography versus intravascular ultrasound-directed stent placement: final results from AVID. *Circulation* 1999; 100(Suppl. I):I–234(Abstract).

30. Stone GW, St. Goar F, Fitzgerald PJ *et al*. The optimal stent implantation trial – final core lab angiographic and ultrasound analysis. J Am Coll Cardiol 1997:29 (Suppl. A); 369A (Abstract).

31. Stone GW, Bailey S, Roberts D *et al*. Long-term results following maximal stenting using ultrasound guided focal balloon stent overexpansion – the second Optimal Stent Implantation study. Circulation 1998; 98 (Suppl. I):826 (Abstract).

32. Mintz GS, Potkin BN, Keren G *et al*. Intravascular ultrasound evaluation of the effect of rotational atherectomy in obstructive atherosclerotic coronary artery disease. Circulation 1992; 86:1383–93.

33. Kovach JA, Mintz GS, Pichard AD *et al*. Sequential intravascular ultrasound characterization of the mechanisms of rotational atherectomy and adjunct balloon angioplasty. J Am Coll Cardiol 1993; 22:1024–32.

34. Radke PW, Hoffmann R, Haager PK, Janssens U, vom Dahl J, Klues HG. Predictors of recurrent restenosis after rotational atherectomy of diffuse in-stent retenosis at 6 month angiographic follow-up: a serial intravascular ultrasound study. Circulation 1998; 98(Suppl. I):3772 (Abstract).

35. Sharma SK, Duvvuri S, Dangas G *et al*. Rotational atherectomy for in-stent restenosis: acute and long-term results of the first 100 cases. J Am Coll Cardiol 1998; 32:1358–65.

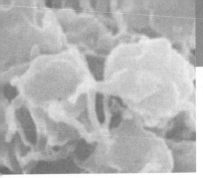

10

Pressure wire and related technologies

MICHAEL CUSACK

KEY POINTS

- Coronary angiography frequently underestimates the true significance of coronary stenoses, even where quantitative coronary angiography (QCA) is used.

- Intra-coronary data derived by both the pressure and the doppler wire systems have been shown to correlate well with both non-invasive ischaemia detection and the presence of disease found on intravascular ultrasound (IVUS) examination.

- Following coronary intervention the myocardial fractional flow reserve (FFR) and the relative coronary flow velocity reserve (rCVR) can determine whether a satisfactory physiological result has been obtained.

- Coronary intervention may be safely deferred for intermediate stenoses where the FFR or CVR suggest that the lesion is not physiological significant.

- Measurement of the index of microcirculatory resistance (IMR) allows quantitative assessment of the coronary microcirculation.

INTRODUCTION

The limitations of coronary angiography to assess the functional significance of coronary stenoses have been recognised for more than 20 years.[1] Large intra- and inter-observer variability occurs when coronary angiograms are interpreted which accounts for the frequent dissociation between clinical and angiographic findings. Morphological assessment of a coronary lesion does not necessarily reflect the impairment of flow by the stenosis. This dichotomy may occur as the resistance of a coronary stenosis will vary in relation to the fourth power of the luminal radius. Thus a relatively small change in vessel radius, beyond angiographic resolution, may result in a significant alteration in flow. The resistance of a lesion to flow will also be influenced by the length of the stenosis. Furthermore, whether ischaemia is induced by any epicardial stenosis will be determined to a significant extent by the size of the perfused territory that lies beyond the stenosis.

As a result, measurements of coronary flow and pressure have been introduced to improve the functional evaluation of coronary stenoses and interventions.[2] Technical progress has permitted intra-coronary measurements to be made using wires with the same dimensions as those of conventional angioplasty guidewires (0.014 inches in diameter) increasing their ease of application in the catheter laboratory.

This chapter will review the physiological background of both coronary flow and pressure measurement, and will focus on the application of these techniques for diagnostic and therapeutic catheterisation.

PRESSURE MEASUREMENT

Blood flow within the coronary vessels is greatly dependent on the haemodynamic status of the patient and may demonstrate significant variations between individual recordings. To overcome this problem the concept of coronary pressure derived myocardial fractional flow reserve (FFR) has been developed. FFR is defined as the maximum myocardial blood flow in the presence of a stenosis expressed as a proportion of the theoretical maximum flow in the absence of any stenosis (Fig. 10.1). The FFR represents the summation of the severity of the epicardial stenosis, the extent of the perfused territory and the contribution of distal collateral blood flow.

For accurate calculation of the FFR, a steady state of maximal hyperaemia is required to maintain myocardial microvascular resistance at a constant minimal level. In submaximal hyperaemia the FFR will be artificially elevated and the severity of the stenosis underestimated. During maximal hyperaemia, any changes in the measured coronary pressure that are recorded equate to alterations in blood flow within the vessel.

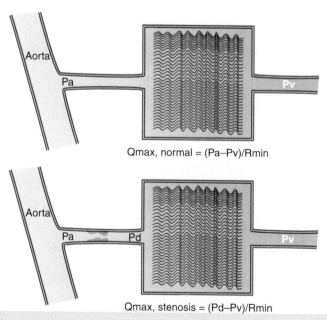

$$Qmax, normal = (Pa-Pv)/Rmin$$

$$Qmax, stenosis = (Pd-Pv)/Rmin$$

Figure 10.1:
Schematic representation of a coronary artery and vascular bed. Myocardial blood flow is equal to the perfusion pressure across the myocardium divided by its resistance. At maximum hyperaemia, resistance to flow (R_{min}) is minimal and constant. Maximum flow in the diseased vessel may, therefore, be expressed as a ratio to that of a normal vessel, i.e. one without a pressure drop, by the equation: $FFRmyo = (P_d - P_v)/(P_a - P_v)$

AO, aorta: P_a, P_d and P_v mean aortic, distal coronary and central venous pressure; Qmax, normal, theoretical maximum achievable myocardial flow if the artery were normal; Qmax, stenosis, maximal achievable flow in the presence of a stenosis. Adapted from Pijls and De Bruyne.[22]

The standard means for inducing hyperaemia is by the administration of adenosine. This is typically infused intravenously for 1–2 minutes (140 mg/kg/min infused via the femoral vein), though it may be used as an intra-coronary bolus dose.[3] Intra-coronary injection of papaverine may also be used.[3] This provides a hyperaemic plateau which lasts for 30–60 seconds though is associated with prolongation of the QT-interval and occasionally ventricular arrhythmia. The distal coronary, aortic and right atrial (RA) pressures are then measured simultaneously via the pressure wire, guide catheter and RA catheter respectively, and the FFR calculated (Fig. 10.1). For simplicity of use, the right atrial pressure is now not often recorded and is taken to have a value of 0mmHg when calculating the FFR. This practice has been demonstrated to reduce the sensitivity of FFR for detecting significant coronary lesions.[4] To compensate for this it is usual to accept values of FFR in the 'grey zone' of 0.75 to 0.80 as potentially indicative of ischaemia.

As measurement of FFR is expressed as a ratio of the proximal to distal coronary pressure within the same vessel, the possible confounding effects of microvascular disease and the contribution of distal collateral vessels are eliminated. Likewise, it is independent of changes in patient haemodynamics, such as heart rate, blood pressure and myocardial contractility.[5] As a normal reference vessel is not required, FFR measurements may be made in multivessel disease. It may also be used to assess the cumulative effect on coronary flow of sequential lesions within a single vessel.

The procedure

There are currently two widely used systems based on a high-fidelity sensor tipped guidewire.[6] Both of these are 0.014 inch wires with the sensor area located 3 cm proximal to the wire tip. With progressive improvement in the performance of these wires they may be used as first-line guidewires during angioplasty.

Before the wire is introduced into the coronary tree the patient is heparinised. Once the guiding catheter is in the coronary ostium, the pressure wire is passed to the catheter tip, where it is calibrated against the pressure transduced from the guiding catheter. The pressure wire is then passed across the lesion to be studied. Maximal hyperaemia is induced and the FFR calculated. As the pressure transducer is 3 cm proximal to the tip of the wire, once the wire has crossed the stenosis the sensor can be pulled back and re-advanced across the stenosis, while the wire tip remains distal to the lesion.

Application of pressure measurement

The primary indication for the use of coronary pressure measurement is to determine whether a coronary stenosis is flow limiting and as a result is responsible for myocardial ischaemia. It is now well established that an FFR below 0.75 is functionally significant and has been found to correlate well with the presence of ischaemia on perfusion scintigraphy, stress echocardiography and exercise testing in a broad spectrum of clinical settings.[5,7,8] However, it may be unreliable in acute ischaemic syndromes due to microvascular injury. Both retrospective and prospective work have demonstrated that lesions with a distal FFR greater than 0.75 may be left untreated without any increase in subsequent adverse events on follow-up.[9,10,11]

A further use of pressure measurement is to determine the precise location of the lesion under assessment by defining the point at which the measured pressure 'steps-up' during pull-back of the wire (Fig. 10.2A and B). A particular area where this has been applied is in the assessment of ostial coronary lesions which may be missed by conventional angiography.

Measurement of the FFR may provide important prognostic information following coronary intervention. An FFR of less than 0.75 implies that the results

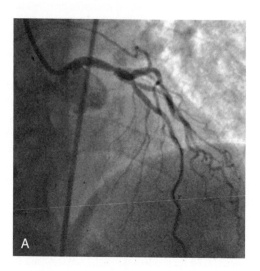

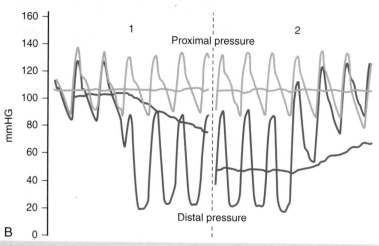

Figure 10.2:
A This patient had significant symptoms of angina. Angiography had demonstrated a moderate stenosis in the distal left main stem. There was a suggestion of disease at the ostium of the LAD though this could not be clearly delineated angiographically. When maximal hyperaemia was induced with an intravenous infusion of adenosine there was a significant reduction in distal pressure in the mid-LAD (FFR 0.49). B During wire advancement (1) and withdrawal (2) the 'step' in the phasic pressure was found to be in the distal LMS/ostium of LAD indicating the presence of a haemodynamically important stenosis in this area.

of the intervention are physiologically unacceptable and would be associated with myocardial ischaemia. An FFR of greater than 0.9 following balloon angioplasty without stenting, has been found to be associated with repeat intervention rates at 6, 12 and 24 months of 12%, 12% and 15% respectively.[12] Where the FFR following angioplasty was less than 0.9 the rates of re-intervention at these time points were 24%, 28% and 30%.[12] Therefore, even where a satisfactory angiographic appearance has been achieved following balloon angioplasty, obstruction to flow detectable physiologically is associated with an unfavourable outcome.

Where a stent has been implanted into a vessel and fully deployed, a pressure drop should no longer be detectable across the treated segment. An FFR across a stent of 0.94 or higher has been found to correlate strongly with optimal stent deployment as determined by intravascular ultrasound (IVUS).[13] The concordance rate between the FFR and IVUS parameters was greater than 90% in this study. In contrast, QCA exhibited low concordance rates with both IVUS and FFR, being 48% and 46% respectively.[13] Where the FFR was determined immediately following stent implantation, those with an FFR greater that 0.95 had a major adverse event rate of 4.9% at six months follow-up.[14] In this study, the event rate rose progressively with successive reductions in post procedural FFR. In those with an FFR between 0.90 and 0.95 the event rate was 6.2%. This rose to 20.3% where the FFR was less than 0.90 and to 29.5% among patients with an FFR under 0.80. These results indicate that the immediate haemo-dynamic result following coronary intervention exerts an important effect on the subsequent clinical outcome. Measurement of coronary pressure may, therefore, be used to determine both whether intervention is indicated and also if a satisfactory result has been achieved.

FLOW MEASUREMENT

Similar advances in guidewire technology to those seen with the pressure transducing wires have made it possible to directly measure flow within coronary vessels using 0.014 inch wires.

In the presence of significant obstruction to flow within a coronary artery, the downstream microvascular resistance falls to maintain a sufficient regional basal blood flow to meet metabolic demands. This resting dilatation of the microvascular bed results in a reduction in the capacity for further vasodilatation above baseline and reduces the potential maximal flow reserve that is available (Fig. 10.3). Thus any hyperaemic stimulus or increase in myocardial oxygen demand results in a smaller absolute increase in blood flow distal to a stenosis compared to that which would be achieved in a region where no stenosis was present.

Unlike the flow characteristics observed in most arterial beds, coronary blood flow has a distinct phasic pattern. Epicardial blood flow is normally reduced during systole as a result of cardiac contraction.[15] The contribution of the systolic component of flow is increased relative to the diastolic component distal to a coronary stenosis.[16] Thus the ratio of distal diastolic to systolic flow velocity encountered in normal vessels differs from that found in those with a significant stenosis. However, the application of this finding to the assessment of the

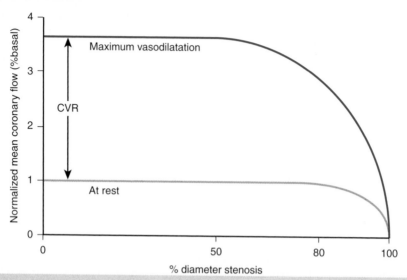

Figure 10.3:
Illustration of the relationship between increasing severity of coronary stenosis produced by extrinsic coronary compression in a canine model and the coronary flow velocity reserved (CVR). Once the degree of vessel stenosis reaches a significant level there is a progressive decline in the CVR available with maximal hyperaemia. Adapted from Gould et al.[23]

haemodynamic significance of coronary stenoses is limited by the differing patterns of flow found in the right and left coronary systems. Also this ratio is sensitive to changes in the contractility of the heart.

As a result of these potentially confounding effects, a doppler derived coronary flow velocity reserve (CVR) has been used to represent the physiological effect of coronary artery stenoses. The CVR is defined as the potential capacity for increased blood flow within both the epicardial coronary vessel and the microvasculature above the resting level (Fig. 10.3). A value of 2.7 +/− 0.6 is typically found for CVR among adults with angiographically normal vessels.[17] This figure is relatively constant in differing myocardial regions, even in cardiac transplants. A CVR of less than 2.0 has been found to correspond to the presence of myocardial ischaemia determined by perfusion scanning, stress echocardiography, or exercise testing.[18] However, in the absence of epicardial coronary disease the CVR may be abnormal when there is disease of the microvasculature.[19] This is typically seen in diabetes mellitus, as a result of ischaemic injury or due to the presence of left ventricular hypertrophy. In the presence of these conditions, the significance of epicardial disease may be overestimated by measurement of CVR alone. When the possibility of microvascular disease exists, the CVR is determined also in a normal reference vessel (CVRreference). The coronary flow velocity reserve in the vessel under investigation may then be expressed relative to that found in the reference vessel:

$$rCVR = CVR_{target}/CVR_{reference}$$

The normal value of rCVR is typically greater than 0.8.[17] As with measurement of the FFR, the rCVR is held to be lesion specific, having removed the contribution of the microvasculature. Both FFR and rCVR have been shown to correlate well with one another across a range of lesion types.[20] In a similar fashion to measurement of FFR, the rCVR prior to intervention has been found to bear a strong relationship to the area stenosis as determined by IVUS.[20] However, immediately following coronary intervention the relationship between rCVR and IVUS measurements becomes less robust.[21] This is in contrast to the strong relationship that exists between FFR and IVUS.

The procedure

Intra-coronary flow velocity is measured with a 0.014 inch guidewire, which has a piezoelectric ultrasound transducer at its tip. Flow velocity is sampled approximately 5 mm from the tip of the wire, the ultrasound beam being approximately 2 mm wide at this point. The wire tip should ideally be positioned coaxially within the artery. However, when the wire is not placed coaxially within the coronary artery, meaningful data may still be obtained. Flow is then recorded both at rest and following the induction of hyperaemia (see Fig. 10.4). This is typically induced by an intra-coronary bolus injection of adenosine, nitrate or papaverine. Assuming that a complete flow velocity profile envelope has been obtained, the mean flow velocity is calculated by dividing the peak velocity by two. The CVR is determined as:

$$CVR = \frac{\text{Mean flow velocity at hyperaemia}}{\text{Mean flow velocity at rest}}$$

Where rCVR is to be measured, this process is repeated in the reference vessel.

Application of flow measurement

The doppler guidewire has similar characteristics to that of a normal angioplasty guidewire and like the pressure wire systems may be used as a first-line wire during PCI. Again, like the pressure wire, the most common clinical application of the doppler wire is in determining the physiological significance of intermediate coronary artery lesions when intervention is contemplated.

The DEBATE I study (Doppler Endpoints Balloon Angioplasty Trial Europe) demonstrated that a CVR of less than 2.5 following angioplasty combined with a residual percentage diameter stenosis (DS) greater than 35% on IVUS correlated positively with clinical recurrence and need for re-intervention at six months.[24] Where a CVR of more than 2.5 was achieved with a satisfactory angiographic result (DS <35%), there was an angiographic restenosis rate and target vessel revascularisation rate of 16% at six months follow-up.[24] These later findings are not dissimilar to those observed with the pressure wire. Improvement in the CVR after intervention may, however, not be immediate. In those patients with an initially impaired CVR following angioplasty, it frequently returns to normal during long-term follow-up.[21] It has been suggested that this relates to delayed recovery of autoregulation in the microvascular bed following removal of an upstream stenosis. When a coronary stent is deployed, however, the CVR is found to normalise immediately in approximately 80% of patients.[25] Stent deployment would be expected to produce a larger, more uniform lumen than balloon angioplasty. It is, therefore, likely that late recovery in CVR following angioplasty relates in part to remodeling of the vessel lumen during follow-up.

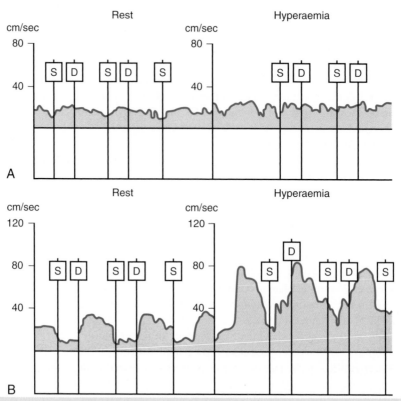

Figure 10.4:
Schematic coronary flow velocities recorded in the mid-portion of the LAD. The systolic (S) and diastolic (D) components of flow are demonstrated. In panel A are the recordings obtained prior to percutaneous intervention. The coronary flow reserve (CFR) at this time was found to be 1.2. CFR within the reference Circumflex vessel was 2.9 resulting in a relative CFR (rCVR) of 0.41. Panel B demonstrates the coronary flow recordings after PCI with stent deployment in the proximal LAD. The CFR has improved to 3.0 and the relative CFR to 1.03 indicating a satisfactory physiological result.

The DEBATE II study group demonstrated a low CVR following stent deployment to be associated with an adverse short-term outcome.[26] This appeared to be related to disturbances in the microvasculature. As with the pressure wire, a suboptimal physiological result following coronary intervention (CVR<2.0) has been found to be predictive of the need for subsequent target lesion revascularisation.[27]

Coronary intervention may be safely deferred where the CVR is greater than 2.0. In a study by Ferrari *et al.* 70 patients with intermediate coronary lesions and an indication for angioplasty due to stable angina and/or ischaemia on non-invasive testing underwent study with the doppler wire.[28] Patients with a CVR of less than 2.0 underwent balloon angioplasty and in those in whom it was greater than 2.0 the intervention was deferred. During 15 ± 6 months follow-up, a major adverse cardiac event rate of 33.3% was observed among those who had undergone angioplasty compared with 9.1% in those in whom it had been deferred. There was, however, a greater prevalence of angina among those managed medically compared to those in the angioplasty group (60% vs. 47%).

In-direct assessment of flow

In addition to pressure transduction, with appropriate software the Radi Pressure Wire™ (Uppsala, Sweden) may be used to record temperature within the coronary vessel. The shaft of the wire monitors temperature dependent electrical resistance allowing it to behave as a proximal thermistor. This development has allowed CVR to be calculated using a thermodilution technique. Typically this is performed by injecting a series of small boluses (3ml) of room temperature saline into the coronary vessel with the Pressure Wire™ sited distally. The time to peak temperature change (transit time) is first recorded for each injection at rest. Maximal hyperaemia is then induced and the procedure repeated. The CVR is calculated by determining the ratio of the mean transit time (T_{mn}) at rest to that during hyperaemia:

$$CVR = \frac{T_{mn} \text{ at rest}}{T_{mn} \text{ at hyperaemia}}$$

In validating this technique a strong correlation has been found between the doppler and thermodilution derived CVR.[29] Interestingly in this study an optimal doppler CVR could be obtained in only 69% of patients whereas a thermal CVR was recorded in 97% of patients.

A value for the CVR may be derived from pressure measurements alone when there is a pressure drop within the vessel at rest:[30]

$$CVR = \frac{\sqrt{\text{pressure drop across stenosis during hyperaemia}}}{\sqrt{\text{pressure drop across stenosis at rest}}}$$

Though a close relationship has been demonstrated between pressure and thermodilution derived CVR, the pressure-derived technique tends to underestimate CVR.[31] This calculation assumes that resistance to flow as a result of friction across a coronary stenosis is negligible.[31] However, it is likely that friction at the vessel wall disrupts laminar flow and is an important component of the pressure gradient recorded within a diseased vessel.[31]

Index of microcirculatory resistance (IMR)

The FFR assesses the effect of epicardial coronary disease on flow and the CVR is altered by both epicardial and microvascular disease (Fig. 10.5). Measurement of IMR allows quantitative assessment of the coronary microcirculation.[32] It is calculated after the mean transit time (T_{mn}) has been determined by bolus injections of saline at hyperaemia:

IMR = Distal Coronary Pressure × T_{mn}

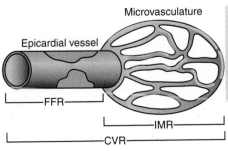

Microvasculature

Epicardial vessel

FFR

IMR

CVR

Figure 10.5: Measurements of FFR are unaffected by the state of the distal microvasculature. The CVR is influenced by resistance to flow within both the epicardial and microvascular vessels and does not distinguish between these. The IMR is specific to the microvasculature in isolation.

Once collateral flow within the microcirculation has been accounted for, microvascular resistance is independent of epicardial coronary disease.[33,34] This technique is not widely used in the clinical setting at the present time. It may in the future, however, become a commonplace technique for the assessment of microvascular damage.

REFERENCES

1. Topol EJ, Nissen SE. Our preoccupation with coronary luminology: the dissociation between clinical and angiographic findings in ischaemic heart disease. Circulation 1995; 92:2333–42.

2. Gould KL, Lipscomb K, Hamilton GW. Physiologic basis for assessing critical coronary stenosis. Instantaneous flow response and regional distribution during coronary hyperemia as measures of coronary flow reserve. Am J Cardiol 1974; 33:87–94.

3. Pijls NH, De Bruyne B (eds) Maximum hyperemic stimuli. In: Coronary pressure. Dortrecht: Kluwer Academic Publishers, 1997, pp. 96–104.

4. Perera D, Biggart S, Postema P et al. Right atrial pressure: Can it be ignored when calculating fractional flow reserve and collateral flow index? J AM Coll Cardiol 2004; 44:438–42.

5. Pijls NH, Van Gelder B, Van der Voort P et al. Fractional flow reserve. A useful index to evaluate the influence of an epicardial coronary stenosis on myocardial blood flow. Circulation 1995; 92(11):3183–93.

6. Pijls NHJ, Kern MJ, Yock PG, De Bruyne B. Practice and potential pitfalls of coronary pressure measurement. Cathet Cardiovasc Interven 2000; 49:1–16.

7. Pijls NH, de Bruyne B, Peels K et al. Measurement of fractional flow reserve to assess the functional severity of coronary-artery stenoses. N Engl J Med 1996; 334(26):1703–8.

8. Wilson RF. Assessing the severity of coronary artery stenoses. N Engl J Med 1996; 334:1735–7.

9. Mates M, Hrabos V, Hajek P et al. Long-term follow-up after deferral of coronary intervention based on myocardial fractional flow reserve measurement. Coron Artery Disease 2005; 16(3):169–740.

10. Berger A, Botman KJ, MacCarthy PA et al. Long-term clinical outcome after fractional flow reserve-guided percutaneous coronary intervention in patients with multi-vessel disease. J AM Coll Cardiol 2005; 46(3):438–42.

11. It is necessary to stent non-ischaemic stenoses? Five year follow-up of the DEFER study. Eur Heart J 2005; 26:(Suppl.1).

12. Bech GJW, Pijls NHJ, De Bruyne B et al. Usefulness of fractional flow reserve to predict clinical outcome after balloon angioplasty. Circulation 1999; 99:883–8.

13. Hanekamp CEE, Koolen JJ, Pijls NHJ, Michels HR, Bonnier HJRM. Comparison of quantitative coronary angiography, intravascular ultrasound, and coronary pressure measurement to assess optimum stent deployment. Circulation 1999; 99:1015–21.

14. Pijls NH, Klauss V, Seibert U et al. Coronary pressure measurement after stenting predicts adverse events at follow-up: a multicenter registry. Circulation 2002; 105(25):2950–4.

15. Sabistorn DC Jr, Gregg DE. Effect of cardiac contraction on coronary blood flow. Circulation 1957; 15:14–23.

16. Goto M, Flynn AE, Doucette JW *et al*. Effect of intra-coronary nitroglycerin administration on phasic pattern and transmural distribution of flow during coronary artery stenosis. Circulation 1992; 85(6):2296–304.

17. Kern MJ, Bach RG, Mechem CJ *et al*. Variations in normal coronary vasodilatory reserve stratified by artery, gender, heart transplantation and coronary artery disease. J Am Coll Cardiol 1996; 28:(5)1154–60.

18. Heller LI, Cates C, Popma J *et al*. Intra-coronary Doppler assessment of moderate coronary artery disease: comparison with 201TI imaging and coronary angiography. FACTS Study Group. Circulation 1997; 96(2):484–90.

19. Strauer BE. The significance of coronary reserve in clinical heart disease. J Am Coll Cardiol 1990; 15(4):775–83.

20. Baumgart D, Haude M, George G *et al*. Improved assessment of coronary stenosis severity using the relative flow velocity reserve. Circulation 1998; 98(1):40–6.

21. van Liebergen RAM, Piek JJ, Koch KT, de Winter RJ, Lie, KI. Immediate and long-term effect of balloon angioplasty or stent implantation on the absolute and relative coronary blood flow velocity reserve. Circulation 1998; 98(20):2133–40.

22. Pijls NH, De Bruyne B. Coronary pressure measurement and fractional flow reserve. Heart 1998; 80:539–42.

23. Gould KL, Lipscomb K. Effects of coronary stenoses on coronary flow reserve and resistance. Am J Cardiol 1974; 34:48–55.

24. Serruys PW, Di Mario C, Piek J *et al*. Prognostic value of intra-coronary flow velocity and diameter stenosis in assessing the short- and long-term outcomes of coronary balloon angioplasty: the DEBATE Study (Doppler Endpoints Balloon Angioplasty Trial Europe). Circulation 1997; 96(10):3369–77.

25. Kern MJ, Dupouy P, Drury JH *et al*. Role of coronary artery lumen enlargement in improving coronary blood flow after balloon angioplasty and stenting: a combined intravascular ultrasound Doppler flow and imaging study. J Am Coll Cardiol 1997; 29(7):1520–7.

26. Albertal M, Voskuil M, Piek JJ *et al*. Coronary flow velocity reserve after percutaneous interventions is predictive of periprocedural outcome. Circulation 2002; 105(13):1573–8.

27. Nishida T, Di Mario C, Kern MJ *et al*. Impact of final coronary flow velocity reserve on late outcome following stent implantation. Eur Heart J 2002; 23(4):331–40.

28. Ferrari M, Schnell B, Werner GS, Figulla HR. Safety of deferring angioplasty in patients with normal coronary flow velocity reserve. J Am Coll Cardiol 1999; 33(1):82–7.

29. Barbato E, Aarnoudse W, Aengevaren WR *et al*. Validation of coronary flow velocity reserve measurements by thermodilution in clinical practice. Eur Heart J 2004; 25(3):219–23.

30. Akasaka T, Yamamuro A, Kamiyama N *et al*. Assessment of coronary flow reserve by coronary pressure measurement: comparison with flow- or velocity-derived coronary flow reserve. J Am Coll Cardiol. 2003; 41(9):1554–60.

31. MacCarthy P, Berger A, Manoharan G *et al*. Pressure-derived measurement of coronary flow reserve. J Am Coll Cardiol 2005; 45(2):216–20.

32. Fearon WF, Balsam LB, Farouque HM *et al*. Novel index for invasively assessing the coronary microcirculation. Circulation 2003; 107(25):3129–32.

33. Fearon WF, Aarnoudse W, Pijls NH *et al*. Microvascular resistance is not influenced by epicardial coronary artery stenosis severity: experimental validation. Circulation 2004; 109(19):2269–72.

34. Aarnoudse W, Fearon WF, Manoharan G *et al*. Epicardial stenosis severity does not affect minimal microcirculatory resistance. Circulation 2004; 110(15):2137–42.

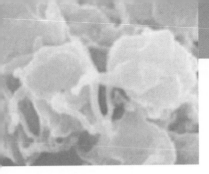

11

Arterial puncture site closure and aftercare

DR JAMES COTTON MD FRCP

KEY POINTS

- Correct management of the access site following percutaneous intervention reduces complications and facilitates early mobilisation and discharge.

- A variety of techniques and devices have been developed to aid sheath removal and haemostasis for cases that are performed by femoral route.

- Manual pressure is probably the 'gold standard' method for sheath removal in terms of safety, but often not practical, therefore, external pressure devices or arterial closure devices need to be employed.

- External pressure or arterial closure devices may allow early mobilisation and be well tolerated, but there is little evidence to suggest that they reduce complications.

INTRODUCTION

It is often said that restenosis is the 'Achilles heel' of percutaneous intervention. With this threat now rapidly receding thanks to drug-eluting stents (see Chapter 13) it is time for the arterial puncture site to step forward as the rightful owner of this classical metaphor.

Any regular PCI operator will have a number of stories of cases where a coronary triumph has been marred or completely overshadowed by a problem relating to the arterial access site. At the time of writing, the femoral artery is by far the most common access site used for percutaneous intervention, with over 80% of all procedures being performed from this site. The reasons are many: the artery is large, easy to cannulate and allows the insertion of large bore sheaths. Moreover the majority of coronary guide catheters are designed for use from the femoral route.

This ease of use comes at a price, however, complications relating to the femoral artery occur in up to 9% of cases, and very rarely may be fatal.[1] A full working knowledge of the correct procedure for sheath removal and groin site aftercare is, therefore, essential for operators using this route.

Whilst much is made of the after-care of the femoral access site, many complications can be avoided by careful arterial puncture. Ideally the anterior wall of the common femoral artery should be punctured below the inguinal ligament, but above the bifurcation of the profunda femoris and the superficial femoral artery. Too high and bleeding complications are difficult to control with manual pressure, too low and the risk of vessel trauma and pseudo aneurism formation increases.

Given that brachial access is no longer a first choice access site and the radial artery is covered in detail elsewhere, the rest of this chapter will focus on the complications relating to, and the closure techniques used for, the femoral artery.

As with all invasive medical procedures, the complication rate from femoral access can be minimised by careful case selection: increased complications are seen in patients with peripheral vascular disease, advanced age, repeat procedures and aggressive anti-thrombotic regimens.[2] Similarly increased operator experience reduces complication rates. Further to this, complications can be limited by selection of the smallest diameter sheath that will allow effective coronary intervention. Downsizing from 8 French is associated with reduced adverse events.[3]

Complications relating to the femoral access site can be haemorrhagic (haematoma, pseudo-aneurism and retroperitoneal bleeding), related to compression from haematomas, embolic or infective. These complications are covered in detail in Chapter 12 (Complications of PCI).

SHEATH REMOVAL

Manual pressure

Whilst the rule that 'the person making the femoral artery puncture should be the person to close it' may not suit all units and operators, the basic tenet that an interventional cardiologist must be an expert in care of the puncture site is a sound one.

There is definitely a 'learning curve' to negotiate when training in femoral sheath removal and an experienced operator will engender far fewer bleeding complications than a novice, and secure the groin site in less time.

As a rule 10–20minutes should be allotted to pressing on a groin. Patients should be well hydrated, have IV access that is functioning well and be comfortable. If the effects of local anaesthesia at the groin site has worn off the site should be re infiltrated. Some units advocate the pre-treatment of all patients with atropine, to avoid unwanted vagal reactions, in addition to intravenous sedation with a benzodiazepine or opiate sedatives. These latter measures may not be required if the patient is comfortable and pain free, however.

Digital pressure is applied at the site of arterial puncture (not the site of skin puncture). Supra-systolic pressure should be applied for one minute, and then released slightly until flow can be felt, but there is no leak from the puncture site. This pressure is maintained for five minutes and then pressure gently released over the next four minutes.

This procedure should lead to effective haemostasis in the majority of cases. If at any point there is bleeding from the site, or formation of a haematoma, the pressure can be increased and the cycle repeated.

Mechanical pressure devices

Manual pressure following the removal of a femoral sheath remains the 'gold standard', however, for many, practical concerns such as staff and resource utilisation mean that mechanical pressure devices have found a niche.

Thankfully sandbags on the groin and pressure bandage techniques to press on the femoral puncture site have largely been replaced by more sophisticated devices. The most commonly used of these is the FemoStop®.

This device has a transparent inflatable pressure element fitted to a rigid beam, which in turn is strapped to the patients lower torso. The inflatable

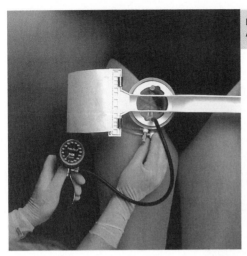

Figure 11.1:
A FemoStop device being deployed.

element allows the degree of pressure to be varied, and visualisation of the compression and puncture sites (Fig. 11.1).

There are conflicting reports as to whether this device reduces complications when compared to manual compression,[4,5] and some evidence that there may be some increased discomfort when compared to the use of a vascular closure device.[6] It is, therefore, important to ensure adequate patient preparation prior to siting a FemoStop (adequate hydration, analgesia and possibly sedation).

The FemoStop major role is, therefore, in reducing manual pressure times, freeing staff for other duties. This is particularly important in patients being treated with aggressive anti-platelet and anticoagulant regimens whereby manual pressing time would be prohibitively long.

Arterial closure devices

Arterial closure devices have been developed as an alternative to manual pressure or external pressure devices in an attempt to reduce haemostasis times, enhance early mobilisation and reduce discomfort for the patient and staff. Early hopes that direct arterial closure would reduce complications and, therefore, lead to safer treatment of the groin site have been largely unsubstantiated, however.[7,8]

The heterogenous nature of the ileo-femoral arterial system and the possibility of occult peripheral vascular disease mandate the use of femoral angiography, simply performed through the femoral sheath, prior to using a closure device. Manual pressure should be used as the closure technique if the puncture is in a heavily diseased artery, in a small vessel or involved in a bifurcation. Obviously closure devices are themselves associated with novel complications, principally failure to prevent haemostasis with subsequent haematoma formation, or peripheral vessel occlusion with distal limb ischaemia.

The three most commonly used devices are the Angioseal, the Vasoseal (both collagen plug devices) and the Perclose suturing device.

One recent meta-analysis of closure device use has suggested that there is no specific advantage or increased risk in using arterial closure devices vs. manual

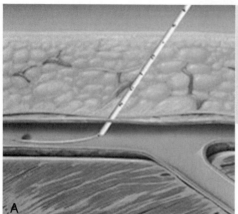

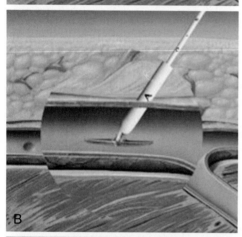

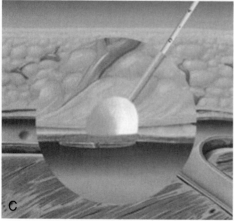

Figure 11.2:
A, The femoral sheath is replaced over a guidewire with a specific introducer sheath. **B,** Thereafter the anchor/collagen introducer is passed into the sheath. **C,** Deployed leaving the 'foot' adjacent to the endoluminal surface and the collagen pressed on the external surface of the artery.

compression in diagnostic cases, but when applied to interventional cases the same was true for Angioseal and Perclose devices, but not Vasoseal. This latter device appeared to have a disadvantage when compared to mechanical compression in the PCI group.[8] A further meta-analysis failed to show conclusively that arterial closure devices are superior to manual compression both in terms of safety and effectiveness.

Angioseal

The Angioseal device seals the femoral puncture site by sandwiching the arteriotomy between an intra luminal absorbable polymer 'anchor' and a collagen sponge on the external surface of the artery. The two are joined by a self tightening suture. The residual components are absorbed at between 60 and 90 days.

The femoral sheath is replaced over a guidewire with a specific introducer sheath (Fig. 11.2a). Therafter the anchor/collagen introducer is passed into the sheath (Fig. 11.2b) and deployed (Fig. 11.2c) leaving the 'foot' adjacent to the endoluminal surface and the collagen pressed on the external surface of the artery.

Perclose

The Perclose device is a semi-automated suture device. This device does not require a thrombin or collagen plug and thereby leaves no foreign material in the lumen. The device is advanced into the femoral artery and the correct depth is signalled by a flush back of blood. Following this a suture 'foot' is deployed into the artery and the sutures advanced and tightened. The excess suture material is then trimmed off with a specific device (Fig. 11.3).

Vasoseal

This system relies on a collagen plug that is positioned against the external aspect of the arteriotomy. The collagen plug then expands in the sheath tract, effecting haemostasis.

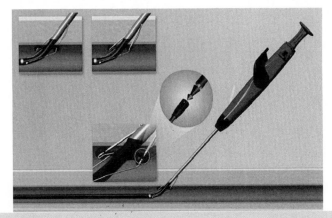

Figure 11.3:
The Perclose device showing deployment of the needles and suture.

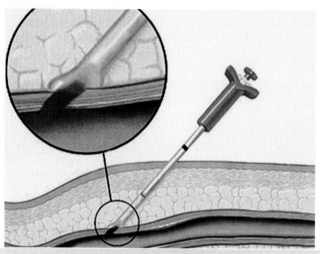

Figure 11.4:
The Vasoseal device ready to be deployed. The inset shows that the plug is accurately located over the arterial puncture

This system does not require an intra-arterial component.

Briefly, a specific arterial locator is passed through the intra-arterial sheath and the sheath removed. A J segment within the artery allows accurate positioning of first a dilator sheath and then the collagen deployment catheter which is used to place the collagen plug on the external surface of the artery (Fig. 11.4).

All three of these devices have found a niche in contemporary interventional practice, however, there are a number of other devices available or in development at the present time.

SUMMARY

Vascular complications can be reduced by careful attention to the puncture site. If this is femoral, manual pressure is considered the gold standard method to achieve haemostasis, but increasingly external pressure devices or arterial closure devices are used.

There is evidence that these devices may improve patient processing and allow early mobilisation, however, the case for these devices improving safety has yet to be fully made.

REFERENCES

1. Nasser T, Mohler ER 3rd, Wilensky RL *et al*. Peripheral vascular complications following coronary interventional procedures. Clin Cardiol. 1995; 18:609–14.

2. Resnic F, Blake GJ, Ohno-Machado L *et al*. Vascular closure devices and the risk of vascular complications after percutaneous coronary intervention in patients receiving glycoprotein IIbIIIa inhibitors. Am J Cardiol. 2001; 88:493–6.

3. Muller DW, Shamir KJ, Ellis SG *et al*. Peripheral vascular complications after conventional and complex percutaneous coronary interventional procedures. Am J Cardiol. 1992 Jan 1; 69(1):63–8.

4. Sridhar K, Fischman D, Goldberg S *et al*. Peripheral vascular complications after intracoronary stent placement: prevention by use of a pneumatic vascular compression device. Cathet Cardiovasc Diagn. 1996 Nov; 39(3):224–9.

5. Benson LM, Wunderly D, Perry B *et al*. Determining best practice: comparison of three methods of femoral sheath removal after cardiac interventional procedures. Heart Lung. 2005 Mar–Apr; 34(2):115–21.

6. Juergens CP, Leung DJ, Crozier JA *et al*. Patient tolerance and resource utilization associated with an arterial closure versus an external compression device after percutaneous coronary intervention. Catheter Cardiovasc Interv. 2004 Oct; 63(2):166–70.

7. Koreny M, Riedmuller E, Nikfardjam M *et al*. Arterial puncture site closing devices compared with standard manual compression after cardiac catheterisation. JAMA; 291:350–7.

8. Nikolsky E, Mehran R, Halkin A *et al*. Vascular complications associated with arteriotomy closure devices in patients undergoing percutaneous coronary procedures – a meta-analysis. J Am Coll Cardiol 2004; 44:1200–9.

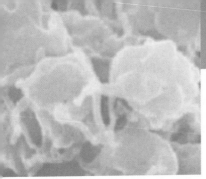

12

Complications of percutaneous coronary intervention

DAVID SMITH

KEY POINTS

- All complications are caused by the operation, but some by the operator.
- Meticulous technique is mandatory.
- Acute vessel closure still occurs.
- Aggressive antiplatelet regimens increase bleeding complications especially retroperitoneal haemorrhage and pericardial tamponade from coronary perforation.
- Infection can happen.
- The arterial access site remains a major potential cause of morbidity.

Any aspect of an angioplasty procedure that prolongs the procedure time or detracts from the well being of the patient can be considered a complication. Some seem more important than others but often it is from an apparently trivial slip that a cascade of events ensues spiraling down towards disaster. Major complications are acute vessel closure, myocardial infarction and possibly death yet they may be caused by a brief lapse of concentration – many a main stem has been dissected with a guide catheter by the casual and abrupt withdrawal of a balloon catheter causing the guide suddenly to be deeply engaged. There is no room for bravado, no place for the slap-dash, attention to detail is everything. Whatever the complication it is the responsibility of you the operator.

GENERAL PRINCIPLES TO AVOID COMPLICATIONS

There are some general principles of angioplasty that in broad terms might be applied to any technical procedure in an attempt to prevent a 'botch up'. What follows is not an exhaustive manual of how to do an angioplasty but a short list of guiding principles one should employ to try to avoid disaster.

Preparation

Prepare appropriately for the case with:

- *Adequate assessment of the angiogram.* Study the lesions carefully, their length, extent of calcification, tortuosity and relationship to branches. Consider the route to the lesion, the distance from the ostium and the bends involved and consider the involvement of side branches, the nature of the distal vessel and the extent and origin of collaterals. Use all views for your assessment. If you are not sure take another picture.
- *Sound procedural strategy.* Based on the assessment of the angiogram select the appropriate guide catheter, wire and predilating balloon or stent diameter and

length. Use QCA to help. Plan what you will do after you have used them, for example, change up for a bigger balloon, change wires for a stiffer wire. Run through the planned procedure using 'what if' scenarios, for example, 'what if it dissects back to ...?' 'what if the branch becomes occluded?', 'what if I cannot pass another stent distally?' and make sure you have the appropriate equipment available to treat them.

- *Adequate preparation of the patient.* Check intravenous access, state of hydration, state of sedation, state of oxygenation if sedated, extent of anticoagulation and anti platelet regimen.

Execution

During the procedure attention to detail is everything.

- Take great care with the arterial puncture – one hole is all that is required!
- *Never* pull, push, inflate or deflate *anything* without fluoroscopy.
- Make sure your guide catheter support is good at the start – if not change guides.
- Instrumentation in the coronary artery should be done gently and carefully – steer the wire, ease the wire, coax the wire – *don't shove it!*
- Remember the catheter system is a co-axial system, movements of the elements are interdependent, therefore, all elements need to be controlled at once. Pay attention to the guide catheter and wire tips even when the action has moved to positioning the balloon or deploying the stent.
- Remember you are working in three dimensions – take advantage of different views to check the position of branches, wires, balloons, stents, etc.
- When it is not going according to plan stay calm. Do not lose your temper. If you cannot think what to do next ask someone else.

Post procedure

Aftercare of the patient is very important. Particular attention should be paid to:

- The arterial puncture site – many a fine piece of coronary work has been ruined by poor care of the arterial puncture site leading to hypotension and subsequent stent thrombosis.
- Control of systemic blood pressure – not too high, not too low.
- Appropriate anticoagulation and anti platelet treatment.

Although adherence to the above guidelines will limit the likelihood of complications it will not eradicate them. Those that occur, however, are likely to be the result of the biological response to the angioplasty process and not the result of operator incompetence.

COMPLICATIONS

Angioplasty necessitates the introduction into the coronary circulation of thrombogenic instruments with the intention of causing vessel wall injury. Dissection of the vessel and exposure of sub intimal prothrombotic tissues are essential components of this process. It is, therefore, not surprising that dissection, thrombosis, subintimal haematoma and spasm are the major contributing factors to the most important of angioplasty complications, acute vessel closure.

Acute vessel closure

Acute closure may be defined as occlusion of the coronary artery occurring during or after the procedure with consequent electrocardiographic and haemodynamic instability. It is the most common cause of peri-procedural myocardial infarction, referral for emergency CABG and death.

Frequency Acute closure occurs in anything from 2% to 13.5% of balloon angioplasty with the majority of reported series suggesting at least 5% established closure and 3% impending closure.[1,2] The frequency has fallen over time to around 1%[3] as stent usage increases, but it still occurs with edge dissections proximal or distal and dissections caused by wires and guide catheters. The majority of abrupt closure occurs in the laboratory but a significant proportion occurs afterwards within the first six hours. Acute closure is rare after 6 hours and very unlikely after 24 hours.

Predictors of acute closure Clinical predictors are insulin dependent diabetes mellitus, female sex and acute coronary syndromes where there is a prothrombotic milieu. Lesion characteristics that predict acute closure are those of very severe stenosis, long lesions (at least twice the luminal diameter), ulcerated lesions, branch point lesions and lesions on a bend of more than 45 degrees. Lesion characteristics have been classified on the basis of angiographic morphology[4] into types A, B1, B2 and C according to risk of failure and risk of acute closure. Lesions of the B2 (more than one B characteristic) and C categories are at high risk of dissection and acute closure (Table 12.1).

Predictors of death with acute closure Acute closure may or may not produce fatal haemodynamic collapse but is more likely to do so in the following circumstances: females, the elderly (>65), those with left main disease, triple vessel disease and/or LV EF<30%. Any vessel closure that results in an acute loss of function of 40% of the myocardium is likely to result in cardiogenic shock and death.

Causes

The role of dissection The major component to acute closure is the intimal dissection that can be caused by the guide catheter, the passage of the wire, the inflation of the balloon or deployment of the stent. Some post mortem and intravascular ultrasound studies have demonstrated, not surprisingly, that dissection occurs in nearly 100% of cases but unfortunately contrast angiography is a relatively insensitive technique for demonstrating it. Angiographic appearances of dissection have been classified into six categories A to F[5] associated with an increasing likelihood of major in-hospital complications from C (persisting extraluminal contrast) 10% risk, D (spiral dissections) 30% risk, E (new persistent intraluminal filling defects) 40% risk to F (occlusive dissection) 70% risk.

The role of thrombus Despite some popular misconceptions it should be noted that it is not possible to identify accurately the material composition of an angiographic filling defect on the angiogram. Dissection flaps can mimic the appearance of thrombus and vice versa while the contribution made by spasm to an angiographic 'train smash' should never be underestimated. Given that the collagens exposed by intimal disruption are highly thrombogenic it can be assumed that any acute closure involving dissection also involves thrombus. Adequate premedication with anti thrombotic agents such as Aspirin and Clopidogrel and appropriate procedural anticoagulation with Heparin will help limit thrombus formation but not preclude it. Once established it may be successfully treated with intra coronary thrombolytics such as urokinase or t-PA although this practice has largely been superceded by the advent of intravenous platelet GP IIb/IIIa receptor blockers such as abciximab that have a surprisingly rapid acute effect on thrombus. These potent anti platelet agents are best applied in the prevention of acute thrombus in high-risk cases by being prescribed in the 24 to 48 hours before angioplasty. Thrombus is more likely to become the dominant problem in acute closure when a stent has been deployed since almost all available stents are made of thrombotic materials. Although type D, E and F dissections can occur both proximal and distal to a newly deployed stent, acute closure of a stented lesion is more likely to be caused by acute thrombosis. It may respond well to mechanical disruption with balloon inflation with concomitant use of IIb/IIIa blockers.

No reflow No reflow is the phenomenon of no antegrade flow in the coronary artery following apparently successful lesion dilatation and in the absence of an identifiable dissection, obstruction or distal vessel 'cut off' suggestive of distal embolisation. The exact mechanism of this phenomenon is unknown but appears to be related to the distal microcirculatory dysfunction. Whilst it may occur during any angioplasty it is more likely to occur in relation to angioplasty in the setting of acute MI (seven times more likely) or unstable angina rather than elective procedures although it also seems more likely in cases of vein graft angioplasty and stenting of particularly bulky lesions. These circumstances have major disruption of the vessel wall as a common factor and this supports the two theoretical causes namely a local humoral effect on the distal vessel or a microembolic effect in the distal microcirculation. The fact that intracoronary Verapimil and Adenosine can be very successful as treatments favours the former theory while the apparent benefit of GP IIb/IIIa receptor blockers and distal protection devices favours the latter. The immediate clinical consequences may be the same as for acute closure and haemodynamic collapse can occur. Bradycardia requiring pacing may ensue particularly with right coronary intervention. Support of the rhythm and circulation (pacing, intra aortic balloon pumping, etc) for a period often results in spontaneous restoration of antegrade flow. Distal protection devices whether filters or extraction devices can be used and may have a role in limiting no reflow and although anecdotally they are successful the trial evidence does not support a definite advantage. There is data to support their use in angioplasty of saphenous vein grafts.[6]

Spasm Spasm of the dilated segment is a common feature and responds to intracoronary nitroglycerin (100–300 micrograms) while recoil is not abolished by nitrates and may take up to three months to disappear.

Coronary perforation

Coronary perforation was a rare complication with balloon angioplasty with rates approximately 0.1%, however, the later technologies which are inherently more aggressive such as directional atherectomy, excimer laser angioplasty and rotablation have all led to an increase in perforation rates up to 10% in some circumstances. Even stents, which act as a vessel wall scaffold and may be used to treat perforation can at times cause perforation especially if the 'bigger is better', therefore, 'biggest is best' approach is used and the stent is over dilated.

Acute sequelae The majority of coronary perforations do not lead to haemopericardium and pericardial tamponade but it is a possibility and emergency surgery with drainage of the pericardium and repair of the vessel may be required. Alternative means of managing uncomplicated perforations range from using long inflations with a perfusion balloon catheter, the deployment of a stent or, probably the best option, a covered stent. There is increasing likelihood of haemopericardium occurring with coronary perforation as antiplatelet regimens become more aggressive. Patients pretreated with Aspirin, low molecular weight Heparin, Clopidogrel and IIb/IIIa receptor blockers are at considerable risk from coronary perforation sometimes even after an apparently innocuous movement of the wire let alone after overinflation of an oversized stent.

Late sequelae Small perforations that appear haemodynamically stable and are safely left may in time result in pseudoaneurysm formation with its own potential complications of rupture and distal embolisation.

Stent complications

The advent of stents and their increasingly widespread use has undoubtedly provided a huge improvement in intravascular intervention but at the same time it has brought to the practice of angioplasty a plethora of new complications.

Stent handling Stents may be self expanding or balloon expandable. Most fall into the latter group. Originally balloon expandable stents were mounted by hand and crimped onto the dilating balloon just prior to delivery. Poor crimping could lead to damage, displacement or dislodging of the stent particularly when passing it in or out of the guiding system. All stents are now ready mounted with sophisticated techniques that ensure that the stent is well attached to the balloon for manipulations prior to deployment but releases contact after deployment. Nevertheless stents may still be damaged by poor handling. The lifting of one strut of the leading edge of the stent as it is introduced into the guiding catheter can go unnoticed until the stent will not easily exit the guide, traverse the proximal coronary section or cross the lesion.

It is even possible to damage them when removing them from their packaging. Great care should be used at all times with minimal handling of the stent itself. Despite these very effective techniques for stent mounting it is still possible to dislodge a stent from the balloon altogether (stent embolisation).

Stent embolisation   This term is used to describe the loss of the stent from the delivery system. The dislodging may occur at the guide catheter tip, when traversing the coronary artery proximal to the lesion or in the lesion itself. It can also occur in more complex stenting such as bifurcation stenting when manipulating one stent through the struts of another.

Great care should be taken when the stent exits or re-enters the guide. Manoeuvering of the guide catheter will often straighten the guide tip to allow the stent and its delivery catheter to become co-axial and permit uneventful passage in either direction.

Unnoticed proximal coronary lesions or calcification can cause the stent to be held up or displaced as it traverses the artery towards the target lesion. A different angiographic view or intravascular ultrasound (IVUS) of this section may reveal the problem and appropriate adjustment to the strategy may be made. If the hold up can be overcome by force alone – often possible if the guide is secure – there is a considerable risk of damage to that section of coronary artery and it should be inspected carefully afterwards and treated if necessary to pre-empt any occlusive dissection.

Hold up at the lesion may also cause displacement or embolisation of the stent especially if it is not securely mounted. Adequate predilation is the key. Often high pressures are required to disrupt the plaque sufficiently to allow the stent through and for the passage to be sufficiently easy that fine adjustments to the position of the stent are possible prior to deployment.

Embolisation of the stent within the coronary artery can be a lot more problematic than if it is lost in the wider circulation when in general they rarely cause problems. Nevertheless strenuous efforts at stent retrieval should be made. If the stent is lost in the coronary artery but is still on the guide wire retrieval can often be achieved with a very low profile balloon inflated enough to secure the stent which can then be withdrawn. The stent can either be secured by the balloon being inflated within it, a method that still may cause problems as the stent will not be very securely attached to the balloon, or brought to a position on the balloon catheter shaft proximal to the balloon so that when the balloon is slightly inflated the stent is secure and cannot come off the balloon catheter. If withdrawal of an embolised stent is not possible the stent may be deployed where it is. If the stent is lost from the wire a second wire and balloon may be passed alongside and the stent crushed into the side wall of the coronary artery. Other means of retrieving stents include snares which may be fashioned from long wires doubled over and introduced into a 5 or 6F catheter or specifically designed devices which are available on the market.

Recrossing stents   Recrossing stents is a potentially complicated procedure which needs to be performed with great care. It may be necessary to re-cross a deployed stent if lesions beyond require treating. When sequential lesions are being treated it may be necessary to treat the proximal lesions first in order to gain access to the distal ones. Sometimes distal lesions only become apparent after deploying the first stent such as in acutely occluded (primary angioplasty) or chronically occluded arteries. It may also be necessary to treat a dissection that occurs distal to the stent. Even if the wire is still in place across the proximal stent passage of a balloon or second stent may be held up. This particularly occurs if the stent has not been fully deployed and there is a protruding strut but even if full deployment has been achieved hold up may occur and it is especially likely to occur at a bend. The proximal LAD and proximal right coronaries are frequently at an angle of greater than 90 degrees to the tip of the guide catheter and stents in these positions pose a problem. Part of the reason is that the guide wire naturally assumes a position on the outside of the arterial bend and thus lies firmly against the stent (this is particularly the case with the stiffer wires) and it is relatively easy for the tip of a balloon catheter or the strut of a passing stent to catch. Various manipulations, however, may allow passage. The wire may be withdrawn until the more floppy section is in place within the stent or a very small inflation of the balloon catheter may provide enough of a buffer to keep the balloon/stent away from the wall of the artery.

Inadequate stent deployment Intravascular ultrasound examinations of deployed stents have revealed that often, despite excellent angiographic appearances, the stent is not fully deployed. The balloon on which the stent is mounted may have a nominal pressure of six atmospheres, in other words at six atmospheres the balloon reaches its nominal dimensions, but this pressure may not be enough to expand the entire stent adequately. The remaining protruding strut or struts may be responsible for early restenosis. In an attempt to circumvent this problem very high pressures may be used and specific high pressure non-compliant balloons have been developed for this purpose. However, high pressure inflations increase the risk of balloon rupture.

Balloon rupture

Balloon rupture may occur with or without stents and may result from rough handling of the balloon before introducing it into the guide catheter or during manual mounting of a stent. It may also result from the lesion characteristics if, for example, there is jagged calcification. It is recognised by spontaneous reduction in inflation pressure, by release of contrast in the vessel during inflation and by blood appearing in the balloon catheter when negative pressure is applied. Most commonly the rupture is a pinhole perforation but it is this that probably causes the most dangerous consequence of balloon rupture namely dissection. The very high pressures in the balloon force a tiny but powerful jet of contrast into the vessel wall causing the dissection. Sudden explosive bursting of a balloon has been known to cause vessel perforation. Other consequences of balloon rupture include air embolism and trapping of the burst balloon when it becomes enmeshed in the partially deployed stent. Balloon rupture is best avoided by careful handling of balloon and stent and by using only specifically designed balloons to attain high pressures. If it does occur it is important to monitor and treat any complications and, if a stent is involved, to return with another balloon to ensure full deployment of the stent.

Complex stent manipulations

With progressively smaller balloon and stent profiles smaller vessels can be treated and bifurcations tackled with new techniques. (See chapter X.) There are many different described techniques for bifurcations and all but the 'shotgun' approach (two stents deployed side by side in the parent and daughter vessels) run the risk of trapping or 'jailing' bits of equipment. If the side branch is wired and the parent vessel stented the wire is 'jailed' behind the stent; using 'crush' techniques the wire or even the stent balloon can be jailed and in any of the techniques stents may become stuck fast and risk embolisation. Two stent deployment systems within one guide catheter can also cause problems with wires or balloons becoming twisted or stuck in the guide, any movement of one affecting the other and thus making accurate stent deployment difficult. With any of these manoeuvers it is very important to think through the equipment before tackling the lesion. Make sure you know the dimensions of the different components and are certain that they will fit. Carefully go through the procedure before doing it to make sure that events are executed in the right order. It can be one of the most troublesome complications to have part of a delivery system, a wire or balloon, stuck deep in the coronary circulation and almost invariably surgery is required to solve the problem.

Drug-eluting stents

Drug-eluting stents (DES) designed to reduce in stent restenosis may cause complications for three reasons. Since the metallic stent is coated with polymer they are necessarily bigger with a higher profile and, therefore, able to become stuck. Lesions are more likely to require adequate predilation. If inadequately deployed they may prevent remodeling and cause aneurysm formation. High pressure inflations are recommended to ensure proper apposition of the stent to the vessel wall. Lastly they have been implicated in sub-acute and late stent thrombosis. Although initial review of the literature suggested no significant association,[7,8] more recent data on this topic is discussed in Chapter 8.

Myonecrosis

Although abrupt vessel closure may lead to acute infarction with associated ECG changes of Q waves it is quite common for there to be a measured rise in creatine kinase (CK) or Troponin without any apparent ECG abnormalities in an otherwise uncomplicated procedure. This may be as frequent as 5–30% of angioplasty procedures. It is not clear exactly why this occurs but it may result from inadvertent small side branch occlusion and it does appear to be related to total balloon inflation time. Despite mechanisms not being fully elucidated studies have clearly demonstrated that such enzyme rises are associated with increased mortality and later cardiac morbidity.[9]

Bleeding complications

Bleeding is a very important complication of angioplasty that can impact in a number of ways to cause serious morbidity or death. Hypotension stemming directly from hypovolaemia or indirectly from the vaso vagal reaction to haematoma may result in cerebral or myocardial ischaemia or induce thrombosis in the otherwise successfully treated artery. Haematomata also provide a site for infection.

Bleeding complications tend to be noticed after the procedure but blood loss may be occurring during the procedure from the catheters during equipment exchanges and during blood sampling both of which should be kept to a minimum. Care should also be taken to ensure that only one puncture of the artery is made and that haemostasis of any additional punctures is achieved before proceeding with the angioplasty.

Bleeding may occur at the arterial puncture site, at a distant accidental puncture site or spontaneously at a remote site, for example, intracerebral or gastrointestinal due to heavy anticoagulation.

Local haemorrhage Large local haemorrhage, enough to require transfusion, is not uncommon and may occur in as many as 10% of patients. The patients characteristics associated with bleeding are age, female sex, diabetes, hypertension and obesity. The procedural characteristics are those involving devices that require larger catheters such as directional atherectomy, rotational atherectomy and the use of intra aortic balloon pumping. An independent predictor of haemorrhage is the use of post procedural Heparin. The site of such bleeds is usually the arterial puncture site and can normally be controlled with manual compression. Clamping devices such as the FemoStop may be used but need to be applied carefully by experienced staff to be effective. It is important to catch haemorrhage early before a large haematoma has developed as compression can become difficult and ineffective once there is a large boggy mass. This especially applies to clamping devices. No confidence should be placed in the use of sandbags as effective compression devices. A number of closure devices are available employing either some form of collagen plug or some form of suture closure. Studies do not show a conclusive benefit in terms of reduction of complications using these devices. Whatever method you choose great care is required to execute the technique correctly to limit complications.

Retroperitoneal haemorrhage Bleeding into the retroperitoneal area may not be obvious and a high index of suspicion is required to make the diagnosis. Unexplained hypotension and hypovolaemia should be investigated aggressively and, if no cause is found, attributed to retroperitoneal haemorrhage until proved otherwise. The diagnosis can be confirmed with abdominal ultrasound or CT examination. Retroperitoneal haemorrhage is dangerous and can readily and rapidly lead to shock and, therefore, requires early treatment. Anticoagulation should be stopped and reversed if necessary with Protamine and fresh frozen plasma despite the risk of acute coronary closure in certain patients. Hypovolaemia should be promptly corrected.

Surgical intervention is rarely indicated. The widespread use of aggressive anti platelet regimens makes retroperitoneal haemorrhage more likely. A recent retrospective analysis found the incidence of retroperitoneal haemorrhage to be 0.74%.[10]

Arterial complications

Pseudoaneurysm The most common arterial complication is a femoral artery pseudoaneurysm. This has been reported to occur in up to 9% of cases but the incidence depends very much on how hard you look. The diagnosis can be made by noting the presence of a tender pulsatile femoral arterial swelling with a bruit. The diagnosis can be confirmed with colour flow Doppler examination which may pick up clinically undetectable pseudoaneurysms. Pseudoaneurysms may resolve spontaneously particularly in patients who are not anticoagulated but they may increase in size especially in anticoagulated patients. Increased painful swelling may compress the femoral nerve and may rupture and they should, therefore, be treated. Surgical repair has been largely superceded by Doppler guided compression repair which has a reported success rate of 84%.[11]

Arteriovenous fistulae Arteriovenous fistulae occur most commonly when both the artery and vein of the same side have been cannulated. This is particularly the case if the vein runs superficial to the artery. Most heal spontaneously but are also amenable to compression treatment as for pseudoaneurysm. In cases where a femoral venous cannula is required as well as an arterial one, AV fistulae are avoided if the puncture sites are made 1 cm or more apart.

Thrombosis and embolism Both thrombosis of the femoral artery and distal embolisation are relatively rare comprising 4–6% of vascular complications. They are readily recognised providing appropriate observations are made and they are readily treated with surgical intervention unless the distal embolism is small in which case a conservative approach with systemic Heparin will suffice. They are more commonly associated with cases involving the use of the intra aortic balloon pump in which case the balloon should be removed.

Infection

Infection from diagnostic cardiac catheterisation from the femoral route is extremely rare. Despite sterile equipment and a sterile technique it is almost certainly the brevity of the procedure that accounts for this. Coronary angioplasty on the other hand may involve the femoral sheath remaining *in situ* for long periods and in the presence of some local haematoma. Nevertheless significant infections secondary to angioplasty-related bacteraemia is still rare occurring in approximately 0.2% of cases. Even then the infection tends to be local causing a septic endarteritis most commonly with a S.aureus.

Unlike diagnostic catheterisation or previously practiced angioplasty current coronary intervention frequently involves leaving foreign bodies in the patient. Stenting is nearly 100% of cases in some centres and the use of arterial closure devices is common. The potential for causing systemic infection, which may be fatal[12] should not be overlooked and a scrupulous sterile technique should always be employed.

Radial artery access Many of the above complications are less likely if the radial artery is used although spontaneous bleeding including retroperitoneal haemorrhage can still occur.

REFERENCES

1. Ferguson JJ Barasch E, Wilson JM *et al.* The relation of clinical outcome to dissection and thrombus formation during coronary angioplasty. J Invas Cardiol.1995; 7:10.

2. Detre KM, Holmes DR, Holubkov R *et al.* Incidence and consequences of peri-procedural occlusion: The 19851986 NHLBI PTCA Registry: Circ. 1990; 82:739–750.

3. Almeda FQ, Nathan S, Calvin JE *et al.* Frequency of abrupt vessel closure and side branch occlusion after percutaneous coronary intervention in a 6.5-year period (1994 to 2000) at a single medical center. Am J Cardiol. 2002; 89(10):1151–5.

4. Guideline for percutaneous transluminal coronary angioplasty; a report of the ACC/AHA task force on assessment of diagnostic and therapeutic procedures. J Am Coll Cardiol 1988; 12:529.

5. Huber MS, Mooney JF, Madison J *et al.* Use of a morphological classification to predict clinical outcome after dissection from coronary angioplasty. Am J Cardiol 1991; 68:467–71.

6. Baim DS, Wahr D, George B *et al.* Randomized trial of a distal embolic protection device during percutaneous intervention of saphenous vein aorto-coronary bypass grafts. Circulation. 2002; 105(11):1285–90.

7. Bavry AA, Kumbhani DJ, Helton TJ *et al.* Risk of thrombosis with the use of sirolimus-eluting stents for percutaneous coronary intervention (from registry and clinical trial data). Am J Cardiol. 2005; 95(12):1469–72.

8. Bavry AA, Kumbhani DJ, Helton TJ *et al.* What is the risk of stent thrombosis associated with the use of paclitaxel-eluting stents for percutaneous coronary intervention?: a meta-analysis. J Am Coll Cardiol. 2005; 45(6):941–6.

9. Califf RM, Adelmeguid AE, Kuntz RE *et al.* Myonecrosis after revascularisation procedures. JACC 1998; 31:241–51.

10. Schaub F, Theiss W, Busch R *et al.* Management of 219 consecutive cases of post catheterisation pseudoaneurysm. JACC 1997; 30:670–5.

11. Farouque HM, Tremmel JA, Raissi Shabiri F *et al.* Risk factors for the development of retroperitoneal hematoma after percutaneous coronary intervention in the era of glycoprotein IIb/IIIa inhibitors and vascular closure devices. JACC 2005; 45:363–8.

12. Alfonso F; Moreno R; Vergas J. Fatal infection after rapamycin eluting coronary stent implantation. Heart. 2005; 91(6):e51.

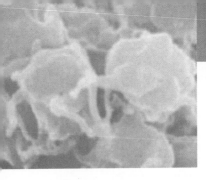

13

Restenosis and in-stent restenosis

NEZAR M. FALLUJI, MD, MPH,

DAVID J. MOLITERNO, MD

KEY POINTS

- Percutaneous coronary intervention (PCI) has become the dominant revascularization modality for obstructive coronary artery disease while restenosis is the 'Achilles heel' of balloon angioplasty.

- Restenosis occurs at a rate of 40–50% angiographically and 20–30% clinically following balloon angioplasty.

- The use of bare metal stents (BMS) reduced the incidence of acute vessel closure and restenosis substantially.

- A new form of restenosis, namely in-stent restenosis (ISR) following BMS implantation, is responsible for a large proportion of repeat PCI procedures.

- The use of drug-eluting stents (DES) has lowered the incidence of ISR further, with clinical restenosis rates less than 10% in contemporary practice.

PATHOPHYSIOLOGY

Vascular injury during coronary intervention, leads to a complex reparative process that may become excessive and cause restenosis. Renarrowing after PCI develops over weeks to months post-procedure, in contrast to de novo coronary lesions, which develop over years, likely reflecting the difference in the underlying mechanisms and the extent of inflammation involved with each lesion type. The process of restenosis can be broadly categorized into four interrelated facets:

1. Vascular elastic recoil occurs within minutes to hours following balloon angioplasty. The underlying mechanism is related to a 'spring-like' rebound of the arterial segment, or it may simply reflect the persistence of a temporarily displaced atherosclerotic plaque. Elastic recoil is reduced with atherectomy and eliminated with stent placement.
2. Thrombus formation, before or after angioplasty, contributes to restenosis by lumen occupation. Furthermore, activated platelets within the thrombus secrete a host of substances from their alpha-granules (Fig. 13.1), which promote vasoconstriction, chemotaxis, mitogenesis, and activation of neighboring platelets, mediating the growth of fibromuscular tissue (neointima). Use of proper antiplatelet agents and anticoagulation therapy during PCI should limit this mechanism of restenosis, though no supportive data exist to establish a role for anti-thrombotics to reduce restenosis.
3. Neointimal hyperplasia predominates the luminal narrowing beyond the acute phase after PCI and is the major underlying mechanism of restenosis following coronary stent placement. Following PCI-mediated vascular injury a reparative process is orchestrated by coagulation and inflammatory factors

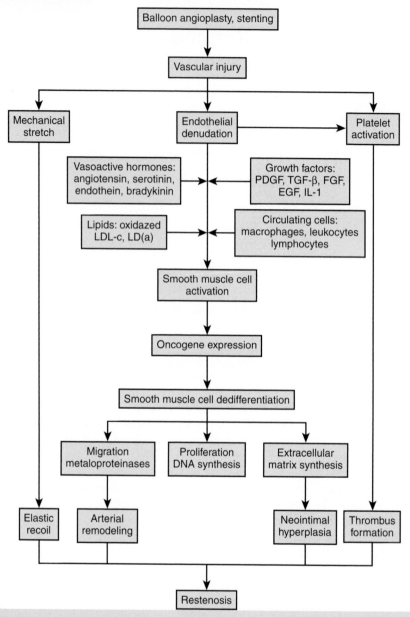

Figure 13.1:
Mechanisms of restenosis following PCI. Source: Chan AW and Moliterno DJ, Clinical Evaluation of Restenosis. In Atherothrombosis and Coronary Artery Disease, edited by V. Fuster, EJ Topol, and EG Nabel, p. 1416 (Figure 93.2).

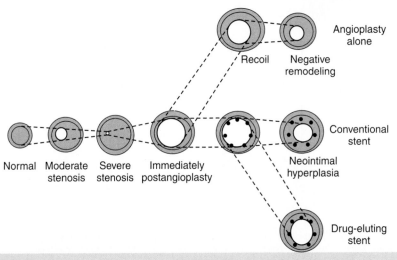

Figure 13.2:
Vascular remodeling following PCI. Source: Chan AW and Moliterno DJ, Clinical Evaluation of Restenosis. In Atherothrombosis and Coronary Artery Disease, edited by V. Fuster, EJ Topol, and EG Nabel, p. 1417 (Figure 93.3).

and cells, which results in smooth muscle cell proliferation and extracelluar matrix formation.

4. Arterial remodeling during the reparative process can result in an increase, decrease, or no change in the cross-sectional area of the artery lumen. This so-called Glagov phenomenon (Fig. 13.2)[1], combined with neointimal hyperplasia, represents the final wave of the restenotic process. The restenotic process is usually complete within 3–6 months after balloon angioplasty and atherectomy, but can extend up to 6–12 months following stent placement. As such, the time course for restenosis after stents is delayed, relative to that for balloon angioplasty, by 1–3 months. Hence, patients who are free of restenosis at nine months after coronary stent placement are likely to have long-term patency within the index lesion. DES contain a polymeric coating that allows sustained (several weeks) release of anti-inflammatory and antiproliferative drugs, which inhibit neointimal growth.

While elastic recoil and thrombus formation can lead to acute vessel closure and acute restenosis, the concept of restenosis primarily refers to neointimal hyperplasia and vascular remodeling over months, which result from an inflammatory reparative processes following PCI-induced vascular injury.

DEFINITIONS OF RESTENOSIS

Angiographic restenosis
Various definitions for angiographic restenosis have been used. 50% or greater dichotomous diameter stenosis at follow-up angiography is a widely used criterion in clinical trials. However, reporting of the minimum luminal diameter (MLD) may avoid variation of restenosis rates reported in clinical trials due to

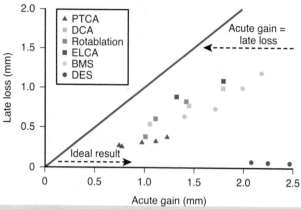

Figure 13.3:
Late Loss Index for various PCI devices. The loss index for DES is compared to that of other PCI devices. DES has an almost ideal profile that would produce a large immediate gain and have a low loss index. Balloon angioplasty has the lowest loss index but produces a relatively smaller immediate gain. Atherectomy produces a large immediate gain but has the highest loss index. BMS = bare metal stents, DCA = directional coronary atherectomy, DES = drug-eluting stents, ELCA = excimer laser coronary angioplasty, PTCA = percutaneous transluminal coronary angioplasty. Source: updated with permission Moliterno DJ and Topol EJ, Restenosis: Epidemiology and Treatment. In Textbook of Cardiovascular Medicine, 2d ed., edited by EJ Topol, p. 1719 (Figure 83.5).

inconsistent definitions of angiographic restenosis. The difference between pre-procedural MLD and immediate post-procedural MLD is defined as *acute gain*, and the difference between post-procedural MLD and MLD at follow-up is termed to *late loss*. Acute gain is lowest with PTCA, followed by atherectomy, and stenting (highest acute gain). Late loss is usually proportional to acute gain, such that the *late loss index*, defined as late loss divided by the acute gain, is similar after revascularization with PTCA, atherectomy, or stents (Fig. 13.3).

While visual methods of assessing angiographic stenosis severity are prone to interobserver and intraobserver variability, the use of quantitative coronary angiography (QCA) is highly reproducible, and is the standard technique employed in most contemporary research trials. QCA is usually unreliable for assessing bifurcation lesions and in the absence of disease-free reference segments.

Clinical restenosis

Since angiographic definitions for restenosis are somewhat arbitrary, the importance of restenosis becomes clinically relevant only when it is linked to symptom(s) or functional parameter(s). Because the process of restenosis is usually gradual, and the newly formed lesion is 'stabilized' with fibrous tissue and smooth muscle cells, recurrent angina is the most common presenting feature, whereas myocardial infarction (MI) and sudden death are less frequent. Chest pain is reportedly present in 25–93% of patients six months following balloon angioplasty, with an average of approximately 50%.[2] The proportion of patients presenting with recurrent chest pain who have restenosis demonstrable at angiography ranges from 48–92%. Hence, the positive predictive value (PPV) of symptoms alone is only modest.

Clinical restenosis is roughly correlated with the need for repeat revascularization (repeat PCI or bypass surgery). Traditionally, target lesion revascularization (TLR) has been used in many of the interventional trials designed to test various pharmacology, while target vessel revascularization (TVR) has been used in device trials in which the effect of the device on the vessel beyond the target lesions also needs to be considered. More recently, the term target vessel failure (TVF) has also become popular, and it refers to TVR plus death or myocardial infarction due to restenosis or reocclusion of the target vessel.

PREDICTORS FOR RESTENOSIS

Many identifiable restenosis predictors were derived from large pharmacological trials related to PCI. Predictors for restenosis after balloon angioplasty, stenting, and brachytherapy modestly differ. Risk factors can be categorized into those related to the patient, the lesion, and the procedure, as summarized in Table 13.1.

PRESENTATION AND EVALUATION OF RESTENOSIS

Regardless of the PCI device used, most patients who have clinical restenosis experience return of angina. As mentioned, myocardial infarction or death due to restenosis per se is unusual.[3] Atypical chest pain or pain different from the patient's angina is unlikely to be secondary to restenosis. Similarly, early angina (that is, within the first couple months after PCI) is usually related to incomplete revascularization, whereas angina presenting much beyond nine months is usually due to lesions other than the index lesion.[3] The incidence of silent restenosis is variable since the definition of angiographic restenosis is somewhat arbitrary. Absence of any symptom may be related to less severe coronary obstruction, diabetes, non-viable myocardium, or abundant collateralization. The importance of silent restenosis in clinical practice remains questionable, as the available data are limited and inconsistent.

Recurrent angina within nine months of PCI is an ACC/AHA Class I indication for repeat coronary angiography.[4] In asymptomatic patients or those with atypical symptoms following PCI, use of non-invasive tests is the recommended evaluation method. A stress test (exercise or pharmacological) with nuclear scintigraphy or echocardiography carries relatively less risk, cost, and time (compared with routine coronary angiography), and it provides physiologic assessment of the restenotic lesion.[5] When stress testing is believed to be unreliable and the myocardium at risk is large, angiography is preferable.

PREVENTION OF RESTENOSIS

Historically, and mostly prior to the development of DES, many classes of drugs were tested to prevent restenosis following PTCA, including antiplatelets, anticoagulants, calcium channel blockers, statins, corticosteriods, thromboxane antagonists, and prostacycline analogues. While animal studies were promising, these various classes of drugs failed to show a positive effect in clinical studies. Growth factor inhibitors (such as trapidil, angiopeptin and cilostazol) may be the exception as they have shown encouraging results that may warrant further investigation.

TABLE 13.1 - PREDICTORS FOR RESTENOSIS

CLINICAL FACTORS:	Balloon Angioplasty φ	Bare Metal Stents	Brachytherapy	Drug-eluting stents
ACD-D genotype	x	x		
Acute coronary syndrome	x	x		
Age	x			
Arterial hypertension		x		
Diabetes mellitus	x	x	x	x
Elevated high-sensitivity C-reactive protein (hsCRP)	x	x		
End-stage renal disease	x			
Glycoprotein PlA polymorphism		x		
History of restenosis	x	x	x	x
Hypercholesterolemia	x			
Male sex	x			
Multi-site angioplasty	x			
Prior myocardial infarction	x			
Tobacco use		x		
Variant angina	x			
LESION MORPHOLOGY:				
Angulated lesion (>45 degrees)	x			
Bifurcation lesion	x			
Calcification	x			
Chronic total occlusion	x	x	x	x
Collateral vessels	x			
Early restenosis (<3 months)	x			
Left anterior descending	x	x		
Long lesion	x	x	x	x
Ostial location	x			
Proximal location	x			
Saphenous vein grafts	x	x	x	x
Severe pre-procedural stenosis or small minimal luminal diameter	x	x	x	
Small vessel diameter	x	x	x	x
Thrombus	x			
PROCEDURAL CHARACTERISTICS:				
Abrupt closure (coronary flow velocity reserve <2.0–2.5 or fractional flow reserve <0.9)	x			
Dissection	x			
Duration of balloon inflation	x			
Final cross-sectional area by intra-vascular ultrasound		x		
Final minimal lumen diameter	x	x	x	
Geographic miss			x	
Re-stenting			x	
Stent design		x		
Stent length		x		
Stent material (gold-coated)		x		

φIncludes non-stented cases that have undergone atherectomy or eximer laser angioplasty.

Source: Chan AW and Moliterno DJ, Clinical Evaluation of Restenosis. In Atherothrombosis and Coronary Artery Disease, edited by V. Fuster, EJ Topol, and EG Nabel, p. 1416

While pharmacological agents failed to reduce restenosis following PTCA, the use of coronary BMS resulted in significant reductions in both acute vessel closure and restenosis (when compared to PTCA), and the use of DES has further reduced the incidence of angiographic and clinical restenosis to less than 10%.

TREATMENT OF RESTENOSIS

For patients who develop restenosis, repeat revascularization is most often the best treatment for symptom relief. Intracoronary stent placement is the appropriate strategy for lesions not previously treated with stents, provided the anatomy is suitable. Most patients with single-vessel restenosis undergo a second PCI, whereas patients with restenosis in multiple vessels may undergo percutaneous or surgical revascularization. This is influenced by several factors including left ventricular function, history of primary CABG, and diabetes.

PTCA

Balloon angioplasty as a treatment for restenosis is associated with a particularly high rate (40–50%) of recurrent restenosis. In a multicenter randomized restenosis stent study, 383 patients with clinical and angiographic restenosis following prior balloon angioplasty were randomized to repeat PTCA versus Palmaz-Schatz stent placement. In this study of non-complete lesions, repeat PTCA was associated with a 32% rate of angiographic restenosis at six months.[6] With ISR, repeat PTCA is effective when used for management of focal lesions with angiographic restenosis rates as low as 20% at six month.[7-8] For more diffuse restenotic lesions, however, repeat PTCA is associated with a six-month angiographic restenosis rate >50%.[9]

Atherectomy

Several small case series documented the safety of rotational atherectomy to treat restenosis. In a non-randomized registry of 304 patients, the combined use of atherectomy and balloon angioplasty was associated with a reduced rate of one-year clinical events (death, MI, TLR) when compared with balloon angioplasty or atherectomy alone (38% vs. 52% vs. 60%, respectively).[11] However, in the multicenter ARTIST trial, 298 patients with ISR were randomly assigned to PTCA or rotational atherectomy; atherectomy was associated with a higher rate of angiographic restenosis (65% vs. 51%) and incidence of composite clinical events (death, MI, TLR) (20% vs. 9%), primarily due to a greater rate of repeat revascularization at six months.[12] Similarly, the use of excimer laser and rotational atherectomy in treating in-stent restenotic lesions has been disappointing (one-year TLR rates of 26% and 28%, respectively). These debulking devices cause a greater late lumen loss, so-called device taxing, implying that remodeling or neointimal proliferation are not favorably reduced.[13]

Stenting

Bare metal stents By reducing elastic recoil and vascular remodeling, and by compressing the plaque and scaffolding the vessel lumen, BMS has resulted in a significant reduction in acute vessel closure and restenosis. ISR secondary to neointimal hyperplasia remains a significant problem with BMS, however, with 20–30% angiographic and 10–15% clinical restenosis.[14,15]

Drug-eluting stents Sirolimus (rapamune) is a macrocyclic lactone with antibiotic, immunosuppressive, and anti-proliferative actions. Biologically it induces cell-cycle arrest and affects proliferation and migration of smooth muscle cells. In the RAVEL trial, which was the first randomized controlled trial of sirolimus-eluting stents (SES) versus BMS, SES reduced ISR at six months by more than 50% when compared to BMS (0 vs. 27%)[16], and at one-year follow up, the overall rate of cardiac events (mostly TVR) was lower with SES (6% vs. 29%).

Paclitaxel interferes with function of the microtubules responsible for proper chromosome segregation during cell division. In the TAXUS II trial, 536 low-risk patients were randomly assigned to a BMS or a paclitaxel-eluting stent (PES).[17] At six months, PES were associated with significant reductions in ISR (3.5% vs. 19.1%) and TLR (3.9% vs. 13.3%). In a meta-analysis of all randomized clinical trials of sirolimus-versus paclitaxel-eluting stents the rate of angiographic restenosis in patients with SES was 9.3% and the rate of TLR was 5.1%. The rate of angiographic restenosis in patients with PES was 13.1% and the rate of TLR was 7.8%.[18]

TREATMENT OF ISR

The conventional, mechanical treatments of ISR (PTCA, cutting balloons, repeat stenting with a BMS, or atherectomy) have been disappointing, with recurrent rates of restenosis averaging 30–50% for focal disease and 50–70% for diffuse disease. The mainstay of treatment for ISR recently involved balloon angioplasty with intracoronary brachytherapy. More recently, the use of DES for ISR has emerged.

Brachytherapy

Gamma and beta radiotherapy have been studied for treatment of ISR. During spontaneous decay of nuclei of certain elements, radiation is emitted in the form of either gamma radiation (electromagnetic energy carried by photons which may penetrate more than 10 mm of human tissue) or beta particles (electrons carrying a wide range of energy and traveling within 2–3 mm of human tissue). By affecting DNA in the actively dividing cells, brachytherapy inhibits smooth muscle proliferation and neointima formation. Use of brachytherapy in management of restenosis and ISR has been evaluated in multiple clinical trials and registries, with both gamma (SCRIPPS, GAMMA-1, WRIST, SVG WRIST, and LONG WRIST) and beta (BETA WRIST, START, and INHIBIT) radiation. The effect of brachytherapy is not always consistent or curative. While infrequent, both thrombosis (perhaps due to inadequate re-endothelialization) and restenosis (possibly from paradoxical neointimal stimulation of an adjacent vessel segment) have been reported following brachytherapy. Overall, brachytherapy has reduced the rate of recurrent restenosis by about 40–50%. Figure 13.4 summarizes the results of the noted effects of beta and gamma radiation on TLR.

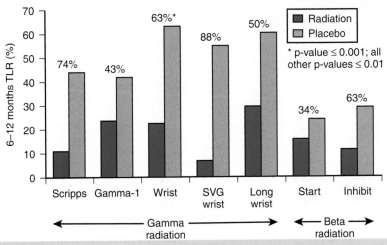

Figure 13.4:
Brachytherapy. Cumulative incidence of target lesion revascularization required after intracoronary radiotherapy using gamma-radiation and beta-radiation. Percentages indicate percent reduction with therapy; all differences were statistically significant. Source: Chan AW and Moliterno DJ, In-Stent Restenosis: Update on Intracoronary Radiotherapy, Cleveland Clinic Journal of Medicine 2001: 68; 796–803.

DES for ISR

Use of DES in the management of ISR was evaluated in small observational studies that suggested benefit. These were soon followed by the ISAR-DESIRE trial, which randomized 300 patients with ISR to treatment with SES, PES or PTCA.[19] DES resulted in a significant reduction (≥50%) in the primary end point of angiographic restenosis at six months (14.3% SES, 21.7% PES, and 44.6% PTCA). TVR rate was reduced significantly as well (8% SES, 19% PES, and 33% PTCA).

When restenosis occurs with DES, it may often be a consequence of local vessel injury during the procedure, polymer peeling, non-homogeneous drug elution, gaps in stent coverage, or inadequate stent expansion. In addition to suboptimal stent placement technique, Table 13.2 lists the variables that have been associated with ISR in sirolimus-eluting stents.[20]

CABG for ISR

Limited data exist regarding the use of CABG in the treatment of ISR. In a retrospective analysis of 510 patients with documented first occurrence of ISR, patients who were managed with CABG (n = 117) had a reduced rate of TVR (8%) and major adverse cardiovascular events (23%) at a mean follow up of 19 months, when compared to PCI.[21] This study, however, was done before the widespread use of DES. Further investigations are needed to compare the use of CABG versus multivessel PCI with DES in the management of ISR.

TABLE 13.2 - TVR PREDICTORS AMONG 1,726 PATIENTS FROM THE GERMAN CYPHER REGISTRY

VARIABLES	ADJUSTED OR (95% CI)	P-VALUE
Target vessel coronary bypass graft	2.43 (1.41–4.18)	0.001
2- or 3-vessel disease	1.69 (1.05–2.72)	0.030
Hypertension	1.66 (0.99–2.79)	0.056
Additional implantation of BMS	1.49 (0.71–3.13)	0.230
Renal insufficiency	1.41 (0.80–2.48)	0.230
Indication of in-stent restenosis	1.40 (0.94–2.07)	0.095
Chronic total occlusion	1.39 (0.73–2.68)	0.320
Ostial lesion	1.28 (0.79–2.07)	0.320
Diabetes mellitus	1.14 (0.76–1.71)	0.530
Total length of SES (per 10 mm)	1.07 (0.90–1.26)	0.450

Source: Zahn R, et al. American Journal of Cardiology 2005; 95:1302-8.

REFERENCES

1. Glagov S, Weisenberg E, Zarins CK, et al. Compensatory enlargement of the human atherosclerotic coronary arteries. NEJM 1987; 316:1371–5.

2. Simonton CA, Mark DB, Hinohara T, et al. Late restenosis after emergent coronary angioplasty for acute myocardial infarction: comparison with elective coronary angioplasty. J AM Coll Cardiol. 1988; 11:698–705.

3. Holmes DR, Vlietstra RE, Smith HC, et al. Restenosis after percutaneous transluminal coronary angioplasty: a report from the PTCA registry of the national Heart, Lung and Blood institute. Am J Cardiol. 1984; 53:77c–81c.

4. Ryan TJ, Antman EM, Brooks NH, et al. 1999 Update: ACC/AHA guidelines for the management of patients with acute myocardial infarction: executive summary and recommendations. Circulation 1999; 100:1016–30.

5. Takeuchi M, Miura Y, Toyokawa T, et al. The comparative diagnostic value of dobutamine stress echocardiography and thallium stress tomography for detecting restenosis after coronary angioplasty. J Am Soc Echocardiography 1995; 8:696–702.

6. Erbel R, Haude M, Hopp HW, et al. Coronary-artery stenting compared with balloon angioplasty for restenosis after initial balloon angioplasty. Restenosis Stent Study Group. N Engl J Med. 1998 Dec 3; 339(23):1672–8.

7. Bauters C, Banos JL, Van Belle E, et al. Six-month angiographic outcome after successful repeat percutaneous intervention for in-stent restenosis. Circulation 1998; 97:318–21.

8. Reimers B, Moussa I, Akiyama T, et al. Long term clinical follow up after successful repeat percutaneous intervention for stent restenosis. J Am Coll Cardiol 1997; 30:186–92.

9. Eltchaninoff H, Koning R, Tron C, et al. Balloon angioplasty for the treatment of coronary in-stent restenosis: Immediate results and 6-month angiographic recurrent restenosis rate. J Am Coll Cardiol 1998; 32:980–4.

10. Morice MC, Serruys PW, Sousa JE, et al. A randomized comparison of a sirolimus-eluting stent with a standard stent for coronary revascularization. N Engl J Med 2002 Jun 6; 346(23):1773–80.

11. Goldberg SL, Berger P, Cohen DJ, *et al*. Rotational atherectomy or balloon angioplasty in the treatment of intra-stent restenosis: BARASTER multicenter registry. Cathet Cardiovasc Intervent 2000; 51:407–13.

12. Vom Dahl J, Dietz V, Silber S, *et al*. Rotational atherectomy does no reduce recurrent in-stent restenosis: results of the angioplasty versus rotational atherectomy for the treatment of diffuse in-stent restenosis trail (ARTIST). Circulation 2002; 105:583–8.

13. Mehran R, Dangas G, Mintz G, *et al*. Treatment of in-stent restenosis with excimer laser coronary angioplasty versus rotational atherectomy: Comparative mechanisms and results. Circulation 2000; 101:2484–9.

14. Fischman DL, Leon MB, Baim DS, *et al*. A randomized comparison of coronary-stent placement and balloon angioplasty in the treatment of coronary artery disease. Stent Restenosis Study Investigators. N Engl J Med 1994 Aug 25; 331(8):496–501.

15. Serruys PW, de Jaegere P, Kiemeneij F, *et al*. A comparison of balloon-expandable-stent implantation with balloon angioplasty in patients with coronary artery disease. Benestent Study Group. N Engl J Med 1994 Aug 25; 331(8):489–95.

16. Serruys PW, Degertekin M, Tanabe K, *et al*. Intravascular ultrasound findings in the multicenter, randomized, double-blind RAVEL (RAndomized study with the sirolimus-eluting VElocity balloon-expandable stent in the treatment of patients with de novo native coronary artery Lesions) trial. Circulation 2002 Aug 13; 106(7):798–803.

17. Colombo A, Drzewiecki J, Banning A, *et al*. Randomized study to assess the effectiveness of slow- and moderate-release polymer-based paclitaxel-eluting stents for coronary artery lesions. Circulation 2003 Aug 19; 108(7):788–94.

18. Kastrati A, Dibra A, Dipl Stat S, *et al*. Sirolimus-eluting stents vs. Paclitaxel-eluting stents in patients with coronary artery disease. A meta-analysis of randomized trials. JAMA 2005 Aug17; 294(7):819–25.

19. Kastrati A, Mehilli J, von Beckerath N, *et al*. Sirolimus-eluting stent or paclitaxel-eluting stent vs balloon angioplasty for prevention of recurrences in patients with coronary in-stent restenosis: a randomized controlled trial. JAMA 2005 Jan 12; 293(2):165–71.

20. Zahn R, Hamm CW, Scheinder S, Incidence and predictors of target vessel revascularization and clinical event rates of the sirolimus-eluting coronary stent (results from the prospective multicenter German Cypher Stent Registry). Am J of Cardiology 2005 Jun 1; 95(11):1302–8.

21. Moustapha A, Assali AR, Sdringola S, *et al*. Percutaneous and surgical interventions for in-stent restenosis: long-term outcomes and effect of diabetes mellitus. J Am Coll Cardiol 2001 Jun 1; 37(7):1877–82.

Section Two

Adjunctive Technology in Percutaneous Coronary Intervention

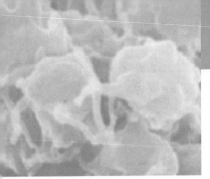

14

Rotational and directional atherectomy

MARK DE BELDER AND BABU KUNADIAN

KEY POINTS

- Coronary atherectomy and atheroma ablation devices were introduced to overcome the acute failings of balloon angioplasty and in an attempt to reduce restenosis.

- Directional coronary atherectomy was introduced before stenting emerged as the dominant technique of PCI.

- In general, stenting is easier and is associated with results as good as or better than those seen with DCA, even when performed optimally.

- DCA is associated with a higher incidence of peri-procedural CK release.

- There are a number of lesion subsets associated with less than ideal results with stenting (even with DES); directional atherectomy using new catheter designs may still have a role in some of these.

- Rotablation is difficult, but is an excellent technique for dealing with resistant fibrotic or calcific tissue.

- Rotablation is the only technique that enables good results in concentric 'napkin-ring' calcification.

INTRODUCTION

The major limitations of balloon angioplasty involved acute problems (failure to achieve a satisfactory dilatation of a lesion as well as acute complications, including dissection of the vessel) and short- to medium-term restenosis. Failure to achieve a reasonable dilatation occurred in very fibrotic and calcified lesions, and in other vessels related to the bulk of focal disease and elastic recoil of the vessel. Certain anatomic situations were also difficult to treat, including aorto-ostial lesions and bifurcations. With the latter, plaque shift from one arm of the bifurcation to another could only partially be overcome using kissing balloon techniques. Dissections occurred particularly in calcified lesions, eccentric bulky lesions, lesions on bends or in tortuous segments of the vessel and in patients with very diffuse disease.

Although stenting has become the default method of PCI, the understanding in the early and mid-1980s of the components of acute failure and restenosis led to two major lines of development – atherectomy and ablative methods as well as methods of scaffolding the vessel. The new technologies that emerged included the directional atherectomy device and two methods of ablation, namely laser techniques and rotablation. Although some of the scenarios when these devices were used can now be treated with stents, certain clinical and anatomic scenarios exist where the use of ablative methods are essential to allow optimal delivery and expansion of stents and in some cases they may be the only means of achieving percutaneous dilatation of a lesion. One of the worst clinical situations to occur in the current era favouring direct stenting is the delivery of a stent to a previously unrecognised undilatable lesion. Only experience, recognition of a number of clinical clues that this situation might be met, and the ability to use ablative technologies can prevent this. This chapter will review the use of atherectomy devices and coronary rotablation.

DIRECTIONAL ATHERECTOMY

This is now largely a historical review, as directional coronary atherectomy (DCA) is now used very infrequently. Many of the devices previously available are no longer manufactured but Guidant (Guidant, Santa Rosa, CA) continues to manufacture the Flexi-Cut™ device and the FoxHollow SilverHawk™ device (FoxHollow Technologies, Redwood City, CA, USA) is also available.

Directional coronary atherectomy was developed by John Simpson to enable debulking of lesions. It was argued that excision of atheromatous material would overcome many of the limitations of balloon dilatation alone, allowing for better dilatation of the lesion with less dependence on stretch (and thus barotrauma), more controlled dilatation (and thus fewer dissections), and that there would, as a result, be better acute clinical results with less restenosis. The initial registries appeared favourable, but the results of several randomised trials were disappointing. The major studies of DCA are listed in Table 14.1. In particular, the use of DCA resulted in a relatively high peri-procedural release of cardiac enzymes, and clinical results were either only marginally better or in some cases appeared worse.[13-15] There are several reasons why early registry experience is not always translated into clinical benefit in a multi-centre randomised trial. These include the performance of a trial before the technique has been adequately developed, designing a trial that partially reflects the learning curve of operators with only limited experience of the technique and, perhaps most importantly, the fact that early registry experience is obtained in carefully selected patients by operators who have the greatest experience of the technique. Moreover, the original concepts of why DCA might be favourable might have been countered by the stimulus to restenosis caused by cutting into the plaque.

Although the CAVEAT and CCAT trials did not establish a clear benefit from DCA, possibly because of inadequate debulking and a higher complication rate compared to balloon angioplasty alone, the OARS, BOAT, ABACAS and GUIDE II studies suggested that optimal debulking, with attempts to reduce residual plaque volume to a minimum (aided if necessary by IVUS guidance), would result in lower restenosis rates. A residual angiographic percent diameter stenosis after DCA (with or without adjunctive balloon angioplasty) of <10–15% was aimed for. However, the higher CK release during procedures remains an issue and given that DCA is more technically demanding, the emergence of stenting as an easier-to-use technique with equal or better results has resulted in a major reduction in the number of DCA procedures being performed worldwide. However, when only BMS were available, the Japanese START study suggested that DCA could still be considered as an alternative to stenting as it achieved a lower rate of restenosis with no differences in clinical events.[8]

Several generations of devices were produced by Devices for Vascular Intervention (acquired initially by Guidant Ltd and subsequently by FoxHollow). Following the original AtheroCath®, sequential improvements were seen in the

TABLE 14.1 - MAJOR STUDIES OF THE ROLE OF DCA

STUDY	TITLE	REF
CAVEAT	Coronary Angioplasty Versus Excisional Atherectomy Trial	1
CCAT	Canadian Coronary Atherectomy Trial	2
CAVEAT-II	As CAVEAT, but for saphenous vein graft lesions	3
OARS	Optimal Atherectomy Restenosis Study	4
BOAT	Balloon vs. Optimal Atherectomy Trial	5
ABACAS	Adjunctive Balloon Angioplasty following Coronary Atherectomy Study	6
GUIDE II	Guidance by Ultrasound Imaging for Decision Endpoints	7
START	STent versus directional coronary Atherectomy Randomized Trial	8
SOLD	Stenting after Optimal Lesion Debulking Study	9
Bramucci Registry	DCA before stenting	10
AtheroLink Registry	DCA before stenting	11
AMIGO	Atherectomy before Multilink Improves luminal Gain and clinical Outcomes	12

SCA-1™, SCA-EX™, Short-Cutter™, the GTO®, the Bantam™ and the Flexi-Cut™ devices, with improved debulking capability and use even in partially calcified lesions. The original devices needing 10F sheaths and guide catheters gave way to 8F-compatible devices. Currently, only the Flexi-Cut™ device is available (Fig. 14.1). The technique requires stiffer than average guide catheters such as the Viking XT™ range (Guidant) with stiff wires such as the Iron Man™ (Guidant).

The device is inserted into the vessel, rotated until the cutting window is lined up with the side of the vessel containing the bulk of the lesion, the cutter is then drawn back and the balloon on the side of the device opposite to the window is then inflated at low pressure. The balloon stabilises the device and pushes the

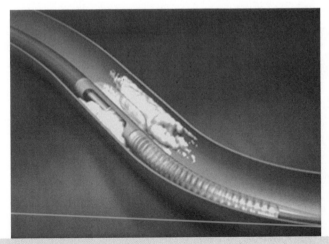

Figure 14.1:
Directional atherectomy.

cutting window against the plaque. The device is then activated and the rotating cup-shaped cutter is advanced, slicing off the atheroma and pushing it forward into the collection nosecone. The balloon is then deflated, the device rotated slightly and further excisions made until adequate atherectomy has been performed. Different sized catheters are available for different vessels and lesions. In smaller vessels, the development of ischaemia during the procedure sometimes requires withdrawal of the device back into the guiding catheter between cuts. This is less of a problem with the Flexi-Cut™ device.

More recently, the FoxHollow SilverHawk™ Plaque Excision System has been introduced (Fig. 14.2), which has the advantage of being 6 F compatible and it does not have a contra-lateral balloon opposite the cutting window but instead a unique hinge design.[16] This potentially reduces barotrauma. Three tip lengths are available with different collection chambers, allowing for a number of clinical scenarios in coronary cases, and the device can be used in vessels ranging from 1.5 to 3.5 mm in diameter. Catheters designed for peripheral vascular cases are also available. The carbide blade allows for excision of calcified plaque. Like the earlier DCA devices, the shaved plaque is stored in the nosecone of the device, allowing its retrieval. These atherectomy devices are the only available tools that allow for retrieval of human atheromatous tissue for research purposes. Another device is the Arrow-Fischell Pullback Atherectomy Device (Arrow Medical Devices Co, Reading, Pennsylvania, US).[17,18]

Debulking with atherectomy, especially when aggressive, has been associated with a higher rate of vessel perforation (0.5–1.3%) than with ballooning alone, and there is also a small risk of aneurysmal formation during follow up, although this has not been associated with adverse clinical events. Whether this could be a problem if DCA were used before implantation of a DES (some of which are associated with negative vessel remodelling during follow up) is not known. Groin complications were slightly higher when using larger guide catheters.

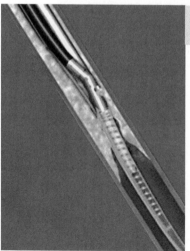

Figure 14.2:
The FoxHollow SilverHawk™ device.

Although stenting has emerged as the dominant method of PCI, there are still some anatomical situations where stenting is technically difficult or may not achieve optimal results, and stenting itself has produced the problem of how to deal with in-stent restenosis. The latter is due entirely to neointimal proliferation within the stent, but inadequate stent expansion (which thereby reduces the size of the lumen that can accommodate the proliferative tissue) has been recognised to be one of the major determinants of sub-optimal clinical results. DCA enthusiasts have, therefore, continued to use this technique in difficult anatomy, and have also explored the role of debulking prior to stent implantation. Again, early registry evidence was favourable but the randomised multi-centre AMIGO trial could find no benefit from this technique, although benefit was seen in the subset of patients where aggressive debulking (<20% residual stenosis) was achieved prior to stenting. Although certain groups have suggested that the benefits only emerge with aggressive debulking prior to stent implantation, this has become a somewhat academic exercise with the emergence of DES.

The lesions for which some operators continue to use DCA rather than stenting include eccentric lesions, ostial stenoses, bifurcations, in-stent restenoses, and some continue to use the technique of aggressive debulking prior to stenting (especially for left main stem lesions). Its use in these lesions has been reviewed recently.[19] Although the use of DES has seen a major reduction in the use of DCA, these lesions remain difficult to treat and results with DES are less favourable than with more straightforward lesions.

ROTATIONAL ATHERECTOMY (ROTABLATION)

Rotablation is probably a more appropriate name for this technique as it results in virtual emulsification of the atheromatous plaque rather than being a method of excising atheroma. It utilises a high-speed rotating elliptically shaped burr, the front face of which is coated with 2000 to 3000 diamond microchips (30–50 μm in diameter). As the burr meets the plaque, the latter is fragmented into particles 5–10 μm in diameter (smaller than red cells) which are washed downstream, pass through the coronary capillary bed and then enter the venous circulation and are removed from the circulation by the reticulo-endothelial system (Fig. 14.3).

There are two major principles of action of this device. The first is through orthogonal displacement of friction, whereby high-speed rotation (at speeds of 140 000 to 150 000 rpm) reduces the longitudinal friction between the burr and the guide wire and eases passage down the vessel. The second is referred to as 'differential cutting' with elastic or soft tissue deflecting away from the burr whereas inelastic tissue cannot deflect and is therefore ablated. The technique minimises wall stretch and thus barotrauma and it was hoped that this would result in a lower restenosis rate. However, this has not been found in clinical practice and the deleterious effects of the heat it generates probably counter any advantage the rotablator might have in this regard. Although rotablation is not, then, a means of reducing restenosis, it allows for successful treatment of lesions that cannot be adequately treated by balloon angioplasty. It is not a technique for removal or fragmentation of soft thrombus.

Since its introduction, the technique has changed somewhat. Modifications include the use of a verapamil/nitrate flush solution used down the guide catheter

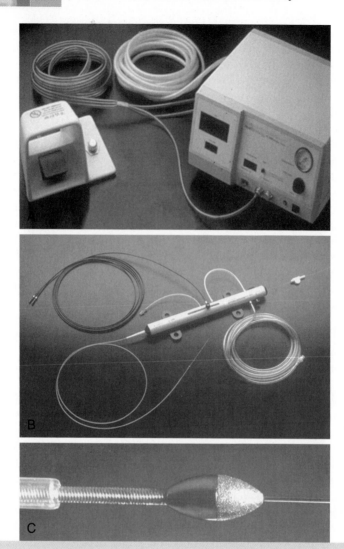

Figure 14.3:
The Rotablator: A The Rotablator console and foot-pedal B The Rotablator device – burr catheter and advancer C The Rotablator burr.

whilst rotablation is performed, a Rotaglide™ lubricant that reduces friction and disperses heat, shorter runs with only gentle advancement into the plaque using a pecking technique that allows for as much coronary perfusion during each run, lower burr speeds, avoidance of drops in speed of >5000 rpm, and up-front use of a glycoprotein IIb/IIIa inhibitor.[20,21] Many operators do not use the latter though until after rotablation in particularly difficult, angulated and heavily calcified vessels because of the small risk of perforation of the vessel, but instead consider its use during the remainder of the procedure once the rotablation is completed. For lesions in dominant right or circumflex coronary arteries, significant bradycardia or heart block can occur. The patients should be well hydrated, atropine pre-treatment should be considered and in some cases it is wise to insert a pacing electrode. Right ventricular pacing electrodes (especially if a glycoprotein IIb/IIIa inhibitor is used) can result in cardiac tamponade if an apical electrode perforates the ventricle, and it is probably wiser to select either a septal position for the pacing electrode or use a flotation pacing catheter.

The burrs come in sizes between 1.25 and 2.5 mm in diameter. They pass along a specialised stainless steel stiff guide wire with a floppy end. The guide wires are harder to torque than other angioplasty wires, and if there is some difficulty placing the wire, a conventional floppier wire can be used with a low profile over-the-wire (OTW) balloon catheter. Having crossed the lesion with the latter, the initial wire can be exchanged for the longer exchange-length rotablator wire. The OTW balloon can then be removed and a burr advanced.

The technique is demanding and must be performed carefully to achieve procedural success without complications. Rotablating at too high a speed and with too much forward force can result in larger particles of atheroma being released and activation of platelets (both of which can contribute to a slow-flow phenomenon and downstream myocardial damage). In addition, excess heat may be generated (a stimulus to restenosis).

MAJOR STUDIES OF ROTABLATION

The major studies of rotablation are listed in Table 14.2.[20–31] The earlier studies compared balloon angioplasty with rotablation (and laser technology in the ERBAC trial) in relatively complex lesion subsets and small vessels. In ERBAC, 685 patients with complex lesions were randomised between rotablation, excimer laser angioplasty or balloon angioplasty. Procedural success was highest in the rotablator arm but there was no difference overall in complications. Further revascularisation at six months was required least frequently with balloon angioplasty. In the COBRA study, procedural success rates were similar in both

TABLE 14.2 - MAJOR STUDIES IN ROTABLATION		
STUDY	**TITLE**	**REF**
SARS	San Antonio Rotablator Study	20
Rota ReoPro	Rotational atherectomy with ReoPro	21
ERBAC	Excimer laser, Rotational atherectomy and Balloon Angioplasty Study Comparison	22
COBRA	Comparison of Balloon vs. Rotational Angioplasty	23
DART	Dilation vs. Ablation Revascularization Trial	24
NACI Registry	New Approaches to Coronary Intervention registry	25
STRATAS	STudy to determine Rotablator And Transluminal Angioplasty Strategy	26
CARAT	Coronary Angioplasty and Rotablator Atherectomy Trial	27
BARASTER	Balloon Angioplasty or Rotational Atherectomy in the treatment of in-STEnt Restenosis	28
ELCA/ROTA, ISR	Excimer Laser Coronary Angioplasty vs. ROTational Atherectomy in treatment of In- Stent Restenosis	29
ROSTER	ROtational atherectomy verSus balloon angioplasty for diffuse in-stent Restenosis trial	30
ARTIST	Angioplasty versus Rotational atherectomy for Treatment of diffuse In-Stent Restenosis Trial	31

arms of the study, and restenosis rates were similar although there was more late loss in the rotablator arm. These studies, performed in the pre- and early stenting era, did not provide compelling evidence to use rotablation in the majority of complex lesions (B2 and C category). A number of nonrandomized studies have looked at the role of the rotablator in lesions such as chronic total occlusions, ostial lesions, and bifurcation lesions. In general, there is no evidence to suggest any benefit, although it may be necessary to use the device in individual resistant, fibrotic or calcified lesions. There is no particular advantage of using the device in small vessels (as shown in DART).

Although these trials did not suggest routine use of rotablation in such lesions, it is generally accepted that the device has an important role in heavily calcified vessels. Identification of calcium on fluoroscopy does not reveal the nature and site of the calcification in the vessel wall. Studies using IVUS, however, have revealed significant variations, with calcification in the medial and adventitial walls rarely causing a major problem with dilatation of a stenosis whereas superficial calcium with an arc >270 degrees, and especially with a thick concentric band of calcification ('napkin-ring' calcification) can be totally resistant to balloon dilatation even at very high pressures. Less extensive calcification can sometimes be dilated but it can be extremely difficult to pass and fully deploy stents in these circumstances. Some operators have attempted to use the Cutting Balloon® (Boston-Scientific, San Diego, CA) in these circumstances although this technique was not designed for this purpose. Others use the FX miniRAIL balloon® (Guidant) that uses the guide wire and an additional wire running alongside the balloon to act as fulcrum points to incise the lesion (allowing dilatation in some vessels at lower pressure) or to act as a pressure point to try and crack calcified segments and thereby achieve dilatation. Whether extensive or relatively localised, superficial calcification is a risk factor for vessel dissection with balloon dilatation and there is a small risk of vessel perforation. This has to be taken into account when considering the small risk of perforation with the rotablator device, although this risk is probably falling with the change of strategy whereby the procedure is most commonly performed with small burrs (see below). There are no randomised trials of patients with heavily calcified lesions undergoing rotablation versus other techniques, mainly because it is impossible to design a trial when the operators know that treatment, with balloon angioplasty, for example, will either fail or given only a modest dilation at best. Prior to the emergence of stenting, many interventionists did not treat these lesions and, instead, patients were referred for coronary surgery. A number of non-randomized series have demonstrated good results with acceptable complication rates.

The issue of the optimal method to use rotablation was the subject of the STRATAS and CARAT studies. Two techniques were considered – a simpler technique utilising sufficient plaque ablation to allow successful dilatation with ballooning at reasonably low pressure ('facilitated angioplasty') versus more aggressive debulking using sequential burrs (final burr:artery ratio >0.7) and then finishing with either no ballooning or ballooning at very low pressure (to avoid deep tissue injury and thereby minimise the stimulus to restenosis). These trials did not show the hoped-for lower restenosis rate with the more aggressive technique, which was associated with a higher release of CK and other complications. Nowadays, rotablation using small burrs (burr:artery ratio <0.6) is most often used to remove difficult calcification and to alter vessel compliance prior to ballooning (and nowadays stenting). Use of the larger burrs has reduced significantly and most operators use a single 1.5 or 1.75 mm burr (reserving the 1.25 mm burr for those with a very tight or heavily calcified lesion). There are, however, individual cases that have such deep napkin-ring calcification that sequential burrs are necessary to achieve a satisfactory lumen. If there is any doubt about whether a lesion might be heavily calcified, it is advisable to inspect it first with IVUS. One tip is that if the IVUS catheter cannot cross the lesion, it needs rotablating.

Although stenting can now be performed in some calcified vessels, it may be extremely difficult to pass the stent down to and across the lesion (often requiring support catheters, stiff guide wires and the use of a 'buddy wire'), and even if stent expansion is possible, full stent expansion may not be. Cases with inadequate stent expansion have a higher restenosis rate than cases with full stent expansion. For this reason, those able to use the rotablator often use the device to partially change the compliance of the vessel prior to stenting thus allowing optimal stent expansion ('rotastenting'). It is argued by some that inadequate expansion of the stents in the era of DES is less important given that they are designed to minimise neointimal proliferation, but the counter arguments include a concern that difficult deployment of a DES may damage the stent coating and thus reduce its anti-proliferative efficacy. In addition, imperfect apposition of the stent to the vessel wall may be one factor that predisposes to late thrombosis. Although there is no compelling evidence to use debulking devices in general prior to stenting, better results will probably be seen with rotastenting in calcified lesions compared to stenting alone. Further research is necessary but, currently, interventionists fall into those who believe in pre-stent preparation of the vessel with the rotablator in such cases, and those who are inexperienced in the technique who use atherotomy devices (such as the Cutting Balloon®) and very high pressure dilatation of the stent after it is deployed.

Because of sub-optimal results of balloon angioplasty for the treatment of diffuse in-stent restenosis, a number of centres investigated the role of debulking with atherectomy or ablative devices prior to ballooning. Although early registry data was reasonably encouraging (as with the BARASTER registry), and the single centre ROSTER randomised trial suggested benefit with the rotablator with relatively aggressive debulking, the larger ARTIST randomised trial failed to demonstrate any benefit from this technique and there were more complications in the rotablator arm. Although this was in part related to inadequate debulking, most centres do not use this technique routinely for this purpose.

Complications with rotablation are lower with the less aggressive debulking technique but there is an incidence of Q wave infarction (1–1.3%), CK-MB >3 times the upper limit of normal in 4–6%, dissection (10–13%), abrupt closure (1.8–11.2%), the slow flow phenomenon (1.2–7.6%), perforation (0–1.5%) and severe spasm (1.6–6.6%). Many of these can be avoided by correct technique using smaller burrs. If they occur, they can be managed with post-rotablation ballooning and stenting (including the use of covered stents in the case of perforation), and generous administration of intra-coronary nitrates, verapamil or adenosine. If tamponade occurs, emergency pericardiocentesis and sometimes surgical bailout is necessary. If severe slow flow or spasm occurs, it is wise to abandon the rotablator and to use balloon angioplasty and stenting as appropriate, as continued rotablation in these circumstances greatly increases the chances of perforation. Particular care with the rotablator must be used in very angulated or heavily calcified lesions. In these cases it is sensible to start with the smallest 1.25 mm burr and to concentrate on optimal technique. In cases with poor left ventricular function it might be necessary to use an intra-aortic balloon pump prior to starting. The device is not necessary in very soft lesions, it is not designed as a thrombus removal device, and it should not be used in the body of vein grafts with friable disease.

The rotablator device continues to have a niche role but it is not required in the majority of cases. Because of this, training in the technique is difficult, and there are many operators who do not feel comfortable using it on an infrequent basis. For this reason, interventionalists should be encouraged to refer difficult cases requiring the rotablator to those with more experience. If an inexperienced operator is faced with a totally resistant lesion then a more experienced operator who is happy to use the rotablator, if available, should become involved with the case. If an operator experienced in rotablation is not available, it is better in many cases to stop the procedure rather than proceeding with very aggressive high-pressure ballooning (which can have unfortunate consequences). The patient can then be referred on to an interventionist who has the necessary rotablator skills.

REFERENCES

1. Topol EJ, Leya F, Pinkerton CA, et al. A comparison of directional atherectomy with coronary angioplasty in patients with coronary artery disease. The CAVEAT Study Group. N Engl J Med. 1993; 329:221–7.

2. Adelman AG, Cohen EA, Kimball BP, et al. A comparison of directional atherectomy with balloon angioplasty for lesions of the left anterior descending artery. N Engl J Med. 1993; 329:228–33.

3. Holmes DR Jr, Topol EJ, Califf RM, et al. A multicenter, randomised trial of coronary angioplasty versus directional atherectomy for patients with saphenous vein bypass graft lesions. CAVEAT-II Investigators. Circulation 1995; 91:1966–74.

4. Simonton CA, Leon MB, Baim DS, et al. "Optimal" directional atherectomy: final results of the Optimal Atherectomy Restenosis Study (OARS). Circulation 1998; 97:332–9.

5. Baim DS, Cutlip DE, Sharma SK, et al. Final results of the Balloon vs Optimal Atherectomy Trial (BOAT). Circulation 1998; 97:322–31.

6. Suzuki T, Hosokawa H, Katoh O, et al. Effects of adjunctive balloon angioplasty after intravascular ultrasound-guided optimal directional coronary atherectomy: the result of

Adjunctive Balloon Angioplasty after Coronary Atherectomy Study (ABACAS). J Am Coll Cardiol. 1999; 34:1028–35.

7. The GUIDE Trial Investigators. IVUS-determined predictors of restenosis in PTCA and DCA: final report from the GUIDE trial, phase II. (abstr). J Am Coll Cardiol. 1996; 29 (Suppl.):156A.

8. Tsuchikane E, Sumitsuji S, Awata N, *et al*. Final results of the Stent versus Directional Coronary Atherectomy Randomized Trial (START). J Am Coll Cardiol. 1999; 34:1050–7.

9. Moussa I, Moses J, Di Mario C, *et al*. Stenting after optimal lesion debulking (SOLD) registry. Angiographic and clinical outcome. Circulation 1998; 98:1604–9.

10. Bramucci E, Angoli L, Merlini PA, *et al*. Adjunctive stent implantation following directional coronary atherectomy in patients with coronary artery disease. J Am Coll Cardiol. 1998; 32:1855–60.

11. Hopp HW, Baer FM, Ozbek C, Kuck KH, Scheller B. A synergistic approach to optimal stenting: directional coronary atherectomy prior to coronary artery stent implantation – the AtheroLink Registry. AtheroLink Study Group. J Am Coll Cardiol. 2000; 36:1853–9.

12. Stankovic G, Colombo A, Bersin R, *et al*. for the AMIGO Investigators. Comparison of directional coronary atherectomy and stenting versus stenting alone for the treatment of de novo and restenotic coronary artery narrowing. Am J Cardiol. 2004; 93:953–8.

13. Harrington RA, Lincoff AM, Califf RM, *et al*. Characetristics and consequences of myocardial infarction after percutaneous coronary intervention: insights from the Coronary Angioplasty Versus Excisional Atherectomy Trial (CAVEAT). J Am Coll Cardiol. 1995; 25:1693–9.

14. Lefkovits J, Blankenship JC, Anderson KM, *et al*. Increased risk of non-Q wave myocardial infarction after directional atherectomy is platelet dependent: evidence from the EPIC trial. J Am Coll Cardiol. 1996; 28:849–55.

15. Bittl JA, Chew DP, Topol EJ, Kong DF, Califf RM. Meta-analysis of randomised trials of percutaneous transluminal coronary angioplasty versus atherectomy, cutting balloon atherotomy, or laser angioplasty. J.Am.Coll.Cardiol. 2004; 43:936–42.

16. Orlic D, Reimers B, Stankovic G, Corvaja N, Chieffo A, Airoldi F, Spanos V, Favero L, Di Mario C, Colombo A. Initial experience with a new 8 French-compatible directional atherectomy catheter: immediate and mid-term results. Catheter Cardiovasc Interv. 2003; 60:159–66.

17. Fischell TA, Drexler H. Pullback atherectomy (PAC) for the treatment of complex bifurcation coronary artery disease. Cathet Cardiovasc Diagn. 1996; 38:218–21.

18. Veinot JP, Ma X, Jelley J, O'Brien ER. Preliminary clinical experience with the pullback atherectomy catheter and the study of proliferation in coronary plaques. Can J Cardiol. 1998; 12:1457–63.

19. Repetto A, Ferlini M, Ferrario M, Angoli L, Bramucci E. Directional coronary atherectomy in 2005. Ital Heart J. 2005; 6:494–7.

20. Kiesz RS, Rozek MM, Ebersole DG, Mego DM, Chang CW, Chilton RL. Novel approach to rotational atherectomy results in low restenosis rates in long, calcified lesions: long-term

results of the San Antonio Rotablator Study (SARS). Catheter Cardiovasc Interv. 1999; 48:48–53.

21. Kini A, Reich D, Marmur JD, Mitre CA, Sharma SK. Reduction in periprocedural enzyme elevation by abciximab after rotational atherectomy of type B2 lesions: results of the Rota ReoPro randomised trial. Am Heart J. 2001; 142:965–9.

22. Reifart N, Vandormael M, Krajcar M, *et al.* Randomized comparison of angioplasty of complex coronary lesions at a single center. Excimer Laser, Rotational Atherectomy, and Balloon Angioplasty Comparison (ERBAC) Study. Circulation 1997; 91–8.

23. Dill T, Dietz U, Hamm CW, *et al.* A randomised comparison of balloon angioplasty versus rotational atherectomy in complex lesions (COBRA study). Eur Heart J. 2000; 21:1759–66.

24. Mauri L, Reisman M, Buchbinder M, *et al.* Comparison of rotational atherectomy with conventional balloon angioplasty in the prevention of restenosis of small coronary arteries: results of the Dilatation vs Ablation Revascularization Trial Targeting Restenosis (DART). Am Heart J. 2003; 145:847–54.

25. Brown DL, George CJ, Steenkiste AR, *et al.* High-speed rotational atherectomy of human coronary stenoses: acute and one-year outcomes from the New Approaches to Coronary Intervention (NACI) registry. Am J Cardiol. 1997; 80:60K–7K.

26. Whitlow P, Bass T, Kipperman R, *et al.* Results of the study to determine rotablator and transluminal angioplasty strategy (STRATAS). Am J Cardiol. 2001; 87:699–705.

27. Safian R, Feldman T, Muller D, *et al.* Coronary angioplasty and Rotablator atherectomy trial (CARAT): immediate and late results of a prospective multicentre randomised trial. Catheter Cardiovasc Interv. 2001; 53:213–20.

28. Goldberg SL, Berger P, Cohen DJ, *et al.* Rotational atherectomy or balloon angioplasty in the treatment of intra-stent restenosis: BARASTER multicenter registry. Catheter Cardiovasc Interv. 2000; 51:407–13.

29. Mehran R, Dangas G, Mintz GS, *et al.* Treatment of in-stent restenosis with excimer laser coronary angioplasty versus rotational atherectomy: comparative mechanisms and results. Circulation 2000; 101:2484–9.

30. Sharma SK, Kini A, Mehran R, Lansky A, Kobayashi Y, Marmur JD. Randomized trial of tototational atherectomy versus balloon angioplasty for diffuse in-stent restenosis (ROSTER). Am Heart J. 2004; 147:16–22.

31. vom Dahl J, Dietz U, Haager PK, *et al.* Rotational atherectomy does not reduce recurrent in-stent restenosis results of the angioplasty versus rotational atherectomy for treatment of diffuse in-stent restenosis trial (ARTIST). Circulation 2002; 105:583–8.

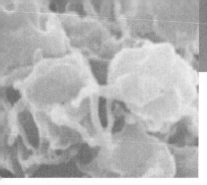

15

PCI in the presence of significant intraluminal thrombus

MAN FAI SHIU

KEY POINTS

■ The number of devices developed for reducing thromboembolic complications has increased over the last decades and have been shown to be successful in PCI of degenerative vein grafts but the main goal of such devices is in the setting of acute myocardial infarction.

■ Early observational studies have shown angiographic and limited clinical benefit for some devices to date. There is a lack of randomized trials showing outcome benefit in terms of improved survival or reduction in major adverse events. It could be that some of the devices are still new and there is a learning curve as with all new techniques.

■ At present it is very much up to individual operators to choose whether to perform thrombectomy prior to balloon angioplasty and/or stent implantation, and which devices is used.

■ It is likely that in the long run some devices will be recognized as a useful adjunctive device for thrombus laden lesions since PCI without prior thrombectomy continues to be associated with increased complications.

Intraluminal thrombus is common in and around the culprit lesion in acute coronary syndromes (ACS). In primary PCI for AMI thrombus is invariably present. Similarly, in failed thrombolysis (Rescue PCI) total or subtotal occlusion of the culprit lesion by thrombus is commonly seen. In the setting of NSTEMI a mixture of thrombus and platelet clumps may be present though these are often not obvious on angiography. Despite the use of intensive anti-coagulant and anti-platelet therapy PCI in the acute setting of the whole spectrum of ACS results in an increased risks of procedural complications and it is believed that this is related to the presence of intra-coronary thrombus.[1]

The cause of such complications is sometimes easy to recognize. During wire and balloon crossing, and in particular once balloon inflation starts thrombo embolic events may exhibit as a sudden reduction in antegrade flow. Often distal embolisation is seen with typical blunt occlusion of distal branches though at times the only feature is extremely slow filling of the whole coronary system, with no evidence of any obstruction at the site of the original lesion. This 'no-reflow' phenomenon often occurs after apparently straightforward stent deployment. The mechanism is believed to be disruption of loosely attached thrombus by the stent struts, leading to micro- and macroemboli.

At present there is no one generally accepted device to deal with the problem of intraluminal thrombus. Given the overall high success rate of PCI in ACI settings most operators simply ignore the presence of intraluminal presence. While such a simple approach can lead to a satisfactory result, there is no doubt that the higher the thrombus load the greater the likelihood of serious complications. Indeed at times there is so much intracoronary thrombus that it is not possible to locate the culprit lesion. This leads to use of multiple stents or excessively long stents to cover the whole affected territory with undesirable consequences. The sheer amount of thrombus trapped between the stent and the vessel wall can be a setting for subacute stents thrombosis.

ASSESSING THE NEED FOR THROMBECTOMY

Ideally thrombectomy is undertaken before much mechanical disturbance to the thrombus. However it is not always possible to avoid. In the majority of procedures, at least initial crossing of the lesion with an angioplasty wire is necessary. The decision to perform thrombectomy is ideally made from the initial angiogram but it is not always possible to do so.

The typical appearances of a thrombus laden vessel are often unmistakable, especially if the vessel is not completely occluded. Large right coronary arteries, due to the paucity of side branches compared to the left system, appear to favor large accumulation of thrombus (Fig. 15.1). A completely occluded vessel, in the context of an acute ischemic presentation with related ECG changes pointing to a culprit vessel would suggest a thrombotic occlusion but the amount of intraluminal thrombus is impossible to ascertain. Decision for thrombectomy is best postponed until after lesion crossing with an 0.014 wire, and better still, after passage of a balloon catheter without actual dilatation. This often allows sufficient antegrade filling to reveal the extent of thrombus load (Fig. 15.2). Additional decisions regarding thrombectomy may depend on the characteristic of the device. For most devices, a highly tortuous vessel proximal to the lesion, and the distance of the target lesion are hurdles for access. Thrombo-extraction for lesions involving significant side branches are associated with complications such as side branch occlusion or perforation. The latter is due to a tendency for branch points such as the LAD/diagonal junction to be relatively fixed, and luminal diameters to change abruptly, both important mechanical factors for vessel trauma in any form of significant device manipulation.

THROMBECTOMY SYSTEMS

Thrombectomy systems differ from distal protection system in that they remove thrombus actively before balloon dilatation and stent implantation (and at times after). These can be broadly separated into either simple aspiration catheters or devices which actively agitates or disrupt the thrombus during aspiration (Table 15.1).

Evidence for the use of these devices has mostly come from observational studies of safety and efficacy. A number of randomized studies have shown clinical benefit. As the size of these studies is small outcome benefit in terms of improved survival is absent, and as the setting is often acute, reduction in myocardial infarction is difficult to establish. However, surrogate endpoints such as improved post-procedural flow grade or minimal lesion diameter have been used to show benefit.[1] Examples are the SAFER study (filter wire in the setting of diffusely diseased vein grafts)[2] and the X-amine ST study (X-Sizer in Acute Myocardial Infarction). These are outnumbered by negative studies that show either no benefit or actual increase in adverse clinical outcome. Therefore, there is no evidence to recommend initial use of these devices. Nevertheless it is probably wise to have the experience and access to one or two devices since there are occasions where the thrombus load is such that without some form of thrombectomy simple stenting is unlikely to bring about a satisfactory outcome.

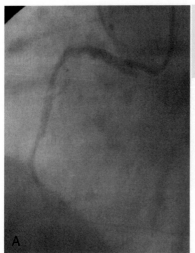

Figure 15.1:
A RCA angiogram showing extensive thrombotic occlusion in a patient with recent non-ST elevation myocardial infarction. B RCA after thrombectomy with the X-Sizer followed by stent implantation.

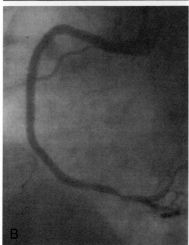

THE PROXIS SYSTEM (VELOCIMED)

Description: The Proxis system comes in a single pack with no additional console. Apart from the device catheter there is a connecting system that allows aspiration at the distal end of the guiding catheter (Fig. 15.3). No external or battery power is required. The aspiration lumen is also the lumen through which the usual PCI equipment is passed through.

Preparation and use: After target vessel engagement, the device catheter is passed just a short distance into the coronary artery or vein graft. Following a contrast injection a balloon at the tip of the catheter is inflated to occlude the proximal segment of the vessel. The segment remains angiographically visible to allow wire crossing and lesion stented with or without balloon pre-dilatation. Once that is done the PCI equipment is removed and debris is aspirated through the central channel of the catheter. Usually, about 6ml of blood is aspirated and the occlusion

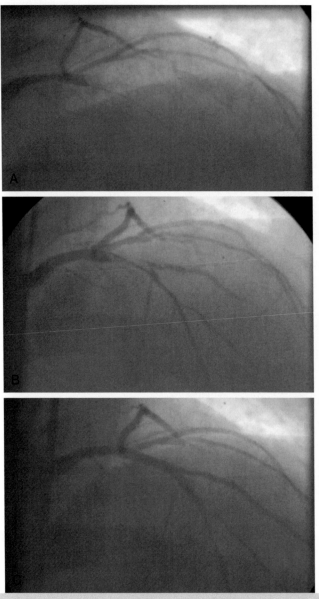

Figure 15.2:
A Left coronary angiogram in a patient with an acute anterior infarction showing no antegrade filling of LAD despite wire crossing of lesion. B Following balloon passage through occlusion without dilatation of lesion. C End result following thrombectomy with X-Sizer and stent implantation.

TABLE 15.1 - CURRENTLY AVAILABLE THROMBECTOMY SYSTEMS

SIMPLE ASPIRATION	ASPIRATION WITH DISRUPTION OF DEBRIS
Rescue	X-Sizer
Percusurge	Angiojet
Proxis	Triactive
Export	Rinspirator
Pronto	

balloon deflated. The procedure can be repeated more than once and the central lumen is sufficiently large to accommodate most standard PCI wires, balloons and stents.

Clinical studies: The efficacy of the Proxis system has been evaluated in both vein grafts and native vessels in the FASTER clinical trial. One unique feature of this system is that the target vessel is occluded proximally at the start of the procedure without any initial wire or balloon crossing, reducing the likelihood of thrombus embolisation.

Percusurge GuardWire System (Medtronic)
Description: The Percusurge GuardWire System consists of three parts: (1) a distal inflation device in the form of a balloon mounted on a 0.014 inch wire (guard wire); (2) an adaptor device to seal the inflation channel; and (3) a 5F (1.7 mm) aspiration catheter (Export). No external power is required and conventional guiding catheters can be used.

Preparation and use: The target lesion is crossed with the guard wire, which has a flexible tip similar to conventional PCI wires (0.014"). The distal balloon is

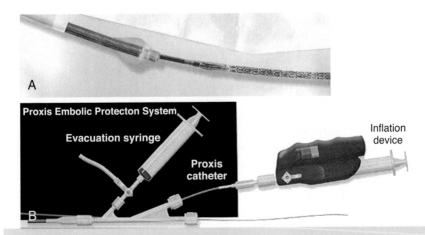

Figure 15.3:
A The illustration shows the tip of the Proxis system with the occlusive balloon inflated. A stent catheter is through the main lumen. B Connections of Proxis inflation module to main catheter.

inflated to completely occlude the vessel as confirmed by contrast injection via the guiding catheter. The balloon can be inflated from 3 to 6 mm for this purpose. The guard wire is then 'sealed' using an adaptor device to maintain distal balloon occlusion. Conventional balloon pre-dilatation (if necessary) and stent implantation is performed using this wire. Coronary stasis is obligatory during this stage. After stent deployment the 5 F aspiration catheter is advanced over the wire past the stented segment until it is just proximal to the inflated occlusion balloon. Between 20 and 40 ml of blood is then aspirated. The Export catheter is removed and the adaptor device is re-attached to deflate the occlusion and restore antegrade flow.

Clinical outcome studies The safety and efficacy of the Percusurge device was confirmed in a large randomized trial of PCI for saphenous vein grafts (the SAFER trial).[2] This is one of the few studies in this field showing clinical end point benefit. At 30 days combined end points of death, AMI and emergency CABG and TVR were lower (9.6% vs. 16.5%, $p = 0.004$). However, a subsequent trial in acute myocardial infarction involving native coronary vessels (the Emerald trial) with 501 randomized patients failed to show clinical benefit in this setting.[4] Various explanations have been offered for the lack of success for clinical end points despite apparent thrombus removal. Balloon occlusion of the target vessel during the procedure and the lack of protection of side branches proximal to the balloon are problems for any distal occlusion device.

Export system The Export catheter is a further development from this device, keeping the aspiration element but dispensing with the distal occlusion balloon. It is too early to say if this will address some of the issues.[5]

Rescue device The Rescue device is very similar to the export catheter. It is a monorail system over a conventional 0.014" wire. The catheter gauge is 4.5 F allowing use in a 7 F guiding catheter. Aspiration is with the help of a console which generates up to 0.8 atm and debris is collected in an in line filter. The devices have been compared, in a non-randomized trial, with conventional stenting in acute myocardial infarction. In a study of 109 patients there was evidence of improved TIMI grade flow at the end of the procedure, but no clinical outcome benefit.[6]

Diver CE device (Invatec) The main innovation in this device, which superficially resemble the above two systems, is that instead of a single aspiration hole the end of the catheter has a main end hole and three additional side holes, apart from the wire channel. This allows more effective aspiration and can still be accommodated inside a 6 F guiding catheter as a rapid exchange system. In a randomized trial of 100 patients in acute myocardial infarction the result showed a greater degree of myocardial blush and more ST segment resolution compared to conventional PCI.[7]

Triactive device (Kensey Nash) This is another balloon occlusion system but with active flush and aspiration. The system is a little more elaborate and

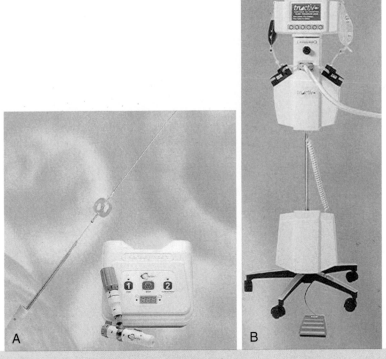

Figure 15.4:
A The Triactive System with balloon occlusion wire inside the aspiration catheter. B The floor-standing externally powered flush/aspiration module.

requires external power to allow longer flush/aspiration than with simple manual syringe suction (Fig. 15.4).

As with the Percusurge the distal occlusion balloon is mounted on the 0.014" wire which then functions as the conventional PCI wire. The balloon stent procedure is performed while antegrade flow is arrested. The main difference from the Percusurge is in the debris removal. Instead of an aspiration catheter a flushing catheter is passed to a position close to the occlusion balloon. Aspiration is through the conventional guiding catheter and the flush/aspiration is controlled by the externally powered device which ensures that the flushing rate does not exceed the aspiration rate. This is to prevent embolism of debris into the aorta. At present the system has mainly been used in vein grafts but there is no reason why it cannot be applied to native vessels in due course.

Rinspiration system (Kerberos) This system uses a single, double lumen catheter that flushes and aspirates simultaneously without distal occlusion. The concept is to aspirate faster than the infusion rate thereby avoiding excessive distal embolization. No external power is regained. A hand operated double syringe system provides the necessary flush/aspiration action maintaining a fixed ratio of flush and aspiration flow rate. Antegrade flow is not stopped

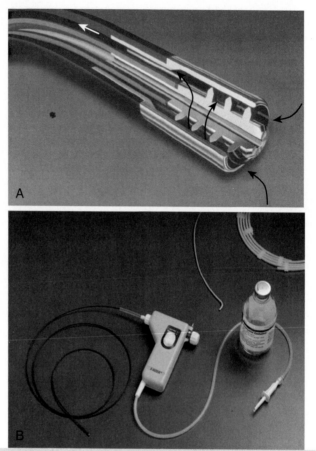

Figure 15.5:
A Illustration of the helical cutter at the tip of the X-Sizer catheter. B The X-Sizer system showing the one piece catheter with controller and vacuum bottle for suction.

and flushing is via a number of side holes and aspiration via a distal end hole, distal embolism is theoretically kept to a minimum.

The X-Sizer (eV3 Inc.)
Description The device is a single disposable unit in the form of an over-the-wire catheter directly attached to a drive unit and connected to a vacuum bottle (Fig. 15.5). The catheter has a central lumen for standard 0.014" PCI wires and an outer lumen for debris removal. There is a choice of two catheter sizes, 1.5 mm and 2.0 mm that require 6 F and 8 F guides, respectively. The motor unit drives an Archimedes-type screw blade located at the tip of the catheter. Compared to other rotational devices such as the Rotablator the speed of rotation is relatively slow at approximately 2000 rpm. The cutting action of the screw shred the debris while the vacuum from the aspiration bottle removes it. The system is not intended to excise atheromatous lesions or calcified material. A safety cutout switch prevents the cutter from exerting undue torque. Should the

rotation stall a reverse button on the motor unit allows the cutter to be freed as negative aspiration is maintained. The vacuum bottle would typically allow removal of about 300 ml of blood/debris.

Preparation and use The lesion is first crossed with a exchange length 0.014" wire and the tip of the wire placed as distally as possible for adequate support during subsequent device maneuver. The device unit is connected to a vacuum bottle and rotation/aspiration should be tested by activating the unit with the tip of the catheter in saline (activation without tip immersion can lead to rapid loss of vacuum). The wire channel is flushed and the catheter introduced into the target vessel. Rotation/aspiration should be activated as the catheter tip is seen to approach the target lesion. Advancement through the target area should be slow and without undue force.[4] A typical procedure involves 2–3 minutes of aspiration with 30–60 ml of blood removed (less time in the case of the large 2 mm device). If necessary, the vacuum bottle can be changed without removal of the catheter from the artery.

Due to the close fitting of the device and guiding catheter, contrast injection for lesion visualization is not possible unless a larger guiding catheter is used (that is, 7 F guide for 1.5 mm device). The catheter is completely removed before a check angiogram is performed. Being an over the wire system this device is difficult to use without an assistant operator.

Clinical outcome studies An early randomized trial was conducted in the United States involving non-acute MI patients with either diseased CABG or native coronary arteries with a strong suggestion of thrombus. This showed angiographic efficacy of thrombectomy and a reduction in one of the clinical end points, namely significant myocardial infarction as indicated by cardiac enzyme rise. A more recent trial (the X-Amine ST trial) focused on 201 patients with acute myocardial infarction in the primary PCI setting. Compared with conventional PCI use of the X-Sizer before balloon and stents showed improved outcomes in terms of greater ST segment resolution and a lower incidence of slow flow or distal embolization. (6% vs. 19.8%, $p<0.0056$).[3]

Angiojet thrombectomy system (Proxis Medical)
Description The system uses a number of very high pressure fluid jets to break up thrombus aspirate the debris utilizing the Venturi effect. A mains powered external compressor is required. The disposable components are the aspiration catheter and connecting ports. There are two coronary catheter sizes that allow 6 F or 7 F size guiding catheters.

Preparation and use An exchange length PCI 0.14" wire is used to cross the target lesion and the thrombectomy catheter is introduced as for other over-the-wire devices. Once in the vessel aspiration can be started. As the tip of the catheter is smooth the catheter can be used to advance past tight stenoses for aspiration of distal thrombus. The system can be used in saphenous vein grafts, native coronary vessels and there is a larger catheter for peripheral vessels up to 8 mm in diameter.

Clinical outcome studies A recently published randomized trial in an acute myocardial infarction setting failed to show any clinical benefit despite effective thrombus aspiration with the Angiojet due to an increased peri-procedural complication rate with a higher mortality in the device group.

REFERENCES

1. Van't Hof AWJ, Liem A, Suryapranata H, *et al.* on behalf of the Zwolle Myocardial Infarction Study Group: Angiographic assessment of myocardial reperfusion in patients treated with primary angioplasty for acute myocardial infarction: Myocardial blush grade. Circulation 1998; 97: 2302–6.

2. Baim DS, Wahr D, George B, *et al.* on behalf of the Saphenous vein graft Angioplasty Free of Emboli Randomized (SAFER) Trial Investigators: Randomized trial of a distal embolic protection device during percutaneous intervention of saphenous vein aorto-coronary bypass grafts. Circulation 2002; 105:1285–90.

3. Lefebre T, Garcia E, Reimers B, *et al.* on behalf of the X AMINE ST Investigators: X-Sizer for thrombectomy in acute myocardial infarction improves ST-segment resolution. J Am Coll Cardiol 2005; 46:246–52.

4. Stone GW, Webb J, Cox DA, *et al.* for the Enhanced Myocardial Efficacy and Recovery by Aspiration of Lberated Debris (EMERALD): Distal microcirculatory protection during percutaneous coronary intervention in acute ST segment elevation myocardial infarction: A randomized controlled trial. JAMA 2005; 293:1063–72.

5. Yang Ch-T, Hwang J-J, Lin L-Ch, Kao H-L: Initial thrombosuction with subsequent angioplasty in primary coronary intervention-comparison with conventional strategy. Int J Cardiol 2005; 102:121–6.

6. Kondo H, Suzuki T, Fukutomi T, *et al.* Effects of percutaneous coronary arterial thrombectomy during acute myocardial infarction on left ventricular remodelling. Am J Cardiol 2004; 93:527–31.

7. Burzotta F, Trani C, Romagnoli E, *et al.* Relation between thrombus burden, efficacy of thrombus removal, and myocardial perfusion in patients treated with a new thrombus-aspirating device (The Diver CE). Am J Cardiol 2004; 94(S6A):42E.

8. San Martin M, Goicolea J, Ruiz-Salmeron R, *et al.* Coronary perforation as apotential complication derived from coronary thrombectomy with the X-Sizer device. Cathet Cardiovasc Intervent 2002; 56:378–82.

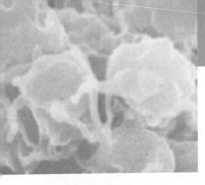

16

Cutting balloon angioplasty

ROGER K.G. MOORE AND RAPHAEL A. PERRY

KEY POINTS

- Incisional dilatation reduces barotrauma and hoop stress and vessel wall injury.

- Cutting balloon angioplasty (CBA) is similar in success to plain old balloon angioplasty (POBA) and can be used in the majority of cases.

- CBA is an ideal treatment for resistant and ostial lesions and is effective in small vessel stenoses.

- There is emerging data that vessel preparation with CBA compared to POBA prior to stent implantation may result in reduced in-stent restenosis.

INTRODUCTION

Since Andreas Grüntzig's first published series of angioplasty cases there has been an exponential rise in the complexity of coronary artery disease deemed treatable by percutaneous revascularisation. This has been enabled by the equally rapid change in the technology and number of devices available to the cardiologist. The principal driving force behind all these developments have been to conquer the two areas that have limited the application of PTCA, now affectionately known as POBA (plain old balloon angioplasty) namely acute vessel closure/coronary dissection and restenosis. Coronary artery stenting has addressed to a significant extent these two Achilles' heels of POBA but has its own drawbacks with the problem of in-stent restenosis that has not been entirely resolved even in the DES era.

POBA[3] increases luminal size by controlled barotrauma causing plaque rupture and vessel wall expansion. It is established that while the final angiographic result of POBA is related to the extent and force of balloon dilatation it is the extent of vessel wall trauma that determines acute vessel closure and also initiates the mechanism that when exaggerated leads to restenosis. Part of the difficulty is that the balloon frequently exerts its maximal force on the more normal parts of the vessel wall causing stretching which is prone to early recoil and damaging normal endothelium rather than cracking more organised fibrous plaque.

The Barath cutting balloon[1] was designed specifically to address the problems of barotrauma-related complications of POBA. The device is a non-compliant balloon which when expanded has three or four longitudinally mounted microtomes on the external surface. The balloon material is folded to shield the blades and protect the vessel wall as the catheter is passed to and from the lesion. When the balloon is expanded at the site of a coronary lesion the blades produce controlled incisions into plaque rather than a random dissection. This allows the balloon barotrauma pressure to be evenly distributed and force to be applied to plaque at least as effectively as to normal parts of the vessel wall. The reduction in hoop stress and lower pressures used to achieve an angiographically acceptable result (maximum of 6–8 atmospheres) are the main factors put forward as being likely to reduce both acute complications and restenosis.

Intravascular ultrasound (IVUS) studies have demonstrated that the different mechanism of lesion dilation with CBA achieves similar luminal dimensions to POBA but with larger plaque reduction and less vessel expansion in noncalcified lesions.[2] In contrast in calcified lesions CBA achieves larger lumen gain than POBA with similar proportional effects on plaque compression and vessel expansion. The virtual absence of vessel recoil would appear to be a significant factor in reducing the restenosis rates.

PRACTICAL POINTS

The Flextome Cutting Balloon (Boston Scientific, US) is the latest incarnation of the original Barath design (Fig. 16.1) and is sized from 2.0 to 4.0 mm in quarter sizes. The deflated profile is from 0.041 to 0.046", the atherotome lengths are either 6, 10 or 15 mm and the distal shaft is 3.2 F (Fig. 16.2). The changes to balloon material and the incorporation of flex points every 5 mm for the 10 and 15 mm atherotomes has improved flexibility although its ability to cross areas of excessive tortuosity is inevitably inferior to the performance of modern compliant balloons. As with many interventional devices there are relative indications and contraindications, which are varied, in everyday use. Clear contraindications to its use are extensive vessel calcification and visible intraluminal thrombus. In practical terms excessive tortuosity and long lesions present difficulties though repeated inflations of the shorter balloon can achieve a good result. If there is difficulty crossing a lesion predilatation with a small balloon to allow passage of the cutting balloon is accepted practice. Once positioned across the lesion inflation should be undertaken slowly to reach 6 atmospheres at 30 seconds and inflation maintained for up to 2 minutes

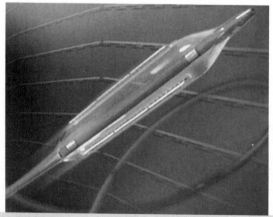

Figure 16.1:
Flextome Cutting Balloon (Boston Scientific).

Over-the wire catheter

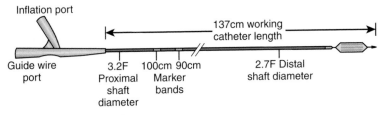

Inflation port

Guide wire port

3.2F Proximal shaft diameter

100cm 90cm Marker bands

137cm working catheter length

2.7F Distal shaft diameter

Monorail™ catheter

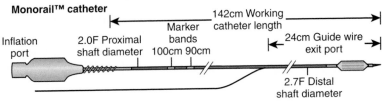

Inflation port

2.0F Proximal shaft diameter

Marker bands 100cm 90cm

142cm Working catheter length

24cm Guide wire exit port

2.7F Distal shaft diameter

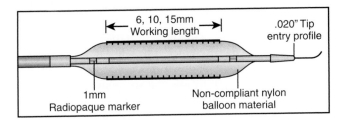

6, 10, 15mm Working length

.020" Tip entry profile

1mm Radiopaque marker

Non-compliant nylon balloon material

Atherotome

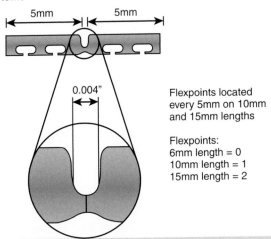

5mm   5mm

0.004"

Flexpoints located every 5mm on 10mm and 15mm lengths

Flexpoints:
6mm length = 0
10mm length = 1
15mm length = 2

Figure 16.2:
Flextome Cutting Balloon dimensions.

provided patients can tolerate this. The slow unfolding of the microtomes prevents vessel damage and allows the movement of the artery to assist incision. It is important to allow full deflation to ensure involution of the microtomes prior to withdrawing the balloon. If full expansion is not achieved up to 8 atmospheres pressure may be applied. The balloon/artery ratio should be 1.2:1 and in practical terms this means using one-quarter size more than the normal vessel segment. The final appearance may be 'stent-like' but up to a 30% residual stenosis is counted as an acceptable result and it is well observed that further positive remodelling takes place after initial dilatation such that follow-up angiograms not infrequently look better than the final result. Small controlled linear dissections are not uncommon and provided there is no change in the appearance over 5–10 minutes, acute vessel closure is extremely unlikely.[3] As stenting is undertaken in 90% lesions acute closure is not a clinical issue and small linear dissection may allow better stent expansion.

CLINICAL DATA

The hypothesis that controlled 'surgical' expansion using CBA would induce less vessel wall injury and reduce neointimal hyperplasia was explored by the CUBA investigators.[4] This study examined the clinical effectiveness as a primary treatment in 304 patients randomised to CBA or POBA and demonstrated that restenosis rates were significantly lower at six months in the CBA arm (CBA 30% vs POBA 42%; p=0.03). These promising early findings, however, were not confirmed by the pivotal multi-center Global trial,[5] which randomised 1,238 patents to either CBA or POBA. The study was limited to simple A/B1 lesions and used a single CBA inflation at a balloon artery ratio of 1.1:1. Restenosis rates were identical in the two groups (CBA 31.4% vs POBA 30.4%; p=0.75) with significantly more coronary perforations in the CBA group (CBA 5 vs POBA 0; p=0.03).

The results of the Global trial combined with the widespread use of coronary stenting has, therefore, confined CBA as a primary interventional procedure to a variety of specific areas. These are principally in small vessel coronary disease, resistant or ostial lesions and as a treatment of the burgeoning problem of in-stent restenosis. There is, however, increasing interest in the use of CBA in vessel preparation prior to stent implantation as a method of providing optimal stent deployment.

SMALL VESSEL PTCA

The CAPAS study randomised 232 patients (248 type B or C lesions) with a reference vessel diameters of <3 mm to CBA or POBA.[6] The success rate was high with a stent implant rate of 6% in CBA and 11% in POBA. Angiographic follow-up was 95% complete and showed a significant reduction in restenosis after CBA (22% vs 41%; p <0.01). Although there was a reduction in TVR after CBA this did not reach statistical significance (22% vs 29%). A further randomised trial by Ergene and colleagues[7] although small, confirmed similar findings with a restenosis rate significantly lower after CBA (27% vs 47%; p <0.05) and observed significantly fewer dissections after CBA. Iijima et al.[8] corroborated these findings in a retrospective comparison of 316 patients, with lesions in

<2.5 mm vessels, treated with POBA, CBA and BMS. The CBA group demonstrated greater acute gain than POBA and lower late loss than both other techniques with a significantly lower binary stenosis rate (CBA 31%, POBA 46.5%, Stent 43.9%; p=0.048).

It would appear that CBA is safe and effective in small vessel coronary disease and it is clear that POBA and BMS has a low long-term success in this setting. Subgroup analysis, however, of the TAXUS IV trial has shown an improvement in binary restenosis with DES in comparison with bare metal of up to 38% in smaller vessels and further evaluation of the long term complications of DES use in this context will be needed before determination of the best treatment options for small vessel coronary disease can be made.

OSTIAL AND RESISTANT LESIONS

The outcome of POBA of ostial lesions at whatever site is poor.[9] Cutting balloon angioplasty has been reported in a wide variety of both aorto-ostial lesions of SVGs and the right coronary artery and of the ostia of major branches of the coronary tree though few series have been compiled.

Aortic ostial lesions contain more fibrous and elastic components in comparison to lesions within the coronary tree and these lesions can be both resistant to plaque rupture and prone to substantial elastic recoil following POBA. The stronger radial force and more organised lesion disruption properties of CBA would, therefore, appear to offer a potential advantage in predilation prior to stent implantation in this area. Muramatsu and colleagues[10] reported 37 patients undergoing CBA to ostial stenoses and compared them to a comparable group of patients having POBA with no patient being stented. The initial angiographic success rate was higher in the CBA group (95% vs 85%) with a much higher incidence of serious dissections following POBA 6.5% vs 0% for CBA. Angiographic restenosis occurred in 41% of CBA patients and 53% of POBA cases. Oversizing the cutting balloon led to a reduced restenosis rate of 31% but a higher dissection rate. A small series of patients reported by Kurbaan et al.[11] showed the benefits of combined cutting balloon and stenting in ostial lesions. In these eight patients initial high pressure (18 atmospheres) ballooning led to a modest improvement in stenosis from 82% to 68% but adjunctive CBA left a residual stenosis of 44% which after stenting was reduced to 10%. During clinical follow up there was no evidence of restenosis. Combined CBA and stenting, therefore, appears the most appropriate treatment for aorto-ostial lesions although this strategy has not been tested in a randomised controlled trial.

Branch ostial lesions combine the problems of resistance and elastic recoil with added difficulty of potential plaque shift into the main vessel. Chung and colleagues investigated the role of CBA in comparison to BMS for ostial disease in 2.5–3 mm vessels in a nonrandomised retrospective study.[12] Although the use of stents offered significantly enhanced acute gain, binary restenosis was lower in the CBA group at six months (CBA 41%, Stent 63%; p=0.05). Interestingly with CBA the MLD within the native vessel remained unaltered both immediately and at six-month follow up whilst significant lumen loss was seen at both time points in the stenting group, lending support to the theory of less plaque shift with CBA.

CBA has been demonstrated to be superior to POBA in the treatment of bifurcation lesions in retrospective analysis with increased procedural success (92% vs 76%; p=0.035), reduced bail out stenting (8% vs 24%; p=0.035) and reduced binary stenosis at three months (40% vs 67%; p=0.026). The incidence of restenosis with CBA is, therefore, comparable with bare metal stenting strategies but is likely to be inferior to the use of DES particularly with the utilization of final kissing balloon techniques.[13]

IN-STENT RESTENOSIS

Although stenting has significantly reduced the incidence of vessel restenosis and need for TVR when restenosis does occur within a stent the rate of re-restenosis remains high with repeat high-pressure ballooning having a recurrence rate of greater than 50%.[15] IVUS studies have shown that in-stent restenosis is principally due to neo-intimal proliferation and hyperplasia as there is little scope for vessel recoil after stent deployment. It was, therefore, proposed that atherectomy by removing tissue would be the treatment of choice with or without adjunctive ballooning. However the results of atherectomy for restenosis have been disappointing with one year TLR rates of 26–31% with an average late loss of approximately 1 mm.[15] The only randomised trial of rotablation (ARTIST) demonstrated a superior effect of POBA to rotational atherectomy and low-pressure adjunctive ballooning for in-stent restenosis.[16]

IVUS studies have demonstrated that the mechanism of lumen enlargement for balloon angioplasty in restenosis is equally dependent on stent expansion and extrusion of neo-intimal tissue through stent struts.[17] The theoretical advantage for CBA over POBA in this setting is its greater ability to extrude tissue by separating the neo-intimal tissue into quadrants during balloon expansion as demonstrated in a recent IVUS study.[18] It should be added that CBA also offers a practical advantage over POBA due to the avoidance of balloon displacement on inflation due to the ability of the blades to anchor the device on the slippery hyperplastic tissue surface. Initial clinical experience was encouraging with Adamian and colleagues[19] retrospectively reporting 181 consecutive matched patients undergoing treatment for in-stent restenosis using POBA, high speed rotational atherectomy (HSRA) and CBA. In this study the final MLD was similar in all three groups with lower MACE at follow up found in the CBA group. With both angiographic re-restenosis and TVR significantly lower in the CBA group compared to HSRA and POBA. These finding were supported by other small observational studies demonstrating lower angiographic restenosis rates[18] with CBA for in-stent restenosis in comparison to POBA and reduced TVR.[20]

These promising initial results, however, have not been replicated in subsequent randomised trials. The RESCUT[21] (REStenosis CUTting balloon evaluation study) was a multicenter, prospective trial in which 428 patients with a wide range of ISR subtypes were randomised to either POBA or CBA. At 30 days and seven months no differences in clinical outcomes were discernable with a 7 month TLR rate in the CBA arm of 13.5% in comparison to 13.1% in the POBA arm (p=0.99). Angiographic characteristics were also comparable with no differences found in late loss (CBA 0.56 mm, POBA 0.62 mm; p=0.42) or binary restenosis (CBA 29.8%, POBA 31.4%; p=0.82). One issue in the trial was the low rate of ISR with POBA. Also the trial design did not allow additional high pressure POBA in the CBA group which would be usual practice. The equivalence of the two techniques in terms of MACE and angiographic outcome in restenotic lesions would appear to be confirmed by the second randomised trial in this area. REDUCE II (REstenosis reDUction by Cutting balloon Evaluation) randomised 416 to CBA and POBA and although the study is yet to be published early reports suggest that binary stenosis and TLR rates are not significantly different between the two arms of the study at six months follow up. Despite this disappointing data interest has remained in the combination of CBA with intravasular brachytherapy in the treatment of ISR supported by pooled nonrandomised data that has consistently reported good angiographic results in terms of late loss and binary restenosis. Unfortunately this combination, however, failed to demonstrate benefit in angiographic characteristics at seven months over brachytherapy and POBA in a recent randomised clinical trial (BETACUT).[22]

The use of DES for ISR has shown promise in small observational trials[23,24] and supported in a recently published retrospective matched comparison[25] of DES treated lesions with a control group consisting of individuals from RESCUT. The use of DES in this report was associated with a benefit in angiographic characteristics at six months with significant differences seen in acute lumen gain (CBA 1.36 mm, DES 1.69 mm; p<0.001), late loss (CBA 0.56 mm, DES 0.35mm; p=0.028) and binary restenosis (CBA 29.8%, POBA 12.8%; p=0.016).

CBA use in the treatment of ISR offers procedural advantage over POBA in terms of reduced balloon slippage and reduced incidence of distal edge dissection but has failed to show benefit in clinical or angiographic characteristics in short- and medium-term follow up. Although direct randomised data in still not available for DES vs CBA in this setting it would appear that DES is likely to offer a significant advantage over CBA alone in the treatment of ISR.

VESSEL PREPARATION PRIOR TO STENTING

Stent placement has made enormous impact on the need for reintervention but stent implantation alone does not guarantee long-term procedural success. Unless the stent is fully deployed with complete lesion coverage there remains a risk of both restenosis and sub acute thrombosis. This is particularly a problem in the presence of calcified or fibrotic lesions where inadequate vessel wall preparation can lead to under expansion despite both high pressure deployment and aggressive post dilation with a non-compliant balloon. Even in the era of DES the majority of target vessel failure has been attributed to stent under expansion.[26] Vessel wall preparation using CBA is a straight forward method of increasing vessel compliance during stent deployment. CBA expands the lesion using low pressure dilatation and longitudinal incisions weakening areas that will then allow correct strut apposition and expansion.

The use of CBA for vessel preparation prior to stent implantation has been tested in REDUCE III, a large multicentre trial that randomised 520 patients to predilation with either CBA or POBA and these groups were further randomised to IVUS guided coronary stenting. At six-month follow up the IVUS guided CBA arm demonstrated significant lower restenosis than the other techniques (CBA IVUS 10.7%, CBA 18%, POBA IVUS 20%, POBA 18%; p=0.016). Failure to use CBA was an independent predictor of restenosis. In an era of concern for subacute and late thrombosis in DES this improvement in BMS results has increasing relevance. The question as to whether CBA has a role in reducing MACE post DES implantation has jet to be tested.

REFERENCES

1. Barath P, Fishbein MC, Vari S, Forrester JS. Cutting balloon: a novel approach to percutaneous angioplasty. Am J Cardiol. 1991; 68:1249–52.

2. Okura H, Hayase M, Hosokawa H et al. Acute lumen gain after cutting balloon angioplasty in calcified and non calcified lesions: intravascular ultrasound analysis of the REDUCE study. JACC February 1999; 33(2) Suppl. A:101A;886–3.

3. Martai V, Martin V, Carcia J, Guiteras P, Auge JM. Significance of angiographic coronary dissection after cutting balloon angioplasty. Am J Cardiol. 1998; 81:1349–52.

4. Mainar V, Auge JM, Dominguez J et al. Randomised comparison of cutting balloon vs conventional balloon angioplasty: final report and the in-hospital results of the CUBA study. Circulation 1997; 96(8) Suppl.:1526–7.

5. Mauri L, Bonan R, Weiner BH, Legrand V, Bassand JP, Popma JJ, Niemyski P, Prpic R, Ho KK, Chauhan MS, Cutlip DE, Bertrand OF, Kuntz RE. Cutting balloon angioplasty for the prevention of restenosis: results of the Cutting Balloon Global Randomized Trial. Am J Cardiol. 2002; 90:107–983.

6. Izumi M, Tsuchikane E, Fumamoto F et al. One year clinical and 3-month angiographic follow-up of cutting balloon angioplasty versus plain old balloon angioplasty randomised study in small coronary artery (CAPAS). JACC 1999; 33(2) Suppl. A:47;810–15.

7. Ergene O, Seyithanogula BY, Tastan A et al. Comparison of angiographic and clinical outcome after cutting balloon and conventional balloon angioplasty in vessels smaller than 3 mm in diameter: a randomized trial. J Invasive Cardiol. 1998; 10:70–5.

8. Iijima R, Ikari Y, Wada M, Shiba M, Nakamura M, Hara K. Cutting balloon angioplasty is superior to balloon angioplasty or stent implantation for small coronary artery disease. Coron Artery Dis. 2004(7):435–40.

9. Topol EJ, Ellis SG, Fishman J, Leimgruber P, Myler RK, Stertzer SH, O'Neill WW, Douglas JS, Roubin GS, King SB 3rd. Multicenter study of percutaneous transluminal angioplasty for right coronary artery ostial stenosis. J Am Coll Cardiol. 1987 Jun; 9(6):1214–18.

10. Muramatsu T, Tsukahara R, Ho M et al. Efficacy of cutting balloon angioplasty for lesions at the ostium of the coronary arteries. J Invas Cardiol. 1999; 11:201–6.

11. Kurbaan AS, Kelly PA, Sigwart U. Cutting balloon angioplasty and stenting for aorto-ostial lesions. Heart. 1997 Apr; 77(4):350–2.

12. Chung CM, Nakamura S, Tanaka K, Tanigawa J, Kitano K, Akiyama T, Matoba Y, Katoh O. Comparison of cutting balloon vs stenting alone in small branch ostial lesions of native coronary arteries. Circ J. 2003 Jan; 67(1):21–5.

13. Ge L, Airoldi F, Iakovou I, Cosgrave J, Michev I, Sangiorgi GM, Montorfano M, Chieffo A, Carlino M, Corvaja N, Colombo A. Clinical and angiographic outcome after implantation of drug-eluting stents in bifurcation lesions with the crush stent technique: importance of final kissing balloon post-dilation. J Am Coll Cardiol. 2005 Aug 16; 46(4):613–20.

14. Baim DS, Levine MJ, Leon MB, Levine S, Ellis SG, Schatz RA. Management of restenosis within the Palmaz-Schatz coronary stent (the U.S. multicenter experience. The U.S. Palmaz-Schatz Stent Investigators. Am J Cardiol. 1993 Feb 1; 71(4):364–6.

15. Almeda FQ, Klein LW. Cutting balloon angioplasty: to cut is to cure? J Invasive Cardiol. 2002 Dec; 14(12):725–7.

16. vom Dahl J, Dietz U, Haager PK, Silber S, Niccoli L, Buettner HJ, Schiele F, Thomas M, Commeau P, Ramsdale DR, Garcia E, Hamm CW, Hoffmann R, Reineke T, Klues HG. Rotational atherectomy does not reduce recurrent in-stent restenosis: results of the angioplasty versus rotational atherectomy for treatment of diffuse in-stent restenosis trial (ARTIST). Circulation. 2002 Feb 5; 105(5):583–8.

17. Mehran R, Mintz GS, Popma JJ, Pichard AD, Satler LF, Kent KM, Griffin J, Leon MB.Mechanisms and results of balloon angioplasty for the treatment of in-stent restenosis. Am J Cardiol. 1996 Sep 15; 78(6):618–22.

18. Muramatsu T, Tsukahara R, Ho M, Ito Y, Hirano K, Ishimori H, Matushita M, Nakano M. Efficacy of cutting balloon angioplasty for in-stent restenosis: an intravascular ultrasound evaluation. J Invasive Cardiol. 2001 Jun; 13(6):439–44.

19. Adamian MG, Marisco F, Brigouri C et al. Cutting balloon treatment for in stent restenosis, a matched comparison with conventional angioplasty and rotational atherectomy. Circulation. 1999; 100:1–305.

20. Nakamura M, Anzai H, Asahara T et al. Cutting balloon angioplasty for stent restenosis. Jpn J Intero Cardiol. 1999; 14:15–20.

21. Albiero R, Silber S, Di Mario C, Cernigliaro C, Battaglia S, Reimers B, Frasheri A, Klauss V, Auge JM, Rubartelli P, Morice MC, Cremonesi A, Schofer J, Bortone A, Colombo A; RESCUT Investigators.Cutting balloon versus conventional balloon angioplasty for the treatment of in-stent restenosis: results of the restenosis cutting balloon evaluation trial (RESCUT). J Am Coll Cardiol. 2004 Mar 17; 43(6):943–9.

22. Schluter M, Tubler T, Lansky AJ, Kahler S, Berger J, Mathey DG, Schofer J. Angiographic and clinical outcomes at 8 months of cutting balloon angioplasty and beta-brachytherapy for native vessel in-stent restenosis (BETACUT): Results from a stopped randomized controlled trial. Catheter Cardiovasc Interv. 2005 Oct 7; 66(3):320–6.

23. Sousa JE, Costa MA, Abizaid A, Sousa AG, Feres F, Mattos LA, Centemero M, Maldonado G, Abizaid AS, Pinto I et al. Sirolimus-eluting stent for the treatment of in-stent restenosis: a quantitative coronary angiography and three-dimensional intravascular ultrasound study. Circulation. 2003; 107:24–27.

24. Degertekin M, Lemos PA, Lee CH, Tanabe K, Sousa JE, Abizaid A, Regar E, Sianos G, van der Giessen WJ, de Feyter PJ et al. Intravascular ultrasound evaluation after sirolimus

eluting stent implantation for de novo and in-stent restenosis lesions. Eur Heart J. 2004; 25:32–8.

25. Airoldi F, Rogacka R, Briguori C, Chieffo A, Carlino M, Montorfano M, Mikhail G, Iakovou I, Michev I, Vitrella G, Albiero R, Colombo A. Comparison of clinical and angiographic outcome of sirolimus-eluting stent implantation versus cutting balloon angioplasty for coronary in-stent restenosis. Am J Cardiol. 2004; 94(10):1297–300.

26. Takebayashi H, Kobayashi Y, Mintz GS, Carlier SG, Fujii K, Yasuda T, Moussa I, Mehran R, Dangas GD, Collins MB *et al.* Intravascular ultrasound assessment of lesions with target vessel failure after siroli-mus eluting stent implantation. Am J Cardiol 2005; 95: 498–502.

27 Ozaki Y, Yamaguchi T, Suzuki T, Nakamura M, Kitayama M, Nishikawa H, Inoue T, Hara K, Usuba F, Sakurada M, Awano K, Matsuo H, Ishiwata S, Yasukawa T, Ismail TF, Hishida H, Kato O. Impact of cutting balloon angioplasty (CBA) prior to bare metal stenting on restenosis. Circ J. 2007 Jan; 71(1):1–8.

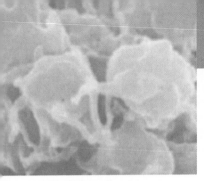

17

Intracoronary brachytherapy

PRAMOD KUCHULAKANTI, MD
AND RON WAKSMAN, MD

KEY POINTS

■ Coronary vascular brachytherapy (VBT), using beta and gamma emitters, has revolutionized the treatment of in-stent restenosis (ISR).

■ ISR continues to be a challenge to the interventional cardiology community, despite several advancements in stent technology, including DES.

■ VBT is the only Food and Drug administration (FDA) approved technology to treat ISR thus far.

INTRODUCTION TO RADIATION BIOLOGY AND SYSTEMS

Radiation inhibits smooth muscle cell (SMC) proliferation and intimal hyperplasia by intervening in the cell cycle to cause cell death to radiosensitive cells, especially those undergoing mitosis following vascular injury. Radiation acts by absorbing into the target molecules such as DNA, RNA, or enzymes, by interacting with these molecules via formation of highly reactive free radicals, or by inducing programmed cell death, called apoptosis. Radiation may reduce restenosis by inhibiting the first wave of cell proliferation in the adventitia and the media, by inducing favorable remodeling,[1] and by suppression of macrophages and adventitial myofibroblasts.[2,3]

Among several isotopes developed for the use in VBT, only the gamma emitter ^{192}Ir, beta emitters ^{90}Sr/^{90}Y, ^{32}P, ^{188}Rh, and ^{99}W found clinical application. The main platforms that deliver radiation are catheter-based systems such as line source wires, radioactive seeds, radioactive gas and liquid filled balloons, or stents. The latter are no longer used because they created the problem of narrowing at the ends of the stent – the 'candy-wrapper effect'.

^{192}Ir is administered by the CheckMate system (Cordis Corporation, Miami, FL), which requires manual loading of the radioactive seeds. The AngioRad system (Vascular Therapies, Norwalk, CT) uses a flexible, 30 mm ^{192}Ir wire source. The Galileo system (Guidant Corporation, Irvine, CA) administers ^{32}P with automated stepping technology and a centering balloon. The RDX system (Radiance Medical, San Diego, CA) also administers ^{32}P, however, the isotope is incorporated directly into the balloon material of the PTCA-type catheter. ^{90}Sr/Y is administered by BetaCath system (Novoste Corporation, Norcross, GA), which employs a hydraulic technique to deliver the radioactive seeds. ^{188}Re is obtained from the ^{188}W/^{188}Re radionuclide generator as a solution which is injected into the coronary dilatation balloon and can be applied at the target by inflating the balloon.

EXPERIMENTAL FOUNDATION OF BRACHYTHERAPY

Brachytherapy evolved into clinical practice based on firm and elaborate experimental animal data. These involved external beam radiation by Schwartz et al.,[4] catheter based systems by several investigators utilizing gamma radiation with [192]Ir (Waksman et al. at Emory University,[5,6] Wiedermann et al. at Columbia University,[7,8] and Raizner et al. at Baylor University[9]), using beta radiation with ^{90}Sr/Y (Verin et al.[11], Waksman[12]), and beta radiation with ^{32}P by Raizner et al. All these investigators have shown reduction in neointimal hyperplasia in the irradiated arteries utilizing doses ranging from 6-56 Gy.

Further experiments have been conducted using radioactive stents by Fischell et al.[13] Hehrlein et al.,[14,15] Laird et al.[16,17] Radioactive stents, which were implanted in an atherosclerotic pig model, failed to show superiority over control non-radioactive stents with any of the treated doses at six months.[17]

Waksman et al.,[18] Weinberger et al.,[19] Robinson et al.,[20] Makkar et al.,[21] and Kim et al.[22] used liquid isotope-filled balloons to irradiate porcine coronaries. The emitters used for this technology were [133]Xenon, [188]Re (14 Gy), and [166]Ho (9, 18 Gy). These pre-clinical studies showed reduction in neointimal tissue as assessed by IVUS and histomorphometry. The concept of the radioisotope filled balloons is attractive because it has the advantages of centering and ease of use; however, a potential leakage hazard is of great concern.

Long-term animal studies utilizing beta and gamma emitter sources were disappointing Although salutary effects were reported by Wiedermann and Waksman in six-month studies utilizing gamma and beta radiation, data with beta emitters (^{32}P and ^{90}Sr/Y) were associated with increased mortality, thrombosis, and neointima formation compared to control. Few of the observations in long-term animal studies are reproduced in humans such as late thrombosis, delayed restenosis, and inferior results with additional stenting. The discrepancy between the long-term animal results and the human results at 3–5 years follow up can be explained by the differences in the species, normal porcine coronary artery versus atherosclerotic human coronary artery, and the age of the animals.

CLINICAL TRIALS

Several series of clinical trials were conducted to understand the safety, efficacy, and durability of VBT mainly in the US and Europe. While both gamma and beta radiations were studied for the treatment of ISR, only beta sources were studied for de novo lesions. Detailed discussion of the clinical trials is out of scope for this chapter, but a brief summary of the landmark clinical trials conducted thus far with gamma and beta emitters is presented. Salient features of the studies published in major journals are shown in Table 17.1.

Clinical trials of gamma radiation

The first study of intracoronary radiation in human coronary arteries was conducted in 1994 by Condado et al. in which 21 patients (22 lesions – two-thirds being de novo lesions) were treated with ^{192}Ir after routine balloon angioplasty. On angiographic follow up at six months, a binary restenosis rate of 28.6% was

TABLE 17.1 - RESULTS OF MAJOR CLINICAL TRIALS WITH GAMMA AND BETA RADIATION PUBLISHED IN PEER REVIEWED JOURNALS, ARRANGED IN CHRONOLOGICAL ORDER

STUDY NAME	NO. OF PTS (RADIATION)	YEAR	ISOTOPE	DOSE (GY)	IN-STENT LATE LOSS (MM)	IN-STENT RESTENOSIS (%)	TLR (%)	TVR (%)	MACE (%)
Gamma Radiation Studies									
SCRIPPS	55 (26)	1997	^{192}Ir	≥8–<30	0.38±1.06	8.3	12	n/a	15
WRIST	130 (65)	2000	^{192}Ir	15–18	0.22±0.84	19	13.8	26	29
GAMMA-1	252 (131)	2001	^{192}Ir	≥8–<30	0.73±0.79	21.6	24.4	31.3	28.2
ARTISTIC	26 (26)	2001	^{192}Ir	12–18	n/a	19	7.6	n/a	15
WRIST PLUS	120 (120)	2001	^{192}Ir	14	0.58±0.57	26	20.8	23.3	23.3
SVG WRIST	120 (60)	2002	^{192}Ir	15–18	0.23±0.75	15	17	28	32
WRIST 12	120 (120)	2002	^{192}Ir	14	n/a	n/a	12.6	14.3	13.4
LONG WRIST	120 (120)	2003	^{192}Ir	15	0.67±0.88	34	39	n/a	42
LONG WRIST	120 (120)	2003	^{192}Ir	18 (*)	0.48±0.88	25	19.6	n/a	21.7
High Dose					0.27±0.74	23	19.6	n/a	19.6
WRIST 21	47 (47)	2005	^{192}Ir	21	0.33 ± 0.7	17.4	15.2	28.3	28.3
Beta Radiation Studies									
BERT	23 (23)	1998		12–16	0.005	10	8.6	13	13
Beta WRIST	50 (50)	2000	^{90}Y	20.6	0.37±0.8	22	28	34	34
PREVENT	105 (80)	2000	^{32}P	16–24	0.2±0.6	8	6	21	26
4R	50 (50)	2001	^{188}Rh	15	0.37±0.65	10.4	–	–	2
Dose Finding Study Group	183 (181)	2001	^{90}Y	9	0.37±0.7	28.6	–	13.3	13.3
				12	0.25±0.1	21.4	–	8.8	11.1
				15	0.21±0.09	15.9	–	10.8	10.8
				18	0.18±0.12	15	–	11.1	15.5
START	476 (244)	2002	^{90}Sr/^{90}Y	18–23	0.21±0.61	14.2	13.9	17	19.1
INHIBIT	332 (166)	2002	^{32}P	20	0.41±69	34	8	19	21
BRITE I	32 (32)	2002	^{32}P	20	-0.005±0.41	0	3	3	3
BRIE	149 (149)	2002	^{32}P	14–18	0.26	9.9	n/a	15.4	28.2

TABLE 1 - RESULTS OF MAJOR CLINICAL TRIALS WITH GAMMA AND BETA RADIATION PUBLISHED IN PEER REVIEWED JOURNALS, ARRANGED IN CHRONOLOGICAL ORDER

STUDY NAME	NO. OF PTS (RADIATION)	YEAR	ISOTOPE	DOSE (GY)	IN-STENT LATE LOSS (MM)	IN-STENT RESTENOSIS (%)	TLR (%)	TVR (%)	MACE (%)
SVG BRITE	49 (49)	2003	^{32}P	20 (**)	n/a	11.8	4.2	8.3	12.5
					n/a	25	36	36	48
ECRIS	225 (113)	2003	^{188}Rh	22.5	0.11±0.54	6.3	1.8	8	14.2
RENO	1098 (1098)	2003	^{90}Sr/^{90}Y	16–25	n/a	24.5	–	7.6	18.7
BRIDGE	112 (54)	2004	^{32}P	20	0.43±0.75	12.7	3.7	11.1	25.9
Tungsten WRIST	30 (30)	2004	^{199}W	18–25	0.14±0.88	11	13	23	23

*upper row – patients with onr month dual antiplatelet therapy and lower row with six months therapy

** upper row de novo lesions and lower row with ISR lesions

reported,[23] which remained the same at five years. Angiographic complications included four aneurysms (two procedure related and two occurring within three months). At three and five years, all aneurysms except one remained unchanged and no other angiographic complications were observed.[24]

Gamma radiation for in-stent restenosis

The efficacy of ^{192}Ir in reducing clinical and angiographic restenosis in patients with in-stent restenosis was confirmed by a number of studies, including two single-center trials, SCRIPPS and WRIST; and multicenter trials, GAMMA-1 and -2; and ARTISTIC.

SCRIPPS trials Scripps Coronary Radiation to Inhibit Proliferation Post-Stenting (SCRIPPS) was the first randomized trial to evaluate the safety and efficacy of intracoronary γ radiation as adjunctive therapy to stents. Follow up at six months and three years showed significantly lower restenosis rates in the ^{192}Ir group – 17% and 33%, respectively, compared to placebo (54% and 63%). A subgroup analysis of the 35 patients enrolled due to ISR showed a 70% reduction in the recurrence rate in the irradiated group compared to placebo.[25,26] There were no evident clinical complications resulting from the radiation treatment, and clinical benefits were maintained at five years, with a significant reduction in the need for target lesion revascularization (TLR).[27]

SCRIPPS II for ISR in diffuse lesions (30–80 mm), SCRIPPS III with prolonged antiplatelet therapy (6–12 months of Plavix®), and SCRIPPS IV to evaluate higher doses (17 Gy versus 14 Gy) followed the original SCRIPPS study and have shown, respectively, that radiation is effective for diffuse lesions, that prolonged platelet therapy reduces late thrombosis and additional stenting is to be avoided, and that optimization of radiation dose improves the outcomes further in diffuse lesions.

Washington Radiation for In-Stent restenosis Trial (WRIST) series Original WRIST was the first study to evaluate the effectiveness of radiation therapy in patients with ISR. In this study, 130 patients (100 with native coronaries and 30 with saphenous vein grafts) with ISR lesions (up to 47 mm in length) were randomized to receive either ^{192}Ir or placebo. At six months, the radiation group showed a reduction in restenosis (19% vs. 58% in placebo) and 79% and 63% reduction in the need for revascularization and MACE, respectively, compared to placebo.[28] Extended follow up of these patients showed durable beneficial effect of radiation at one year, three years[29] and five years[30] in MACE rates compared to placebo. MACE rates were significantly lower at five years follow up, albeit at the expense of repeat revascularization procedures suggesting that radiation may delay, in part, the biological processes and that a late catch-up phenomena or late thrombosis will reduce the long-term benefit of radiation.

Other landmark trials in this series were SVG-WRIST which evaluated the effect of radiation therapy in patients with diffuse ISR lesions in saphenous vein grafts,[31] Long WRIST in patients with diffuse ISR in native coronary arteries (lesion length 36 to 80 mm),[32] Long WRIST High Dose which tested the efficacy of an 18 Gy dose of radiation, WRIST Plus and WRIST 12 which tested the efficacy of prolonged Clopidogrel therapy (up to 6 months and 12 months, respectively) to reduce the incidence of late thrombosis, and WRIST 21 which tested whether escalation of radiation dose to 21 Gy would improve the clinical outcomes beyond Long WRIST High Dose. These studies have demonstrated superiority of radiation therapy in the treatment of ISR in vein graft disease (SVG-WRIST) and diffuse lesions (Long WRIST). The Long WRIST High Dose registry showed that a 3 Gy increase in the dose, from 15 to 18 Gy, provided additional reduction in MACE rates.[33] The strategy of prolonged antiplatelet therapy for six months in WRIST Plus reduced thrombosis rates from 9.6% to 2.5% – levels comparable to non-irradiated controls.[34] WRIST 12 has demonstrated further reduction in MACE and TLR with 12 months of Clopidogrel therapy.[35] Based on these observations, it has become standard practice to provide at least 12 months of Clopidogrel therapy for patients undergoing radiation therapy for ISR. Further escalation of dose from 18 Gy to 21 Gy was studied in WRIST 21 but has not been shown to improve the results. Hence, a dose of 18 Gy may be sufficient to treat ISR with γ radiation.

GAMMA trials GAMMA-1, a multicenter, randomized trial conducted with IVUS-guided dosimetry, showed significant reductions in the in-stent and in-lesion restenosis rates compared to 50.5% and 55.3% in the control group. The greatest benefit was obtained in patients with long lesions and/or diabetes. In this study, it was observed that the late thrombosis phenomenon was more frequent in patients treated with radiation therapy than with placebo (5.3% vs. 0.8%). All patients in the ^{192}Ir group who presented with late thrombosis had new stents placed within the in-stent target lesion at the time of the procedure.[36] This trial demonstrated the efficacy of intracoronary gamma radiation for the prevention of ISR recurrence, and increased awareness regarding the correlation between late thrombosis and an increased risk of myocardial infarction (MI).

Gamma-2, a registry of 125 patients including complex lesions such as calcific lesions requiring rotablation, used a fixed dose of 14 Gy at 2 mm from the center of the source and showed a reduction of 52% and 40% in in-stent and in-lesion restenosis, respectively, and a reduction of 48% and 36% in TLR rates and MACE rates, respectively.[37]

ARTISTIC I and II Angiorad Radiation Technology for In-Stent restenosis Trial In native Coronaries (ARTISTIC) examined the usage of the AngioRad system in patients with ISR in native coronary arteries. At three years, the cumulative MACE rate was 24.1% in placebo patients and 22.8% in the AngioRad group.[38] ARTISTIC II used the same system in 236 patients and tested the efficacy as measured by a composite clinical end-point at nine months after radiation. These results were compared to the historical control group of 104 patients from the ARTISTIC I and WRIST studies. The Kaplan-Meier estimate of freedom from target vessel failure (TVF) for the placebo group was 52% while in the irradiated group it was 85.5%.[39]

Clinical trials of beta radiation

Large-scale clinical studies testing the effectiveness of beta radiation for de novo, restenotic and ISR lesions, and vein grafts have paralleled the encouraging results of gamma radiation.

Beta Radiation for ISR

BETA WRIST In this study, beta radiation was shown to be effective in the treatment of ISR in 50 patients. These patients demonstrated a 58% reduction in the rate of TLR and a 53% reduction in TVR at six months compared to the historical control group of WRIST.[40] The clinical benefit was maintained at two-year follow up with a reduction in TLR (42 % vs. 66%), TVR (46% vs.72%), and MACE (46 % vs. 72%) compared to placebo. This study showed that the efficacy of beta and gamma emitters for the treatment of ISR appeared similar at longer-term follow up.

START and START 40/20 In the START (Stents And Radiation Therapy) Trial, 476 patients were randomized to either placebo or an active radiation train 30 mm in length using the BetaCath system.[41] Late thrombosis as a complication of brachytherapy was first recognized during this trial and antiplatelet therapy was prolonged to at least 90 days.

During multiple studies of radiation, including START, the medical community became aware of the mismatch between the interventional injury length and radiation length – the so-called 'geographic miss' phenomenon – with the potential to compromise clinical outcome.[42]

To verify the benefits of extending the radiation margins by 10 mm (5 mm at each end) to ensure coverage of injured segment, START 40/20, a 207-patient registry that mirrored START was conducted. Compared to the control arm of START, patients in START 40/20 had a reduction of 44% in restenosis in the analysis segment, 50% reduction in TLR, 34% reduction in TVR, and 26% reduction in MACE. This registry demonstrated no deleterious effects of adding 10 mm of length to the source train, but there was a lack of a relationship between 'geographic miss' and clinical or angiographic outcomes for ISR.

INHIBIT and GALILEO INHIBIT INHIBIT (Intimal Hyperplasia Inhibition with Beta In-stent Trial) examined the efficacy of the Galileo system for the treatment of ISR in 332 patients.[43]

At nine months, treatment with ^{32}P reduced binary restenosis by 67% and 50% in the stented and analysis segments, respectively. There were no differences in the edge effect rates between the active and control-treated groups.

At nine months, ^{32}P significantly reduced rates of TLR and MACE. Tandem positioning to cover diffuse lesions >22 mm with ^{32}P was safe and effective. Galileo INHIBIT was an international, multicentered registry of 120 patients with ISR in which ^{32}P was delivered at 20 Gy at 1 mm into the vessel wall. There was a reduction in the primary clinical end point defined as MACE-TLR by 49% and reduction in angiographic endpoint of binary restenosis by 74% in the stented segment and by 27% in the analysis segment.[44] The thrombosis rate was low, 1.5%, and similar to the control group, 1.2%.

Balloon catheter-based beta radiation Trials for ISR

BRITE, BRITE-II, 4R, and CURE Beta radiation using the Radiance system was administered in 32 patients in the feasibility study called BRITE (Beta Radiation to prevent In-sTent rEstenosis). Seventy percent of the dose was administered when the balloon was inflated. At six months, TVR (3%), MACE (3%), and in-stent binary restenosis rates (0%) were the lowest reported to-date in any vascular brachytherapy series.[45] The BRITE II study evaluated the efficacy of beta radiation using the RDX system in 429 patients randomized to either radiation (n=321) or placebo (n=108).The RDX system demonstrated safety characterized by high technical success rates (>95%), low periprocedural complications (<1%), and low 30-day MACE (<1%). The most prevalent location of restenosis was within the radiated vessel outside the injured zone despite lower rates of geographic miss (8.5%).[46] The RDX system demonstrated a very low ISR rate (10. 9% vs. 46.1%) and proved to optimize the results when compared to historical studies.

4R, a South Korean registry evaluated β-radiation therapy with ^{188}Re-MAG$_3$-filled balloon following rotational atherectomy for diffuse ISR in 50 patients. The mean dose was 15 Gy and the mean irradiation time was 201.8 ± 61.7 seconds. No adverse events occurred during the follow up period. The six-month binary angiographic restenosis rate was 10.4%. Two potential limitations of this technology included reduced dosing at the balloon margins (edge effect) and the risks of balloon rupture with radiation spill. In the event of balloon rupture using ^{188}Re, concomitant administration of potassium perchlorate may mitigate thyroid uptake.[47]

The Columbia University Restenosis Elimination (CURE) study evaluated liquid ^{188}Re injected into a perfusion balloon. Thirty patients were treated with balloon alone and 30 patients were stented (with subsequent ^{188}Re therapy). The delivered dose was 20 Gy to the balloon surface with a dwell time of 6.9 ± 2.2 minutes. At 12 months follow up in the first 37 patients, the rate of TLR-free survival was 75%.[48]

RENO and BRIE Registry Novoste (RENO) is a registry of 1098 consecutive patients using the Novoste BetaCath system. Six-month follow up data showed non-occlusive restenosis in 18.8% of patients, total occlusion in 5.7%, and a MACE rate of 18.7% (1.9% deaths from any cause, 2.6% from acute MI, 13.3% from TVR by PCI and 3.3% from TVR by CABG).[49] The Beta Radiation in Europe (BRIE) study evaluated the safety and efficacy of the BetaCath system in patients with up to two discrete lesions, de novo and restenotic, in different vessels. The binary in-stent restenosis was 9.9%, excluding total occlusions, was 4.9%.[50] This study highlights the full potential of brachytherapy, provided late total occlusions are minimized by prolonged antiplatelet therapy.

Tungsten WRIST In a feasibility study using Tungsten (^{199}W) wire dose range (18–25 Gy), in 30 patients with ISR in native coronaries, Waksman *et al.* have shown the safety and comparable results to other beta and gamma sources.[51]

Beta radiation for de novo lesions Several clinical studies were undertaken to test the effectiveness of beta radiation for de novo lesions concurrent to the trials of ISR. Important early studies included the Geneva trial,[52] the dose-finding study BERT (Beta Energy Restenosis Trial) which used ^{90}Y,[53] and the Proliferation REeduction with Vascular ENergy Trial (PREVENT)[54] that utilized ^{32}P.

BERT BERT was a feasibility study of 23 patients with de novo lesions using the Novoste system.[53] No complications or adverse events were noticed at 30 days and at nine months follow up. Three patients underwent repeat revascularization to the target lesion. The Canadian arm of this study included 30 patients, and at six months follow up, the angiographic restenosis rate was 10% with negative late loss and late loss index.[55] The European arm of BERT (BERT 1.5) was conducted at the Thoraxcenter in Rotterdam, The Netherlands in an additional 30 patients who were treated successfully with balloon angioplasty. Angiographic restenosis in this cohort was higher than reported in the US and Canadian trials. Overall, the restenosis rate based on 64 of the 80 patients in the BERT series is 17%, and the late loss and late loss indexes were below 5%. Over 50% of the patients had larger minimal lumen diameter (MLD) at follow up compared to control, and a sub study of IVUS demonstrated vessel remodeling at the irradiated site.[56]

PREVENT PREVENT was a randomized study of 105 patients with de novo (70%) or restenotic (30%) lesions. Angiographic restenosis at six months was 8.2% (target site) and 22.4% (target site plus adjacent segments) compared to 39.1% and 50.0% in the control group, respectively.[54] The one-year MACE (death, MI, and TLR) was less in radiation group though not statistically significant. The occurrence of MI due to thrombotic events after discharge occurred in seven patients who received radiation therapy and in none in the control group.

DOSE-FINDING STUDY GROUP This was the only study which tested optimization of dose in a randomized fashion to 9, 12, 15, and 18 Gy using Yttrium-90 in 183 patients. Stenting after radiation was required in 47% of patients because of residual stenosis or major dissection. At six-month angiographic follow up, a significant dose-dependent benefit was evident. Thrombosis or late occlusion of the target vessel occurred in 3.3% of patients who were treated with only balloon angioplasty and in 14.3% patients who received new stents. This study demonstrated a marked reduction in restenosis in non-stented arteries after administration of 18 Gy of beta radiation, especially in patients who underwent plain balloon angioplasty, suggesting that beta radiation therapy should be evaluated as an adjunctive to PTCA.[57]

BETA-CATH In this large randomized study, 1455 patients with sub optimal results after balloon angioplasty were treated with a stent and then assigned to ^{90}Sr/Y or placebo treatment.[58] In patients treated with balloon angioplasty alone, radiated patients (n=264) tended to have lower TVF (14.2%) compared to placebo patients (20.4%, n=240). In the 452 patients treated with extended antiplatelet therapy who received a new stent, there were no differences in the 240-day TVF rate. Comparison of placebo and radiation treatment from pooled PTCA and stent groups (antiplatelet therapy ≥60 days) showed similar eight-month TLR and TVF-MACE.

An interesting point in this study was the low TVF in the irradiated balloon-only group. This was attributed to a reduction in angiographic restenosis within the initial lesion site in these patients (21.4% vs. 34.3% in placebo group), although the restenosis rates were similar in the analysis segment (treated segment + the radiation margins). The loss of benefit at the treatment margins is attributable to 'geographic miss' due to the relatively short treatment length in the study. This was the first to identify the higher-than-expected rate of late stent thrombosis when radiation was used with new stent implantation.

SVG BRITE This study examined the RDX system using a ^{32}P emitter at a dose of 20 Gy at 1 mm from the balloon surface in saphenous vein grafts of 49 patients; 24 of whom were treated for de novo lesions. New stents were implanted in most patients with de novo lesions. The outcome of the patients with de novo lesions was encouraging with only 8% TVR and 12% angiographic restenosis rate.[59]

ECRIS EndoCoronary-Rhenium-Irradiation-Study (ECRIS) was a randomized trial in which 225 patients (71% de novo lesions) were randomly assigned to receive β-irradiation using ^{188}Re-filled balloon catheter or no additional intervention. Clinical and procedural data did not differ between the groups except that there was a higher rate of stenting in the control group (63%) compared with the rhenium-188 group (45%). After six months of follow up, late loss was significantly lower in the irradiated group compared with the control group, both of the target lesion (0.11±0.54 versus 0.69±0.81 mm) and of the total segment (0.22±0.67 versus 0.70±0.82 mm). This was also evident in the subgroup of patients with de novo lesions and independent from stenting. Binary restenosis rates and TVR were significantly lower after rhenium-188 brachytherapy compared with the control group.[60]

BRIDGE The BRIDGE study is a multicenter, randomized, controlled trial of 112 patients which evaluated the acute and long-term efficacy of intravascular brachytherapy with ^{32}P (20 Gy at 1 mm in the coronary wall) immediately following direct stenting in de novo lesions. TVR and MACE rates at one year in the irradiated group (20.4% and 25.9%, respectively) were higher than in the control group (12.1% and 17.2%, respectively).[61]

Clinical trials with radioactive emitting stents In contrast to brachytherapy using removable sources, radioactive stents (permanent implants) have beta emitting atoms (^{32}P) on the stent surface and emit beta particles that are absorbed by neointimal tissue to a depth of 1–2 mm into the vessel wall over longer periods of time. The first clinical trials included IRIS, the Milan dose-finding study, and the Vienna experience. In IRIS (Isostent for Restenosis

Intervention Study) pilot trials, ^{32}P radioactive Palmaz-Schatz stents were developed with varying radioactivities and were implanted with a high rate of technical success but limited by an angiographic restenosis rate (stent and edges) of 40% at six months follow up.[62] The Milan dose-finding study showed that activities >3 µCi (^{32}P stents 0.75–12 µCi) profoundly inhibited intimal hyperplasia, however restenosis still occurred in >40% of lesions at the stent edges, that is, the 'candy wrapper' effect.[63,64] These findings were replicated in the Vienna study using high activity (6–21 µCi) stents.[65] An effort to circumvent edge restenosis by 'hot' and 'cold' end stents failed to prevent edge effect with an angiographic restenosis rate of 33% in 56 implanted stents.[66] In summary, while radioactive stents effectively inhibit intrastent neointimal hyperplasia, the problem of edge restenosis has not been solved with either less aggressive stent implantation or modification of the stent ends. Currently there is no indication for their clinical use.

Beta versus gamma brachytherapy While contemporaneous clinical trials to-date have demonstrated comparability of clinical efficacy of beta and gamma brachytherapy,[67] beta systems have several inherent advantages, such as reduced radiation exposure to operators and catheterization laboratory personnel, less shielding requirements, and easier handling of sources that have lead to more widespread acceptance of this technology. Potential limitations of beta sources in larger vessels (for example, vein grafts, peripheral arteries and renal access grafts) may be offset by the use of sources with higher activity, centering mechanisms, and appropriately longer dwell times.

Limitations to brachytherapy Although clinical trials using vascular brachytherapy for both coronary and peripheral applications have demonstrated positive results in reducing restenosis rates, these trials have also identified two major complications related to the technology – late thrombosis and edge stenosis. Late thrombosis is probably due to the delay in healing associated with radiation. It has been estimated that late thrombosis can be remedied through prolonged administration of antiplatelet therapy following intervention. The main explanation for the occurrence of edge effect is a combination of low dose at the edges of the radiation source and an injury created by the device for intervention, which is not covered by the radiation source. It is shown that wider margins of radiation treatment to the intervening segment significantly reduce the edge effect.

Peripheral brachytherapy Since the manifestation of coronary atherosclerosis and peripheral artery disease is primarily evident in older patient populations, and because patients in the baby boomer generation are nearing their 60s, the full impact of peripheral and coronary atherosclerosis in the US is upon us. Whereas coronary vascular procedures increase at a rate of 8% per year, there is greater growth in the frequency of peripheral procedures, estimated at 19% per year.

Restenosis in the peripheral arterial system Restenosis following PTA is mainly seen in small and medium peripheral arteries, such as the saphenous femoral-popliteal arteries (SFA) and renal arteries, with diffuse atherosclerotic disease. The mechanisms for a high rate of recurrence after intervention in the peripheral arterial system (PAS) are mainly attributed to exuberant healing response with smooth muscle proliferation,[68,69] early and late recoil after balloon angioplasty,[70,71] mechanical problems with stents, such as stent fractures and crushing, in-stent restenosis, and aggressive progression of the atherosclerotic disease.

Radiation systems for the peripheral vascular system   The vessel size of the PAS favored the use of gamma radiation due to the penetration characteristics of the emitter. The majority of investigational work performed in the PAS used Ir-192 in doses of 14–18 Gy prescribed at 2 mm from the source center. Several radiation systems for peripheral endovascular brachytherapy have been suggested and are under development and testing.

External radiation   External beam radiation is a viable option for the treatment of peripheral vessels. It allows a homogenous dose distribution with the possibility of fractionation.

External radiation is currently used in a few centers for the treatment of in-stent restenosis of the SFA. Preliminary reports are encouraging, although caution should be applied to this strategy because of the potential for radiation injury to the nerve, vein, and the skin. Preliminary attempts with external radiation for the treatment of AV dialysis grafts failed to reduce the restenosis rate. This unsuccessful attempt was attributed to the conservative use of low doses and thrombosis of these grafts. Using sterotactic techniques to localize the radiation to the target area may improve the results of this approach.

Catheter-based gamma systems   The most common catheter-based system used for SFA application is the MicroSelectron HDR system (Nucletron-Odelft, Delft, The Netherlands), which uses a computerized, high-dose rate afterloader system that delivers a 3 mm stepping, 10 Ci activity of Ir-192 into a closed-lumen radiation catheter. The Peripheral Brachytherapy Centering Catheter (Paris, Guidant Corporation, Indianapolis, IN) is a 7 F, double-lumen catheter with multiple centering balloons near its distal tip that enable the catheter to be in the center of the lumen of large peripheral vessels during inflation. The Paris catheter is no longer available. The only closed-end lumen catheter available is the one used for oncology applications.

Catheter-based beta systems   The only catheter-based beta system available is the BetaCath system, with a source train of up to 60 mm, which can be pulled back to allow coverage of long lesions. The main limitation of the system is the penetration of the beta emitter, which is weakened significantly beyond 5 mm. This system can be used for below-the-knee applications or for other small vessels, including in-stent renal stenosis. It is recommended to perform the radiation prior to the intervention to ensure better centering and a higher dose to the treated proliferating tissue.

Clinical trials

Superficial femoral artery Liermann and Schopohl were the first to perform VBT for the treatment of in-stent restenosis in the peripheral arteries. Known as the Frankfurt Experience, this pilot study was conducted in 30 patients with ISR in their SFAs.[72–75] Patients underwent atherectomy and PTA followed by endovascular radiation using the MicroSelectron HDR afterloader and a noncentering catheter with Ir-192. No adverse effects from the radiation treatment were reported at up to seven-year follow up. The five-year patency rate of the target vessel was 82%, with only 11% stenosis within the treated segment reported. Late total occlusion developed in 7% of the treated vessels after 37 months.

The Vienna experience A series of studies was conducted at the University of Vienna. The majority were randomized studies targeting the SFA with or without stents using the MicroSelectron HDR afterloader with or without a centering catheter utilizing different doses.

Vienna I was a pilot study with an indication of radiation safety after PTA that showed only 60% patency at one year.[76] The Vienna II trial had 113 patients with de novo or recurrent femoropopliteal lesions who were randomized to PTA + brachytherapy (n=57) or PTA alone (n=56). The primary end point of cumulative patency rates at 12-month follow up was higher in the PTA + brachytherapy group (63.6%) compared to the PTA group (35.3%). The patients from this study were followed-up to 36 months and demonstrated durability of the results.[77] In Vienna III, a centering catheter that was used for the same patient population with a dose of 18 Gy showed a restenosis rate of 23.4% in the irradiated group compared to 53.3% in the placebo arm.[78] Vienna IV was a pilot study examining radiation with stenting of the SFA; and Vienna V was a randomized study for similar indications. Both Vienna IV and V demonstrated an increase rate of subacute and late thrombosis when stents were combined with radiation, with up to 16.7% in the radiation group versus 4.3% in the control stenting without radiation. Once thrombosis was controlled, the radiation group had less restenosis.[79]

The PARIS trials The Paris Radiation Investigational Study (PARIS) is the first FDA-approved, multicenter, randomized, double-blind, control study involving 300 patients following PTA to SFA stenosis using a gamma radiation [192]-Ir source. Utilizing the MicroSelectron HDR afterloader, a treatment dose of 14 Gy is delivered via a centered segmented end-lumen balloon catheter. The primary objectives of this study are to determine angiographic evidence of patency and a reduction of >30% of the restenosis rate of the treated lesion at six months. A secondary endpoint is to determine the clinical patency at 6 and 12 months by treadmill exercise and by the ankle-brachial index (ABI). In the feasibility phase of PARIS, 40 patients with claudication were enrolled. The mean lesion length was 9.9±3.0 cm with a mean reference vessel diameter of 5.4±0.5 mm. The six-month angiographic follow up was completed on 30 patients; 13.3% of them had evidence of clinical restenosis.[80]

Due to poor enrolment, only 203 patients with claudication and femoropopliteal disease were enrolled in the study. After successful PTA, a segmented centering balloon catheter was positioned to cover the PTA site. The patients were transported to the radiation oncology suite and randomized to receive either radiation therapy using the MicroSelectron HDR afterloader with Ir-192 at a dose of 14 Gy at 2 mm into the vessel wall (105 patients), or treatment with a sham control in 98 patients. Patients were followed for 12 months, with clinic visits at 1, 6, and 12 months and follow up angiography at 12 months. The restenosis rate at follow up was similar in both groups (28.6% brachytherapy vs. 27.5% placebo). There was no significant difference in MLD, late loss, or the number of total occlusions. Exercise ABI, resting ABI, and maximum walking time were not different between treatment groups. For patients older than 65 years, maximum walking times at 6 and 12 months were better in the brachytherapy group. In the subgroups of patients with diabetes, male patients, or patients receiving Clopidogrel or who have a proximal/medial lesion, maximum walking time in the brachytherapy group was better than in the placebo at 6 months but not different at 12 months.

More studies to support the effectiveness of gamma radiation for in-stent restenosis were recently published by Krueger et al.[81] In this study, 30 patients who underwent PTA for de novo femoropopliteal stenoses were randomly assigned to undergo 14 Gy centered endovascular irradiation (irradiation group, n=15) or no irradiation (control group, n=15). Intra-arterial angiography was performed 6, 12, and 24 months after treatment; and duplex ultrasonography was performed the day before and after PTA and at 1, 3, 6, 9, 12, 18, and 24 months later. Baseline characteristics did not differ significantly between the two groups. Mean absolute individual changes in degree of stenosis, compared with the degrees of stenosis shortly after PTA in the irradiation group versus in the control group were $10.6\% \pm 22.3$ versus $39.6\% \pm 24.6$ ($P < .001$) at 6 months, $2.0\% \pm 34.2$ versus $40.6\% \pm 32.6$ ($P = .002$) at 12 months, and $7.4\% \pm 43.2$ versus $37.7\% \pm 34.5$ ($p = .043$) at 24 months. The rates of target lesion restenosis at six months ($p=.006$) and 12 months ($p=.042$) were significantly lower in the irradiation group. The authors concluded that endovascular radiation was effective for patients who were treated with angioplasty for de novo femoropopliteal lesions.

Restenostic lesions and VBT   The effectiveness of VBT for restenotic SFA lesions was examined in another randomized study reported by Zehnder et al. In this study, gamma radiation was used at a dose of 12 Gy. The primary endpoint was >50% restenosis at 12 months assessed by duplex Doppler. The recurrence rate in the radiation arm was 23% versus 42% in the PTA alone group.[82] This study demonstrated that VBT can be effective in restenotic lesions.

Brachytherapy and Probucol   In another randomized four-arm study for patients with PTA lesions, patients were randomized to VBT, VBT and probucol, probucol alone, or placebo. The recurrence rate in the radiation arm alone was 17%, VBT and probucol was 20%, probucol alone was 27%, and the placebo group was 42%. This study confirms prior observations regarding the effectiveness of VBT for the treatment of SFA lesions without additional benefit of probucol when compared to PTA alone.[83]

Studies with Beta Radiation for SFA stenosis Two studies that utilized the Corona system were the MOBILE study that targeted in-stent restenosis lesions and the LIMBER (Limb Ischemia Treatment and Monitoring post Vascular Brachytherapy to prevent Restenosis) study.

Drug-eluting stents and brachytherapy

Evidence is favorable for the efficacy of DES to reduce restenosis in de novo lesions and experience is growing with other lesions including in-stent restenosis of BMS. In the randomized ISAR-DESIRE study, Kastrati *et al.* reported restenosis rates of 14.3% with sirolimus-eluting stents and 21.7% with paclitaxel-eluting stents.[84] Recent randomized and non randomized studies comparing vascular brachytherapy and DES confer that DES are showing similar safety and efficacy profile when compared to vascular brachytherapy. In the SISR trial there was reduction in target lesion revascularization in the DES group compared with VBT although this study borrowed patients from the historical Gamma 1 and Gamma 2 it appears that DES are effective as vascular brachytherapy even for diffuse ISR lesions.[85,86] Thus the role of vascular brachytherapy in the coronary arteries remained for the treatment of DES restenosis. The RESCUE (Radiation for drug Eluting Stent in Coronary FailUrE) study was an international registry of patients who present with ISR of a previously placed coronary DES and assigned to treatment with either beta or gamma radiation following PCI. Eight months follow up data in 61 patients showed 6 (10%) MACE and similar TLR and TVR.[87]

Although DES reduced significantly the rate of TLR in coronary arteries, recent series of more complex lesions and subset of patients reports restenosis rates of up to 10% with over 2 000 000 DES implanted annually. Thus we anticipate that nearly 100 000 patients will present with DES restenosis. The encouraging results from the RESCUE trial combined with evidence-based historical data from previous brachytherapy trials will keep this technology in vogue.

REFERENCES

1. Waksman R, Rodriquez JC, Robinson KA, *et al.* Effect of intravascular irradiation on cell proliferation, apoptosis and vascular remodeling after balloon overstretch injury of porcine coronary arteries. Circulation 1997; 96:1944–1952.

2. Rubin P, Williams JP, Riggs PN, *et al.* Cellular and molecular mechanisms of radiation inhibition of restenosis. Part I: role of the macrophage and platelet-derived growth factor. Int J Radiat Oncol Biol Phys 1998; 40:929–941.

3. Wang H, Griendling KK, Scott NA, *et al.* Intravascular radiation inhibits cell proliferation and vascular remodeling after angioplasty by increasing the expression of p21 in adventitial myofibroblasts. Circulation 1999; 100: I-700.

4. Schwartz RS, Koval TM, Edwards WD, *et al*. Effect of external beam irradiation on neointimal hyperplasia after experimental coronary artery injury. J Am Coll of Cardiol 1992; 19:1106–1113.

5. Waksman R, Robinson KA, Crocker IR, *et al*. Endovascular low-dose irradiation inhibits neointima formation after coronary artery balloon injury in swine. A possible role for radiation therapy in restenosis prevention. Circulation 1995; 91:1533–1539.

6. Waksman R, Robinson KA, Crocker IR, *et al*. Intracoronary radiation before stent implantation inhibits neointima formation in stented porcine coronary arteries. Circulation 1995; 92:1383–1386.

7. Wiedermann JG, Marboe C, Amols H, *et al*. Intracoronary irradiation markedly reduces restenosis after balloon angioplasty in a porcine model. J Am Coll Cardiol 1994; 23:1491–1498.

8. Wiedermann JG, Marboe C. Amols H, *et al*. Intracoronary irradiation markedly reduces neointimal proliferation after balloon angioplasty in swine: persistent benefit at 6-months follow up. J Am Coll Cardiol 1995; 25:1451–1456.

9. Mazur W, Ali MN, Khan MM, *et al*. High dose rate intracoronary radiation for inhibition of neointimal formation in the stented and balloon injured porcine models of restenosis: angiographic, morphometric and histopathological analyses. Int J Radiot Oncol Biol Phy 1996; 36:777–788.

10. Wiedermann JG, Leavy JA, Amols H, *et al*. Effects of high dose intracoronary irradiation on vasomotor function and smooth muscle histopathology. Am J Physiol 1994; 267 (Heart Circ Physiol.36):H125–132.

11. Verin V, Popowski Y, Urban P, *et al*. Intra-arterial beta irradiation prevents neointimal hyperplasia in a hypercholesterolemic rabbit restenosis model. Circulation 1995; 92:2284–2290.

12. Waksman R, Robinson KA, Crocker IR, *et al*. Intracoronary low-dose beta-irradiation inhibits neointima formation after coronary artery balloon injury in the swine restenosis model. Circulation 1995; 92:3025–3031.

13. Fischell TA, Kharma BK, Fischell DR, *et al*. Low dose beta particle emission from stent wire results in complete localized inhibition of smooth muscle cell proliferation. Circulation 1994; 90:2956–2963.

14. Hehrlein C, Kniser S, Kollum M, *et al*. Effects of very low dose endovascular irradiation via an activated guidewire on neointima formation after stent implantation. Circulation 1995; 92:I-69.

15. Hehrlein C, Gollan C, Donges K, *et al*. Low dose radioactive endovascular stent prevent smooth muscle cell proliferation and neointimal hyperplasia in rabbits. Circulation 1995; 92:1570–1575.

16. Laird JR, Carter AJ, Kufs WM, *et al*. Inhibition of neointimal proliferation with low-dose irradiation from a beta-particle-emitting stent. Circulation 1996; 93:529–536.

17. Carter AJ, Laird JR, Bailey LR, *et al*. Effects of endovascular radiation from a beta-particle-emitting stent in a porcine coronary restenosis model. A dose-response study. Circulation 1996; 94:2364–2368.

18. Waksman R, Chan RC, Vodovotz Y, *et al*. Radioactive 133-xenon gas-filled angioplasty balloon: A novel intracoronary radiation system to prevent restenosis. J Am Coll Cardiol 1998; 31:356A.

19. Weinberger J. Solution-applied beta emitting radioisotope (SABER) system: Handbook of Vascular Brachytherapy, 1st Ed, Waksman R, Serruys P, London, 1998, Martin Dunitz Ltd.

20. Robinson KA, Pipes DW, Bibber RV, *et al*. Dose response evaluation in balloon injured pig coronary arteries of a beta emitting [186]Re liquid filled balloon catheter system for endovascular brachytherapy. Advances in Cardiovascular Radiation Therapy II, Washington DC, 1998, March 8–10.

21. Makkar R, Whiting J, Li A, Cordero H, *et al*. A beta-emitting liquid isotope filled balloon markedly inhibits restenosis in stented porcine coronary arteries. J Am Coll Cardiol 1998; 31:350A.

22. Kim HS, Cho YS, Kim JS, *et al*. Effect of transcatheter endovascular holmium-166 irradiation on neointimal formation after balloon injury in porcine coronary artery. J Am Coll Cardiol 1998; 31:277A.

23. Condado JA, Waksman R, Gurdiel O, *et al*. Long-term angiographic and clinical outcome after percutaneous transluminal coronary angioplasty and intracoronary radiation therapy in humans. Circulation 1997; 96:727–732.

24. Condado JA, Waksman R, Saucedo JF, *et al*. Five-year clinical and angiographic follow up after intracoronary iridium-192 radiation therapy. Cardiovasc Radiat Med 2002; 3:74–81.

25. Teirstein PS, Massullo V, Jani S, *et al*. Catheter-based radiotherapy to inhibit restenosis after coronary stenting. N Engl J Med 1997; 336:1697–7703.

26. Teirstein PS, Massullo V, Jani S, *et al*. Two-year follow up after catheter-based radiotherapy to inhibit coronary restenosis Circulation 1999; 99:243–247.

27. Grise MA, Massullo V, Jani S, *et al*. Five-Year Clinical Follow Up After Intracoronary Radiation, Results of a Randomized Clinical Trial. Circulation 2002; 105:2737–2740.

28. Waksman R, White RL, Chan RC, *et al*. Intracoronary radiation therapy for patients with in-stent restenosis: 6-month follow up of a randomized clinical study. Circulation 1998; 98:17, I-651:3421.

29. Ajani AE, Waksman R, Sharma AK, *et al*. Three-year follow up after intracoronary gamma radiation therapy for in-stent restenosis. Original WRIST. Washington Radiation for In-Stent Restenosis Trial. Cardiovasc Radiat Med 2001; 2:200–204.

30. Waksman R, Ajani AE, White RL, *et al*. Five-Year Follow Up After Intracoronary Gamma Radiation Therapy for In-Stent Restenosis. Circulation 2004; 109:340–344.

31. Waksman R, Ajani AE, White RL, *et al*. Intravascular Gamma Radiation For In-Stent Restenosis In Saphenous-Vein Bypass Grafts. N Engl J Med 2002; 346:1194–1199.

32. Waksman R, Cheneau E, Ajani AE, *et al*. Intracoronary Radiation Therapy Improves the Clinical and Angiographic Outcomes of Diffuse In-Stent Restenotic Lesions Results of the Washington Radiation for In-Stent Restenosis Trial for Long Lesions (Long WRIST) Studies. Circulation 2003; 107:1744–1749.

33. Javed MH, Mintz GS, Waksman R, *et al.* Serial intravascular ultrasound assessment of the efficacy of intracoronary γ radiation therapy for preventing recurrence of very long, diffuse, in-stent restenosis lesions Circulation. 2000; 104:856–859.

34. Waksman R, Ajani AE, White RL, *et al.* Prolonged antiplatelet therapy to prevent late thrombosis after intracoronary gamma-radiation in patients with in-stent restenosis: Washington Radiation for In-Stent Restenosis Trial plus 6 months of clopidogrel (WRIST PLUS). Circulation 2001; 103:2332–2335.

35. Waksman R, Ajani AE, Pinnow E, *et al.* Twelve Versus Six Months of Clopidogrel to Reduce Major Cardiac Events in Patients Undergoing γ-Radiation Therapy for In-Stent Restenosis. Washington Radiation for In-Stent restenosis Trial (WRIST) 12 Versus WRIST PLUS. Circulation. 2002; 106:776–778.

36. Leon MB, Teirstein PS, Moses JW, *et al.* Localized intracoronary gamma-radiation therapy to inhibit the recurrence of restenosis after stenting. N Engl J Med 2001; 344:250–256.

36. Kim HS, Ajani AE, Waksman R. Vascular brachytherapy for in-stent restenosis. J Interv Cardiol 2000; 13:417–423.

37. Waksman R, Bhargava B, Chan RC, *et al.* Intracoronary radiation with gamma wire inhibits recurrent in-stent restenosis. Cardiovasc Radiat Med 2001; 2:63–68.

38. Kereikas DJ, Waksman R, Mehra A, *et al.* Multi-center experience with a novel Ir-192 vascular brachytherapy device for in-stent restenosis: final results of the AngioRad™ T radiation therapy for in-stent restenosis intracoronaries II (ARTISTIC II) trial. J Am Coll Cardiol 2003; 41:49A.

39. Waksman R, White RL, Chan RC, *et al.* Intracoronary beta radiation therapy inhibits recurrence of in-stent restenosis. Circulation 2000; 101:1895–1898.

40. Popma JJ, Suntharalingam M, Lansky AJ. Randomized trial of 90Sr/90Y beta-radiation versus placebo control for treatment of in-stent Restenosis Circulation 2002; 106:1090–1096.

41. Kim HS, Waksman R, Cottin Y, *et al.* Edge stenosis and geographical miss following intracoronary gamma radiation therapy for in-stent restenosis. J Am Coll Cardiol 2001; 15:1026–1030.

42. Waksman R, Raizner AE, Yeung AC, *et al.* Use of localized intracoronary beta radiation in treatment of in-stent restenosis: the INHIBIT randomized controlled trial. Lancet 2002; 359:551–557.

43. Waksman R on behalf of the Galileo INHIBIT and INHIBIT investigators. Manual stepping of 32P fl-emitter for diffuse in-stent restenosis lesions, tandem versus single position. Clinical and Angiographic Outcome from a Multicenter Randomized study. Presented at AHA 2001.

44. Waksman R, Buchbinder M, Reisman M, *et al.* Balloon-Based Radiation Therapy for Treatment of In-Stent Restenosis in Human Coronary Arteries: Results From the BRITE I Study. Cathet Cardiovascular Intervent 2002; 57:286–294.

45. Waksman R on behalf of the BRITE II investigators. Balloon based radiation for coronary in-stent restenosis: 9 months results from the BRITE II study. Presented at ACC 2003.

46. Park S-W, Kong M-K, Moon DH, *et al.* Treatment of diffuse in-stent restenosis with rotational atherectomy followed by radiation therapy with a rhenium-188-mercaptoacetyltriglycine-filled balloon. J Am Coll Cardiol 2001; 38:631–637.

47. Weinberger J, Giedd KN, Simon AD, et al. Radioactive beta-emitting solution filled balloon treatment prevents porcine coronary restenosis. Cardiovasc Radiat Med 1999; 1:252–256.

48. Urban P, Serruys P, Baumgart D, et al. A multicentre European registry of intraluminal coronary beta brachytherapy. Eur Heart J 2003; 24:604–612.

49. Serruys PW, Sianos G, van der Giessen W, et al. Intracoronary β-radiation to reduce restenosis after balloon angioplasty and stenting. The Beta Radiation in Europe (BRIE) Study. Eu Heart Journal 2002; 23:1351–1359.

50. Waksman R, Ajani AE, Dilcher CE, et al. Intracoronary Radiation Therapy Using a Novel Beta Emitter for In-Stent Restenosis: Tungsten WRIST. J Am Coll Cardiol. 2004; 43:A90.

51. Verin V, Urban P, Popowski Y, et al. Feasibility of intracoronary beta-irradiation to reduce restenosis after balloon angioplasty. A clinical pilot study. Circulation 1997; 95:1138–1144.

52. King SB III, Williams DO, Chougule P, et al. Endovascular beta-radiation to reduce restenosis after coronary balloon angioplasty. Results of the beta energy restenosis trial (BERT). Circulation 1998; 97:2025–2030.

53. Raizner AE, Oesterle SN, Waksman R, et al. Inhibition of restenosis with β-emitting radiotherapy report of the proliferation reduction with vascular energy trial (PREVENT) Circulation 2000; 102:951–958.

54. Bonan R, Arsenault A, Tardif JC, et al. Beta Energy Restenosis trials, Canadian Arm. Circulation 1997; 96: I-219.

55. Gijzel AL, Wardeh AJ, van der Giessen WJ, et al. B-energy to prevent restnosis: the Rotterdam contribution to the BERT 1.5 trial – 1 yr. Follow up. Eur Heart J 1999; 370 (abstract 1945).

56. Verin V, Popowski Y, deBruyne B, et al. Endoluminal beta-radiation therapy for the prevention of coronary restenosis after balloon angioplasty. N Engl J Med 2001; 344:243–249.

57. Results from Late-breaking clinical trails sessions at ACC 2001. J Am Coll Cardiol 2001; 38:595–612.

58. Stone GW, Mehran R, Midei M, et al. Usefulness of beta radiation for de novo and In-Stent restenotic lesions in saphenous vein grafts. J Am Coll Cardiol 2003; 92:312–314.

59. Höher M, Wöhrle J, Wohlfrom M, et al. Intracoronary _-Irradiation with a Rhenium-188–Filled Balloon Catheter A Randomized Trial in Patients with De Novo and Restenotic Lesions. Circulation 2003; 7:3022–3027.

60. Serruys PW, Wijns W, Sianos G, et al. Direct stenting versus direct stenting followed by centered beta-radiation with IVUS-guided dosimetry and long-term antiplatelet treatment; results of a randomized trial (the BRIDGE trial). J Am Coll Cardiol 2004; 44:528–537.

61. Moses J. IRIS trials low activity 32P stent. Advances in cardiovascular radiation therapy III, Washington DC 1999; 387–388 (abstract).

62. Albeiro R, Adamian M, Kobayashi N, et al. Short and intermediate -term results of (32) P radioactive beta emitting stent implantation in patients with coronary artery disease: The Milan Dose-Response Study. Circulation 2000; 101:18–26.

63. Albiero R, Nishida T, Adamian M, *et al*. Edge restenosis after implantation of high activity (32)P radioactive beta-emitting stents. Circulation 2000; 101:2454–2457.

64. Wexberg P, Siostrzonek P, Kirisits C, *et al*. High activity radioactive BX -stents for reduction of restenosis after coronary interventions: the Vienna P-32 dose response study. Circulation 1999; 100:I-156.

65. Wardeh A, Wijns W, Albiero R, *et al*. Angiographic follow up after 32-P beta emitting radioactive "cold ends" Isostent implantation. Results from Aalst, Milan and Rotterdam. Circulation 2000; 102: II-442 (abstract).

66. Shirai K, Lansky AJ, Mintz GS, *et al*. Comparison of the angiographic outcomes after beta versus gamma vascular brachytherapy for treatment of in-stent restenosis. Am J Cardiol. 2003; 92:1409–13.

67. Haude M, Erbel R, Issa H, *et al*. Quantitative analysis of elastic recoil after balloon angioplasty and after intracoronary implantation of balloon-expandable Palmaz-Schatz stents. J Am Coll Cardiol. 1993; 21:2634.

68. Consigny PM, Bilder GE. Expression and release of smooth muscle cell mitogens in arterial wall after balloon angioplasty. J Vasc Med Biol. 1993; 4:1–8.

69. Mintz GS, Popma JJ, Pichard AD, *et al*. Arterial remodeling after coronary angioplasty. A serial intravascular ultrasound study. Circulation. 1996; 94:35–43.

70. Isner JM. Vascular remodeling. Honey, I think I shrunk the artery. Circulation. 1994; 89:2937–2941.

71. Liermann DD, Bottcher HD, Kollath J, *et al*. Prophylactic endovascular radiotherapy to prevent intimal hyperplasia after stent implantation in femoropopliteal arteries. Cardiovasc Intervent Radiol. 1994; 17:12–16.

72. Bottcher HD, Schopohl B, Liermann D, *et al*. Endovascular irradiation–a new method to avoid recurrent stenosis after stent implantation in peripheral arteries: technique and preliminary results. Int J Rad Oncol Biol Phys. 1994; 29:183–186.

73. Liermann D, Kirchner J, Schopohl B, *et al*. Brachytherapy with iridium-192 HDR to prevent restenosis in peripheral arteries: an update. Herz. 1998; 23:394–400.

74. Sidawy AN, Weiswasse JM, Waksman R. Peripheral vascular brachytherapy. J Vasc Surg. 2002; 35:1041–1047.

75. Minar E, Pokrajac B, Ahmadi R, *et al*. Brachytherapy for prophylaxis of restenosis after long-segment femoropopliteal angioplasty: pilot study. Radiology. 1998; 208:173–179.

76. Minar E, Pokrajac B, Maca T, *et al*. Endovascular Brachytherapy for Prophylaxis of Restenosis After Femoropopliteal Angioplasty: Results of a Prospective Randomized Study. Circulation. 2000; 102:2694–2699.

77. Pokrajac B, Schmid R, Poetter R, *et al*. Endovascular brachytherapy prevents restenosis after femoropopliteal angioplasty: results of the Vienna-3 multicenter study. Int J Radiat Oncol Biol Phys. 2003; 57(suppl): S250.

78. Wolfram RM, Pokrajac B, Ahmadi R, *et al*. Endovascular brachytherapy for prophylaxis against restenosis after long-segment femoropopliteal placement of stents: initial results. Radiology. 2001; 220:724–729.

79. Waksman R, Laird JR, Jurkovitz CT, *et al*. Intravascular radiation therapy after balloon angioplasty of narrowed femoropopliteal arteries to prevent restenosis: results of the PARIS feasibility clinical trial. J Vasc Interv Radiol. 2001; 12:915–921.

80. Krueger K, Zaehringer M, Bendel M, *et al*. De novo femoropopliteal stenoses: endovascular gamma irradiation following angioplasty – angiographic and clinical follow up in a prospective randomized controlled trial. Radiology. 2004; 231:546–554.

81. Zehnder T, von Briel C, Baumgartner I, *et al*. Endovascular brachytherapy after percutaneous transluminal angioplasty of recurrent femoropopliteal obstructions. J Endovasc Ther. 2003; 2:304–311.

82. Greiner, Gallino, Mahler, *et al*. The effects of probucol and brachytherapy on restenosis after angioplasty of the femoropopliteal arteries a randomized multicenter trial. Submitted for publication 2004.

83. Kastrati A, Mehilli J, Beckerath N, *et al*. Sirolimus-Eluting Stent or Paclitaxel-Eluting Stent vs Balloon Angioplasty for Prevention of Recurrences in Patients With Coronary In-Stent Restenosis: A Randomized Controlled Trial. JAMA 2005: 293;165–171.

84. Werner GS, Emig U, Krack A, *et al*. Sirolimus-eluting stents for the prevention of restenosis in a worst-case scenario of diffuse and recurrent in-stent restenosis. Catheter Cardiovasc Interv 2004;63:259–64.

85. Iofina E, Haager PK, Radke PW, *et al*. Sirolimus- and paclitaxel-eluting stents in comparison with balloon angioplasty for treatment of in-stent restenosis. Catheter Cardiovasc Interv 2005; 64:28–34.

86. Kuchulakanti P, Torguson R, Canos D, *et al*. Optimizing Dosimetry with High Dose Intracoronary Gamma Radiation (21 Gy) for Patients with Diffuse In-Stent Restenosis Cardiovasc Revasc Med, 2005; 6:108–112.

87. Torguson R, Sabate M, Deible R, *et al*. Intravascular Brachytherapy versus drug eluting stents for the treatment of patients with DES Restenosis. Am J Cardiol. 2006; 98:1340–1344.

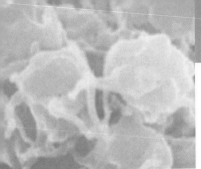

18

Laser use in percutaneous coronary intervention

SADIA KHAN AND PETER SCHOFIELD

KEY POINTS

- Laser guidewires have a limited application for interventional cardiology.

- Excimer laser catheters may be useful for treating coronary lesions which can be crossed with a guidewire but not with a balloon catheter.

- Laser balloon angioplasty may be useful for treating immediate vessel recoil or severe dissection. However, the introduction of coronary stents has essentially obviated the need for laser balloon angioplasty.

- Transmyocardial laser revascularisation (TMLR) improves symptoms and exercise capacity in patients with refractory angina who are not suitable for conventional revascularisation. The procedure, however, involves significant morbidity and mortality.

- Percutaneous myocardial revascularisation (PMR) is an effective treatment for patients with severe angina due to disease, which is not amenable to treatment, by angioplasty or bypass grafting. The periprocedural mortality and morbidity is less than TMLR.

INTRODUCTION

Laser is an acronym for 'light amplification by stimulated emission of radiation' and describes the process by which an intense monochromatic coherent light beam is produced. This beam can be delivered to a small area with great precision through fibreoptics allowing tissue to be ablated by a combination of mechanical and chemical methods. These properties suggest that lasers would find clinical application in some of the challenges of interventional cardiology such as guidewire passage through chronic occlusions, dissection following balloon angioplasty and restenosis. The ability to create channels in myocardium with great precision has also been used for myocardial laser revascularisation, both percutaneously and via thoracotomy, in patients with chronic refractory angina.

The presence of a chronic total coronary artery occlusion continues to be a major problem for interventional cardiology. Around 10% of all attempted coronary angioplasties are performed for chronic total coronary occlusion.[1] The procedural success rate is lower for patients with chronic total occlusions who undergo coronary angioplasty when compared with patients who have stenosed, but patent, vessels. Depending to some extent on the nature of the occlusion and its duration, the success rate is usually in the order of 50–70%[2,3] – this is clearly much lower than for stenosed vessels. Failure to treat a chronic total occlusion may be due to the inability to cross the lesion with a guidewire or to inability to advance the balloon catheter across the lesion once the wire has crossed successfully. When treating a chronic total occlusion, the conventional technique uses a stiff guidewire and advancement of the balloon catheter close to the tip of the guidewire for additional rigidity. A variety of technologies have been introduced without a major improvement in the success rates. These include guidewires with olive-shaped tips, drills of various velocities, radio frequency heat applicators and laser devices. Two laser technologies will be considered further: first the laser guidewires and second the over-the-wire Excimer laser catheter.

LASER GUIDEWIRES

An Argon laser heated balltip (hot tip) guidewire has been used for the initial passage through chronic total occlusions.[4] In some cases, it has been successful when conventional systems had failed. Vessel perforation is a possible complication of the technique. Further developments in hot tip recanalisation have not occurred and this technology is now rarely used.

The results of the bare Argon laser instrument Lastac are again comparable to those achieved with less costly mechanical means, although the cases undertaken may have been slightly more complex.[5] A beneficial mechanical component is undoubtedly present with these catheters, which have many of the features which may be useful when treating chronic total occlusions (e.g. stiffness, bluntness). Randomised prospective trials against conventional technologies have not been carried out and this equipment now has very limited application.

EXCIMER LASER CATHETER

Excimer laser coronary angioplasty may help to solve some of the problems associated with treating chronic total occlusions. The technique requires the passage of a guidewire through the lesion, which clearly is not always possible. Once the guidewire has been advanced to the distal vessel, the Excimer laser catheter can be used to ablate tissue.

The Excimer laser system can be used with over-the-wire multifibre catheters of different diameters. Generally, the larger the diameter of the vessel being treated, the larger the diameter of the laser catheter utilised. Once the occlusion has been crossed with a conventional guidewire, the laser catheter is usually advanced to a position about 5 mm proximal to the lesion. The laser treatment is then initiated and during laser ablation the catheter is advanced slowly – at about 1 mm per second or less. Following the initial laser procedure, an acceptable angiographic result may have been achieved, or it may be necessary to sequentially increase the catheter size, or it may be necessary to use conventional angioplasty technology (i.e. balloon catheters and coronary stents). Periprocedural medications include aspirin, heparin (bolus dose), intravenous nitrate and calcium channel blockers.

In the Excimer Laser Coronary Angioplasty Registry, 172 chronic total occlusions were treated in 162 patients (10.3% of the 1569 patients entered). Once a guidewire crossed an occlusion, the overall laser success rate for treatment of chronic total occlusions was 83%. The extent of stenosis decreased from 100% to 55 *b+ 26%.[6] In 74% of patients, adjunctive percutaneous balloon coronary angioplasty was used after laser treatment. A final procedural success, defined as less than 50% residual stenosis and no major complication (death, myocardial infarction or CABG) was achieved in 90%. Major complications were infrequent: one death, 1.9% myocardial infarction and 1.2% requirement for emergency bypass surgery. The results suggest that Excimer laser angioplasty may be useful for treating chronic total occlusions that can be crossed with a guidewire but not with the balloon catheter. A role has also been suggested when the occlusion has been confirmed to be extremely long.[6]

Excimer laser angioplasty continues to develop, particularly as an adjunct to conventional balloon angioplasty or coronary stenting in the treatment of chronic total occlusions. The data suggest that failure of laser angioplasty occurs because of low catheter flexibility and the need for good guidewire support when treating total occlusions – once the catheter has reached the target area, the morphology of the lesion seems to be of only minor importance for the success of the procedure.[7] An alternative strategy when treating totally occluded arteries, which can be crossed with a guidewire, but not the balloon catheter is to use the Rotablator system. This technology, which uses a high-speed rotational burr, produces ablation of tissue. By using burrs of increasing diameter, the lesion may be successfully treated by the rotablator technique alone. Frequently, coronary balloon angioplasty or coronary stenting are required after the initial rotablator therapy. Currently there are no randomised studies comparing Excimer laser angioplasty with Rotablator in the treatment of chronic total occlusions which can be crossed with a guidewire but not a balloon catheter.

LASER BALLOON ANGIOPLASTY

Conventional balloon coronary angioplasty improves luminal dimensions by producing fracture of the atheromatous plaque and by stretching the plaque-free wall. It is associated with dissection of the media and the formation of intimal flaps. These changes create local flow abnormalities which are associated with varying degrees of mural thrombus formation. In the vast majority of cases, dissection and thrombus formation do not result in acute vessel occlusion. During the next few months, however, the vascular reponse to injury may lead to restenosis. The aim of the laser balloon angioplasty is to create a large, smooth vascular lumen, which may lead to better short- and long-term results than conventional balloon angioplasty. In theory, this could potentially be achieved by thermal welding of dissection flaps, the elimination of vascular recoil, the elimination of coronary vasospasm, the reduction in platelet activation and the inhibition of smooth muscle cell proliferation.[8]

Laser balloon angioplasty, therefore, permits the application of heat (generated by the laser source) and pressure (by balloon inflations) to thermally weld tissue during coronary angioplasty. The system uses an Nd: YAG laser and a modified coronary balloon angioplasty catheter. The dose of laser is usually delivered over a period of around 20 seconds, which results in adventitial temperatures of between 90 and 110*b∞C. The technique is very similar to conventional balloon angioplasty. The laser balloon catheter is positioned over a 0.014" guidewire. Once the balloon is in the appropriate location, it is inflated to low pressure (usually about 4 atmospheres) and the programmed laser dose is delivered over around 20 seconds. The balloon inflation is continued for an additional 20–40 seconds while the temperature of the arterial wall returns to normal. It is unusual for further balloon dilatation to be necessary in order to improve the immediate angiographic result.

Laser balloon angioplasty has been shown to be effective in the management of acute failure of balloon coronary angioplasty, due to either immediate vessel recoil or severe dissection with impaired flow ('impending closure'). Despite this early success rate, however, the late angiographic restenosis rate of laser balloon angioplasty is very similar to conventional balloon angioplasty.[8] This is despite laser balloon angioplasty producing larger vessel lumens in the acute stage. With the introduction of coronary stents, the potential role for laser balloon angioplasty seems to have been taken over. The use of coronary stents will usually solve the acute problem of vessel recoil or severe dissection resulting in threatened occlusion. In addition, coronary stents are associated with a lower angiographic restenosis rate. Therefore, there would now appear to be no role for the technique of laser balloon angioplasty.

In the vast majority of patients with angina pectoris due to coronary artery disease, antianginal medication, balloon coronary angioplasty/coronary stenting, or CABG can achieve successful treatment. Some patients, however, have angina refractory to medical therapy and have diffuse disease in the distal part of their coronary circulation, which is not amenable to treatment by either coronary angioplasty/stenting or coronary artery bypass surgery. Such patients have often undergone several revascularisation procedures in the past. In this group of patients, who present a difficult management problem, new laser techniques have been utilised in recent years. These include transmyocardial laser revascularisation (TMLR) and percutaneous myocardial revascularisation (PMR).

TRANSMYOCARDIAL LASER REVASCULARISATION (TMLR)

This is a technique that creates transmural channels in ischaemic myocardium using laser ablation. Before the advent of coronary angioplasty and coronary artery bypass surgery, attempts were made at direct transmyocardial revascularisation.[9,10] A variety of tubes and needles were used to create transmural channels, with limited success in terms of clinical improvement. The concept was based on the knowledge of myocardial sinusoids and the thebesian system. These communications were thought to allow the direct perfusion of the myocardium by blood from the left ventricle. Other techniques included the creation of myocardial neovascularisation by internal thoracic artery implantation directly into the myocardium.[11] In principle, TMLR incorporates the direct perfusion and neovascularisation of these other techniques. Although the exact mechanism of action of TMLR is unknown, suggestions include direct perfusion through patent channels, denervation produced by the surgical procedure and new vessel formation (angiogenesis).[12] At the moment, the most likely mechanism for symptomatic improvement seems to be angiogenesis.

The technique of TMLR is usually carried out through a left anterolateral thoracotomy. The pericardium is opened and dissected free of the heart and the area of reversible ischaemia is exposed. This is determined pre-operatively by myocardial perfusion scanning (nuclear techniques or positron emission tomography). There is no requirement for cardiopulmonary bypass. The original laser used was the high energy carbon dioxide system (The Heart Laser, PLC Medical Systems). The laser probe is placed on the surface of the heart and fired when the ventricle is maximally distended with blood and electrically quiescent.

The laser energy is absorbed by the blood within the left ventricle and this produces an acoustic image analogous to steam which is readily visible on transoesophageal echocardiography. Clearly, this appearance on the echocardiogram denotes transmyocardial penetration. The channels created by the CO_2 laser are approximately 1 mm in diameter and are created in a distribution of approximately one per square centimetre (Fig. 18.1). Haemorrhage from the channel is controlled with direct finger pressure or an epicardial suture if pressure is not adequate. TMLR can also be performed using a Holmium:YAG laser or an Excimer laser.

Uncontrolled studies using the CO_2 laser have suggested an overall improvement both subjectively and objectively following TMLR. In a USA multicentre, uncontrolled phase II clinical trial, based on 200 patients, the operative mortality was 9%.[12] All patients had angina refractory to medical therapy, documented evidence of reversible ischaemia by radionuclide scanning and were untreatable by conventional forms of revascularisation. There was a significant improvement in the Canadian Cardiovascular Score (CCS) for angina at 3, 6 and 12 months following the procedure. Taking a decrease of two CCS classes as a clinically significant improvement, 75% of those assessed post-operatively achieved this. In addition, there was a significant decrease in the number of perfusion defects in the treated left ventricular wall. Patients who had at least one year of follow up experienced a significant decrease in the number of admissions for angina from 2.5 per patient-year before treatment to 0.5 per patient-year in the year following surgery.

In a registry report from European and Asian centres performing TMLR using the carbon dioxide laser, the operative mortality was 9.7%.[13] Benefit in terms of improvement in exercise performance was clinically significant, but less impressive than in the US uncontrolled study and less than benefits observed following other revascularisation procedures. Less than 50% of patients achieved an improvement of at least two angina classes compared with the 75% in the USA study. Complications of the technique include peri-operative bleeding and

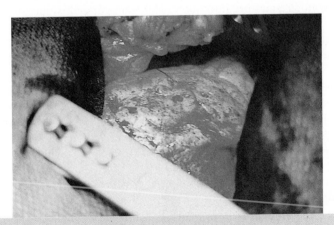

Figure 18.1:
Shows channels created at the time of TMLR surgery.

infection, left ventricular failure in the early post-operative period and cardiac arrhythmias – both supraventricular and ventricular.

TMLR is still a new technology which is being used more widely in Europe, the USA and Asia. It is clear that the benefits of the procedure in terms of improvements in angina and exercise tolerance will need to be sufficient to justify the peri-operative morbidity and mortality if the procedure is to become universally accepted. The results of a USA multicentre randomised controlled trial of TMLR against medical management have been submitted to the Food and Drug Administration Advisory Committee. They initially recommended non-approval for use in the USA due to the lack of a definitive explanation for the underlying mechanism, although many other well accepted techniques in clinical practice still lack full insight into the pathophysiological mechanism. In addition, there were concerns about the conduct of the trial in that the design allowed cross-over from medical therapy to TMLR and follow up data was incomplete. A follow up submission was eventually approved. There have been two large randomised controlled trials of TMLR – one from the US and one from the UK. The US trial randomised 198 patients to continued medication or TMLR plus medication.[14] There was a high cross-over rate from medical therapy to TMLR and the 12-month data only includes 64 patients from the TMLR group and 23 from the control group. An improvement of at least two angina classes was found at 12 months in 72% of the TMLR group and 13% of control patients. There was an operative mortality of 3% for TMLR with no significant difference in survival at 12 months between the two groups. The results of the UK trial were less favourable.[15] In this study 188 patients with severe angina associated with coronary artery disease unsuitable for conventional revascularisation were randomised to continued medication or TMLR plus medication. There were no cross-overs and almost complete follow-up data. At 12 months, the CCS angina score decreased by at least two classes in 25% of the TMLR patients and 4% of the control group. There was a peri-operative mortality of 5% for TMLR with no significant difference in survival at 12 months between the two groups. The morbidity associated with the TMLR procedure included wound/respiratory infection (33%) transient arrhythmia (usually atrial fibrillation) (15%) and left ventricular failure (12%). Exercise capacity measured using treadmill exercise times and 12 minutes' walk distance, was greater in the TMLR patients, although the difference between the two groups did not reach statistical significance. TMLR, therefore, seems to produce symptomatic improvement in this patient population, although an increase in exercise capacity has not been consistently demonstrated. Since the subjective improvement seems to be greater than the objective measurements, there are reservations regarding the widespread introduction of TMLR into clinical practice. It carries a peri-operative mortality of between 3% and 10% as well as a significant procedural morbidity.

PERCUTANEOUS MYOCARDIAL REVASCULARISATION (PMR)

With further developments in technology, it became possible to perform direct myocardial laser revascularisation using a percutaneous approach. A Holmium: YAG laser was developed in order to deliver energy directly to the endocardial surface of the left ventricular cavity (percutaneous myocardial revascularisation, CardioGenesis). Clearly, from the patient's point of view, this technique is much less invasive. It obviates the need for a general anaesthetic and thoracotomy with a consequent reduction in the length of hospital stay. Following TMLR, the mean length of stay is between 10 and 12 days, whereas patients can normally be discharged from hospital 24 to 48 hours after PMR.

With the CardioGenesis PMR system, access to the left ventricle is gained via a 9 F sheath introduced into the right femoral artery. The equipment essentially consists of a 'guiding catheter', a 'laser catheter' (which has a right angle bend towards its tip) and a 'laser fibre', which is passed through the laser catheter (Fig. 18.2). It is essential that the patient and the X-ray table do not move once the views in which to work have been selected. The two views typically selected are 40 degrees right anterior oblique and 50 degrees left anterior oblique, often with up to 10 degrees of cranial angulation. Whilst a biplane facility is preferred, the procedure can be easily carried out on single-plane equipment, although it may take slightly longer. The 'guiding catheter' is advanced to the left ventricular cavity and pre-procedure left ventricular angiograms are performed in the two selected views. In addition, pre-procedure coronary angiograms are usually carried out in the same projections. Both the coronary angiograms (at end-diastole) and the left ventricular angiograms (at end-diastole) are traced onto acetate sheets fixed over the viewing screens (Fig. 18.3). These then act as 'maps' during the procedure. The area or areas to be treated are determined prior to the procedure using myocardial perfusion scanning. Reversible ischaemia may be present in the inferior, anterior, or lateral walls, or may involve the interventricular septum or left ventricular apex. All of these sites are accessible for treatment.

The 'laser catheter' is advanced through the 'guiding catheter'which has been positioned within the left ventricle. The 'guiding catheter' is available in a variety of curves and the one selected depends on the size and shape of the left ventricular cavity as well as the area to be treated. By manipulating the 'guiding catheter' and/or the 'laser catheter' all sites within the left ventricle can be accessed. Once in the appropriate position, the 'laser fibre' is advanced through the 'laser

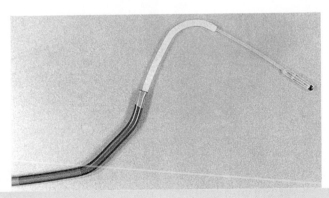

Figure 18.2:
The guiding catheter/laser catheter/laser fibre.

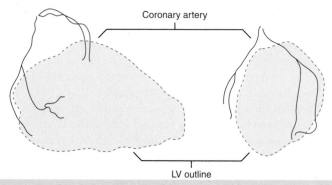

Figure 18.3:
Road map showing left ventricular (LV) outline and coronary arteries pre-procedure.

catheter' until there is contact with the endocardial surface of the left ventricle. This can often be felt, but can be seen as the laser catheter 'backs away' from the left ventricular wall and frequently ventricular ectopics are produced. Usually the right anterior oblique view is preferred for demonstrating contact with the anterior and inferior walls, and the left anterior oblique view for contact with the lateral and septal walls. The 'laser fibre' should be perpendicular to the left ventricular wall (Fig. 18.4). The laser is then activated, which typically produces 3 mm of penetration into the left ventricular myocardium: the 'laser fibre' is then advanced slightly and re-activated, which produces a channel of around 6 mm in total into the wall. The laser fibre is then withdrawn into the laser catheter and a new site is selected by manipulating the 'guiding catheter' and/or the 'laser catheter'. Clearly, it is important to determine prior to the procedure that the part of the left ventricle to be treated is at least 8 mm thick, using transthoracic echocardiography, to reduce the risk of left ventricular perforation. The apex of the left ventricle is usually thinner than the rest of the ventricle, and, therefore,

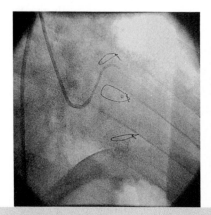 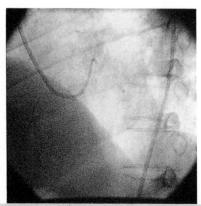

Figure 18.4:
Laser fibre against the left ventricular (LV) wall. Right anterior oblique projection (left) and left anterior oblique projection (right).

most operators will only be using one 'burst' of laser energy rather than two (that is, only 3 mm deep channel) when treating the apical area. When a channel is created, the site is recorded by marking it on the acetate sheet in the two views. Typically, channels are created at about 1 cm intervals. When treating the anterior and inferior walls, the 'map' of channels is usually best demonstrated in the left anterior oblique view, whereas for the lateral and septal walls, the right anterior oblique view is preferred (Fig. 18.5). A total of 10–15 channels are typically created in each of the areas demonstrated to have evidence of reversible ischaemia (inferior, anterior, lateral or septal).

The patients are given a bolus of intravenous Heparin (10 000 units) prior to the procedure. During manipulation of the 'guiding catheter' and/or 'laser catheter' it is quite common to induce ventricular ectopics, couplets or triplets and even non-sustained ventricular tachycardia. The rhythm disturbance is usually resolved by repositioning the catheters. Transient left bundle branch block can be induced during catheter manipulation. Therefore, if the patient has pre-existing right bundle branch block, it is advisable to position a temporary pacing wire prior to the procedure.

PMR is not used at the moment if there is evidence of left ventricular thrombus, if there is evidence of significant aortic stenosis or if there is severe peripheral vascular disease. The latter two exclusions produce problems of access to the left ventricular cavity. In addition, patients are unsuitable if the area intended for PMR treatment is less than 8 mm in thickness. Patients can usually be discharged from hospital the day after the PMR procedure.

The results of a multicentre randomised prospective trial of PMR (PACIFIC trial) were reported in 1999.[16] The patients included in the study had angina refractory to medical therapy, associated with coronary artery disease and were not suitable for conventional forms of revascularisation. They had evidence of reversible myocardial ischaemia on myocardial perfusion scans and left ventricular ejection fractions of at least 30%. The study included 221 patients from several US sites and one UK site. Subjects were randomised to medication alone (n=111) or to PMR in addition to usual medication (n=110). At six-month follow up there was a mean reduction of 1.4 CCS angina classes in the PMR

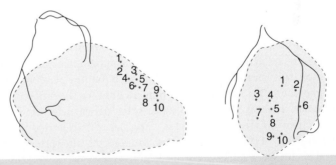

Figure 18.5:
Map of channels after procedure. Right anterior oblique projection (left). Left anterior oblique projection (right).

group compared with 0.125 in the control group (p=0.001). There was also a 30% increase in treadmill exercise time at six months in the PMR group compared with 5% in the control group, from baseline valves of a little over 400 seconds (p <0.001). Notably, there were no peri-procedural deaths in the PMR group. The morbidity associated with the procedure was also low. Of the 110 patients who underwent PMR, one developed cardiac tamponade requiring percutaneous drainage and one developed atrioventricular block requiring permanent pacing. In an uncontrolled longitudinal study there was a significant improvement in angina class and increase in exercise time three months and six months following PMR.[17] A randomized sham-controlled study using this PMR system was reported last year.[18] This study, known as the BELIEF (Blinded Evaluation of Laser Intervention electively For Angina Pectoris) study, recruited 82 patients with refractory angina in CCS class 3 or 4. It was designed to assess whether the improvement in symptoms of angina following PMR were attributable to placebo effect and clinician bias. The cohort recruited to this study was similar to the patients in the PACIFIC study. Patients were randomized to PMR with optimal medical therapy (n=40) or optimal medical therapy plus a sham procedure (n=42). Both the treating clinician and the patient were blinded to group allocation. There was one death in the sham group attributed to myocardial infarction. Follow up was completed in 79 patients at 6 and 12 months, with the primary outcome being improvement in CCS class. At both these timepoints, significantly more PMR patients improved by two or more CCS classes (40% vs 12% at 6 month, p<0.01 and 35% vs 14% at 12 months, p=0.04). There was no significant difference in exercise parameters, however, the trial was not powered to detect this. There was an improvement in angina specific health-related quality of life (p<0.05) as measured by the Seattle Angina Questionnaire. This data supports the conclusions reached in the unblinded trials of PMR as to improvement in angina scores using the Cardiogenesis laser system. They are, however, contrary to the negative findings of the single-blinded DIRECT (Direct myocardial laser revascularisation In Regeneration of Endomyocardial channels) trial. This study was reported in abstract form at the Transcatheter Cardiovascular Therapeutics conference in 2000. The subjects were randomized to placebo (n=102), low dose laser treatment (n=98) or high dose laser treatment (n=98). There was no difference in the groups at 6 or 12 months as regards to exercise parameters or angina scores. The laser used in this study was the Biosense DMR system which differs from the Cardiogenesis system in that electromechanical mapping of the left ventricular cavity is used to identify areas to be treated by laser as opposed to angiographic and perfusion data, and in that the DMR laser is a 'contact' system such that the depth of the channels created is significantly less. These factors may account for the differences between these two studies. There is also data to suggest that patient selection for PMR has a significant effect on treatment success. Stone et al.[19] reported a prospective multicentre study of 141 patients who were randomized after attempted PCI of a chronic total occlusion in a native coronary artery (with no other lesions needing PCI or CABG) to optimal medical management with or without PMR. Angina improved significantly in both groups but there was no difference between the groups (p=0.86) nor was a difference found in exercise parameters in the

71 patients of the 141 recruited who completed baseline and six-month tests (p=0.73). Although this patient group also suffered CCS class 3/4 angina they were potentially revascularisable by CABG and are less likely to have the diffuse coronary artery disease of those patients in the BELIEF and PACIFIC studies above. The evidence discussed above suggests that PMR using the Cardiogenesis laser system is an effective treatment for patients with chronic refractory angina which is not controlled by conventional means, and that PMR is likely to be preferred to TMLR in patients who have no other revascularisation option, since it is much less invasive and is likely to have a lower morbidity and mortality. TMLR may, however, still have a useful role – perhaps as an adjunct to coronary artery bypass surgery. There are many patients who have obstructed coronary vessels, some of which are suitable for bypass grafting and some of which are not. In these patients a combination of bypass grafting to some territories and TMLR to other regions may be the optimal therapy. This is currently a Class II recommendation for TMLR treatment in the Society of Cardiothoracic Surgeons Practice Guidelines.[20] Similarly PMR may be undertaken in conjunction with coronary angioplasty/stenting in the future – for example, with angioplasty/stenting of the LAD artery and PMR of the inferior wall since the right coronary artery is diffusely diseased. It is likely that the use of laser myocardial revascularisation, whether TMLR or PMR, will increase in the coming years.

REFERENCES

1. Ketre K, Holubkov R, Kelsey S et al. Percutaneous transluminal coronary angioplasty in 1985–88 and 1977–81. The National Heart, Lung, and Blood Institute Registry. N Engl J Med 1988; 318:265–70.

2. Hamm CW, Kupper W, Kuck K, Hofmann D, Bleifield W. Recanalisation of chronic, totally occluded coronary arteries by new angioplasty systems. Am J Cardiol 1990; 66:1459–63.

3. Bell MR, Berger PB, Bresnahan JF, Reeder GS, Bailey KR, Holmes DR. Initial and long-term outcome of 354 patients after coronary balloon angioplasty of total coronary artery occlusions. Circulation 1992; 85:1003–11.

4. Bowes RJ, Oakley GD, Fleming JS et al. Early clinical experience with a hot tip laser wire in patients with chronic coronary artery occlusion. J Invas Cardiol 1990; 2:241–5.

5. Mast EG, Plokker HW, Ernst JM et al. Percutaneous recanalisation of chronic total occlusions: experience with the direct Argon laser assisted angioplasty system (LASTAC). Herz 1990; 15:241–4.

6. Holmes DR, Forrester JS, Litvack F et al. Chronic total obstruction and short-term outcome: the Excimer laser coronary angioplasty registry experience. Mayo Clin Pro 1992; 68:5–10.

7. Baumbach A, Haase K, Karsch K. Usefulness of morphologic parameters in predicting the outcome of coronary Excimer laser angioplasty. Am J Cardiol 1991; 68:1310–15.

8. Safian RD, Reis GJ, Pomerantz RM. Laser balloon angioplasty: potential clinical applications. Herz 1990; 15:299–306.

9. Sen PK, Udwadia TE, Kinare SG *et al.* Transmyocardial acupuncture: a new approach to myocardial revascularisation. J Thorac Cardiovasc Surg 1965; 50:181–9.

10. Khazei All, Kime WP, Papadopoulous C *et al.* Myocardial canalization: a new method of myocardial revascularisation. Ann Thorac Surg 1968; 6:163–71.

11. Vineberg A. Clinical and experimental studies in the treatment of coronary artery insufficiency by internal mammary artery implant. J Int Coll Surg 1954; 22:503–18.

12. Horvath KA, Cohn LH, Cooley DA. Transmyocardial laser revascularisation: results of a multicentre trial with transmyocardial laser revascularisation used as sole therapy for end-stage coronary artery disease. J Thorac Cardiovasc Surg 1997; 113:645–54.

13. Burns SM, Sharples ID, Tait S *et al.* The transmyocardial laser revascularisation international registry report. Eur Heart J 1999; 20:31–7.

14. March RJ. Transmyocardial laser revascularisation with the CO_2 laser: one year results of a randomised controlled trial. Semin Thorac Cardiovasc Surg 1999; 11:12–18.

15. Schofield PM, Sharples LD, Caine N *et al.* Transmyocardial laser revascularisation in patients with refractory angina: a randomised controlled trial. The Lancet 1999; 353:519–24.

16. Oesterle SN, Yeung A, Ali N *et al.* The CardioGenesis percutaneous myocardial revascularisation (PMR) randomised trial: initial clinical results. J Am Cardiol 1999; 33(2)Suppl. A:380A (Abstract).

17. Lauer B, Junghans U, Stahl F, Kluge R, Oesterle S, Schuler G. Catheter-based percutaneous myocardial laser revascularisation in patients with end-stage coronary artery disease. Eur Heart J 1998; (19 Abstract suppl.):589 (Abstract).

18. Salem M, Rotevatn S, Stavnes S, Brekke M, Vollset SE and Nordrehaug JE. Usefulness and Safety of Percutaneous Myocardial Laser Revscularisation for Refractory Angina Pectoris. Am J Cardiol 2004: 93:1086–91.

19. Stone GW, Terstein PS, Rubenstein R, Schmidt D, Whitlow P, Kosinski E, Mishkel G and Power GA. A Prospective, Multicenter, Randomised Trial of Percutaneous Transmyocardial Laser Revascularisation in Patients with Nonrecanalizable Chronic Total Occlusions. JACC 2002; 39:1581–7.

20. Bridges CR, Horvath KA, Nugent WC, Shahian DM, Haan CK, Shemin RJ, Allen KB, and Edwards FH. The Society of Thoracic Surgeons Practice Guidelines Series: Transmyocardial Laser Revascularization. Ann Thorac Surg 2004; 77:1494–1502.

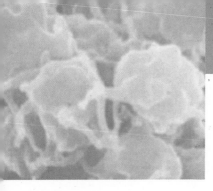

19

Circulatory support in percutaneous coronary intervention

ADAM DE BELDER BSC MD MRCP

KEY POINTS

■ Intra-aortic balloon pumping may be a useful adjunct to angioplasty for:

  – patients with poor LV function;

  – 'failed' thrombolysis;

  – cardiogenic shock; and

  – ischaemic arrhythmias.

■ Meticulous technique for insertion and removal with adequate nursing and technical support is essential to minimise complications associated with use of a balloon pump.

■ IABP is best used prophylactically in 'high-risk' patients rather than waiting for problems to arise.

INTRODUCTION

Coronary angioplasty can be hairy for the patient and the operator. Certain groups of patients can be considered to be at prohibitively high risk for coronary angioplasty. Typically, these patients have markedly impaired left ventricular function, a single target vessel supplying a large area of viable myocardium, or both, and the cardiac surgeons are not interested. While angioplasty is generally well tolerated in the low risk setting, transient coronary occlusion induced by balloon inflations in these high risk patients, may impose an intolerable ischaemic burden on marginally compensated myocardium and lead to haemodynamic collapse.

It is logical to propose that any reduction in risk that can be achieved in high risk patients is worth the effort.

It is sometimes difficult to predict which patients will run into trouble in the catheter laboratory, but the following conditions should make one raise an eyebrow before putting your gloves on:

● cardiogenic shock;
● poor LV function;
● ischaemic arrhythmias; and
● unstable refractory angina.

There are a number of techniques available to support the myocardium under these circumstances.[1] Most of them are confined to the dustbin of history, but some are worthy of a mention.

Anterograde coronary perfusion There are a number of catheters designed to maintain anterograde coronary perfusion driven by central aortic pressure, in the presence of transient coronary occlusion. They are of limited benefit, particularly when there is systemic hypotension. Coronary stenting has also revolutionised the management of occlusive dissections.

Coronary haemoperfusion Various techniques are described to provide haemoperfusion during coronary artery occlusion. After withdrawal of the sidearm of an oversized arterial sheath, blood is heparinised and reinfused using either hand injection, roller pump or power injector to provide adequate flow rates. The main limitation to this technique is that blood cannot be perfused to sidebranches that are occluded by the angioplasty balloon.

Perfluorocarbon coronary perfusion Fluosol is a biologically inert perfluoro-carbon emulsion with a high oxygen carrying capacity and a low viscosity, and has been used as a distal coronary perfusate during coronary angioplasty. There is little convincing evidence that it has any clinical benefit, which, in addition to the preparation time and cost, has limited the use of fluosol in this setting.

Coronary sinus retroperfusion Oxygenated blood is delivered via the coronary sinus to the great cardiac vein during ventricular diastole; a 10 mm balloon 1 cm from the coronary sinus distal tip inflates and deflated with each cardiac cycle, preventing escape of retroperfused blood into the right atrium.
There are disadvantages to this technique:

- It is only really feasible for LAD angioplasty, as the right coronary and circumflex vessels usually drain into the right atrium, ventricle or a portion of the coronary sinus.
- Coronary sinus cannulation is not easy, and setting up retroperfusion can take time.
- There is little data about the degree of myocardial protection offered during high risk angioplasty.

Cardiopulmonary support Total circulatory support with cardiopulmonary bypass can now be performed percutaneously. This does require the use of large stiff cannulae (18–20 Fr) inserted into the femoral vein and artery. This has limited its use due to a very high femoral access site complication rate.

Intra-aortic balloon pump The one device that has survived and is in regular use is the intra-aortic balloon pump (IABP).

History A failing heart poses a therapeutic dilemma – the increased aortic pressure required for adequate myocardial perfusion produces an unfavourable increase in afterload on the failing left ventricle. Ross[2] pointed out that peripheral vasoconstrictors often made the failing heart worse and proposed that mechanical assistance to the circulation would help.
Since then a number of means to temporarily support the circulation have been devised all with the same purpose to provide diastolic augmentation with increased coronary perfusion and to decrease left ventricular work

In 1961, Clauss *et al.* reported the use of a 'proportioning pump' placed on the arterial side of the circulation.[3] The original paper highlighted the potential benefits and many of the problems associated with the use of such a device. In dog experiments, they elegantly demonstrated that the greatest and most consistent relief of heart work, with the highest diastolic perfusion were achieved by very accurate timing of counterpulsation in co-ordination with direct arterial pressure measurement, or even triggered to the electrical output from the ECG machine. They showed the inefficiency of the pump with improper synchronisation with the cardiac cycle.

The first paper to report the use of balloon inflation (using CO_2) as a means of providing aortic counterpulsation came from Moulopoulos *et al.*[4] Using a human cadaver, the balloon catheter was inserted into the ascending aorta of a patient 30 mins after death, and radio-opaque dye injected which showed movement of dye toward the coronary tree, augmented by the balloon.

In 1967, Nachlas and Siedband reported that intraaortic counterpulsation in a dog model diminished the size of experimentally-induced myocardial infarction.[5] Kantrowitz and colleagues[6] described the use of a helium-filled balloon placed within the aorta to support the failing heart in a number of patients. One of these patients died but not before substantial physiological data had been obtained to support its use.

Since then, improvements have made the IABP a standard piece of equipment for most catheterisation laboratories. The following section describes how to use the device safely, and then I have reviewed the relevant literature to decide in what situations the IABP might be helpful.

Insertion technique for placing the IABP It is important to establish that the patient has good peripheral circulation mainly to determine if limb ischaemia develops.

Ideally, an IABP should be inserted in the appropriate surroundings with easy access to imaging and where strict sepsis can be maintained. It is possible to insert balloon pumps at the bedside, but it is not ideal.

Choosing the size of balloon is important. Generally, balloon capacity varies between 34 and 40cc helium, and are now available in as small as 8 French gauge. The principle is to use bigger balloon capacity on taller patients (>5'6"). If possible, I insert the IABP without a sheath, as this reduces the risk of limb ischaemia.

The femoral artery is approached using the Seldinger technique. The femoral artery is dilated over a J-tipped guide wire. If the procedure is performed without a sheath, the IABP is inserted directly over the wire. The slender polyurethane balloon is very low profile and has a blunt end. Passage of the IABP into the femoral artery is best done with gentle manual rotation as the balloon enters the femoral artery. The tip of the balloon is radio-opaque – this helps position it within the descending aorta, with the distal tip placed just below the origin of the left subclavian artery.

The IABP has only two connections. The first is for the measurement of arterial pressure, and the other is to attach to a console that shuttles helium in and out of the balloon for rapid inflation and deflation.

Augmentation is best achieved with timing of the inflation/deflation to the arterial waveform, but timing can also accurately be co-ordinated with the ECG waveform.

Thrombosis is a potential problem with a large artificial structure within the aorta, and I like to anticoagulate my patients with Heparin to keep an ACT of approximately 200 seconds.

It is always sensible to monitor patients with staff well used to looking after sick cardiac patients. In addition, technical support from perfusionists or similar staff helps prevent complications and optimises the effectiveness of the device.

Removal of the IABP   Once the decision to withdraw the IABP is made, the rate of augmentation is gradually decreased. Once augmentation is decreased to 1 in 4 or 1 in 8, the device can be removed. The Heparin is tailed off such that when the ACT is <150 seconds, the balloon can be taken out. It is important to aspirate the balloon before removal. Manual pressure is then applied to the groin, until haemostasis is achieved.

COMPLICATIONS

Patients requiring an IABP tend to have a higher incidence of concomitant disease, and it is not uncommon for problems to arise with peripheral ischaemia. It is, therefore, very important to assess limb vessel patency before placement and have regular checks during placement.

Other complications have been reported, such as aortic dissection and traumatic injury to the femoral artery, but these are fortunately rare.

WHICH PATIENTS WOULD BENEFIT FROM IABP TO COVER AN ANGIOPLASTY PROCEDURE?

Patients with AMI

In 1994, the Randomised IABP trial[7] enrolled 182 patients from 11 centres – all patients had to have an occluded infarct-related vessel at initial angiography presenting with typical chest pain within the previous 24 hours. All subsequently had restored IRA patency with primary angioplasty (n=106), intracoronary thrombolysis (n=25) or rescue angioplasty following failed thrombolysis (n=51). Following restoration of IRA flow, the patients were randomised to IABP for 48 hours (n=96) or standard care (n=86). The primary endpoint was IRA reocclusion at 5–7 days with repeat angiography, which occurred in 162 (89%) of the original cohort. The IABP group had an 8% reocclusion rate against 21% for the control group. The composite secondary endpoint (inhospital death, CVA, reinfarction, emergency revascularisation or recurrent ischaemia) was 13% for the IABP group and 24% in the controls (p<0.05). There were no differences between the groups with respect to bleeding complications and requirement for vascular repair. This is the only trial that suggests an IABP for allcomers with AMI might benefit from balloon pumping. Subsequent trials have not been so striking.

Brodie *et al.*[8] reported their experience with the IABP in the management of 1490 patients undergoing primary angioplasty for AMI from 1984–1997. Catheter laboratory events occurred in 88 (5.9%) patients (VF, CP arrest, prolonged hypotension). Retrospective analysis of this group compared the incidence of these events with or without an IABP. There were fewer adverse events in the IABP group compared with no IABP:

- cardiogenic shock (14.5% vs 35.1%, n=119);
- CHF or low ejection fraction (0% vs 14.6%, n=119); and
- in all high risk patients combined (11.5% vs 21.9%, n=238)

There are obvious limitations to this study with selection bias, but it suggests that patients who have low BP or malignant arrhythmias during an acute MI should be considered for prophylactic use of an IABP.

IABP AS ADJUNCTIVE THERAPY TO RESCUE ANGIOPLASTY AFTER FAILED THROMBOLYSIS FOR ANTERIOR AMI

This was a nonrandomised study[9] of 60 patients who had successful reperfusion performed to a blocked LAD after unsuccessful thrombolysis. The results are presented as a before (n=20 group A) and after (n=40 group B) the decision to prophylactically insert an IABP. Before discharge all patients had a repeat angiogram.

		Group A		Group B
Reinfarction	3		1	
Reocclusion		2		0
In-hospital mortality	20%		5%	
LVEF		no difference	44.3±8.2%	to
			51.0±14.21%	p<0.01

This is a small non-randomised study, but supports the possibility that IABP as adjunctive therapy to PTCA for rescue angioplasty reduces reocclusion and improves left ventricular function

USE OF IABP IN 'HIGH RISK' PATIENTS WITH AMI

Within the PAMI-II trial was a subgroup randomisation concerning the use of IABP in 'high risk' patients.[10] These were defined as patients who were:

- age >70 years;
- three vessel disease;
- LVEF <45%;
- vein graft occlusion;
- malignant arrhythmia; and
- suboptimal PTCA result.

This group were randomised to receive 36–48 hours of IABP (n=211) or traditional care (n=226).

There was no significant difference in death, reinfarction, infarct-related artery reocclusion, stroke or new-onset heart failure or sustained hypotension seen between the two groups.

It might be argued that any beneficial effects of IABP were not seen because of the soft inclusion criteria for 'high risk' patients. Whatever, this paper would not support the blanket use of IABP for so-called 'high risk' patients with AMI.

AMI – CARDIOGENIC SHOCK TREATED WITH THROMBOLYSIS AND IABP INSERTION

This was a retrospective analysis of 335 patients with cardiogenic shock over a ten-year period from two community hospitals in the USA.[11] 46 patients underwent thrombolysis within 12 hours of acute infarction with established cardiogenic shock (27 underwent IABP, 19 did not). There was a remarkable community hospital survival rate in the IABP group (93% vs 37%) with a significant improvement in overall hospital and one-year survival rate (67% vs 32%).

They also emphasized the benefit of using the IABP when transferring high risk patients for revascularisation.

It has been difficult to enrol patients with cardiogenic shock into prospective randomised studies, and there is no definitive study to direct practice. However, I feel there is sufficient evidence to warrant a strategy of IABP support and revascularisation by PTCA in these patients who otherwise have a very grim outlook.

Patients with poor left ventricular function undergoing PTCA This is a group who, I believe, benefit most from the use of prophylactic balloon pumping, yet there are no randomised studies examining this issue. A retrospective analysis of 28 patients undergoing 'high risk' angioplasty with IABP support with a mean LV ejection fraction of 24%, showed that despite systolic BP falling to <70mmHg in 39% cases, the augmented diastolic pressure was >90mmHg at all times. There were no deaths or myocardial infarctions complicating these procedures, but three patients required surgical repair of the femoral artery.[12]

There is a need for a robust prospective randomised trial to answer this important question – it seems highly logical to use an IABP under these circumstances, but perhaps the added co-morbidity form the procedure may preclude it.

There seems little doubt that in patients undergoing angioplasty to the last remaining conduit, which perhaps supply collaterals to other areas of a heart, which is already significantly impaired, the use of an IABP is sensible.

There are a number of interventional cardiologists who have never used an IABP on the grounds that it is:

- cumbersome;
- a potential threat to the peripheral circulation;
- of little clinical value; and
- inconvenient ('by the time the balloon pump is in, I could have done the angioplasty').

More fool them. I have heard a number of stories where the cardiologist has mourned the fact that an IABP was not inserted before a case. Occasionally, its insertion can help a dire situation, but its presence when trouble starts is gratefully received.

CASE REPORT 1 A 53-year-old presented with chest pain at rest. He reported a myocardial infarction 15 years ago since when he had been free of symptoms. On admission he was hypotensive and tachycardic. His resting ECG showed left bundle branch block.

He underwent urgent angiography. This revealed poor left ventricular function (EF – 20%). The LAD was chronically occluded. The circumflex was free of significant disease, and the right coronary artery revealed a critical lesion at the ostium and in the proximal segment. (Fig. 19.1A)

He developed ventricular tachycardia with loss of output requiring multiple DC shocks. After restoration of sinus rhythm, a 40cc 8 French IABP was placed via the left femoral artery, which settled the ST segment shift and venticular ectopy. Angioplasty with stenting was performed to restore blood flow to the right coronary artery (Fig. 19.1B) after which there were no further complications.

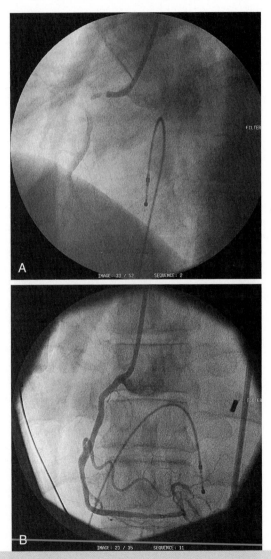

Figure 19.1:
A, Angiogram revealing critical lesion at the ostium of the right coronary artery and in the proximal segment. B, After IABP, angioplasty and stenting.

CASE REPORT 2 A 68-year-old man presented with severe chest pain and was in cardiogenic shock. Seventeen years previously he had four vein coronary artery vein grafts applied. Over the last three years, he had developed mild angina which had responded to medical therapy.

A coronary angiogram revealed poor LV function (EF – 15–20%). All his native vessels were occluded (Fig. 19.2A). Three of the vein grafts were occluded. A vein graft supplied the LAD, which back-filled the distal right coronary artery.

A 40cc 8 French IABP was placed via the left femoral artery and the balloon augmentation set to 1:1. The native circumflex artery was reopened and

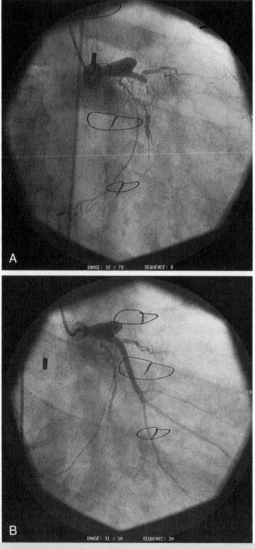

Figure 19.2:
A, Coronary angiogram revealing poor LV function. B, After IABP, angioplasty and stenting.

a stent inserted at the site of occlusion (Fig. 19.2B). He made a good recovery with resolution of his shock and complete alleviation of his angina. He remains well.

REFERENCES

1. Lincoff AM, Popma JJ, Ellis SG, Vogel RA, Topol EJ. Percutaneous support devices for high risk or complicated coronary angioplasty. J Am Coll Cardiol 1991; 17:770–780.

2. Ross J Jr. Left ventricular contraction and the therapy of cardiogenic shock. Circulation 1967; 35:611–613.

3. Clauss RH, Birtwell WC, Albertal G et al Assisted circulation. I. The arterial counterpulsator. J Thoracic & Cardiovasc Surg 1961; 41:447–458.

4. Moulopoulos SD, Topaz S, Kolff WJ. Diastolic balloon pumping (with carbon dioxide) in the aorta – A mechanical assistance to the failing circulation. Am Heart J 1962; 63:669–675.

5. Nachlas MM, Siedband MP. The influence of diastolic augmentation on infarct size following coronary artery ligation. J Thoracic Cardiov Surg 1967; 53:698–706.

6. Kantrowitz A, Tjønneland S, Freed PS et al. Initial clinical experience with intraaortic balloon pumping in cardiogenic shock. JAMA 1968; 203:113–117.

7. Ohman EM, George BS, White CJ et al. Use of aortic counterpulsation to improve sustained coronary artery patency during acute myocardial infarction: results of a randomised trial. Circulation 1994; 90:792–799.

8. Brodie BR, Stuckey TD, Hansen C, Muncy D. Intra-aortic balloon counterpulsation before primary percutaneous transluminal coronary angioplasty reduces catheterization laboratory events in high-risk patients with acute myocardial infarction. Am J Cardiol 1999; 84:18–23.

9. Ishihara M, Sato H, Tateisha H et al. Intraaortic balloon pumping as adjunctive therapy to rescue coronary angioplasty after failed thrombolysis in anterior wall acute myocardial infarction. Am J Cardiol 1995; 76:73–75.

10. Stone GW, Marsalese D, Brodie BR et al. A prospective, randomized evaluation of prophylactic intraaortic balloon counterpulsation in high risk patients with acute myocardial infarction treated with primary angioplasty. J Am Coll Cardiol 1997; 29:1459–1467.

11. Kovack PJ, Rasak MA, Bates ER, Ohman EM, Stomel RJ. Thrombolysis plus aortic counterpulsation: improved survival in patients who present to community hospitals with cardiogenic shock. J Am Coll Cardiol 1997; 29:1454–1458.

12. Kahn JK, Rutherford BD, McConahay DR et al. Supported 'high risk' coronary angioplasty using intraaortic balloon pump counterpulsation. J Am Coll Cardiol 1990; 15:770–780.

Section Three

Percutaneous
Coronary
Intervention in
Problematic Clinical
and Lesion Subsets

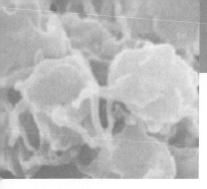

20

Percutaneous coronary intervention for acute myocardial infarction

JUHANA KARHA, MD AND SORIN J. BRENER, MD

KEY POINTS

- Primary PCI is the reperfusion strategy of choice in the management of acute STEMI.

- With short time delays, primary PCI is superior to fibrinolytic therapy even if the patient has to be transported to another medical center.

- Today, the performance of primary PCI routinely involves stenting to reduce risk of restenosis.

- Preliminary evidence suggests that use of DES is safe and effective. The utility of DES in primary PCI is evaluated in an ongoing clinical trial.

- Adjunctive pharmacotherapy includes Aspirin, Clopidogrel, Abciximab, and intravenous Heparin. Once stabilized, all patients also need aggressive risk factor modification, including therapy with statin drugs.

- Currently there is no role for distal embolic protection devices unless the culprit conduit is a sapheous vein graft.

- Future investigation will need to assess the maximum time delays of transport for primary PCI with different patient subsets.

- Targets of future investigation include the identification of the optimal myocardial protection strategy before and after reperfusion, the duration of dual anti-platelet therapy after PCI, and the concomitant revascularization of non-infarct territories.

INTRODUCTION

Acute ST-elevation myocardial infarction (STEMI) is caused by a thrombotic occlusion of an epicardial coronary artery. Ischemic injury to the affected myocardium eventually leads to irreversible myocardial necrosis. The resultant myocardial dysfunction is a powerful predictor of poor subsequent prognosis. Other pathophysiological mechanisms behind the poor outcome associated with acute STEMI include embolization of atherothrombotic material to the myocardial microvasculature, ventricular tachyarrhythmias, conduction disturbances, mitral valve regurgitation, and rarely, free wall or ventricular septal rupture. Important therapeutic measures include rapid evaluation and intensive monitoring of the patient, administration of anti-platelet and anti-thrombin medications, and immediate administration of reperfusion therapy. The main management paradigm is predicated on the open artery hypothesis, which states that early, sustained, and complete restoration of antegrade blood flow in the epicardial culprit artery is associated with reduced infract size and improved survival. Longer time intervals from symptom onset to ultimate opening of the artery (referred to as ischemic time) correlate with higher mortality (Fig. 20.1). Thus, the initial assessment of the patient with acute STEMI should establish the presence of any contra-indications to reperfusion therapy. The two reperfusion

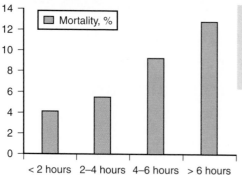

Figure 20.1:
Among patients with pre-PCI culprit artery TIMI flow grade 0-1, the symptom-onset to balloon time is correlated with mortality (p=0.001). Adapted from DeLuca G, et al. J Am Coll Cardiol 2003 42 991–997.

strategies are primary PCI and fibrinolytic therapy. Although theoretically possible, emergency CABG surgery is, in practice, rarely performed.

Primary PCI vs. Fibrinolytic therapy The two reperfusion strategies, primary PCI and fibrinolytic therapy, each have certain advantages. Primary PCI offers the opportunity to not only restore blood flow to the affected myocardium, but also to eliminate any residual stenosis at the site of the thrombotic lesion. Furthermore, other flow-limiting stenoses may also be identified and, if indicated, relieved. On the other hand, primary PCI is not available at most medical facilities at all times of day and week. Its outcome is highly dependent on the skill of the operator and the catheterization laboratory personnel, and the cost of the therapy is considerable. Fibrinolytic therapy is easy and quick to administer, widely available, and less expensive. On the other hand, it often does not provide durable reperfusion with higher risk of future reinfarction and need for revascularization procedures. Intra-cranial hemorrhage, although a rare complication, is often devastating.

Multiple clinical trials have compared primary PCI with fibrinolytic therapy with the goal of establishing the preferred strategy. A meta-analysis of these trials demonstrated that primary PCI is the superior reperfusion strategy (Table 20.1 and Fig. 20.2).[1] The field of interventional cardiology has seen the emergence of multiple advances since many of these comparative studies were conducted. First, as compared with balloon angioplasty, the implantation of intracoronary stents during angioplasty alleviated, but did not eliminate, the difficult problem of restenosis. To further reduce the risk of in-stent restenosis, drug-eluting stents (DES) with anti-proliferative activity were developed. These sirolimus- or paclitaxel-eluting stents have radically reduced the rate of in-stent restenosis in clinical practice. These sirolimus- or paclitaxel-eluting stents have radically reduced the rate of in-stent restenosis in clinical practice. A number of small clinical trials have evaluated the safety and efficacy of DES compared with bare-metal stents in primary PCI. In general, use of DES was associated with a similar rate of death or reinfarction and a reduced rate of repeat revascularization up to 1 year from randomization. (Laarman GJ, Suttorp MJ, Dirksen MT, et al. Paclitaxel-Eluting versus Uncoated Stents in Primary Percutaneous Coronary Intervention. *N Engl J Med* 2006; 355:1105-1113; Spaulding C, Henry P, Teiger E, et al. Sirolimus-Eluting versus Uncoated Stents in Acute Myocardial Infarction.

TABLE 20.1 - SUMMARY OF THE 23 RANDOMISED TRIALS OF PRIMARY ANGIOPLASTY VERSUS THROMBOLYTIC THERAPY

Patients' characteristics	Symptom duration (h)	Number randomised to PTCA (n = 3872)	Number randomised to thrombolysis (n = 3867)	Stents used	Glycoprotein IIb/IIIa antagonists used	Thrombolytic agent used, administration time	TIME TO TREATMENT (MIN) PTCA	TIME TO TREATMENT (MIN) Thrombolytic therapy
Streptokinase trials (n=1837)								
Zijlstra[8] Age ≤ 75 years, ST↑	<6	152	149	No	No	1.5 million U SK, 1h	62*	30*
Riberio[9] Age < 75 years, ST↑	<6	50	50	No	No	1.2 million U SK, 1h	238	179
rinfeld[10] ST↑	<12	54	58	No	No	1.5 million U SK, 1h	63†	18†
Zijlstra[11] ST↑, low risk	<6	47	53	No	No	1.5 million U SK, 1h	68*	30*
Akhras[12] ST↑	<12	42	45	No	No	1.5 million U SK, 1h	NA	NA
Widimsky[13]** ST↑, LBBB	<6	101	99	Yes	No	1.5 million U SK, 1h	80†	70†
de Boer[14] Age ≥ 76 years; ST↑	<6	46	41	Yes	No	1.5 million U SK, 1h	59*	31*
Widimsky[5] ST↑	<12	429	421	Yes	Yes	1.5 million U SK, 1h	277†§	245†§
Fibrin-specific trials (n=5902)								
DeWood[16] Age ≤ 76 years; ST↑	<12	46	44	No	No	Duteplase, 4h	126*	84*
Grine[17] ST↑	<12	195	200	No	No	t-PA, 3h	60†	32†
Gibbons[13] Age < 80 years; ST↑	<12	47	56	No	No	Duteplase, 4h	45†	20†
Ribichini[19,20] Age < 80 years; inferior MI, anterior ST↓	<6	55	55	No	No	Accelerated t-PA	40†	33†
Garcia[21,22] anterior MI	5	95	94	No	No	Accelerated t-PA	84*	69*
GUSTO IIB[23] ST↑, LBBB	<12	565	573	No	No	Accelerated t-PA	114†	72†
Le May[24] ST↑, LBBB	<12	62	61	Yes	Yes	Accelerated t-PA	77†¶	15†
Bonnefoy[25] ST↑	<6	421	419	Yes	Yes	Accelerated t-PA	190†	130†
Schomig[26] ST↑	<12	71	69	Yes	Yes	Accelerated t-PA	65*§	30*¶
Vermee[27]** Age <80 years; ST↑	<6	75	75	Yes	No	Accelerated t-PA	100†	85†
Andersen[28] ST↑	<12	790	782	Yes	NA	Accelerated t-PA	NA	NA

Continued

245

TABLE 20.1 · SUMMARY OF THE 23 RANDOMISED TRIALS OF PRIMARY ANGIOPLASTY VERSUS THROMBOLYTIC THERAPY—cont'd

Patients' characteristics	Symptom duration (h)	Number randomised to PTCA (n = 3872)	Number randomised to thrombolysis (n = 3867)	Stents used	Glycoprotein IIb/IIIa antagonists used	Thrombolytic agent used, administration time	TIME TO TREATMENT (MIN) PTCA	Thrombolytic therapy
Kastrati[29]	ST↑, LBBB	<12	81	81	Yes	Yes	Accelerated t-PA	75*¶	35*¶
Aversano[30]	ST↑	<12	225	226	Yes	Yes	Accelerated t-PA	102*¶	46*¶
Grines[31]	ST↑	<12	71	66	Yes	Yes	Accelerated t-PA	155*	51*
Hochman[7]	Cardiogenic shock	<36	152	150	Yes	Yes	Accelerated t-PA	75†¶	6168†¶‖

LBBB=left bundle branch block; MI=myocardial infarction; NA=data not available; SK=streptokinase; ST↑=elevation; ST↓=depression; t-PA=tissue-type plasminogen activator; accelerated t-PA=32–15 mg intravenous bolus, followed by an infusion of 0.75 mg/kg bodyweight over 30 min (maximum 50 mg) and then 0.50 mg/kg bodyweight over 60 min (maximum 35 mg) for a maximum dose of 100 mg. ¶68% of patients in the Grines Study[31] and 70% of patients in the Hochman study[7] received accelerated t-PA. *From admission. †From randomisation. §Average time. ‡From symptom onset to reperfusion. ¶Median time. ‖Time to the permitted delayed revascularisation procedure (percutaneous or surgical) in the initial medical stabilisation group. **Both the PRAGUE[13] and the LIMI[27] trials included a third group of individuals, who had thrombolytic therapy followed by transfer for subsequent PTCA (n=100 and n=74 patients, respectively); these 174 patients were excluded from our analyses.

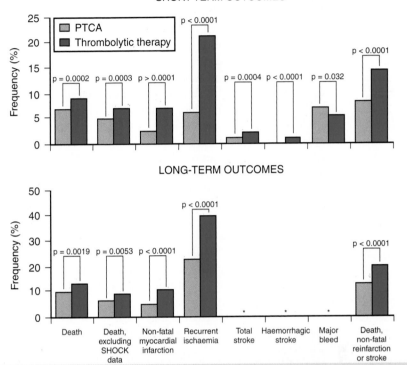

SHORT-TERM OUTCOMES

LONG-TERM OUTCOMES

Figure 20.2:
Short-term and long-term clinical outcomes in individuals treated with primary PTCA or thrombolytic therapy. * = data not available. Reproduced with permission from Keeley EC, *et al*. Lancet 2003; 361: 13–20, Figure 2.

N Engl J Med 2006; 355:1093-1104 (a large dedicated randomized trial is ongoing).

Anti-platelet therapy The interplay between platelets and the coagulation cascade is critically important in the pathophysiology of acute STEMI, as the atherosclerotic plaque ruptures and thrombotic occlusion of the artery ensues. Medications targeting these two systems have, therefore, been a focus of investigation. The use of Aspirin (acetylsalicylic acid) in treatment of myocardial infarction (MI) has a long history. The meta-analysis performed by the Fibrinolytic Therapy Trialists demonstrated the marked benefit that Aspirin has in reducing mortality following myocardial infarction. The standard practice is to administer aspirin upon the diagnosis of MI. Although no good evidence exists guiding the selection of Aspirin dose, most cardiologists prefer 325 mg, initially given in a chewable form. The patient should continue Aspirin therapy indefinitely after the MI (most likely a daily dose of 81 mg is optimal).

Adenosine diphosphate (ADP) receptor blockade with a thienopyridine compound has an important role in interventional cardiology. The Clopidogrel for the Reduction of Events During Observation (CREDO) trial demonstrated in patients undergoing PCI (with bare metal stenting) that Clopidogrel use beyond the traditional one month (through one year) was associated with further clinical benefit.[2] These findings were consistent with the clinical benefit of long-term Clopidogrel therapy seen in the PCI-Clopidogrel in Unstable angina to prevent Recurrent Events (CURE) study, which also predated the era of drug-eluting stenting.[3] Many recent reports have documented a persistent risk for stent thrombosis years after implantation of DES. (Bavry AA, Kumbhani DJ, Helton TJ, et al. Late thrombosis of drug-eluting stents: a meta-analysis of randomized clinical trials. *Am J Med* 2006; 119:1056–1061.) Their use in the setting of STEMI is particularly concerning because of the mandatory prolonged treatment with dual anti-platelet therapy. (Spertus JA, Kettelkamp R, Vance C, et al. Prevalence, Predictors, and Outcomes of Premature Discontinuation of Thienopyridine Therapy After Drug-Eluting Stent Placement: Results From the PREMIER Registry. *Circulation* 2006; 113:2803–2809. At this point it is unclear what the optimal duration of Clopidogrel therapy is following PCI. It appears that following BMS placement it is safe to discontinue Clopidogrel after one month of therapy, but that longer therapy may offer further benefit. Following DES placement, until further evidence is available, Clopidogrel should probably be continued for at least 1 year, and potentially indefinitely to guard against late stent thrombosis. Clearly, much more information is required before firm recommendations can be made about this issue.

The administration of a Clopidogrel loading dose prior to PCI reduces ischemic complications. The required time interval between the loading dose and the PCI, as well as the amount of the loading dose, are insufficiently defined. (Sabatine MS, Cannon CP, Gibson CM, et al. Effect of Clopidogrel Pretreatment Before Percutaneous Coronary Intervention in Patients With ST-Elevation Myocardial Infarction Treated With Fibrinolytics: The PCI-CLARITY Study. *JAMA* 2005; 294:1224–1232.) This is less of an issue in primary PCI as one cannot anticipate the procedure. Similar to the open questions regarding Clopidogrel loading, it is unclear what (if any) re-loading of Clopidogrel is required in case of patients already on a maintenance dose of Clopidogrel (75 mg daily).

The platelet glycoprotein IIb/IIIa receptor antagonists (IIb/IIIa inhibitors) are routinely used with primary PCI. A sizable body of evidence exists for the benefit that abciximab, the first of these compounds, has in reducing ischemic endpoints following PCI. The patient populations that have been studied also include patients with acute STEMI. Topol and colleagues recently performed a pooled analysis of five trials (RAPPORT, ISAR-2, ADMIRAL, CADILLAC, and ACE) and demonstrated that compared with placebo, abciximab use is associated with a reduction in the combined endpoint of death, reinfarction, or TVR (Fig. 20.3).[4] At 30 days the event rates were 4.8% vs. 8.8%, respectively (odds ratio 0.54, p<0.05) and this benefit extended up to six months follow up. Based on these data, the administration of abciximab is now common in many laboratories as adjunctive to primary PCI. Starting abciximab upon diagnosis of acute STEMI, that is, *prior* to arrival to the catheterization laboratory might offer further incremental benefit. This hypothesis will have to be evaluated in future studies.

In summary, a patient with acute STEMI who undergoes primary PCI with the placement of a DES would receive on the day of the procedure Aspirin 325 mg,

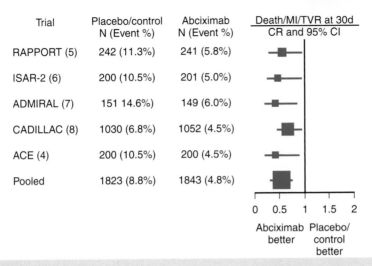

Trial	Placebo/control N (Event %)	Abciximab N (Event %)	Death/MI/TVR at 30d CR and 95% CI
RAPPORT (5)	242 (11.3%)	241 (5.8%)	
ISAR-2 (6)	200 (10.5%)	201 (5.0%)	
ADMIRAL (7)	151 14.6%)	149 (6.0%)	
CADILLAC (8)	1030 (6.8%)	1052 (4.5%)	
ACE (4)	200 (10.5%)	200 (4.5%)	
Pooled	1823 (8.8%)	1843 (4.8%)	

```
        0   0.5   1   1.5   2
       Abciximab  Placebo/
         better    control
                   better
```

Figure 20.3:
Death, reinfarction, and TVR at 30 days. Two trials included stroke in the composite endpoint (ACE, CADILLAC), but the incidence was quite low. Reproduced with permission from Topol EJ, et al. J Am Coll Cardiol 2003; 42: 1886–1889, Figure 1A.

a Clopidogrel loading dose, and Abciximab. Upon hospital discharge he or she would then likely take daily aspirin 81 mg and Clopidogrel 75 mg for at least one year.

Anti-thrombin therapy Anti-coagulation with intravenous unfractionated Heparin (UFH) has been used for decades in the treatment of acute ischemic coronary syndromes. Although the data supporting this practice are not particularly robust, considerable consensus exists in support of heparin's use on the basis of the pathophysiology of the thrombotic occlusion leading to myocardial infarction. During coronary angioplasty the advancement of guidewires, balloon catheters, and other devices into the coronary arteries requires anticoagulation to prevent iatrogenic thrombosis. This has traditionally been achieved with intravenous UFH with the target activated clotting time (ACT) of >250 seconds. Thus, most commonly, upon the diagnosis of acute STEMI, the patient receives a weight-based bolus + infusion of heparin, and further heparin may be administered in the catheterization laboratory during primary PCI to achieve the desired target ACT.

In the last decade low molecular weight Heparins have been introduced into clinical practice in the management of venous thrombosis. They are superior to UFH in their more predictable bioactivity without the need to monitor the level of anticoagulation. The administration is simpler with subcutaneous injections, likely reducing the possibility of a dosing error. However, the use in patients with severe renal insufficiency may lead to supratherapeutic levels and is not recommended. The low molecular weight Heparin enoxaparin has been studied in the medical management of ACS and has been found to be superior to UFH with respect to both safety and efficacy endpoints. The recent Superior Yield of the New Strategy of Enoxaparin, Revascularization and Glycoprotein IIb/IIIa inhibitors (SYNERGY) trial in patients with non-ST-elevation acute coronary syndromes who were treated with an invasive strategy of early coronary angiography and PCI (if indicated) compared enoxaparin with UFH.[5] No significant difference was noted in the primary endpoint between the two study groups. The 30-day rate of death or MI was 14.0% in the enoxaparin group and 14.5% in the UFH group. At this time, primary PCI in the United States is being performed largely with unfractionated Heparin as the antithrombotic agent. However, some operators in Europe use enoxaparin in PCI for unstable coronary syndromes, including acute STEMI.

Bivalirudin, a direct thrombin inhibitor, has recently been introduced to clinical practice during elective low-to-intermediate-risk PCI. The Randomized Evaluation in PCI Linking Angiomax to Reduced Clinical Events (REPLACE)-2 trial of 6,010 stable patients undergoing PCI established that a strategy of bivalirudin (plus bailout IIb/IIIa inhibitor) was non-inferior to UFH plus IIb/IIIa inhibitor with respect to ischemic outcomes, and superior in terms of bleeding complications.[6] Thus, many operators are using bivalirudin as the antithrombotic regimen in elective PCI. Similar results were obtained in the setting of acute coronary syndromes. (Stone GW, White HD, Ohman EM, et al. Bivalirudin in patients with acute coronary syndromes undergoing percutaneous coronary intervention: a subgroup analysis from the Acute Catheterization and Urgent Intervention Triage strategy (ACUITY) trial. *Lancet* 2007; 369:907–919.) However, little data exist on its use in patients with acute STEMI undergoing angioplasty, and it is not recommended in primary PCI.

Embolic protection devices Downstream embolization of atherosclerotic debris is inevitable in angioplasty. This results in an increased incidence of no-reflow, post-procedural myonecrosis, and microvascular dysfunction, all associated with poorer long-term outcome. Much interest has recently focused on mechanical solutions for this challenging problem. The various embolic protection devices (EPD) are positioned proximal or distal to the site of angioplasty with the goal of preventing debris from reaching the microvasculature. The three main design types of the multitude of EPDs either in commercial use or in development are filters and proximal or distal occlusive balloons. The challenges with the use of EPD include deliverability of the device in cases of severe stenosis or tortuosity, absence of a suitable landing zone, the presence of any side branches between the lesion and the device (that might receive the debris before it reaches the EPD), initial embolization with the manipulation of the wire before the placement of the EPD, and imperfect collection with some debris reaching past the EPD and into the microvasculature.

Angioplasty on degenerated saphenous vein grafts is associated with significant embolization burden, and thus served as a good clinical testing setting for the hypothesis that distal embolic protection would improve clinical outcomes. The Saphenous vein graft Angioplasty Free of Emboli Randomized (SAFER) trial randomized 801 patients undergoing PCI on a vein graft to the use of PercuSurge GuardWire™ balloon occlusion device vs. standard guidewire.[7] The patients in the EPD group had a lower incidence of post PCI myocardial infarction (8.6% vs. 14.7%, p=0.008) and no-reflow phenomenon (3% vs. 9%, p=0.02) compared to the control patients. These findings established the utility of distal embolic protection in vein graft angioplasty.

Encouraged by the SAFER trial results, the use of EPD in angioplasty for acute myocardial infarction (n=501) was evaluated in the Enhanced Myocardial Efficacy and Recovery by Aspiration of Liberated Debris (EMERALD) trial.[8] Patients were randomized to GuardWire Plus™ balloon occlusion and aspiration system vs. standard therapy, and visible debris was recovered in 73% of the interventions in the EPD group. However, there was no difference in microvascular function (as detected by ST-segment resolution), infarct size, or major adverse cardiac events between the two groups. Given that primary PCI carries with it a high risk of distal embolization, the EMERALD trial results suggest that embolic protection does not have the same benefits in native coronary artery PCI as those observed in vein graft angioplasty. However, it is possible that improvements in device design might make EPD a beneficial therapy in native coronary artery angioplasty in the future.

Facilitated PCI Attempting to combine the strengths of primary PCI and fibrinolytic therapy in a single strategy led to the concept of 'facilitated' PCI. This refers to the administration of full- or reduced-dose fibrinolytic agent, alone or along with a glycoprotein inhibitor, followed by immediate angiography and PCI (if indicated). This strategy would realize the benefit of early reperfusion (fibrinolytic therapy), prime the coronary lesion for PCI (glycoprotein inhibitor), and achieve full and sustained reperfusion (PCI). The trial data on this strategy show that although angiographic endpoints are slightly better with the combination therapy compared to full-dose fibrinolytic therapy, the clinical outcomes are similar. The Global Use of Strategies to Open Occluded Coronary Arteries (GUSTO)-V trial compared standard-dose reteplase to half-dose reteplase and abciximab, without mandatory angiography, and found that the 30-day mortality was similar in the two groups. The reduced incidence of non-fatal MI and urgent revascularization in the combination group was counterbalanced by a higher rate of non-intracranial bleeding complications.[9] A meta-analysis of 17 such trial did not suggest of benefit for the facilitated approach compared with regular primary PCI. (Keeley EC, Boura JA, Grines CL. Comparison of primary and facilitated percutaneous coronary interventions for ST-elevation myocardial infarction: quantitative review of randomised trials. *Lancet* 2006; 367:579–588.)

Rescue PCI Fibrinolytic therapy fails to achieve reperfusion in at least 25% of patients. These patients are then often managed with rescue PCI. The trials that sought to compare PCI to conservative therapy among patients who had failed to reperfuse with fibrinolytic therapy had major difficulties with enrollment. This was due to the strong sentiment that exists in the cardiology community that such patients should be managed with immediate coronary angiography and an attempt to revascularize the culprit artery. The RESCUE 1 trial documented no significant difference in 30-day mortality in patients treated with rescue angioplasty vs. those not treated with rescue angioplasty

(5.1% vs. 9.6%), although there was significant reduction in the incidence of recurrent ischemia and heart failure.[10] However, more recent post-hoc analyses in the era of stenting and IIb/IIIa inhibition have demonstrated that rescue angioplasty is associated with improved long-term survival compared to conservative management.[11, 12] The Middlesbrough Early Revascularization to Limit INfarction (MERLIN) trial demonstrated a reduced need for revascularization at 30 days among patients in the rescue angioplasty group, but was underpowered to detect a survival benefit.[13] Similar results were obtained in the Rescue Angioplasty after Failed Thrombolytic Therapy for Acute Myocardial Infarction (REACT) trial. (Gershlick AH, Stephens-Lloyd A, Hughes S, et al. Rescue Angioplasty after Failed Thrombolytic Therapy for Acute Myocardial Infarction. *N Engl J Med* 2005; 353:2758-2768. Thus, based on these data, transfer for rescue PCI is the preferred paradigm of care for patients who fail to achieve reperfusion with the administration of fibrinolytic therapy. Another increasingly common practice pattern is routine immediate angiography following fibrinolytic therapy (that is, even for patients who have successfully reperfused).

Transport for primary PCI

A controversial area in the management of acute STEMI is whether patients who present to facilities without primary PCI capability should be treated with immediate fibrinolytic therapy or be transferred to another center to undergo primary PCI. As discussed above, when primary PCI can be performed quickly (that is, the medical center where the patient presents at has the ability to perform primary PCI), it is superior to fibrinolytic therapy. In considering the implications of delaying reperfusion therapy (by the transfer) in order to receive the benefit of the superior strategy, the relevant variable becomes the 'needle-to-balloon' delay. This refers to the delay between the two time points when reperfusion presumably occurs with the two strategies. Investigators have sought to determine the threshold needle-to-balloon delay in various patient subsets. This would be helpful to clinicians as they struggle with the decision of transfer for primary PCI versus administration of fibrinolytic therapy. Several large trials have compared these two strategies. Dalby and colleagues performed a meta-analysis on these trials (Fig. 20.4).[14] It is notable that the mean time to PCI in the transfer groups of these studies ranged between 80 and 122 minutes. The meta-analysis found that the incidence of both reinfarction and stroke were reduced among patients transferred for primary PCI compared to patients who received fibrinolytic therapy (relative risk 0.32, p<0.001; and relative risk 0.44, p=0.015). There was a trend for reduced mortality among the transfer arm (relative risk 0.81, p=0.08). Interestingly, if the CAPTIM trial were excluded (that is, patients who received fibrinolytic therapy at their homes), transfer for PCI was associated with improved mortality compared to fibrinolytic administration (relative risk 0.76, p=0.035).

In a meta-analysis of primary PCI vs. fibrinolysis trials, Nallamothu and Bates discovered that the mortality benefit associated with primary PCI may be lost if door-to-balloon time is delayed by >1 hour compared with fibrin-specific fibrinolytic therapy door-to-needle time.[15] In their analysis, the two

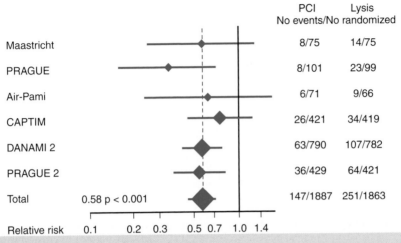

Figure 20.4:
Relative risks for the composite of death/reinfarction/stroke with thrombolysis and transfer for primary PCI in individual trials and the combined analysis. Reproduced with permission from Dalby M, *et al*. Circulation 2003; 108: 1809–1814, Figure 1. Six trials were included in the meta-analysis: PRAGUE, PRAGUE-2, DANAMI-2, Air-PAMI, CAPTIM, and the Maastricht study.

reperfusion strategies became equivalent with regard to mortality after a PCI-related time delay of 62 minutes. The recent ACC/AHA guidelines call for transfer for PCI in patients presenting more than three hours from MI onset and where the estimated first balloon inflation would occur within 60 minutes of when the fibrinolytic agent could be infused (if presentation is within three hours of symptom onset, the two strategies are equivalent).[16] Most operators use an expected needle-to-balloon delay of 1–2 hours as the cut off for transfer.

REFERENCES

1. Keeley EC, Boura JA, Grines CL. Primary angioplasty versus intravenous thrombolytic therapy for acute myocardial infarction: a quantitative review of 23 randomized trials. Lancet 2003; 361:13–20.

2. Steinhubl SR, Berger PB, Mann JT, *et al*. Early and sustained dual oral antiplatelet therapy following percutaneous coronary intervention: a randomized controlled trial. CREDO Investigators. JAMA 2002; 288:2411–20.

3. Mehta S, Yusuf S, Peters R, *et al*. Effects of pretreatment with clopidogrel and aspirin followed by long-term therapy in patients undergoing percutaneous coronary intervention: the PCI-CURE study. Lancet 2001; 358:527–33.

4. Topol EJ, Neumann FJ, Montalescot G. A preferred reperfusion strategy for acute myocardial infarction. J Am Coll Cardiol 2003; 42:1886–9.

5. Ferguson JJ, Califf RM, Antman EM, *et al*. Enoxaparin vs unfractionated heparin in high-risk patients with non-ST-segment elevation acute coronary syndromes managed with an intended early invasive strategy: primary results of the SYNERGY randomized trial. JAMA 2004; 292:45–54.

6. Lincoff AM, Bittl JA, Harrington RA, *et al*. Bivalirudin and provisional glycoprotein IIb/IIIa blockade compared with heparin and planned glycoprotein IIb/IIIa blockade during percutaneous coronary intervention: REPLACE-2 randomized trial. JAMA 2003; 289:853–63.

7. Baim DS, Wahr D, George B, *et al*. Randomized trial of a distal embolic protection device during percutaneous intervention of saphenous vein aorto-coronary bypass grafts. Circulation 2002; 105:1285–90.

8. Stone GW, Webb J, Cox DA, *et al*. Distal microcirculatory protection during percutaneous coronary intervention in acute ST-segment elevation myocardial infarction: a randomized controlled trial. JAMA 2005; 293:1063–72.

9. Reperfusion Therapy for Acute Myocardial Infarction with Fibrinolytic Therapy or Combination Reduced Fibrinolytic Therapy and Platelet glycoprotein IIb/IIIa Inhibition: The GUSTO V Randomized Trial. Lancet 2001; 357:1905–14.

10. Ellis SG, Ribeiro da Silva E, Heyndrickx GR, *et al*. Randomized comparison of rescue angioplasty with conservative management of patients with early failure of thrombolysis for acute anterior myocardial infarction. Circulation 1994; 90:2280–84.

11. Schweiger MJ, Cannon CP, Murphy SA, *et al*. Early coronary intervention following pharmacologic therapy for acute myocardial infarction (the combined TIMI 10B-TIMI 14 experience). Am J Cardiol 2001; 88:831–6.

12. Gibson CM, Cannon CP, Murphy SA, *et al*. Relationship of the TIMI myocardial perfusion grades, flow grades, frame count, and percutaneous coronary intervention to long-term outcomes after thrombolytic administration in acute myocardial infarction. Circulation 2002; 105:1909–13.

13. Sutton AG, Campbell PG, Graham R, *et al*. A randomized trial of rescue angioplasty versus a conservative approach for failed fibrinolysis in ST-segment elevation myocardial infarction: the Middlesbrough Early Revascularization to Limit INfarction (MERLIN) trial. J Am Coll Cardiol 2004; 44:287–96.

14. Dalby M, Bouzamondo A, Lechat P, Montalescot G. Transfer for primary angioplasty versus immediate thrombolysis in acute myocardial infarction. A meta-analysis. Circulation 2003; 108:1809–14.

15. Nallamothu BK, Bates ER. Percutaneous coronary intervention versus fibrinolytic therapy in acute myocardial infarction: is timing (almost) everything? Am J Cardiol 2003; 92:824–6.

16. Antman EM, Anbe DT, Armstrong PW, *et al*. ACC/AHA guidelines for the management of patients with ST-elevation myocardial infarction – executive summary: a report of the American College of Cardiology/American Heart Association Task Force on Practice Guidelines (Writing Committee to Revise the 1999 Guidelines for the Management of Patients With Acute Myocardial Infarction). Circulation 2004; 110:588–636.

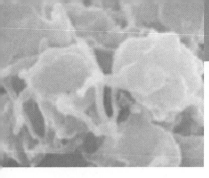

21

Percutaneous coronary intervention in left main stem disease

SEUNG-JUNG PARK, MD, PHD
AND YOUNG-HAK KIM, MD, PHD

KEY POINTS

- Left main coronary artery (LMCA) stenosis might be considered as an attractive target for balloon angioplasty because of its large caliber, short lesion length and lack of tortuosity.

- Unprotected LMCA (ULMCA) bifurcation disease is a very controversial target of PCI. Although there was a favorable initial outcome after ULMCA intervention using BMS in low-risk patients, bypass surgery remains the first choice for treating ULMCA stenosis due to in-stent restenosis.

- Drug-eluting stent implantations are reported to have a procedural success rate of 100%, no deaths, emergent CABG, or myocardial infarction, and 2% TVR rate at one-year follow-up.

- Patients and lesions treated with DES had higher risk profile and complexity such as more multivessel involvement, longer lesions and more bifurcations.

- DES implantation in ULMCA bifurcation showed more favorable long-term outcomes, although location of bifurcation lesions remains a challenge.

- LMCA dissection following coronary angiography or interventional procedure is a rare but serious complication.

INTRODUCTION

Several etiologies can make LMCA stenosis (Table 21.1). LMCA stenosis might be considered as an attractive target for balloon angioplasty because of its large caliber, short lesion length and lack of tortuosity. Histologically, the LMCA has the most elastic tissue of the coronary vessel, accounting for the poor response of the LMCA to simple balloon angioplasty. However, coronary stents have been shown to reduce the immediate need for CABG for abrupt vessel closure and the likelihood of restenosis after balloon angioplasty. At present, new devices are

TABLE 21.1 - ETIOLOGY OF LEFT MAIN CORONARY ARTERY DISEASE
Atherosclerosis
Non atherosclerotic etiologies
Radiation
Takayasu's arteritis
Syphilitic aortitis
Rheumatoid arthritis
Aortic valve disease
Kawasaki disease
Injury after left main coronary intervention or cardiac surgery
Idiopathic

TABLE 21.2 - INITIAL AND LONG-TERM OUTCOMES OF ULMCA STENTING WITH BMS

Low Risk Patients

Authors	Silvestri et al[5]	Black et al.[7]	Park et al.[4]	Tan et al.[6]
Number	93	53	127	89
Technical success, %	100	100	99.2	NA
In-hospital outcomes				
Cardiac death, %	0	1.8	0	0
Myocardial infarction, %	0	0	1	2.3
Emergent CABG, %	0	0	1	0
Long-term				
Duration, month	6	7.3±5.8	25.5±16.7	24
Cardiac death, %	0	1.9	0.8	3.4
Myocardial infarction, %	0.8	0	0	2.3
Target lesion revascularization, %	21	15.4	11.8	31.8

High Risk Patients

Authors	Silvestri et al[5]	Black et al.[7]	Tagaki et al.[9]	Tan et al.[6]
Number	93	39	67	144
Technical success, %	100	100	100	NA
In-hospital outcomes				
Cardiac death, %	9	7.6	0	10.2
Myocardial infarction, %	4	0	3.0	NA
Emergent CABG, %	0	0	3.0	NA
Long-term				
Duration, month	6	7.3±5.8	31±23	24
Cardiac death, %	2	13.8	10.3	29.8
Myocardial infarction, %	0	0	0	18.8
Target lesion revascularization, %	10.5	19.4	19.4	50.0

NA=not available

widely used to overcome the limitations of balloon angioplasty, and may also be useful to treat unprotected LMCA (ULMCA) stenosis in particular groups of patients. Therefore, stenting of ULMCA stenosis is considered as a therapeutic option in selected patients.[1-13]

Left main stenting with bare metal stent

Several studies with BMS evaluated the procedural safety and initial outcome of PCI for ULMCA stenosis as shown in Table 21.2. Careful patient selection may be crucial to produce favorable outcomes. In the later report of ULTIMA registry (n=279), 46% of patients were deemed inoperable or at high surgical risk.[6] Among them, 38 patients (14%) died in hospital. The one-year incidence was 24.2% for all-cause mortality, 20.2% for cardiac mortality, 9.8% for myocardial infarction, and 9.4% for CABG. By multivariate analysis in ULTIMA registry, the independent correlates of all-cause death during and after hospitalization were shown in Table 21.3. Decreasing left ventricular function was related to events in an inverse fashion but not linearly, with an apparent inflection point at the 30% left ventricular ejection fraction (LVEF) cut off level. On the other hand, the low subset of 89 patients form the ULTIMA registry, the one-year actuarial incidence of death was 3.4%, and that of myocardial infarction was 2.3%. Of note, there were no periprocedural deaths in this subgroup, and there were no additional

TABLE 21.3 - CORRELATES OF ALL CAUSE MORTALITY (IN-HOSPITAL AND DURING FOLLOW-UP) AFTER ULMCA INTERVENTION IN THE ULTIMA REGISTRY

EVENT	% OF STUDY POPULATION	HAZARD RATIO	95% CI	P VALUE
Left ventricular ejection fraction ≤ 30%	14.3	4.21	2.27 – 7.81	0.001
Mitral regurgitation grade 3 or 4	4.1	3.66	1.61 – 8.30	0.001
Cardiogenic shock	13.7	3.56	1.73 – 7.34	0.001
Serum creatinine ≥ 2 mg/dL	5.8	3.10	1.30 – 7.39	0.011
Severe lesion calcification	8.9	2.32	1.13 – 4.76	0.022

deaths or myocardial infarction beyond four months after discharge (up to 35 months). Park *et al.* reported the data of ULMCA stenting for selected patients with normal left ventricular function and good surgical candidates.[2,4,10] Procedural success rate was 99.1% and six-month restenosis rate was 19%. From the Asian Pacific Multicenter Registry data, three-year event rates are shown in Fig. 21.1.[10] Other recent studies from single institutions, however, have reported substantially improved outcomes. Silvestri *et al.* reported a one-year mortality of 11% and 7% for the high- and low-risk elective ULMCA stenting, including 47 patients who were considered to be at high risk for CABG (age >75 years, EF <35%) and 93 patients who were considered to be at low risk for CABG (age <75 years, no prior CABG, EF =35%, no renal failure, poor coronary runoff, or respiratory failure.[5]

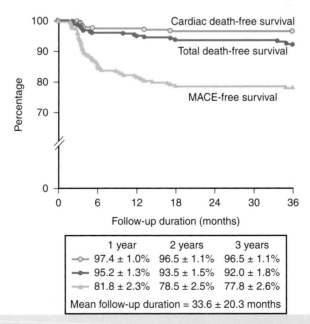

Figure 21.1:
Three-year survival curves of unprotected LMCA stenting for patients with normal left ventricular function from Asian Pacific Multicenter registry. MACE: including total death, myocardial infarction, and TLR.

ULMCA bifurcation disease is a very controversial target of PCI. Park *et al.* reported that elective stenting for ULMCA bifurcation (n=63) in highly selected patients with normal LVEF and large reference vessel might be safe and effective, and has good initial and long-term outcomes.[8] In this report, the procedure was successful in all patients, and major in-hospital events did not occur in any patients. The overall angiographic restenosis rate was 28%.

These results compare favorably to the current standard of care for ULMCA disease, CABG. The Society of Thoracic Surgery reported an in-hospital mortality of 3.9% in patients with left main disease.[14] The Cleveland Clinic Foundation reported 2.3% in-hospital mortality and 11.3% one-year mortality.[15] In low surgical risk patients age (<65 years, New York Heart Association congestive heart failure class =2) the one-year mortality was 5.7%. Although comparing studies by different authors and patient populations is subject to significant limitations, we may at least speculate that the short-term and intermediate event rates in stented and bypassed patients is comparable, at least in centers with expertise and experience in PCI of ULMCA.

TECHNICAL CONSIDERATIONS IN UNPROTECTED LEFT MAIN STENTING

1. Stenting at ostial and shaft lesions

The ostial ULMCA lesion is dilated and stented with the guide tip positioned in the aortic sinus. The proximal end of the stent is left protruding outside the ostium and expanded against the aortic wall as in any standard stenting of an aortic-ostial lesion. We usually deploy the stent slightly to protrude into the aorta (1–2 mm) for treatment of ULMCA ostial lesion. After the deployment of the stent, the stented segment is further dilated with high-pressure balloon inflation to achieve angiographic optimization. The lesion at the mid-shaft can be predilated and then stented as any discrete lesion in other branches.

2. Bifurcation lesion

Due to the technical difficulties, stenting for ULMCA bifurcation disease should be restricted to highly skilled interventionalists working with patients who understand the risk/benefit ratio of the percutaneous approach. During the procedure, occlusion of a side branch as a result of plaque shifting or stent strut can lead to the acute closure of ostium of the LAD artery or left circumflex artery and disastrous clinical events. Park *et al.* reported that stenting with or without debulking for LMCA bifurcation stenosis was performed in selected patients with safety and technical feasibility.[8] Stenting techniques were stenting across the left circumflex ostium, T(Y)-shaped stenting, kissing stenting, or bifurcation stenting. In this study, the left circumflex ostium was covered by a stent without risk of occlusion if it is diminutive or normal, showing that a small or non-diseased left circumflex artery in the vicinity of a stenosis does not prohibit the use of a stent. Furthermore, 54% of patients were successfully treated with stent placement across the left circumflex ostium, suggesting that this technique may be widely used for treatment of LMCA bifurcation lesions. However, progression of the side branch lesion spanned by a stent may be difficult to treat, and a possible risk of side branch occlusion remains an important limitation of this strategy.

ULMCA stenting with drug-eluting stent

Although, there was a favorable initial outcome after ULMCA intervention using BMS in low-risk patients, in-stent restenosis is the most important reason for bypass surgery as the first choice for treating ULMCA stenosis. In-stent restenosis in these patients not only influences long-term survival, but may also make repeat intervention so difficult that surgery is required. Recently, DES remarkably decrease in-stent restenosis in elective patients with relatively simple coronary lesions. Along with these results, some studies reported early clinical experience ULMCA stenting with DES.

1. Outcomes of DES implantation

Until now, three reports in three cardiac centers reported the mid-term outcomes of ULMCA interventions with DES with comparison to the pre-DES era as shown in Table 21.4. At one-year follow up, Park *et al.* reported a procedural success

TABLE 21.4 - COMPARISON OF LESION CHARACTERISTICS AND PROCEDURAL TECHNIQUES BETWEEN THE DES AND PRE-DES ERA

	CHIEFFO ET AL.[12]		VALGIMIGLI ET AL.[13]		PARK ET AL.[11]	
	DES	Pre-DES	DES	Pre-DES	DES	Pre-DES
Patient	85	64	95	86	102	121
Age	63.2±11.7	65.6±11.7	64±12	66±10	60.3±11.1	57.6±11.9
Male	70 (84.3%)	54 (82.3%)	66%	62%	87 (71.9%)	76 (74.5%)
Diabetes mellitus	18 (21.2%)	7 (10.9%)	30%	22%	29 (84.4%)	26 (21.5%)
Ejection fraction, %	51.1±11 *	57.4±12.7	41±14	42±13	60.4±8.4	61.8±6.8
Acute MI	NA	NA	17%	20% *	10 (9.8%)	8 (6.6%)
Cardiogenic shock at entry	NA	NA	9%	12%	0	0
LM plus multivessel involvement (≥2)	NA	NA	80%	69%	59 (58.4%)	13 (10.7%)
Distal location	69 (81.2%) **	37 (57.8%)	65%	66%	72 (70.6%) **	51 (42.5%)
Reference diameter, mm	3.73±0.6 **	4.01±0.7	3.25±0.5	3.37±0.6	3.46±0.65 **	3.98±0.69
MLD, pre, mm	1.34±0.5 *	1.53±0.6	1.09±0.44	1.05±0.59	1.31±0.57	1.35±0.58
Treated lesions	2.9±1.6 **	2.3±1.3	NA	NA	43 (42.2%)	42 (34.7%)
Stent length, mm	24.3±12 **	15.8±8.6	24±13	20±9	26.6±18.1 **	13.3±5.5
DCA, mm	2 (2.3%) **	13 (20.3%)	0 **	6%	3 (2.9%) **	40 (33.1)
MLD, post, mm	3.3±0.6 **	3.8±0.7	2.83±0.49	2.97±0.6	3.36±0.47	4.08±0.57
Bifurcation stenting	51 (74%)	NA	40% *	15%	29 (41%) **	9 (18%)
Culotte	5 (10%)	NA	36%	11	0	0
T technique	4 (8%)	NA	44%	88	1 (3%)	8 (89%)
Crush	30 (59%)	NA	12%	0	11 (38%)	0
Kissing	12 (24%)	NA	8%	0	17 (59%)	1 (11%)

DCA=directional coronary atherectomy, LM=let main, MI=myocardial infarction, MLD=minimal luminal diameter, NA=not available, *p<0.05, **p<0.01, †percentage in patients with bifurcation lesions

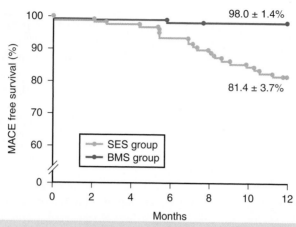

Figure 21.2:
Kaplan-Meier Curves for one-year MACE-free survival in patients treated with sirolimus-eluting stents (SES group) and BMS group. A statistically significant difference was observed between the two groups (p=0.0003). MACE: events including death, myocardial infarction, and TLR.

rate of 100%, no deaths, emergent CABG, or myocardial infarction, and 2% TVR rate in 102 patients with normal left ventricular function who underwent elective ULMCA intervention with sirolimus-eluting stents, despite distal bifurcation involvement in 71% of patients.[11] They showed significant improved one-year outcomes of ULMCA intervention with DES compared with BMS as shown Fig. 21.2. Chieffo *et al.* reported 3.4% mortality rate and 20.8% target lesion revascularization (TLR) rate at 7.6±4.2 months follow-up in a study of 88 consecutive patients who underwent sirolimus-eluting stent implantation.[12] Many patients in this study had complex lesions, including 63 patients with bifurcation lesions and 9 patients with trifurcation lesions. Valgimigli *et al.* included 95 patients with DES implantation and reported 4% mortality and 6% TVR rates in 95 patients during one-year follow-up.[13] In this study, 52 patients received sirolimus-eluting stent and 43 patients received paclitaxel-eluting stent. These three studies consistently observed the benefit of DES over BMS regarding clinical and angiographic outcomes.

2. Technical consideration in DES implantation
Compared to the pre-DES era, the patients and lesions treated with DES had higher risk profile and complexity such as more multivessel involvement, longer lesions and more bifurcations as shown in Table 21.4. Furthermore, complex stenting procedures were more preferred for complete reconstruction of ULMCA bifurcation. Crush technique is a new but widely accepted technique as a useful bifurcation stenting strategy. Nevertheless, DES implantation in ULMCA bifurcation showed more favorable long-term outcomes compared to the pre-DES era.

Location of bifurcation lesions remained challenging in ULMCA intervention even in the DES era. All the cases with target vessel failure in the three reports shown in the Table 21.5 were caused by the restenosis at the ULMCA bifurcation.

TABLE 21.5 - COMPARISON OF INITIAL AND LONG-TERM CLINICAL OUTCOMES BETWEEN THE DES AND PRE-DES ERA

| | CHIEFFO ET AL.[12] | | VALGIMIGLI ET AL.[13] | | PARK ET AL.[11] | |
	DES	Pre-DES	DES	Pre-DES	DES	Pre-DES
Patient	85	64	95	86	102	121
Angiographic outcome						
Follow up rate	NA	NA	NA	NA	84%	82%
MLD, follow up, mm	NA	NA	NA	NA	3.25±0.53 **	2.78±1.11
Late loss, mm	0.58 **	1.08	NA	NA	0.05±0.57 **	1.27±0.90
Restenosis	12 (19%)	15 (30.6%)	NA	NA	6 (7.0%) **	30 (30.3%)
Clinical outcome						
Initial						
Time	In-hospital	In-hospital	30 days	30 days	In-hospital	In-hospital
Death	0	0	10 (11%)	6 (7%)	0	0
MI	5 (5.9%)	5 (7.8%)	4 (4%)	8 (9%)	7 (6.9%)	10 (8.3%)
Stent thrombosis	0	0	0	0	0	0
TVR	0	2 (2.3%)	0	2 (2%)	0	0
Any events	NA	NA	14 (15%)	19 (19%)	7 (6.9%)	10 (8.3%)
Long-term						
Duration, month	6	6	503 (median)	11.7±3.4	30.3±13.7	
Death	3 (3.5%)	9 (14.1%)	14%	16%	0	0
MI	NA	NA	4% **	12%	7 (6.9%)	10 (8.3%)
Stent thrombosis	1 (0.1%)	0	NA	NA	0	0
TVR	16 (18.8%)	19 (30.6%)	6% **	12%	2 (2.0%) **	21 (17.4%)
Any events	NA	NA	24% **	45%	9 (7.9%) **	31 (25.6%)

MI=myocardial infarction, MLD=minimal luminal diameter, NA=not available, TVR=target vessel revascularization, *p<0.05, **p<0.01

Thus, the report by Chieffo *et al.* did not show a statistically significant benefit of DES over BMS regarding TVR. These warrant further studies focusing on the evaluation of the most optimal strategy or the dedicated bifurcated stent to improve outcomes of ULMCA bifurcation intervention with DES.

ADJUNCTIVE DEVICES FOR IMPROVEMENT OF THE OUTCOME OF ULMCA STENTING

1. Intravascular ultrasound

Intravascular ultrasound provides lots of quantitative and qualitative information on coronary artery lesions. It is often difficult to evaluate the actual size of the LMCA on angiography. Often the left main trunk is short and lacks a normal segment for comparison. In addition, contrast in the aortic cusp sometimes obscure the ostium, and 'streaming' of contrast may result in a false impression of luminal narrowing. Furthermore angiography underestimates stenosis severity. IVUS before stenting, therefore, provides useful information about the selection of adequate size of balloons and stents, and the accurate amounts and extent of calcification and contributed to change in treatment modalities in 40% of non-LMCA lesions. Although there is no absolute ultrasound criteria for 'critical' left main stenosis to intervene, suggested IVUS criteria for significant left main disease are >50% diameter stenosis, >60% area stenosis, absolute <7mm^2 in patients with symptoms, or absolute < 6mm^2 in asymptomatic patients. A recent study evaluated 122 patients with intermediate left main disease (~42% diameter stenosis by QCA).[16] In a single center, a small study evaluating the impact of IVUS in ULMCA intervention showed that the incidence of major adverse events was similar as 2 of 24 (8%) in the IVUS group and 7 of 34 (20%) in the non-IVUS group (p=0.18).[17] However, IVUS evaluation may be crucial in ULMCA intervention for precise lesions assessment, which facilitate to select and perform optimal stenting strategy.

2. Debulking atherectomy

Debulking coronary atherectomy (DCA) might facilitate successful stent placement by removing the plaque and potentially reduce restensosis rate by improving acute results. A nonrandomized comparison study using BMS showed that debulking before stenting resulted in significant reduction of angiographic restenosis (p=0.034) and TLR (p=0.049) by univariate analysis.[4] Hu et al. found similar results in 67 low- to high-risk patients with ULMCA stenosis with distal bifurcation involvement treated with IVUS-guided directional atherectomy.[18] The all-cause mortality, angiographic restenosis, and TLR rates at six months were 7%, 24%, and 20%, respectively. However, the benefit may not be maintained in the era of DES. In recent studies with DES shown in Table 21.4, the use of debulking was infrequent compared to the BMS era because of strong inhibition of neointimal production by DES. From these data, therefore, although a strategy of debulking combined with bare metal stenting can significantly reduce complication rates, it may be overtaken by the use of DES. A further research on the effect of DCA in DES era is warranted.

3. Intra-aortic balloon pump

Patients with normal left ventricular function are tolerant to global ischemia during the balloon occlusion. Although intra-aortic balloon pump is not routinely recommended during the procedure, intra-aortic balloon pump should be used for prevention of hemodynamic collapse in patients with severely depressed left ventricular function.

EMERGENCY INTERVENTION FOR UNPROTECTED LMCA STENOSIS

1. Procedure-related complications

The LMCA dissection following coronary angiography or interventional procedure is a rare but serious complication. Careful observation or elective CABG may be a reasonable approach for a non-flow limiting dissection. However, emergent CABG or bail-out stenting should be performed for a flow-limiting dissection of the LMCA. A recent retrospective observational study showed that bail-out stenting for LMCA dissection was successful in all cases (n=10) and had very favorable long-term outcomes.[19]

2. Acute myocardial infarction

Because there is paucity of data reporting outcomes of acute myocardial infarction patients with acute closure of the LMCA, the role of primary angioplasty remains uncertain. Most patients initially presented with cardiogenic shock, requiring aggressive mechanical support. These patients, unlike other forms of acute myocardial infarction, have a high in-hospital mortality and morbidity because of left ventricular pump failure. In the ULTIMA registry, in-hospital cardiac death rate is still very high, occurring in >50% of patients undergoing primary angioplasty because it cannot prevent acute left ventricular failure.[20] However, a recent study showed that 10 surviving patients of 18 patients with LMCA infarction at discharge lived well during 39±22 months except only one case of TLR.[21] Therefore, new approaches, such as early catheter-based reperfusion therapy plus left ventricular assisted device insertion, will be a good alternative to emergent bypass surgery.

FUTURE PERSPECTIVES

The ultimate proof of the relative value of ULMCA PCI and CABG will clearly depend on the results of randomized clinical trials comparing PCI using DES with CABG. These trials will involve a number of technical considerations that could significantly alter angioplasty outcome. Until these trials are performed, judicious selection of appropriate patients will be crucial to define those who are optimal candidates before ULMCA PCI. Nonetheless, until such data becomes available some years hence, we may make some reasonable speculations based on the currently available short-term and long-term data. There are not enough data to recommend routine stenting of ULMCA disease who are otherwise good candidates for CABG. On the other hand, the available results suggest that PCI using a DES may represent an acceptable alternative therapy for ULMCA, and that guidelines might reasonably be re-evaluated based on this published and emerging experience.

CONCLUSIONS

Procedural safety of ULMCA intervention has widely been reported since the pre-DES era. Furthermore, DES implantation achieved profound advancement of mid-term patency of ULMCA stenting. Despite lack of long-term results, these early experiences suggest DES implantation as a default approach in ULMCA stenosis. Current planned and ongoing randomized studies comparing the efficacy of DES with CABG will reveal the more appropriate therapy for ULMCA lesions.

REFERENCES

1. Ellis SG, Tamai H, Nobuyoshi M, et al. Contemporary percutaneous treatment of unprotected left main stenoses: initial results from a multicenter registry analysis 1994–1996. Circulation. 1997; 96:3867–72.

2. Park SJ, Park SW, Hong MK, et al. Stenting of unprotected left main coronary artery stenoses: immediate and late outcome. J Am Coll Cardiol. 1998; 31:37–42.

3. Kosuga K, Tamai H, Ueda K, *et al.* Initial and long-term results of angioplasty in unprotected left main coronary artery. Am J Cardiol. 1999; 83:32–7.

4. Park SJ, Hong MK, Lee CW, *et al.* Elective stenting of unprotected left main coronary artery stenosis: Effect of debulking before stenting and intravascular ultrasound guidance. J Am Coll Cardiol. 2001; 38:1054–60.

5. Silvestri M, Barragan P, Sainsous J, *et al.* Unprotected left main coronary artery stenting: immediate and medium-term outcomes of 140 elective procedures. J Am Coll Cardiol. 2000; 35:1543–50.

6. Tan WA, Tamai H, Park SJ, *et al.* ULTIMA Investigators. Long-Term Clinical Outcomes After Unprotected Left Main Trunk Percutaneous Revascularization in 279 Patients. Circulation, 2001; 104:1609–14.

7. Black Jr A, Cortina R, Bossi I, *et al.* Unprotected left main coronary artery stenting Correlates of midterm survival and impact of patient selection J Am Coll Cardiol. 2001; 37:832–83.

8. Park SJ, Lee CW, Kim YH, *et al.* Technical feasibility, safety and clinical outcome of stenting of unprotected left main coronary artery bifurcation narrowing Am J Cardiol. 2002; 104:1609–14.

9. Takagi T, Stankovic G, Finci L, *et al.* Results and long-term predictors of adverse clinical events after elective percutaneous interventions on unprotected left main coronary artery. Circulation. 2002; 106:698–702.

10. Park SJ, Park SW, Hong MK, *et al.* Long-term (3-Years) outcomes after stenting of unprotected left main coronary artery stenosis in patients with normal left ventricular function. Am J Cardiol. 2003; 91:12–16.

11. Park SJ, Kim YH, Lee BK, *et al.* Sirolimus-eluting stent implantation for unprotected left main coronary artery stenosis: comparison with bare metal stent implantation. J Am Coll Cardiol. 2005; 45:351–6.

12. Chieffo A, Stankovic G, Bonizzoni E, *et al.* Early and mid-term results of drug-eluting stent implantation in unprotected left main. Circulation. 2005; 111:791–5.

13. Valgimigli M, van Mieghem CA, Ong AT, *et al.* Short- and long-term clinical outcome after drug-eluting stent implantation for the percutaneous treatment of left main coronary artery disease: insights from the Rapamycin-Eluting and Taxus Stent Evaluated At Rotterdam Cardiology Hospital registries (RESEARCH and T-SEARCH). Circulation. 2005; 111:1383–9. Society of Thoracic Surgery National Database. ctsnet.org/doc/3037.

14. Ellis SG, Hill CM, Lytle BW. Spectrum of surgical risk for left main coronary stenosis: benchmark for potentially competing percutaneous therapies. Am Heart J. 1998; 135:335–8.

16. Abizaid AS, Mintz GS, Abizaid A, *et al.* One-year follow-up after intravascular ultrasound assessment of moderate left main coronary artery disease in patients with ambiguous angiograms. J Am Coll Cardiol 1999; 34:707–15.

17. Agostoni P, Valgimigli M, Van Mieghem CAG, *et al.* Comparison of early outcome of percutaneous coronary intervention for unprotected left main coronary artery disease in the drug-eluting stent era with versus without intravascular ultrasonic guidance. Am J Cardiol. 2005; 95:644–7.

18. Hu FB, Tamai H, Kosuga K, *et al.* Intravascular ultrasound-guided directional coronary atherectomy for unprotected left main coronary stenoses with distal bifurcation involvement. Am J Cardiol. 2003; 92:936–40.

19. Lee SW, Hong MK, Kim YH, *et al.* Bail-out stenting for left main coronary artery dissection during catheter-based procedure: acute and long-term results. Clin Cardiol 2004; 27:393–5.

20. Marso SP, Steg G, Plokka T, *et al.* Catheter-based reperfusion of unprotected left main stenosis during an acute myocardial infarction (the ULTIMA experience). Am J Cardiol. 1999; 83:1513–17.

21. Lee SW, Hong MK, Lee CW, *et al.* Early and late clinical outcomes after primary stenting of the unprotected left main coronary artery stenosis in the setting of acute myocardial infarction. Int J Cardiol. 2004; 97:73–6.

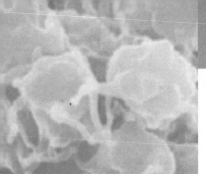

22

Percutaneous coronary intervention for chronic total occlusions

BRENDAN DUFFY, MD, RYAN D. CHRISTOFFERSON, MD, AND PATRICK L. WHITLOW, MD

KEY POINTS

■ A recent expert consensus document has defined chronic total occlusions (CTO) as an atherosclerotic coronary narrowing resulting in complete interruption of antegrade flow with the duration of the occlusion greater than three months.

■ There are age-related histologic changes in plaque composition that are important to development of successful strategies for CTO angioplasty.

■ Retrospective studies have shown an increase in long-term survival with successful CTO angioplasty.

■ In most cases, procedural failure is due to inability to cross the lesion with a guidewire, although other factors such as dissection, thrombus formation, or failure to dilate the lesion once crossed may also contribute.

■ Newer guidewires specifically designed for CTO intervention are stiffer, stronger, and more supportive, combined with greater torque response.

■ Despite the development of improved CTO strategies and new guidewires, up to 40% of cases may still be unsuccessful.

INTRODUCTION

Chronic total occlusions (CTO) are believed to represent the most challenging lesion subset that interventional cardiologists encounter. They have been reported in up to 20–31% of diagnostic angiograms while percutaneous revascularization is only attempted in 11–15% of patients with CTO.[1–3] General misgivings about attempting percutaneous recanalization of CTO stem from prior evidence of poor success rates, high restenosis and reocclusion rates, cost, radiation exposure, and time constraints. However, successful recanalization in patients with viable myocardium has been shown to reduce angina,[4–6] prevent myocardial infarction,[4,7,8] reduce the need for bypass surgery,[4,9,10] and improve survival.[5,9,11] Most recently, DES have reduced restenosis and reocclusion after successful CTO recanalization.[12,13] The availability of DES has fueled a renewed interest in improving procedural success and extending CTO angioplasty to more patients.

As with other percutaneous coronary procedures, patient selection is vital to success. Several clinical and angiographic characteristics have been established as predictors of procedural success, and should be given careful consideration when planning CTO intervention. Once CTO angioplasty is undertaken, recent developments in strategy have enhanced the likelihood of success and have the potential to reduce complications. When traditional guidewires fail, newer guidewires and devices developed specifically for CTO recanalization have improved the procedural success rate of CTO. This chapter will review the histology and pathophysiology of CTO, develop a rationale for patient and lesion selection, outline the factors influencing success or failure, and report on specialized techniques and devices for CTO angioplasty.

PATHOPHYSIOLOGY AND HISTOLOGY

A recent expert consensus document has defined CTO as an atherosclerotic coronary narrowing resulting in complete interruption of antegrade flow with the duration of the occlusion greater than three months.[14] When analyzed microscopically, the histologic appearance of a CTO consists of varying degrees of atheroma, cholesterol, fibrous tissue, calcium, extracellular matrix and neovascular channels. In addition to these findings, there are age-related histologic changes in plaque composition that are important to development of successful strategies for CTO angioplasty. Age-related changes can occur as early as three months after the initial occlusion. It has been shown that lesions between 3 and 12 months do not differ with respect to recanalization feasibility from those that have been present for years.

Cholesterol and foam cell laden intimal plaque composition is more frequent in 'soft' recent CTOs, whereas fibrocalcific intimal or 'hard' plaque is increased with CTO age.[15–17] Indeed, fibrocalcific or 'hard' plaque is more likely to deflect the guidewire and is much more resistant to balloon and stent passage, perhaps explaining the difficulty in crossing 'older' lesions. In reality, most plaque does have histologic features of both more recent and older occlusions, potentially representing a staccato aging process of the plaque. Of note, neovascular channels with surrounding loose fibrous tissue frequently develop within the lesion.[18] Less than 50% of CTO lesions are actually totally occluded with no detectable microvascular channels on histology. The presence of a recanalized neovascular channel correlates with an angiographically tapering lesion and/or a short (~15mm) occlusion.[18] Tapering lesions are considered more favorable for intervention, as these channels enable the guidewire to engage the fibrous cap and navigate the lesion more easily. The extracellular matrix within the plaque of occluded arteries is rich in collagens type I and III, which becomes the target of potential therapy, as infusions of bacterial-derived collagenase have been postulated to improve the success rate in CTO intervention.[19]

In addition to the microscopic appearance of CTO, understanding of the angiographic appearance of a CTO is important for successful long-term patency after CTO intervention. On the macrovascular level, well-developed collaterals by passing the CTO help maintain myocardial viability despite an occluded epicardial artery. A coronary wedge pressure of 45 mmHg can be provided by these collaterals, and this pressure is adequate to prevent resting ischemia.[17] It had been thought that the presence of residual collateral flow and microvascular dysfunction after recanalization was associated with high reocclusion rates; however, Werner *et al.* demonstrated that there is no relationship between collateral blood supply, or coronary flow velocity reserve and target vessel failure. Instead, a low fractional flow reserve after recanalization was associated with a higher risk of reocclusion.[20]

RATIONALE FOR RECANALIZATION AND PATIENT SELECTION

Theoretical advantages to successful CTO recanalization include the reduction in predisposition to arrhythmic events, increased tolerance of future coronary occlusion events,[10,11] improvement in left ventricular function[21] and improved survival.[11] Following successful CTO recanalization there is an improvement in clinical symptoms. Only 7–18% of patients will subsequently undergo bypass surgery following successful recanalization compared to 36–58% should the percutaneous attempt fail.[22] Retrospective studies have shown an increase in long-term survival with successful CTO angioplasty[4,11,23–26] (Table 22.1).

Any decision to attempt a CTO needs to take into account a balance between the clinical and angiographic nuances of the individual patient as well as the operator's technical expertise and limitations. A recent expert consensus document suggests that PCI of a CTO should be undertaken when: (a) the occluded artery is responsible for the patients symptoms, or in asymptomatic patients when there is demonstrable ischemia in the territory of the CTO; (b) the territory supplied by the occluded vessel is viable; and (c) there is a > 60% success rate, <1% projected death rate and a <5% chance of having a myocardial infarction. Alternatively surgical intervention may be preferred when: (a) the left main trunk is involved, (b) three vessel disease is present in patients with insulin dependent diabetes, severe left ventricular dysfunction or chronic renal failure; (c) an occluded LAD is not amenable to PCI; and (d) multiple CTOs are present with a low anticipated success rate.[27] The goal should be complete revascularization of viable myocardium whenever possible.

TABLE 22.1 - LONG TERM SURVIVAL OF ATTEMPTED REVASCULARIZATION OF CTOS

STUDY	PATIENTS	SUCCESSFUL RECANALIZATION	STENT USE	MORTALITY
¶Olivari et al.[4] 1-year f/u	376 patients From Jun 1999 to Jan 2000	73.3%	90%	Procedural Success = 1.05%¶ Procedural Failure = 3.61% P = 0.13
Sureo et al.[11] 10-year f/u	2007 patients From Jun 1980– Dec 1999	74.4%	7%	Procedural Success = 26.5% Procedural Failure = 34.9% P = 0.001
Ramanathan et al.[23] 1-year f/u	963 patients between 1993–2000	73%	Unavailable	Procedural Success = 2%* Procedural Failure = 5.2% P<0.001
Bell et al.[24] 7-year f/u	354 patients Oct 1979 to Sept 1990	69%	None	Procedural Success = 18% Procedural Failure = 25% P = 0.21
Hoye et al.[25] 5-year f/u	874 patients between 1992 to 2002	65%	81%	Procedural Success = 6.5% Procedural Failure = 12% P = 0.02
Aziz et al.[26] 2.4-year f/u	543 patients between Jan 2000 and Jun 2004	69.4%	Unavailable	Procedural Success = 2.5% Procedural Failure = 7.3% P = 0.004

¶CTO length of >15 mm or not measurable, moderate to severe calcification, occlusion for >180 days, and multivessel disease were significant predictors of PCI failure.

*Success and partial success

TABLE 22.2 - COMMON REASONS FOR FAILURE TO REVASCULARIZE A CTO

Inability to cross the lesion with a guidewire
Sub-Intimal dissection
Inability to cross the lesion with a balloon
Inability to dilate the lesion
Dye extravasation
Presence of thrombus

FACTORS INFLUENCING SUCCESSFUL AND UNSUCCESSFUL RECANALIZATION

As there is much to be gained by a successful CTO intervention, much attention has been focused on the determinants of procedural success or failure. In most cases, procedural failure is due to inability to cross the lesion with a guidewire, although other factors such as dissection, thrombus formation, or failure to dilate the lesion once crossed may also contribute (Table 22.2).[28]

The most powerful angiographic predictors of procedural failure appear to be the age and length of the occlusion, although the presence of moderate to severe calcification, a non-tapered stump, or side branch at the occlusion may also portend lower success rates (Table 22.3).

Unfortunately the age of the occlusion is impossible to determine in a significant proportion of cases. Many experts consider a length of 15 mm to be a critical success limit. Favorable anatomic features include a progressively narrowing diameter with a central course, a functional occlusion (which likely represents a CTO with recanalization by microchannels which can be exploited to engage the lesion with the tip of the wire), and an occlusion before or after a side branch. Notably, with greater operator experience and state of the art technology CTOs can be safely and effectively opened regardless of the presence or absence of bridging collaterals,[28] although this remains controversial.[29]

Recently, the importance of traditional angiographic predictors has been called into question by the ACROSS pilot trial, featuring 101 patients from the current era of newer guidewires. In this trial technical and procedural technical characteristics such as fluoroscopic time and the need for multiple guidewires were predictive of success, and traditional anatomic characteristics, such as age and length of occlusion, were not predictors.[30] Successes in guidewire and device technology may have changed the landscape of CTO intervention, necessitating reappraisal of the more traditional predictors of success and failure.

TABLE 22.3 - NEGATIVE PREDICTORS OF A SUCCESSFUL OUTCOME

Length of occlusion >15 mm
Duration of occlusion >3 months
Presence of moderate to severe calcification, tortuosity, or ostial occlusion
A blunt 'cut-off' or non tapered stump
Origin of a side branch at the occlusion
Lack of visibility of the distal vessel

COMPLICATIONS

Although historically thought of as a relatively benign procedure when compared to non-CTO intervention, data from Suero *et al.* suggest a different perspective.[11] When compared to a matched cohort of non-CTO interventions, in-hospital outcomes of death, myocardial infarction, urgent revascularization, and stroke were similar. Coronary dissection rates were actually higher in the CTO interventions. Additionally, in hospital death and urgent revascularization were even higher than for non-CTO intervention if the procedure was unsuccessful. When performing a CTO procedure, care must be taken to preserve the non-diseased vessels proximal to the stenosis, to preserve major collateral vessels, and to prevent thrombus formation, air embolism, guidewire fracture, entrapment and/or perforation. Most guidewire entrapment can be avoided by never rotating the guidewire more than 180 degrees. Maximal dye consumption should be limited to 3–5 ml/kg, and fluoroscopy times should be ≤60 minutes to minimize the risk of contrast induced nephropathy and radiation induced skin injury.

The choice of guidewire may have the most influence on the risk for perforation. Stiffer, hydrophilic wires are more inclined to travel subintimally and cause coronary dissection or perforation, and, therefore, should be used with caution. Coronary dissection carries an increased risk for compromise of collateral channels, or for side-branch or parent vessel closure, leading to periprocedural myocardial infarction. Guidewire only perforation is frequently benign; however, it can lead to hemopericardium, tamponade, and even death. Perforation may occur unrelated to the guidewire, as a result of adjunctive device use, balloon inflation, stent implantation, or atherectomy. In the event of these large perforations, prompt treatment should be instituted with prolonged obstructive balloon inflation proximal to the rupture site. Consideration should be given to placement of a membrane-coated stent. Protamine should be administered concurrent with prolonged balloon inflation, and bedside pericardiocentesis should be performed if there is echocardiographic or clinical evidence of tamponade. Prompt surgical consultation should also be obtained in case hemopericardium cannot be controlled.

SPECIALIZED TECHNIQUES AND TECHNOLOGIES FOR RECANALIZATION

Improvement in guidewire technology is the primary reason for improving CTO angioplasty success rates. Newer guidewires specifically designed for CTO intervention are stiffer, stronger, and more supportive, combined with greater torque response. The optimal strategy for guidewire selection depends upon the characteristics of the lesion. Conventional guidewires often do not have the tip stiffness or push adequate to transverse the fibrous cap. If a conventional guidewire fails to cross easily, newer specialized guidewires have a thicker core and/or gradually taper toward the tip, may aid in traversing the fibrous cap. Additionally, these newer wires may be coated with a hydrophilic polymer that increases the ability to slide the wire within the occlusion after the fibrous cap has been crossed. These newer hydrophilic wires have been shown to improve CTO success rates over conventional wires,[31] but also appear to be more likely to enter a subintimal plane, causing dissection or perforation, particularly in the hands of an inexperienced operator. In general the operator should escalate wire choice going from less to more support, which will result in increased stiffness of the wire. The distal tip bend should have a short radius to allow turning in a small channel. One may consider re-shaping an additional bend 1–2 mm from the guidewire tip, because once inside the occlusion the tip tends to straighten out, losing steerability. A number of guidewires have been developed specifically to tackle CTOs, with variable characteristics that can be exploited depending on lesion morphology (Table 22.4).

As a result of varying lesion characteristics it is frequently necessary to use multiple guidewires to successfully complete the procedure.

Successful CTO angioplasty requires strategic planning. It is important to review the angiographic images carefully. Multiple views of the vessel are generally necessary to adequately assess for lesion characteristics and distal collaterals. Visualization of the distal vessel is critical to ensuring guidewire passage into the true distal lumen. Helpful suggestions for increasing procedural safety and improving procedural success rate include:

- Concomitant use of a contra-lateral injection to visualize the distal vessel via a second arterial sheath.
- Saving a freeze-frame, or 'road-map' of the proximal and distal segments for reference during the procedure.
- Using a parallel-wire technique, e.g. if a false lumen is entered, introduce a second wire and steer it away from the false lumen marked by the first wire.
- Introduction of an over the wire balloon to give adequate support to the guidewire, and allow contrast injection into the distal coronary bed once the guidewire appears to be beyond the lesion.
- Using heparin only until after the wire has crossed the lesion and can be confirmed to be in the distal 'true' lumen because Heparin can be reversed if perforation occurs.

TABLE 22.4 - GUIDEWIRES SUITABLE FOR CROSSING CTOS

WIRE	MANUFACTURER	PROPERTIES
Hi-Torque Pilot 50, 150 and 200	Guidant	Hydrophilic, 0.014″
Cross-IT XT 100, 200, 300 and 400		Tapered tip, 0.010″
		Hydrophilic, 0.014″
Whisper MS		Flexible Hydrophilic, 0.014″
Shinobi	Cordis	Hydrophilic, 0.014″
Shinobi Plus		Stiff, Hydrophilic
PT Graphic	Boston Scientific	Hydrophilic, 0.014″
Choice PT		Hydrophilic, 0.014″
Crosswire NT	Terumo	Hydrophilic, 0.016″
Miracle Brothers 3, 4.5, 6 and 12 gram	Asahi Intecc	Increasing stiffness and torque response, 0.014″
Confianza		Torque responsive, tapered tip down to 0.009″
Confianza Pro		Hydrophilic except 1mm hydrophobic tip, tapered tip to 0.009′ torque responsive

While failure to cross with a balloon occurs in 2–9% of patients, these issues can be resolved by:

- Switching the guide catheter for more back up support, using a long femoral sheath or an 8 Fr guide for extra control, and using an Amplatz catheter for both the RCA and LCA.
- Ensuring coaxial alignment of the guide catheter.
- Placing a 'buddy wire' into a branch that is proximal to the occlusion, in order to increase guide support.
- Inflating a balloon proximal to the lesion, or inside a branch, in order to stabilize the guide catheter.
- Debulking the lesion with rotational atherectomy or excimer laser.
- Utilizing the Tornus® device to twist across the lesion.

Consider calling a halt to the procedure when:

- A large dissection is created by opening false lumen.
- Collaterals are cut off by opening a false lumen.
- All options are exhausted in a pre-determined time frame.
- There is excessive dye consumption or radiation exposure.

Despite the development of improved CTO strategies and new guidewires, up to 40% of cases may still be unsuccessful. This has led to the development of CTO-specific devices, some of which are adaptations of technology designed for peripheral vascular applications. Although several devices have been developed, to date only two devices have achieved United States Food and Drug Administration approval for intractable CTO cases. These devices are the *Safe Cross* system and the *Frontrunner* catheter (Table 22.5).

The Safe-cross system, developed by Intraluminal Therapeutics, Inc. (Carlsbad, CA), combines a 0.014" diameter guidewire with both optical coherence reflectometry guidance technology and controlled radio frequency (RF)

TABLE 22.5 - FDA APPROVED DEVICES FOR USE IN CTOS

Safe Cross RF Guidewire
- Features a steerable 0.014" wire.
- Uses low-coherence light transmitted through an optical fiber within a steerable 0.014" guide wire to detect plaque versus adventitia via back-scattered light.
- Delivers radiofrequency ablation energy, to penetrate the fibrous cap/plaque components.
- Pulses delivered are of low frequency (250–500 kHz) and short duration (100 ms).

Frontrunner Catheter
- Features manually operated reverse biopsy forceps for controlled blunt microdissection taking theoretical advantage of increased adventitial versus plaque elasticity.
- The device is supported by a 4.5 Fr microcatheter.

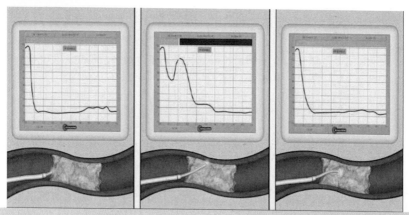

Figure 22.1:
The ILT Safe Cross-RF system with optical coherence reflectometry and radiofrequency ablation Capability. When the tip is in contact with the central plaque the reflectance curve is smooth and the display bar is green (left). When the tip is in close proximity to the wall the curve shows a secondary hump and the display turns red (middle). As the tip is redirected the display turns green again indicating that is safe to deliver radiofrequency energy (right).

energy (Fig. 22.1). A waveform is generated using fiber optic feedback from the lesion, carried through the wire, and displayed on a monitor. The system alerts the operator when the guidewire comes near the wall of the vessel, indicating a need to redirect the wire back into the lumen of the artery. Calcified and fibrous occlusions are more easily crossed using RF energy delivered from the wire tip. Once the wire has crossed the lesion, ordinary balloon angioplasty and stenting are employed to complete the procedure. Preliminary studies regarding the technical success of the procedure show success rates from 52% to 54% in patients with prior failed attempt using conventional guidewires.[32,33] Of note, perforation was detected in 2.6% of patients using this system.

The Frontrunner system, developed by LuMend, Inc (Redwood City, CA), utilizes microforceps on the tip of the guidewire to produce blunt microdissection (Fig. 22.2). This creates a channel through the CTO, which facilitates wire crossing, and conventional angioplasty/stenting. This technique has been used for both coronary and peripheral angioplasty. Initial results from Milan, Italy, on 50 patients, show that the device has modest success rates (53%).[34] However, the device was also associated with an unexpectedly high rate of coronary perforation (18%) and tamponade (4%). There is a learning curve for use of the device, and success rates increased while complication rates decreased over the three years of the study. The original multicenter study of the frontrunner in lesions failing attempts with conventional techniques (>10 minutes fluoroscopy time) reported similar success, 56%.

Aside from the approved devices, additional technology is under development and evaluation, in attempts to enhance the lesion access and wire crossing ability. Developed for calcified or fibrous CTO lesions, the FlowCardia Crosser therapeutic ultrasound system (Sunnyvale, CA) delivers 20 kHz ultrasound pulses, thereby mechanically fragmenting the lesion. It has been studied in 78 patients with conventional wire failure, with a success rate of >60%, and an adverse event rate of 4%.[35] The Venture catheter, from St. Jude, Inc. (Maple

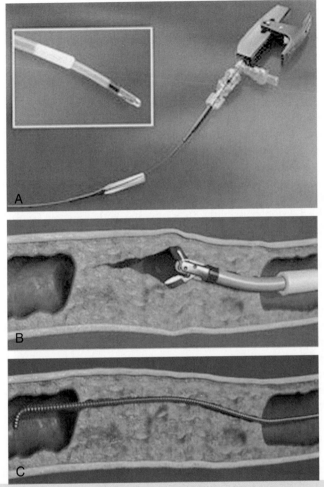

Figure 22.2:
(A) A schematic of the Frontrunner XP® CTO catheter. (B) A diagram of the blunt Micro-dissection technique. (C) Once the micro-channel is complete and the distal cap is crossed a guide-wire can be advanced allowing percutaneous intervention.

Grove, MN), is a steerable wire-control catheter, through which traditional guidewires can be advanced across the lesion. The deflectable tip of this device improves wire positioning and provides additional backup for the wire. Lesion access may be enhanced by another new device, developed by Stereotaxis, Inc. (St. Louis, MO), called the Stereotaxis Niobe Magnetic Navigation System. This device uses magnetically driven wire manipulation to facilitate access to angulated or tortuous arteries. The advantage to magnetic navigation is that the wire is driven from the tip, and so torque is not stored within the wire. This enables the wire to turn at angle unable to be achieved by traditional means. Preclinical studies in CTO are underway.

If severe calcification prevents advancement of conventional balloon or microcatheter after the lesion is crossed by a guidewire, a novel penetration over-the-wire catheter has been developed to remedy this situation. The *Tornus* device, from Asahi, consists of eight braided stainless steel strands that taper over the distal 15 cm of the catheter. If the catheter is advanced over the wire in a counter-clockwise fashion, it will theoretically twist across the lesion. The wire can then be exchanged after successful crossing, and balloon advancement is facilitated. The catheter was recently approved in the United States, and results of early clinical use in ten patients have been reported, showing a success rate of 100%, and no complications.[36]

Vibrational angioplasty has been developed to deliver energy to the wire tip by vibration. This device can be attached to an angioplasty catheter and wire combination, and activation of the device results in a complex reciprocation/lateral movement, as well as standing waves at the wire tip. These movements result in mechanical fragmentation of the lesion. In 99 patients with CTO, the device enabled lesion crossing in 86% of cases, with a similar complication rate to conventional wires.[37]

While mechanical strategies have enhanced the success rate of CTO angioplasty, pharmacologic approaches have been studied as well. Collagenase has been studied as a means to dissolve the fibrous cap, which is composed partially of collagen. Dissolution of the collagen is presumed to soften the lesion and facilitate easier guidewire passage. In 21 patients treated with collagenase infusion, 13 (62%) had a successful procedure, compared to 7 of 24 patients (29%) in the placebo group.[19] The main limitation to this strategy is the time commitment, as the collagenase must incubate for several hours after infusion in the coronary artery prior to attempting to cross the lesion.

Another potential pharmacologic strategy is the infusion of intracoronary thrombolytics to open the thrombus-filled microchannels characteristic of a CTO. This strategy has the potential to enhance success rates by clearing these microchannels, facilitating wire crossing. Prolonged infusion of intracoronary urokinase has been studied in 60 patients with CTO refractory to traditional means, finding a procedural success rate of 50–60% after lytic infusion.[38] Abbas, *et al.* also used intracoronary tPA or tenecteplase to enhance crossing CTO's in 46 of 85 (54%) of attempted cases.[29]

CLINICAL OUTCOMES AND CLINICAL TRIALS

Once the lesion has been dilated, the emphasis switches to keeping the vessel patent. Table 22.6 lists clinical trials demonstrating that BMS is superior to balloon angioplasty, with less restenosis and reocclusion, and lower MACE and target lesion revascularization (TLR) rates.[39–47]

Similar to the success of DES in other complex lesion subsets, the use of DES in CTO angioplasty has demonstrated lower restenosis, reocclusion and MACE rates compared to BMS in several registry studies (Table 22.7).[12,13,48–52]

Additional important data is continuing to emerge regarding the use of DES in CTO lesions. Preliminary results from the first randomized controlled trial of DES versus BMS, called the Prospective Randomized Trial of Sirolimus Eluting and Bare Metal Stents in Patients with Chronic Total Occlusions (PRISON 2) trial, have been reported.[53] In this study, 200 patients were randomized to either sirolimus eluting stent or BMS. At six months, restenosis rates were 11% in the

TABLE 22.6 - CLINICAL TRIALS OF BALLOON ANGIOPLASTY VERSUS BMS

STUDY	ENROLLMENT	NUMBER	STENT	RESULTS
SICCO[39] Stenting in Chronic Coronary Occlusions	Mar 1994 to May 1995	PTCA = 59 Stent = 58 Randomized only after a successful PTCA result	Palmaz-Schatz stents	Restenosis (p<0.01)* Stent group = 32% PTCA group = 74% Reocclusion (p = 0.058) Stent group = 12% PTCA group = 26%
Mori et al.[40]	Jan 1992 to Jun 1995	PTCA = 43 Stent = 53 Randomized only after a successful PTCA result	Palmaz-Schatz stent	Restenosis (p<0.005)* Stent group = 28% PTCA group = 57% Reocclusion (p = 0.04) Stent group = 7% PTCA group = 11%
GISSOC[41] Gruppo Italiano di Studi sulla Stent nelle Occlusioni coronariche	Jun 1992 to May 1995	PTCA = 54 Stent = 56 Randomized only after a successful PTCA result	Palmaz-Schatz stent	Restenosis (p<0.001) Stent group = 32% PTCA group = 68% Reocclusion (p = 0.003) Stent group = 8% PTCA group = 34%
SPACTO[42] Stent vs Percutaneous Angioplasty in Chronic	Jul 1994 to Jan 1997	PTCA = 42 Stent = 43 Randomized only after a successful PTCA result	Wiktor GX stent	Restenosis (p = 0.01)* Stent group = 32% PTCA group = 64% Reocclusion (p=0.01) Stent group = 3% PTCA group = 24%
STOP[43] Stents in Total Occlusions for Restenosis Prevention	Oct 1996 to Sep 1997	PTCA = 42 Stent = 48 Randomized only after a successful PTCA result	AVE microstent	Restenosis (p = 0.032)* Stent group = 42% PTCA group = 71% Reocclusion (NS) Stent group = 8% PTCA group = 17%
TOSCA[44] Total Occlusion Study of Canada	Mar 1996 to May 1997	PTCA = 208 Stent = 202	Heparin-coated 15-mm long PS-153 Palmaz-Schatz coronary stent	Restenosis (p<0.01)* Stent group = 55% PTCA group. = 70% Reocclusion (p = 0.02) Stent group = 11% PTCA group = 20%
PRISON[45] Primary Stenting of Occluded Native Coronary Arteries	Jan 1998- Nov 1999	PTCA=100 Stent=100 Randomized only after a successful PTCA result	NIR stent	Restenosis (p-0.14)* Stent group = 22% PTCA group = 33% Reocclusion (NS) Stent group = 8% PTCA group = 7%
Hancock et al.[46]	May 1994 to Oct 1995	PTCA = 30 Stent = 30 Randomized only after a successful PTCA result	Palmaz Schatz stent	Restenosis (NS)* Stent group = 22% PTCA group. = 40% Reocclusion (p<0.01) Stent group = 29% PTCA group = 7%

Continued

TABLE 22.6 - CLINICAL TRIALS OF BALLOON ANGIOPLASTY VERSUS BMS—cont'd

STUDY	ENROLLMENT	NUMBER	STENT	RESULTS
SARECCO[47] Stent or Angioplasty After Recanalization of Chronic Coronary Occlusions	Mar 1995 to Mar 1997	PTC = 55 Stent = 55 Randomized only after a successful PTCA result	Stent type decided by operator	Restenosis (p = 0.01) Stent group = 26% PTCA group = 62% Reocclusion (p = 0.05) Stent group = 2% PTCA group = 14%

* 6-month follow up

¶ 9-month follow up

§ 4-month follow up

TABLE 22.7 - REGISTRIES OF DES IN CTO INTERVENTION

STUDY	NUMBER	DRUG ELUTING STENT	MACE1 YEAR	6-MONTH ANGIOGRAPHIC RESULT FOR DES
Nakamura *et al.*[12]	60	Cypher Vs matched BMS conrtols	DES group = 3% BMS group =42% P<0.001	Restenosis = 2% Reocclusion = None
RESEARCH* Registry[13] Rapamycin Eluting Stent Evaluated At Rotterdam Cardiology Hospitals	56	Cypher Vs matched BMS control	DES group.= 3.5% BMS group =17.2% p<0.05	Restenosis = 9.1% Reocclusion = 3%
SICTO registry[48] Sirolimus-eluting Stent In Chronic Total Occlusion	25	Cypher No Control	8% (all TVR)	Restenosis = None Reocclusion = None
Werner *et al.*[49]	48	Taxus Vs matched BMS cohort	12.5% DES group 47.9% BMS group p<0.005	Restenosis = 8.3% Reocclusion = 2.1%
Ge *et al.*[50]	122	Cypher Vs matched control	6 month 16.4% DES 35.1 (BMS p<0.001	Restenosis = 9.2% Reocclusion = 2.5%
Buellesfeld *et al.*[51]	45	Taxus No control	15.6%	Restenosis = 13.2% Reocclusion = None
TRUE registry[52]§ Taxus in Real life Usage Evaluation	183	Taxus No control	17.1%	Restenosis = 17% Reocclusion = 0/6%

MACE defined as death, nonfatal myocardial infarction or TVR

*Only 60% of patients had 6 month angiographic follow up

§ 7-month follow up

¶ 6-month follow up

sirolimus group, versus 41% in the bare metal group (p<0.001). Additionally, lower MACE rates were seen in the sirolimus group (4%) than in the bare metal group (20%, p<0.001). The Approaches to ChRonic Occlusions with Sirolimus Stents (ACROSS-Cypher)/ Total occlusion Study of Coronary Arteries (TOSCA 4) study is an ongoing prospective registry enrolling 250 patients with a CTO and will assess the angiographic restenosis at six months following intervention with a sirolimus stent, compared with the BMS cohort form the TOSCA-1 study.

With regards to comparison of sirolimus versus paclitaxel stents, there are some preliminary results in the form of registry data to guide therapy. In the Multicenter registry in Asia study, 922 CTO lesions were studied, and there was no difference in MACE at 30 days, or restenosis at 12 months between groups (396 sirolimus and 526 paclitaxel).[54] These data are similar to those found by Cosgrave et al., who looked at 529 CTO lesions, demonstrating no difference in restenosis or MACE rates at follow up (248 sirolimus and 281 paclitaxel).[55]

CONCLUSIONS

While the current ACC/AHA PCI recommendations[56] do not differentiate between a simple stenotic lesion and CTO, the European Society of Cardiology PCI guidelines[57] recognize the challenges in this lesion subset and give a class IIa recommendation to CTO intervention (class IIa indicates the weight of evidence/opinion is in favor of usefulness/efficacy). Several practical caveats aimed at improving success rates have become commonplace. The operator disposition should be patient and persistent, and there should be a careful and prolonged evaluation of the images before the procedure is undertaken. The use of specialized techniques and familiarity with developing technologies are essential for a successful operator. Continued evidence suggests that a successful outcome results in improved survival, fewer symptoms, and enhanced left ventricular function. Although available clinical data comments on the morbidity and mortality of failed attempts at PCI, there is little data to know the fate of patients with a CTO that was not attempted. This patient subset may potentially benefit from a successful intervention. Therefore, with the adequate operator experience and technical know-how, combined with new tools in the form of advanced guidewires and devices, this patient subset is being greeted with renewed vigor and enthusiasm.

REFERENCES

1. Srinivas VS, Brooks MM, Detre KM, King SB, 3rd, Jacobs AK, Johnston J, Williams DO. Contemporary percutaneous coronary intervention versus balloon angioplasty for multivessel coronary artery disease: a comparison of the National Heart, Lung and Blood Institute Dynamic Registry and the Bypass Angioplasty Revascularization Investigation (BARI) study. Circulation. 2002; 106:1627–33.

2. Williams DO, Holubkov R, Yeh W, Bourassa MG, Al-Bassam M, Block PC, Coady P, Cohen H, Cowley M, Dorros G, Faxon D, Holmes DR, Jacobs A, Kelsey SF, King SB, 3rd, Myler R, Slater J, Stanek V, Vlachos HA, Detre KM. Percutaneous coronary intervention in the current era compared with 1985–1986: the National Heart, Lung, and Blood Institute Registries. Circulation. 2000; 102:2945–51.

3. Christofferson RD, Lehmann KG, Martin GV, Every N, Caldwell JH, Kapadia SR. Effect of chronic total coronary occlusion on treatment strategy. Am J Cardiol. 2005; 95:1088–91.

4. Olivari Z, Rubartelli P, Piscione F, Ettori F, Fontanelli A, Salemme L, Giachero C, Di Mario C, Gabrielli G, Spedicato L, Bedogni F. Immediate results and one-year clinical outcome after percutaneous coronary interventions in chronic total occlusions: data from a multicenter, prospective, observational study (TOAST-GISE). J Am Coll Cardiol. 2003; 41:1672–8.

5. Chung CM, Nakamura S, Tanaka K, Tanigawa J, Kitano K, Akiyama T, Matoba Y, Katoh O. Effect of recanalization of chronic total occlusions on global and regional left ventricular function in patients with or without previous myocardial infarction. Catheter Cardiovasc Interv. 2003; 60:368–74.

6. Seggewiss H, Strick S, Everlien M, Fassbender D, Schmidt HK, Gleichmann U. [The recanalization of the chronically occluded infarct vessel in single-vessel coronary disease. The reduction of cardiac events in long-term clinical follow-up]. Dtsch Med Wochenschr. 1995; 120:1305–11.

7. Melchior JP, Meier B, Urban P, Finci L, Steffenino G, Noble J, Rutishauser W. Percutaneous transluminal coronary angioplasty for chronic total coronary arterial occlusion. Am J Cardiol. 1987; 59:535–8.

8. Ivanhoe RJ, Weintraub WS, Douglas JS, Jr., Lembo NJ, Furman M, Gershony G, Cohen CL, King SB, 3rd. Percutaneous transluminal coronary angioplasty of chronic total occlusions. Primary success, restenosis, and long-term clinical follow-up. Circulation. 1992;85: 106–15.

9. Finci L, Meier B, Favre J, Righetti A, Rutishauser W. Long-term results of successful and failed angioplasty for chronic total coronary arterial occlusion. Am J Cardiol. 1990; 66:660–2.

10. Angioi M, Danchin N, Juilliere Y, Feldmann L, Berder V, Cuilliere M, Buffet P, Anconina J, Cherrier F. [Is percutaneous transluminal coronary angioplasty in chronic total coronary occlusion justified? Long term results in a series of 201 patients]. Arch Mal Coeur Vaiss. 1995; 88:1383–9.

11. Suero JA, Marso SP, Jones PG, Laster SB, Huber KC, Giorgi LV, Johnson WL, Rutherford BD. Procedural outcomes and long-term survival among patients undergoing percutaneous coronary intervention of a chronic total occlusion in native coronary arteries: a 20-year experience. J Am Coll Cardiol. 2001; 38:409–14.

12. Nakamura S, Muthusamy TS, Bae JH, Cahyadi YH, Udayachalerm W, Tresukosol D. Impact of sirolimus-eluting stent on the outcome of patients with chronic total occlusions. Am J Cardiol. 2005; 95:161–6.

13. Hoye A, Tanabe K, Lemos PA, Aoki J, Saia F, Arampatzis C, Degertekin M, Hofma SH, Sianos G, McFadden E, van der Giessen WJ, Smits PC, de Feyter PJ, van Domburg RT, Serruys PW. Significant reduction in restenosis after the use of sirolimus-eluting stents in the treatment of chronic total occlusions. J Am Coll Cardiol. 2004; 43:1954–8.

14. Stone GW, Kandzari DE, Mehran R, Colombo A, Schwartz RS, Bailey S, Moussa I, Teirstein PS, Dangas G, Baim DS, Selmon M, Strauss BH, Tamai H, Suzuki T, Mitsudo K, Katoh O, Cox DA, Hoye A, Mintz GS, Grube E, Cannon LA, Reifart NJ, Reisman M, Abizaid A, Moses JW, Leon MB, Serruys PW. Percutaneous recanalization of chronically occluded coronary arteries: a consensus document: part I. Circulation. 2005; 112:2364–72.

15. Suzuki T, Hosokawa H, Yokoya K, Kojima A, Kinoshita Y, Miyata S, Suzumura H, Kawajiri K. Time-dependent morphologic characteristics in angiographic chronic total coronary occlusions. Am J Cardiol. 2001; 88:167–9, A5–6.

16. Srivatsa SS, Edwards WD, Boos CM, Grill DE, Sangiorgi GM, Garratt KN, Schwartz RS, Holmes DR, Jr. Histologic correlates of angiographic chronic total coronary artery occlusions: influence of occlusion duration on neovascular channel patterns and intimal plaque composition. J Am Coll Cardiol. 1997; 29:955–63.

17. Meier B. Chronic total occlusion. In: Topol E, ed. Textbook of Interventional Cardiology. Philadelphia: W.B. Saunders; 1994:318–38.

18. Katsuragawa M, Fujiwara H, Miyamae M, Sasayama S. Histologic studies in percutaneous transluminal coronary angioplasty for chronic total occlusion: comparison of tapering and abrupt types of occlusion and short and long occluded segments. J Am Coll Cardiol. 1993; 21:604–11.

19. Strauss BH, Goldman L, Qiang B, Nili N, Segev A, Butany J, Sparkes JD, Jackson ZS, Eskandarian MR, Virmani R. Collagenase Plaque Digestion for Facilitating Guide Wire Crossing in Chronic Total Occlusions. Circulation. 2003; 108:1259–62.

20. Werner GS, Bahrmann P, Mutschke O, Emig U, Betge S, Ferrari M, Figulla HR. Determinants of target vessel failure in chronic total coronary occlusions after stent implantation. The influence of collateral function and coronary hemodynamics. J Am Coll Cardiol. 2003; 42:219–25.

21. Sirnes PA, Myreng Y, Molstad P, Bonarjee V, Golf S. Improvement in left ventricular ejection fraction and wall motion after successful recanalization of chronic coronary occlusions. Eur Heart J. 1998; 19:273–81.

22. Meier B. Chronic total occlusion: how do we get there from here? J Invasive Cardiol. 2001; 13:233–5; discussion 262–4.

23. Ramanathan K, Gao M, Nogareda GJ, et al. Successful percutaneous recanalization of a non-acute occluded coronary artery predicts clinical outcomes and survival. Circulation. 2001; 104:415.

24. Bell MR, Berger PB, Bresnahan JF, Reeder GS, Bailey KR, Holmes DR, Jr. Initial and long-term outcome of 354 patients after coronary balloon angioplasty of total coronary artery occlusions. Circulation. 1992; 85:1003–11.

25. Hoye A, van Domburg RT, Sonnenschein K, Serruys PW. Percutaneous coronary intervention for chronic total occlusions: the Thoraxcenter experience 1992–2002. Eur Heart J. 2005; 26:2630–6.

26. Aziz S, Grayson AD, Stables RH, et al. Percutaneous coronary intervention for chronic total occlusions: improved survival for patients with a successful revascularization procedure compared to a failed procedure. Am J Cardiol. 2005; 96:37H.

27. Stone GW, Reifart NJ, Moussa I, Hoye A, Cox DA, Colombo A, Baim DS, Teirstein PS, Strauss BH, Selmon M, Mintz GS, Katoh O, Mitsudo K, Suzuki T, Tamai H, Grube E, Cannon LA, Kandzari DE, Reisman M, Schwartz RS, Bailey S, Dangas G, Mehran R, Abizaid A, Moses JW, Leon MB, Serruys PW. Percutaneous recanalization of chronically occluded coronary arteries: a consensus document: part II. Circulation. 2005; 112:2530–7.

28. Kinoshita I, Katoh O, Nariyama J, Otsuji S, Tateyama H, Kobayashi T, Shibata N, Ishihara T, Ohsawa N. Coronary angioplasty of chronic total occlusions with bridging collateral

vessels: immediate and follow-up outcome from a large single-center experience. J Am Coll Cardiol. 1995; 26:409–15.

29. Abbas AE, Brewington SD, Dixon SR, Boura JA, Grines CL, O'Neill WW. Intracoronary fibrin-specific thrombolytic infusion facilitates percutaneous recanalization of chronic total occlusion. J Am Coll Cardiol. 2005; 46:793–8.

30. Menown I, Kuchela A, Fong P, Chow J, Kandzari DE, Berdan L, Buller CE. Approaches to the Chronic Occlusions Study (ACROSS) Registry. Am J Cardiol. 2004; 92:97E.

31. Saito S, Tanaka S, Hiroe Y, Miyashita Y, Takahashi S, Satake S, Tanaka K. Angioplasty for chronic total occlusion by using tapered-tip guidewires. Catheter Cardiovasc Interv. 2003; 59:305–11.

32. Baim DS, Braden G, Heuser R, Popma JJ, Cutlip DE, Massaro JM, Marulkar S, Arvay LJ, Kuntz RE. Utility of the Safe-Cross-guided radiofrequency total occlusion crossing system in chronic coronary total occlusions (results from the Guided Radio Frequency Energy Ablation of Total Occlusions Registry Study). Am J Cardiol. 2004; 94:853–8.

33. Hoye A, Onderwater E, Cummins P, Sianos G, Serruys PW. Improved recanalization of chronic total coronary occlusions using an optical coherence reflectometry-guided guidewire. Catheter Cardiovasc Interv. 2004; 63:158–63.

34. Dejan Orlic GS, Giuseppe Sangiorgi, Flavio Airoldi, Alaide Chieffo, Iassen Michev, Matteo Montorfano, Mauro Carlino, Nicola Corvaja, Leo Finci, Antonio Colombo,. Preliminary experience with the frontrunner coronary catheter: Novel device dedicated to mechanical revascularization of chronic total occlusions. Catheterization and Cardiovascular Interventions. 2005; 64:146–52.

35. Stone GW, Colombo A, Teirstein PS, Moses JW, Leon MB, Reifart NJ, Mintz GS, Hoye A, Cox DA, Baim DS, Strauss BH, Selmon M, Moussa I, Suzuki T, Tamai H, Katoh O, Mitsudo K, Grube E, Cannon LA, Kandzari DE, Reisman M, Schwartz RS, Bailey S, Dangas G, Mehran R, Abizaid A, Serruys PW. Percutaneous recanalization of chronically occluded coronary arteries: Procedural techniques, devices, and results. Catheter Cardiovasc Interv. 2005; 66:217–36.

36. Tsuchikane E, Katoh O, Shimogami M, Ito T, Ehara M, Sato H, Matsubara T, Suzuki T. First clinical experience of a novel penetration catheter for patients with severe coronary artery stenosis. Catheter Cardiovasc Interv. 2005; 65:368–73.

37. Michalis LK, Rees MR, Davis JA, Pappa EC, Katsouras C, Goudevenos J, Sideris DA. Vibrational angioplasty and hydrophilic guidewires in the treatment of chronic total coronary occlusions. J Endovasc Ther. 2000; 7:141–8.

38. Zidar FJ, Kaplan BM, O'Neill WW, Jones DE, Schreiber TL, Safian RD, Ajluni SC, Sobolski J, Timmis GC, Grines CL. Prospective, randomized trial of prolonged intracoronary urokinase infusion for chronic total occlusions in native coronary arteries. J Am Coll Cardiol. 1996; 27:1406–12.

39. Sirnes PA, Golf S, Myreng Y, Molstad P, Emanuelsson H, Albertsson P, Brekke M, Mangschau A, Endresen K, Kjekshus J. Stenting in Chronic Coronary Occlusion (SICCO): a randomized, controlled trial of adding stent implantation after successful angioplasty. J Am Coll Cardiol. 1996; 28:1444–51.

40. Mori M, Kurogane H, Hayashi T, Yasaka Y, Ohta S, Kajiya T, Takarada A, Yoshida A, Matsuda Y, Nakagawa K, Murata T, Yoshida Y, Yokoyama M. Comparison of results of

intracoronary implantation of the Plamaz-Schatz stent with conventional balloon angioplasty in chronic total coronary arterial occlusion. Am J Cardiol. 1996; 78:985–9.

41. Rubartelli P, Niccoli L, Verna E, Giachero C, Zimarino M, Fontanelli A, Vassanelli C, Campolo L, Martuscelli E, Tommasini G. Stent implantation versus balloon angioplasty in chronic coronary occlusions: results from the GISSOC trial. Gruppo Italiano di Studio sullo Stent nelle Occlusioni Coronariche. J Am Coll Cardiol. 1998; 32:90–6.

42. Hoher M, Wohrle J, Grebe OC, Kochs M, Osterhues HH, Hombach V, Buchwald AB. A randomized trial of elective stenting after balloon recanalization of chronic total occlusions. J Am Coll Cardiol. 1999; 34:722–9.

43. Lotan C, Rozenman Y, Hendler A, Turgeman Y, Ayzenberg O, Beyar R, Krakover R, Rosenfeld T, Gotsman MS. Stents in total occlusion for restenosis prevention. The multicentre randomized STOP study. The Israeli Working Group for Interventional Cardiology. Eur Heart J. 2000; 21:1960–6.

44. Buller CE, Dzavik V, Carere RG, Mancini GB, Barbeau G, Lazzam C, Anderson TJ, Knudtson ML, Marquis JF, Suzuki T, Cohen EA, Fox RS, Teo KK. Primary stenting versus balloon angioplasty in occluded coronary arteries: the Total Occlusion Study of Canada (TOSCA). Circulation. 1999; 100:236–42.

45. Rahel BM, Suttorp MJ, Laarman GJ, Kiemeneij F, Bal ET, Rensing BJ, Ernst SM, ten Berg JM, Kelder JC, Plokker HW. Primary stenting of occluded native coronary arteries: final results of the Primary Stenting of Occluded Native Coronary Arteries (PRISON) study. Am Heart J. 2004; 147:e22.

46. Hancock J, Thomas MR, Holmberg S, Wainwright RJ, Jewitt DE. Randomised trial of elective stenting after successful percutaneous transluminal coronary angioplasty of occluded coronary arteries. Heart. 1998; 79:18–23.

47. Sievert H, Rohde S, Utech A, Schulze R, Scherer D, Merle H, Ensslen R, Schrader R, Spies H, Fach A. Stent or angioplasty after recanalization of chronic coronary occlusions? (The SARECCO Trial). Am J Cardiol. 1999; 84:386–90.

48. Lotan C. Sirolimus eluting stent in chronic total occlusions (SICTO) study. In: Trancatheter Cardiovascular Therapeutics. Washington DC; 2004:1472–5.

49. Werner GS, Krack A, Schwarz G, Prochnau D, Betge S, Figulla HR. Prevention of lesion recurrence in chronic total coronary occlusions by paclitaxel-eluting stents. J Am Coll Cardiol. 2004; 44:2301–6.

50. Ge L, Iakovou I, Cosgrave J, Chieffo A, Montorfano M, Michev I, Airoldi F, Carlino M, Melzi G, Sangiorgi GM, Corvaja N, Colombo A. Immediate and mid-term outcomes of sirolimus-eluting stent implantation for chronic total occlusions. Eur Heart J. 2005; 26:1056–62.

51. Buellesfeld L, Gerckens U, Mueller R, Schmidt T, Grube E. Polymer-based paclitaxel-eluting stent for treatment of chronic total occlusions of native coronaries: results of a Taxus CTO registry. Catheter Cardiovasc Interv. 2005; 66:173–7.

52. Grube E, Zoccai GB, Antoniucci D, et al. Assessing the safety and effectiveness of Taxus in 183 patients with chronic total occlusions: insights from the Taxus in Real life Usage Evaluation (TRUE) registry. Am J Cardiol. 2005; 96:37H.

53. Suttorp MJ. A prospective randomized trial of sirolimus-eluting and bare metal stents in patients with chronic total occlusions. In: Transcatheter Cardiovascular Therapeutics (TCT) 2005. Washington, DC.; 2005.

54. Nakamura S, Jang-Ho B, Cahyadi YH, Udayachalerm W, Tresukosol D, Tansuphaswadikul S. Comparison of efficacy and safety between sirolimus-eluting stent (cypher) and paclitaxel-eluting stent (taxus) on the outcome of patients with chronic total occlusions: multicenter registry in Asia. Am J Cardiol. 2005; 96:38H.

55. Cosgrave J, Iakovou I, Biondi-Zoccai G, Melzi G, Sangiorgi GM, Airoldi F, Chieffo A, Colombo A. Paclitaxel and sirolimus-eluting stents for the treatment of chronic total occlusions. Am J Cardiol. 2005; 96: Dec 15; 96(12):1663–8.

56. Smith SC, Jr., Feldman TE, Hirshfeld JW, Jr., Jacobs AK, Kern MJ, King SB, 3rd, Morrison DA, O'Neill W W, Schaff HV, Whitlow PL, Williams DO, Antman EM, Adams CD, Anderson JL, Faxon DP, Fuster V, Halperin JL, Hiratzka LF, Hunt SA, Nishimura R, Ornato JP, Page RL, Riegel B. ACC/AHA/SCAI 2005 Guideline Update for Percutaneous Coronary Intervention-Summary Article A Report of the American College of Cardiology/American Heart Association Task Force on Practice Guidelines (ACC/AHA/SCAI Writing Committee to Update the 2001 Guidelines for Percutaneous Coronary Intervention). J Am Coll Cardiol. 2006; 47:216–35.

57. Silber S, Albertsson P, Aviles FF, Camici PG, Colombo A, Hamm C, Jorgensen E, Marco J, Nordrehaug JE, Ruzyllo W, Urban P, Stone GW, Wijns W. Guidelines for percutaneous coronary interventions. The Task Force for Percutaneous Coronary Interventions of the European Society of Cardiology. Eur Heart J. 2005; 26:804–47.

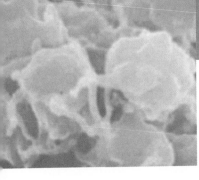

23

Bifurcation lesions

ANTONIO COLOMBO, MD
AND IOANNIS IAKOVOU, MD

KEY POINTS

- Treatment of coronary bifurcation lesions represents a challenging area in interventional cardiology.

- Stenting the main branch with provisional side branch stenting seems to be the prevailing approach.

- In the era of DES various two-stent techniques emerged ('crush') or were re-introduced ('V', 'simultaneous kissing stents', 'T', 'culottes') to allow stenting in the side branch when needed. When appropriately implemented these approaches are associated with favorable results on both branches.

Recent advances in PCI and lately the introduction of DES have led to the dramatic increase in the number of patients treated percutaneously.[1–5] Bifurcation lesions are one of these complex lesion subsets that are now being confronted more frequently.

Repeated studies have shown that treatment of bifurcational lesions has a lower procedural success and higher rate of restenosis[6–8] compared to treatment of standard lesions. Various techniques with the use of one or two stents have been developed to optimize the treatment of this subset of lesions.[6–15] Paradoxically, while stenting of individual lesions has been shown to be superior to balloon angioplasty, stenting of both branches seems to offer no advantage over stenting of the main branch (MB) alone.[8] The recent introduction of DES resulted in a lower event rate and in a reduction of restenosis in comparison with historical controls.[16] However, side branch (SB) ostial restenosis remains an area where further improvement is needed.

DES AND BIFURCATIONS

Two randomized studies and some observational reports addressed the issue of bifurcational lesion treatment with DES.[16–18] The recently published Sirolimus-eluting stent bifurcational study has given us some important initial direction to structure our approach toward the optimal treatment of bifurcational lesions.[15] This study was a 5-center randomized trial to assess feasibility and safety of treatment of patients with sirolimus-eluting stents (Cypher, Cordis/Johnson & Johnson, Warren, NJ) at true bifurcational lesions (>50% stenosis in both main vessel and ostium of side branch) that enrolled 85 patients (86 lesions). Two different strategies were used: Group A – elective use of two Cypher stents and Group B – the implantation of a single Cypher stent in the MB with balloon dilatation across the stent struts for the SB. The protocol allowed the investigators to switch to double stenting if flow impairment or residual ostial stenosis >50% developed in the side branch. Twenty-two out of 43 patients randomized to group B crossed over, resulting in implantation of two stents. The total restenosis rate at six months was 25.7%, and it was not significantly different between the double-stenting (28.0%) and the provisional SB-stenting (18.7%) groups. The majority of the restenosis cases occurred at the ostium of the SB and was focal. In the second randomized study (single center, n=91), Pan et al. compared stenting the MB and balloon dilatation for the SB to stenting for both branches. Similarly to the previous study there were no statistically significant differences between the two strategies.[18]

THROMBOSIS AFTER BIFURCATIONAL STENTING

Pathological studies suggested that arterial branch points are foci of low shear stress and low flow velocity and are sites predisposed to the development of atherosclerotic plaque, thrombus, and inflammation.[19-21] The two or three layers of stent struts (with 'Crush') apposed to the vessel wall, initially raised concerns about possible increased thrombogenicity. Furthermore, delayed endothelization associated with DES may extend the risk of thrombosis beyond 30 days.[22] In the Sirolimus-eluting stent bifurcational study the rate of stent thrombosis was 3.5%. Very recently, we reported a 3.6% rate of cumulative stent thrombosis after DES implantation in bifurcations in a prospective observational cohort study which included 2229 patients treated with both Sirolimus (n=1062 patients) and Paclitaxel-eluting stents (n=1167 patients, Taxus, Boston Scientific, Natick, MA)(23). Treatment of bifurcations was identified an independent predictor of thrombosis. However, there were no significant differences regarding the incidence of thrombosis in bifurcations treated with one versus two stents.[23]

ONE OR TWO STENTS?

As a general approach, operators should only stent the MB but an effective strategy for double stenting should be available. The decision to use one or two stents or sometimes even three (in case of a trifurcation) should be taken as early as possible. An appropriate and timely taken decision will affect the result, save time and cost, and lower the risk of complications. If we take the decision to use one stent (at the MB) there is almost always the possibility to place a second stent on the SB in case the result is not optimal or adequate. This condition is defined as 'provisional stenting'.

In order to decide whether to place one stent or two we have to consider: (1) if the SB is of adequate size, length, and anatomical distribution suitable to be treated with a stent; and (2) if the SB has a stenosis at the ostium over 50%. If the answer is NO to both questions, we will use provisional stenting at the MB, if YES we will place a second stent at the SB.

A number of techniques are available with various levels of complexity and indications: the 'V', the 'Simultaneous Kissing Stents' ('SKS'), 'Crush' and its variations ('reverse' and 'step'), 'T' and its variation ('modified'), and 'Culottes'. The most commonly used techniques for two stent placement are the first three and will be described in detail below.

SELECTION OF GUIDING CATHETER

The selection of the size (6, 7, or 8 Fr) of the guiding catheter comes after having decided to stent the SB or not. Treatment of bifurcations requires frequently simultaneous insertion of two balloons or two stents, therefore, some specific considerations regarding the selection of an appropriate guiding catheter are important. With currently available low profile balloons (i.e. Maverick, Boston Scientific), it is possible to insert two balloons inside a large lumen 6 F guiding catheter. If two stents are needed some limitations need to be known. The two stents can only be inserted, one following the other but not simultaneously in a 6 F guiding catheter. The standard 'Crush' and the 'V' or 'SKS' technique cannot be performed unless a guiding catheter of at least 7 F, with an internal lumen diameter of 0.081" (2.06 mm), for Taxus stent or 8 Fr, with an internal lumen diameter of 0.088" (2.2 mm), for Cypher stent is utilized. A 6 F guiding catheter can be utilized if the operator performs a 'provisional stenting' technique with a second stent (for the SB), which is advanced following positioning of the first stent in the MB. Techniques such as the 'T', the 'reverse Crush', the 'step Crush' (see below for a description for each technique) can all be used with a 6 F guiding catheter. The 'modified T' requires at least 7 F, and the 'Culottes', 'Y', and 'Skirt' require at least 8 Fr guiding catheters.

TWO STENT TECHNIQUES

The 'V' and The 'Simultaneous Kissing Stents' Technique

Description These techniques consist in the delivery and implantation of two stents together. One stent is advanced in the SB, the other in the MB, and the two stents touch each other forming a proximal carina (Fig. 23.1).[24,25] When this carina extends to a considerable length (usually 5 mm or more) into the main vessel then this technique is denoted as 'SKS'.[26] The type of lesions we consider most suitable for this technique are very proximal lesions such as bifurcation lesions located at the left main stem with a left main artery which is short or free of disease. Ideally the angle between the two branches should be less than 90°. The 'V' technique is also suitable for other bifurcations provided the portion of the vessel proximal to the bifurcation is free of disease and there is no need to deploy a stent more proximally.

When performing these techniques it is important to inflate the two delivery balloons sequentially and to post dilate the stents with short balloons in order to minimize any trauma in the proximal segment of the vessel.

Advantages The main advantage of these techniques is that the access to any of the two branches is never lost. In addition, when a final kissing (FK) inflation is performed there is no need to recross any stent.

Disadvantages Theoretical concerns about the risk of thrombosis related to this new carina have not been confirmed in our and other operators' experience.[17,27] If there is a need to place a stent at the proximal segment of a vessel treated with V stenting, two options can be used: (a) a stent is placed proximally leaving a small gap between the kissing stents and the proximal stent; and (b) the kissing

THE "V" OR "SKS" STENT TECHNIQUE

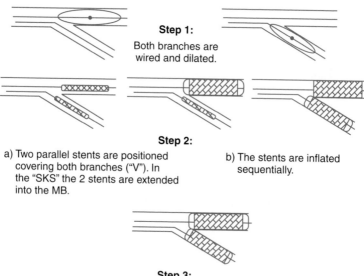

Step 1:
Both branches are
wired and dilated.

Step 2:

a) Two parallel stents are positioned
covering both branches ("V"). In
the "SKS" the 2 stents are extended
into the MB.

b) The stents are inflated
sequentially.

Step 3:
FK balloon inflation using the same pressure for both balloons.
Short balloons should be used to avoid protrusion and proximal trauma.

Figure 23.1:
The 'V' and 'Simultaneous Kissing Stents' Stenting Technique. (Abbreviations: FK = Final Kissing,
MB = Main Branch, SKS= Simultaneous Kissing Stents.)

stent is converted into a 'Crush' with the stent in the MB plastering the other stent
(one arm of the V) in the SB. A wire will then cross the struts into the SB and a
balloon will be inflated toward the SB. Following wire removal from the SB, the
proximal stent will then be advanced towards the MB. In this case we are left
with a short segment of the MB proximal to the bifurcation which has four layers
of struts.

2. THE 'CRUSH' TECHNIQUE AND ITS VARIATIONS

2A. The standard 'crush' technique

Description The 'Crush' technique[13] was introduced at the time of DES
introduction and is described schematically in Fig. 23.2. Two stents are placed in
the MB and the SB with the former more proximally than the later. It is important
to keep the protrusion of the SB stent as minimal as needed with the sole intent
to fully cover the ostium of the SB. The stent of the SB will be deployed and its
balloon and wire will be removed. The stent subsequently deployed in the MB
will flatten the protruding cells of the SB stent hence the denomination 'Crushing'
or 'Crush'. Wire recrossing and dilatation of the SB with a balloon of at least
equal diameter with the stent,[28] and then FK balloon inflation is recommended.
The implementation of FK balloon inflation was done in order to allow better
strut contact against the ostium of the SB and, therefore, better drug delivery.[17,28]
The 'Crush' technique became, therefore, a sort of simplified 'Culottes' technique.

"CRUSH" TECHNIQUE

Step 1:
Both branches are wired and dilated.

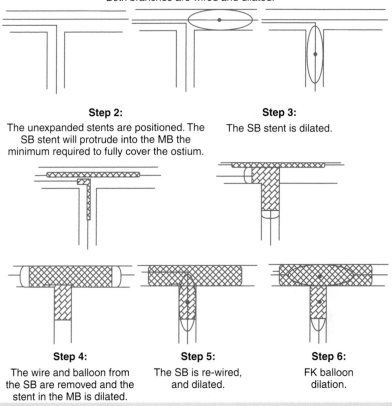

Step 2:
The unexpanded stents are positioned. The SB stent will protrude into the MB the minimum required to fully cover the ostium.

Step 3:
The SB stent is dilated.

Step 4:
The wire and balloon from the SB are removed and the stent in the MB is dilated.

Step 5:
The SB is re-wired, and dilated.

Step 6:
FK balloon dilation.

Figure 23.2:
'Crush' technique (Abbreviations: FK= Final Kissing, MB= Main Branch, SB= Side branch.)

After the implementation of the FK inflation as part of the refinement of the technique, restenosis at the ostium of the SB seems to decrease. The positive aspect is that whenever restenosis occurs, this narrowing is very focal (less than 5 mm in length) and most of the times not associated with symptoms or ischemia. An important element to keep in mind when planning to perform the 'Crush' technique is that the two available DES will reach different maximal opening of their cells.[17,27] The maximal cell diameter will be 3.0 mm for the Cypher stent and 3.7 mm for the Taxus stent. This data should be kept in mind when the SB has a diameter over 3.0 mm.

Advantages The main advantage of the 'Crush' technique is that the immediate patency of both branches is assured. This gain is important when the SB is functionally relevant or difficult to be wired. In addition provides excellent coverage of the ostium of the SB, which is the main disadvantage of the simpler 'T' technique (see below).

Disadvantages The main disadvantage is that the performance of the FK balloon inflation makes the procedure more laborious due to the need to re-cross multiple struts with a wire and a balloon.

There are some theoretical concerns related to the segment with a triple-stent layer and for this reason the amount of overlap should be short.

2B. The 'reverse crush' technique

Description The main reason to perform the 'reverse Crush' is to allow an opportunity for provisional SB stenting. A stent is deployed in the MB and balloon dilatation with FK inflation towards the SB is performed. It is assumed that the result at the ostium or at the proximal segment of the SB is suboptimal in order for the operator to decide to deploy a stent at this site. A second stent is advanced into the SB and left in position without being deployed. Then, a balloon sized according to the diameter of the MB is advanced in the vessel and positioned at the level of the bifurcation paying attention to stay inside the stent previously deployed in the MB. The stent in the SB is retracted about 2 to 3 mm into the MB and deployed, the deploying balloon is removed and an angiogram is obtained to verify that a good result is present at the SB (no further distal stent in the SB is needed). If this is the case, the wire from the SB is removed and the balloon in the MB is inflated at high pressure (12 atm or more). The other steps are similar to the ones described for the 'Crush' technique and involve recrossing into the SB, perform SB dilatation, and FK balloon inflation.

Advantages The main advantage of the 'reverse Crush' technique is that the immediate patency of both branches is assured and that can be performed utilizing a 6 F guiding catheter.

Disadvantages It shares the same disadvantages with the 'standard Crush' and it is more laborious.

2C. The 'step crush' technique

Description The final result is basically similar to the one obtained with the 'standard Crush' technique with the only difference that each stent is advanced and deployed separately in order to use a 6 F guide. First, a stent is advanced in the SB protruding into the MB a few millimetres. A balloon is then advanced in the MB over the bifurcation. Then, the stent in the SB is deployed, the balloon removed, and an angiogram is performed: if the result is adequate, the wire is also removed. The MB balloon is then inflated to crush the protruding SB stent and removed. Subsequently, a stent is advanced in the MB and deployed (usually at 12 atm or more). The next steps are similar to the 'Crush' technique and involve re-crossing into the SB, performing SB stent dilatation and FK balloon dilatation.

Advantages The main reason to utilize this technique is to perform the 'Crush' technique utilizing a 6 F guiding catheter. Operators who perform the radial approach may be particularly interested in this technique.

Disadvantages It shares the same disadvantages with the 'standard Crush'.

3. THE 'T' TECHNIQUE AND ITS VARIATIONS

3A. The 'standard T' technique

Description The classic 'T' technique consists in positioning a stent first at the ostium of the SB being careful to avoid the stent protrusion in the MB (Fig. 23.3). Some operators leave a balloon in the MB to help to further locate the MB. Following deployment of the stent and removal of the balloon and the wire from the SB, a second stent is advanced in the MB. A wire is then re-advanced into the SB and FK balloon inflation is performed.

Advantages It is less laborious than 'Crush'. Unlike the 'V' it can be used for the coverage of proximal to bifurcation lesions.

THE "T" STENTING TECHNIQUE

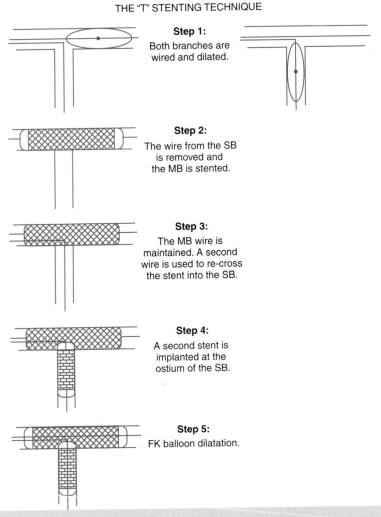

Step 1:
Both branches are wired and dilated.

Step 2:
The wire from the SB is removed and the MB is stented.

Step 3:
The MB wire is maintained. A second wire is used to re-cross the stent into the SB.

Step 4:
A second stent is implanted at the ostium of the SB.

Step 5:
FK balloon dilatation.

Figure 23.3:
The 'T' stenting technique (through the stent). (Abbreviations: FK= Final Kissing, MB= Main Branch, SB= Side branch.)

Disadvantages In almost all of the cases, this technique will lead to incomplete coverage of the ostium of the SB. At the present time in our practice, the above technique has been abandoned, and now there are two reasons to perform the 'T' technique: (1) to place a stent at the ostium of a SB following placement of a stent in the MB because the result at the SB ostium was evaluated as unsatisfactory (provisional SB stenting); and (2) to perform stenting at the ostium of the SB when there is isolated SB ostial stenosis.

3B. The modified 'T' technique

Description Following predilatation, the performance of this technique demands advancement of a stent into the SB first (without deployment of the stent) then a second stent is advanced and positioned (without being yet deployed) across the bifurcation in the MB (Fig. 23.4). The stent in the SB is deployed and following verification of an adequate result, the balloon and the wire are removed from the SB.

THE MODIFIED "T" STENTING TECHNIQUE

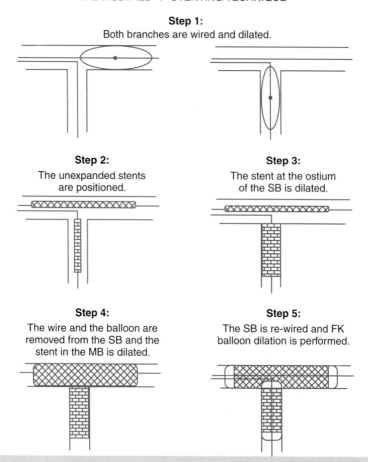

Step 1:
Both branches are wired and dilated.

Step 2:
The unexpanded stents
are positioned.

Step 3:
The stent at the ostium
of the SB is dilated.

Step 4:
The wire and the balloon are
removed from the SB and the
stent in the MB is dilated.

Step 5:
The SB is re-wired and FK
balloon dilation is performed.

Figure 23.4:
The modified 'T' stenting technique. (Abbreviations: FK= Final Kissing, MB= Main Branch, SB= Side branch.)

Then the stent in the MB is deployed usually at 12 atm or more. A wire is then re-advanced into the SB and a FK balloon dilatation is performed (usually at 8 atm). The performance of the modified 'T' technique commits always to stenting the MB and SB and almost always will leave a small gap between the two stents.[12]

Advantages The same as the standard 'T'.

Disadvantages The same as the standard 'T', plus the need for a larger guiding catheter.

4. THE 'CULOTTES' TECHNIQUE

Description The 'Culottes' technique uses two stents and leads to full coverage of the bifurcation at the expense of an excess of metal covering of the proximal end[7] (Fig. 23.5). Both branches are predilated. First a stent is deployed across the most

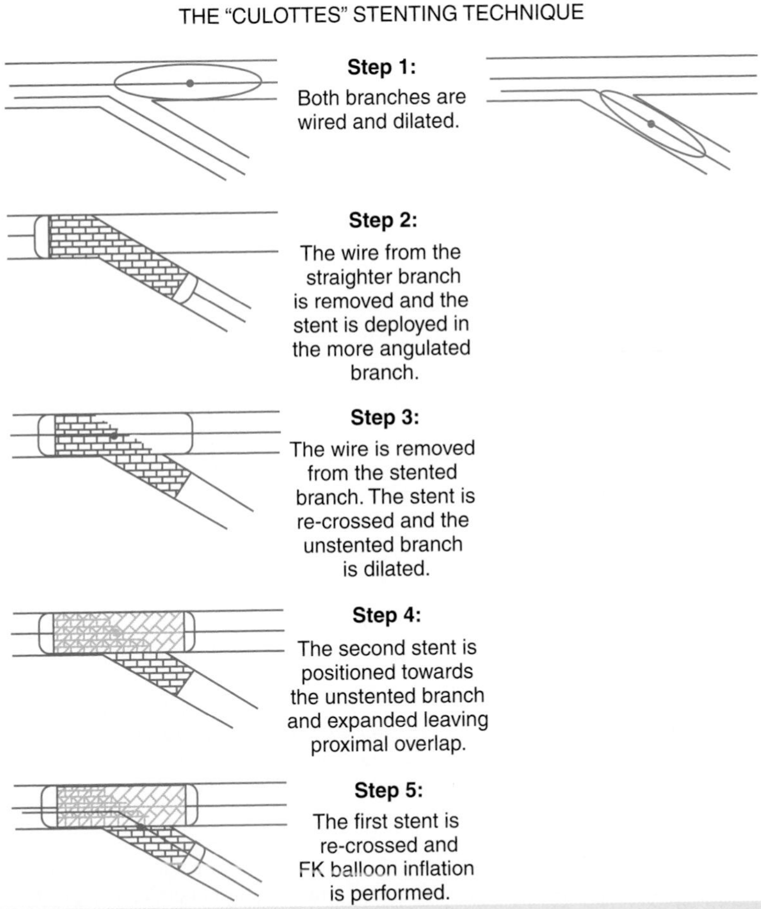

THE "CULOTTES" STENTING TECHNIQUE

Step 1: Both branches are wired and dilated.

Step 2: The wire from the straighter branch is removed and the stent is deployed in the more angulated branch.

Step 3: The wire is removed from the stented branch. The stent is re-crossed and the unstented branch is dilated.

Step 4: The second stent is positioned towards the unstented branch and expanded leaving proximal overlap.

Step 5: The first stent is re-crossed and FK balloon inflation is performed.

Figure 23.5:
The 'Culottes' stenting technique. (Abbreviations: FK= Final Kissing.)

angulated branch, usually the SB. The non-stented branch is then rewired through the struts of the stent and dilated. A second stent is advanced and expanded into the non-stented branch, usually the MB. Finally, FK balloon inflation is performed.

Advantages   This technique is suitable for all angles of bifurcations and provides near perfect coverage of the SB ostium.

Disadvantages   Like 'Crush', it leads to a high concentration of metal with a double-stent layer at the carina and in the proximal part of the bifurcation. The main disadvantage of the technique is that rewiring both branches through the stent struts can be difficult and time consuming.

CONCLUSIONS

The introduction of DES improved the results in bifurcational lesions at the level of both branches. When the SB is not severely diseased or has a small diameter, implantation of a stent in the MB and provisional stenting in the SB is the preferred strategy. Implantation of two stents as initial approach is appropriate when both branches are significantly diseased (diameter stenosis >50%) and of suitable diameter for stenting. A number of techniques are available with various levels of complexity and indications: the 'V', simultaneous kissing stent (SKS), 'Crush', 'T', and 'Culottes'. When restenosis occurs it is most of the time focal and involves the SB; it is unclear if this focal restenosis needs a reintervention.

REFERENCES

1. Colombo A, Iakovou I. Ten years of advancements in interventional cardiology. J Endovasc Ther 2004; 11 Suppl 2:II10–II18.

2. Colombo A, Iakovou I. Drug-eluting stents: the new gold standard for percutaneous coronary revascularisation. Eur Heart J 2004; 25:895–7.

3. Iakovou I, Ge L, Michev I, et al. Clinical and angiographic outcome after sirolimus-eluting stent implantation in aorto-ostial lesions. J Am Coll Cardiol 2004; 44:967–71.

4. Iakovou I, Sangiorgi GM, Stankovic G, et al. Effectiveness of sirolimus-eluting stent implantation for treatment of in-stent restenosis after brachytherapy failure. Am J Cardiol 2004; 94:351–4.

5. Cohen DJ, Bakhai A, Shi C, et al. Cost-effectiveness of sirolimus-eluting stents for treatment of complex coronary stenoses: results from the Sirolimus-Eluting Balloon Expandable Stent in the Treatment of Patients With De Novo Native Coronary Artery Lesions (SIRIUS) trial. Circulation 2004; 110:508–14.

6. Al Suwaidi J, Berger PB, Rihal CS, et al. Immediate and long-term outcome of intracoronary stent implantation for true bifurcation lesions. J Am Coll Cardiol 2000; 35:929–36.

7. Chevalier B, Glatt B, Royer T, Guyon P. Placement of coronary stents in bifurcation lesions by the 'culotte' technique. Am J Cardiol 1998; 82:943–9.

8. Yamashita T, Nishida T, Adamian MG, *et al.* Bifurcation lesions: two stents versus one stent-immediate and follow-up results. J Am Coll Cardiol 2000; 35:1145–51.

9. Pan M, Suarez de Lezo J, Medina A, *et al.* A stepwise strategy for the stent treatment of bifurcated coronary lesions. Catheter Cardiovasc Interv 2002; 55:50–7.

10. Ormiston JA, Webster MW, Ruygrok PN, Stewart JT, White HD, Scott DS. Stent deformation following simulated side-branch dilatation: a comparison of five stent designs. Catheter Cardiovasc Interv 1999; 47:258–64.

11. Fort S, Lazzam C, Schwartz L. Coronary 'Y' stenting: a technique for angioplasty of bifurcation stenoses. Can J Cardiol 1996; 12:678–82.

12. Kobayashi Y, Colombo A, Akiyama T, Reimers B, Martini G, di Mario C. Modified "T" stenting: a technique for kissing stents in bifurcational coronary lesion. Cathet Cardiovasc Diagn 1998; 43:323–6.

13. Colombo A, Stankovic G, Orlic D, *et al.* Modified T-stenting technique with crushing for bifurcation lesions: immediate results and 30-day outcome. Catheter Cardiovasc Interv 2003; 60:145–51.

14. Colombo A. Bifurcational lesions and the 'crush' technique: understanding why it works and why it doesn't-a kiss is not just a kiss. Catheter Cardiovasc Interv 2004; 63:337–8.

15. Carrie D, Karouny E, Chouairi S, Puel J. 'T'-shaped stent placement: a technique for the treatment of dissected bifurcation lesions. Cathet Cardiovasc Diagn 1996; 37:311–13.

16. Colombo A, Moses JW, Morice MC, *et al.* Randomized study to evaluate sirolimus-eluting stents implanted at coronary bifurcation lesions. Circulation 2004; 109:1244–9.

17. Ge L, Airoldi F, Iakovou I, *et al.* Clinical and Angiographic Outcome Following Implantation of Drug-Eluting Stents in Bifurcation Lesions with the Crush Stent Technique: Importance of Final Kissing Balloon Post-dilatation. J Am Coll Cardiol; In Press.

18. Pan M, de Lezo JS, Medina A, *et al.* Rapamycin-eluting stents for the treatment of bifurcated coronary lesions: a randomized comparison of a simple versus complex strategy. Am Heart J 2004; 148:857–64.

19. Glagov S, Zarins C, Giddens DP, Ku DN. Hemodynamics and atherosclerosis. Insights and perspectives gained from studies of human arteries. Arch Pathol Lab Med 1988; 112:1018–31.

20. Honda Y, Fitzgerald PJ. Stent thrombosis: an issue revisited in a changing world. Circulation 2003; 108:2–5.

21. Farb A, Burke AP, Kolodgie FD, Virmani R. Pathological mechanisms of fatal late coronary stent thrombosis in humans. Circulation 2003; 108:1701–6.

22. Virmani R, Guagliumi G, Farb A, *et al.* Localized hypersensitivity and late coronary thrombosis secondary to a sirolimus-eluting stent: should we be cautious? Circulation 2004; 109:701–5.

23. Iakovou I, Schmidt T, Bonizzoni E, *et al.* Incidence, Predictors, and Outcome of Thrombosis after Successful Implantation of Drug-Eluting Stents. JAMA In press.

24. Schampaert E, Fort S, Adelman AG, Schwartz L. The V-stent: a novel technique for coronary bifurcation stenting. Cathet Cardiovasc Diagn 1996; 39:320–6.

25. Colombo A, Gaglione A, Nakamura S, Finci L. "Kissing" stents for bifurcational coronary lesion. Cathet Cardiovasc Diagn 1993; 30:327–30.

26. Sharma SK, Choudhury A, Lee J, *et al.* Simultaneous kissing stents (SKS) technique for treating bifurcation lesions in medium-to-large size coronary arteries. Am J Cardiol 2004; 94:913–17.

27. Ge L, Tsagalou E, Iakovou I, *et al.* In-Hospital And 9-Month Outcome Of Treatment Of Coronary Bifurcational Lesions With Sirolimus-Eluting Stents. Am J Cardiol 2005; 95:757–60.

28. Ormiston JA, Currie E, Webster MW, *et al.* Drug-eluting stents for coronary bifurcations: insights into the crush technique. Catheter Cardiovasc Interv 2004; 63:332–6.

29. Baim DS. Is birfurcation stenting the answer? Cathet Cardiovasc Diagn 1996; 37:314–16.

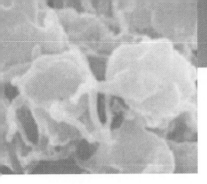

24

Percutaneous coronary intervention in small vessels

PAUL SORAJJA, MD, AND DAVID R. HOLMES, JR, MD

KEY POINTS

- Small vessel disease (<3 mm diameter) encompasses an important proportion of contemporary PCI, ranging from 30 to 50%.

- Patients with small vessel lesions characteristically are older with a greater frequency of female gender, diabetes, multivessel disease, heart failure, peripheral vascular disease, and complex lesion types than patients with disease in larger vessels.

- In the treatment of small vessel lesions, several clinical trials of bare metal stenting versus angioplasty have been performed with disappointing results in most studies.

- The trials of angioplasty versus bare metal stenting highlighted the poor ability of small vessels to accommodate even modest degrees of neointimal proliferation following stent deployment.

- Greater late lumen loss theoretically portends higher rates of restenosis, particularly as small vessel size reduces the ability to accommodate neointimal proliferation.

- Small reference vessel diameter is an independent predictor of restenosis.

- Neointimal response is directly related to the degree of vessel injury.

- Currently available DES have dramatically reduced restenosis in small vessel PCI.

INTRODUCTION

The revascularization of coronary atherosclerosis in small vessels poses unique challenges to the interventionalist. While PCI is the preferred mode of revascularization, the clinical characteristics of these patients and these lesions portend lower angiographic success and poorer subsequent clinical outcomes in comparison to the revascularization of disease in larger vessels. Thus, the treatment of small vessel disease requires a dedicated approach, which is the focus of this chapter.

CLINICAL PROBLEM

Small vessel disease (<3 mm diameter) encompasses an important proportion of contemporary PCI, ranging from 30 to 50% of the >1 million PCI procedures performed annually worldwide. Patients with small vessel lesions characteristically are older with a greater frequency of female gender, diabetes, multivessel disease, heart failure, peripheral vascular disease, and complex lesion types (American Heart Association/American College Cardiology type C) than patients with disease in larger vessels.[1] Given current, worsening epidemiological trends for these morbidities, and the continued aging of the population of patients with coronary atherosclerosis, it is expected that small vessel disease will continue to form an ever-growing portion of the prevailing practice of PCI.

While PCI has been compared to medical therapy and CABG in a large number of clinical studies, none have directly examined the optimal therapy for the population of patients with small vessel disease. Notably, bypass grafting of small vessels, particularly when the LAD is ≤2.0 mm in diameter, has been associated with significantly higher perioperative mortality in several studies.[2,3] This increased risk has been attributed to the potential for increase thrombosis in smaller vessels, technical difficulties of grafting, and poorer graft patency.[2,4] Given these outcomes and the frequent accompanying morbidity of these patients (e.g., prior CABG), the less invasive approach offered by PCI is frequently employed when revascularization is desired.

BALLOON ANGIOPLASTY AND BARE METAL STENTING

Historically, the development of steerable guidewires and low profile devices enabled angioplasty to be performed in both small and large vessels with comparable procedural success.[5] In the late 1980s, failure to cross or dilate lesions and acute complications, such as dissection and persistent acute closure, occurred largely irrespective of vessel size.[5] Later, technological advancements, namely stenting, reduced acute complications, but these improvements were not as evident for smaller vessel PCI because of the reduced availability of stents for these vessel sizes. This shift in device technology has been an explanation for currently lower procedural success rates of small vessel PCI as recently reported in several studies.[1,6] Nonetheless, current reported rates of angiographic and procedural success of small vessel PCI range from 92 to 96%.[1,6,7] Of note, the rates of in-hospital MACE (Q-wave myocardial infarction, emergency CABG, death) are comparable or only slightly higher in comparison to that of patients undergoing treatment for large vessel lesions (Table 24.1).

TABLE 24.1 - PROCEDURAL SUCCESS AND IN-HOSPITAL COMPLICATION RATES FOR SMALL VERSUS LARGE VESSEL PERCUTANEOUS CORONARY INTERVENTION.[1,6,7]

	AKIYAMA ET AL. 1993–96		SCHUNKERT ET AL. 1994–97		AL-SUWAIDI ET AL. 1997–98	
	<3 MM N = 602	≥3 MM N = 696	≤2.5 MM N = 813	>2.5 MM N = 1,493	<3 MM N = 587	≥3 MM N = 1,071
In-hospital MACE						
Death	0.2%	0.2%	3.0%	1.6%*	1.0%	1.3%
Q-wave MI	1.3%	1.1%	0.4%	0.3%	–	–
Non-Q-wave MI	3.7%	2.9%	5.8%	5.0%	–	–
Any MI	–	–	–	–	1.5%	2.1%
CABG	1.8%	1.7%	0.4%	0.3%	1.0%	1.5%
Death, MI, CABG	–	–	3.4%	2.0%*	3.6%	4.8%
Abrupt closure	–	–	–	–	1.9%	1.2%
Procedural success	96%	95%	92%	95%*	93%	95%

MACE, major adverse clinical events; MI, myocardial infarction; *p<0.05 vs. small vessel

The advent of coronary stenting in the 1990s significantly improved both the acute procedural success and rates of restenosis in patients undergoing PCI. These improvements occurred primarily because of the scaffolding effect of stents, with reduction in elastic recoil, improved treatment of procedural complications (e.g. dissection), and amelioration of the adverse effects of subsequent negative vessel remodeling. Neointimal proliferation was not affected, but, in fact, worsened because stenting typically results in more neointimal hyperplasia probably due to greater medial injury than occurs with angioplasty alone. In large vessels, the larger acute luminal gain that occurs with stenting significantly exceeds the degree of subsequent neointimal proliferation, resulting in greater net luminal gain in favor of stenting overall. A number of randomized clinical trials of stenting versus angioplasty verified the beneficial effects of stenting, but they did so primarily for the treatment of lesions in vessels whose diameter was 3.0 mm or more. Because small vessels are limited in their ability to accommodate significant neointimal proliferation, small reference diameter is a strong predictor of clinical restenosis in patients who undergo stenting, in addition to lesion length and the presence of diabetes (Table 24.2).[8,9]

In the treatment of small vessel lesions, several clinical trials of bare metal stenting versus angioplasty have been performed with disappointing results in most studies (Table 24.3 and Fig. 24.1). Nonetheless, these investigations highlighted the importance of stent design, whose relevance to clinical outcome becomes particularly evident in patients with small vessel lesions. Stent design,

TABLE 24.2- IN-SEGMENT RESTENOSIS RATES IN THE SIRIUS ANGIOGRAPHIC SUBSTUDY ACCORDING TO VESSEL SIZE, LESION LENGTH, AND THE PRESENCE OF DIABETES[27]

	LESION LENGTH (MM)		
	<10	10 TO 15	>15
Reference diameter (mm)			
BMS			
Nondiabetics			
<2.5	36.8	40.1	45.7
2.5 to 3.0	27.7	30.6	35.7
>3.0	18.7	20.9	25.0
Diabetics			
<2.5	58.1	61.5	66.8
2.5 to 3.0	47.8	51.3	57.0
>3.0	35.4	38.7	44.3
Sirolimus-eluting stent			
Nondiabetics			
<2.5	8.2	9.4	11.5
2.5 to 3.0	5.6	6.4	7.9
>3.0	3.4	3.9	4.9
Diabetics			
<2.5	17.7	19.8	23.7
2.5 to 3.0	12.4	14.0	17.0
>3.0	7.8	8.9	10.9

TABLE 24.3- PUBLISHED CLINICAL TRIALS OF BALLOON ANGIOPLASTY VERSUS BARE-METAL STENTING.[12-16]

	ISAR-SMART‡		PARK ET AL.		SISA		SISCA		BESMART	
	PTCA	MULTI-LINK	PTCA	NIR	PTCA	BESTENT	PTCA	BESTENT	PTCA	BESTENT
No. patients	200	204	60	60	182	169	71	74	189	192
Reference diameter (mm)	2.37	2.41	2.48	2.55	2.45	2.50	2.38	2.44	2.24	2.23
Lesion length (mm)	11.8	12.5			10.2	10.8	10.8	11.8	9.6	9.1
Cross-over to stent (%)	16.5		20.0		20.3		14.1		22.7	
Post-procedural MLD (mm)	1.98	2.35*	2.14	2.44*	1.84	2.30*	1.79	2.22	1.70	2.06
Late luminal loss (mm)	0.72	1.04*	0.63	1.12*	0.48	0.89*	0.25	0.54	0.57	0.65
6-month restenosis rate (%)	37.4	35.4	30.9	35.7	32.9	28.0	18.8	9.7	47	21
6-month TVR (%)	16.5	20.1	5.0	3.3	20.3	17.8	23.2	9.6*	24.6†	13.0†

Reference diameter, lesion length, minimal lumen diameter (MLD), and late luminal loss are expressed as means. Percutaneous transluminal coronary angioplasty (PTCA); †Target lesion revascularization; ‡Follow-up performed at 7 months in ISAR-SMART. *$p<0.05$ vs. PTCA

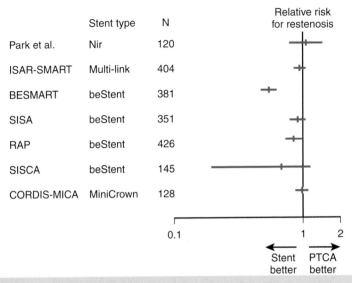

	Stent type	N	Relative risk for restenosis
Park et al.	Nir	120	
ISAR-SMART	Multi-link	404	
BESMART	beStent	381	
SISA	beStent	351	
RAP	beStent	426	
SISCA	beStent	145	
CORDIS-MICA	MiniCrown	128	

Figure 24.1:
Relative risk for 6-month angiographic restenosis calculated for stent versus PTCA in randomized trials. Reprinted from the Journal of the American College of Cardiology, Volume 38, Kastrati *et al.*, Stenting for small coronary vessels: a contestable winner, pages 1604–7, 2001, with permission from Elsevier.

which includes strut thickness, cell type (i.e., open or closed), and stent type (i.e., slotted tube, multicellular, self-expanding, coil), directly influences the degree of neointimal proliferation following deployment.[10] In the ISAR-STEREO 1 and 2 trials, a ~40% reduction in the rate of restenosis occurred in patients who received the thin-strut (50 μm) Multi-link stent versus those who received the thick-strut (140 μm) Multi-link Duet stent or the thick-strut (140 μm) Bx-Velocity stent.[11]

In the studies of angioplasty versus bare-metal stenting in patients with small vessel lesions, the only trials that demonstrated a positive outcome for stenting or a trend towards its benefit were those that utilized the Medtronic BeStent. This stent was composed of relatively thinner struts (0.0030" thickness) and was specifically designed for deployment in small vessels (<3.0 mm). In the BeStent in Small Arteries trial (BESMART), which examined treatment of focal lesions (mean length, 9 to 10 mm) in small vessels (mean reference diameter, 2.2 mm), stenting with the BeStent significantly reduced the six-month rate of binary angiographic restenosis from 47% to 21% (p=0.0001).[12] A unique observation in the BESMART study was that late loss was comparable for either angioplasty or stenting, and helped to maximize the net gain in favor of stenting. Similarly, in the Stenting in Small Coronary Arteries trial (SISCA), late luminal loss with stenting did not exceed the acute luminal gain, resulting in outcomes in favor of stenting. Conversely, in the other studies, late loss after stenting either significantly reduced (Stenting in Small Arteries or SISA study of the BeStent) or altogether eliminated (Nir stent and Multilink stent) the net gain of stenting, resulting in no benefit for reduction in restenosis from elective stenting.[13–6]

In the United States, the only currently available coronary stent specifically designed for small vessel disease is the Multi-link Pixel[tm] (Guidant Corp.). This stent (2.0 to 2.5 mm diameter) has a strut thickness of 0.0039" and is compatible with 5 F systems. In the Italian Registry of the Multi-link Pixel stent, the device was successfully deployed in all lesions (n=243) without major adverse events. Although the mean reference diameter of the treated vessels was 2.1 mm, the rate of TLR remarkably was 7.4% at 6 months.[17] Similar results have been observed in the 150-patient US and Israeli registry, which reported a six-month TLR rate of 8.8%.

DRUG-ELUTING STENTS

The trials of angioplasty versus bare-metal stenting highlighted the poor ability of small vessels to accommodate even modest degrees of neointimal proliferation following stent deployment. Thus, the advent of DES, with their dramatic ability to reduce such proliferation, has generated great enthusiasm for more successful percutaneous intervention of small vessel lesions.

Several recent clinical trials have examined the impact of DES in small vessel PCI. The Sirolimus-Eluting Stent in the Prevention of Restenosis in Small Coronary Arteries (SES-SMART) study randomized 257 patients (mean reference diameter, 2.2 mm) to receive either a sirolimus-eluting Cypher stent or the architecturally similar, bare-metal Bx Sonic stent.[18] Procedural success exceeded 95% for both arms. Treatment with the Cypher stent significantly reduced in-segment late loss (0.16 mm vs. 0.69 mm; p<0.001) and binary in-stent angiographic restenosis (9.8% vs. 53.1%; p<0.001) with an effect consistent across patient subgroups, including diabetics. Similar striking reductions in late loss and binary restenosis for the sirolimus-eluting stent also have been reported in the European and Canadian sirolimus-eluting stent studies (E-SIRIUS and C-SIRIUS), both of which focused on PCI of long lesions in small coronary arteries (Figs. 24.2 and 24.3).[19,20] Importantly, the degree of late loss in the Cypher stent arm of these trials was comparable to that observed in studies of the Cypher stent in large vessels. Of note, in the E-SIRIUS study, multiple or overlapping stents were utilized in 49% and 34%, respectively, with a mean stent length to lesion length ratio of 1.7. In each of the aforementioned randomized studies, 8-month target lesion revascularization rates for patients treated with a sirolimus-eluting stent ranged from 4.0 to 7.0%, a 75% reduction in comparison to patients in the bare-metal stenting arms.

Recently, the Rapamycin-Eluting Stent Evaluated At Rotterdam Cardiology Hospital (RESEARCH) registry reported outcomes for 91 patients (112 de novo lesions) treated with the 2.25 mm diameter sirolimus-eluting stent.[21] This study, whose treated lesions had a mean reference diameter of 1.88 ±0.34 mm, consists of the smallest vessels treated with DES that have been reported thus far. Among the 62 or 70% of patients with follow-up angiography, the mean late lumen loss at seven months was 0.07 ±0.48 mm with a binary angiographic restenosis of 10.7%. Repeat TLR occurred in 5.5% of these patients. Thus, despite the very small size of the vessels examined in the RESEARCH registry, the outcomes were comparable to that reported for the sirolimus-eluting stent arms in the randomized studies of small vessel PCI (SES-SMART, C-SIRIUS, and E-SIRIUS).

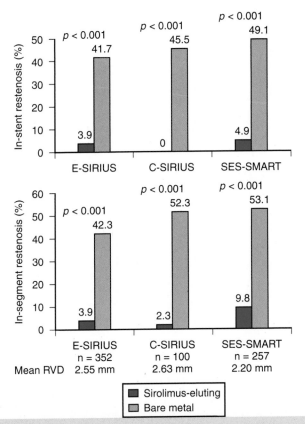

Figure 24.2:
Rates of in-stent (Top) and in-segment (Bottom) angiographic restenosis for studies of the sirolimus-eluting stent in small vessel PCI.[27]

Data on small vessel PCI using the paclitaxel-eluting Taxus stent (Boston Scientific) also have been reported. In the randomized TAXUS-IV trial of the slow-release, polymer-based, paclitaxel-eluting Taxus stent versus the bare-metal Express stent, the mean reference vessel diameter of the 1,314 study patients was 2.75 mm with a mean lesion length of 13.4 mm.[22] Twelve-month TLR rates respectively were 5.6%, 4.3%, and 3.5% for patients who received a 2.5 mm, 2.5 to 3.0 mm, and ≥3.0 mm stent. These rates corresponded to a 68 to 76% relative reduction in target lesion revascularization in comparison to patients who were treated with the Express stent.

To date, there have been no direct comparisons of available drug-eluting platforms for patients undergoing small vessel PCI. Both the sirolimus-eluting and paclitaxel-eluting stents have demonstrated significant improvement over bare-metal platforms with reported rates of target lesion revascularization ranging from 4.0 to 7.0% in patients with vessels <3.0 mm, including patients with very small vessels (RESEARCH registry) and those with long lesions (E-SIRIUS and C-SIRIUS). Nonetheless, in separate angiographic substudies, in-stent late lumen loss has been greater for the Taxus stent, with a range of 0.35 to 0.44 mm for

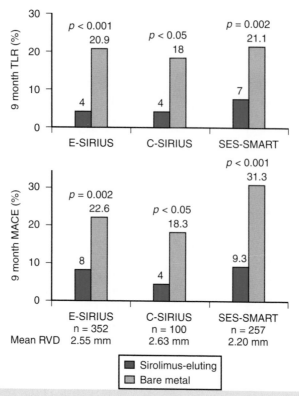

Figure 24.3:
Nine-month target lesion revascularization (TLR, Top) and MACE (MACE, Bottom) rates for studies of the sirolimus-eluting stent in small vessel PCI.[18-20]

different vessel sizes versus 0.15 to 0.22 mm for the Cypher stent. Greater late lumen loss theoretically portends higher rates of restenosis, particularly as small vessel size reduces the ability to accommodate neointimal proliferation.[23] Thus far, significantly discernible differences in reported restenosis rates for small vessel PCI between the Cypher and Taxus stents have not been observed, although these stents have not been examined in this patient population in a randomized fashion.

Technical approach
Certain key observations in studies of small vessel PCI help to formulate the interventional approach in these patients.

1. *Small reference vessel diameter is an independent predictor of restenosis*
   Small reference vessel diameter has been a known predictor of angiographic and clinical restenosis after bare-metal stenting, but this relationship between vessel size and restenosis continues to remain in the era of DES. In the SIRIUS trial, the odds ratio of in-segment, binary angiographic restenosis after multivariate adjustment was 0.54 per 1 mm decrement in reference vessel diameter.[24] Rates of restenosis in small vessels are further augmented in

patients with diabetes and those with long lesions. Thus, patient counseling remains important in the approach to the treatment of these small vessel lesions.

2. *Neointimal response is directly related to the degree of vessel injury* Minimization of medial injury by maintaining a device-to-artery ratio of ≤1.1 helps to reduce the inflammatory response that theoretically leads to subsequent neointimal proliferation. Of note, in a randomized study of PCI in lesions <3.0 mm, there were lower rates of restenosis, TLR, and higher event-free survival for patients who had gradual and prolonged balloon angioplasty versus conventional angioplasty.[25] Direct stenting, when possible, may be performed with rates of procedural success and adverse clinical events that are comparable to that observed with predilatation in small vessel PCI.[26] Of note, in the SES-SMART study, predilatation was mandatory yet low TVR rates were observed.

3. *Greater in-segment late lumen loss has been reported after stenting in small vessels* The absolute amount of in-stent late lumen loss, as a surrogate of neointimal proliferation, is relatively constant for different vessel sizes or only slightly higher for smaller vessels. However, markedly greater in-segment late lumen loss has been reported in PCI of smaller vessels, resulting in greater in-segment restenosis (Fig. 24.4).[27] Thus, avoiding geographic miss and minimizing vessel injury at stent margins, such as may occur with post-dilatation or edge implantation into diseased areas, are of particular importance in small vessel PCI. Notably, in the SES-SMART trial, where predilatation was mandatory, there was no difference in late luminal loss or the loss index between the in-segment and in-stent zones.

4. *Currently available DES have dramatically reduced restenosis in small vessel PCI* In randomized trials that have examined PCI of vessels <3.0 mm, the use of either sirolimus-eluting or paclitaxel-eluting stents reduced angiographic and clinical restenosis by ~75% with 8 to 12-month TLR rates of 4 to 7%. This reduction has been consistent in different patient subgroups, including those with diabetes mellitus, long lesions, and those treated with long stents. Although these trials have examined a limited number of patients, current safety and efficacy data suggest that the use of DES should be considered when possible.

FUTURE FACETS

Providing a significant scaffolding effect while minimizing vessel trauma, inflammation, and neointimal proliferation has been the therapeutic goal in the use of coronary stents. Drug-eluting stents have significantly reduced neointimal proliferation with relative reductions in restenosis that are comparable to that observed in the treatment of large vessel lesions, yet small vessel lesions continue to portend higher absolute rates of in-segment restenosis. While studies of BMS have demonstrated the importance of stent design on clinical outcome, both of the currently available DES utilize platforms designed for deployment in larger vessels.

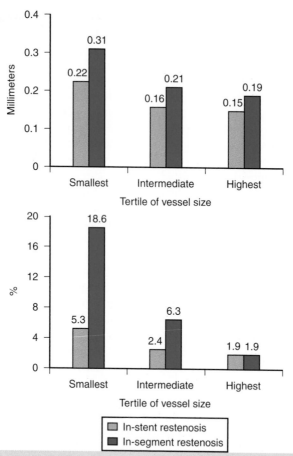

Figure 24.4:
Late-loss and angiographic restenosis for sirolimus-eluting stents grouped by tertile of vessel size. Mean reference vessel diameters for smallest, intermediate, and highest tertiles were 2.3 mm, 2.8 mm, and 3.3 mm, respectively.[27]

Notably, stent strut thickness is 0.0055" for Cypher stents and 0.0052" for Taxus stents. Future directions likely will incorporate devices dedicated for use in small vessel PCI. Cobalt-chromium stents (Guidant's Multilink Vision stent and Medtronic's Driver stent), as an example, have been shown to reduce neointimal proliferation in comparison to nitinol or stainless-steel-based stents, but are currently available only for large vessel stenting. A second example is the 2.0 mm BiodivYsio stent, whose biocompatible, phosphorylcholine coating may illicit less inflammation and serve as a vehicle for local drug delivery.[28] Development of new metal alloys or non-metal scaffolding, biocompatible coating or polymers capable of eluting one or more antiproliferative drugs, and low-profile, flexible designs to facilitate device delivery is continuing. Such devices and other platforms specifically designed for small vessels will continue to advance the ability to successfully perform PCI with improved clinical outcomes for these patients.

REFERENCES

1. Schunkert H, Harrell L, Palacios IF. Implications of small reference vessel diameter in patients undergoing percutaneous coronary revascularization. J Am Coll Cardiol 1999; 34:40–8.

2. O'Connor NJ, Morton J, Birkmeyer JD, Olmstead EM, O'Connor GT. Effect of coronary diameter in patients undergoing coronary artery bypass surgery. Circulation 1996; 93:652–5.

3. Fisher LD, Kennedy JW, Davis KG, *et al.* Association of sex, physical size, and operative mortality after coronary artery bypass in the coronary artery surgery study (CASS). J Thorac Cardiovasc Surg 1982; 84:334–41.

4. Bjork VO, Ekestrom S, Henze A, Ivert T, Landou C. Early and late patency of aortocoronary vein grafts. Scand J Thorac Cardiovasc Surg. 1981; 15:11–21.

5. Savage MP, Goldberg S, Hirshfeld JW, *et al.* Clinical and angiographic determinants of primary coronary angioplasty success. J Am Coll Cardiol 1991; 17:22–8.

6. Al Suwaidi J, Yeh W, Williams DO, Laskey WK, Cohen HA, Detre KM, Kelsey SF, Holmes DR Jr. Comparison of immediate and one-year outcome after coronary angioplasty of narrowing <3 mm with those > or =3 mm (the National Heart, Lung, and Blood Institute Dynamic Registry). Am J Cardiol 2001; 87:680–6.

7. Akiyama T, Moussa I, Reimers B, *et al.* Angiographic and clinical outcome following coronary stenting of small vessels. A comparison with coronary stenting of large vessels. J Am Coll Cardiol 1998; 32:1610–18.

8. Kereiakes DJ, Linnemeier TJ, Baim DS, *et al.* Usefulness of stent length inpredicting in-stent restenosis (the MULTI-LINK stent trials). Am J Cardiol 2000; 86:336–41.

9. Mauri L, O'Maly J, Ho KKL, *et al.* The relative contributions of stented lesion length, non-stented lesion length and excessive stent length on coronary restenosis complications for spot stenting. Circulation 2002; 106:11–481.

10. Escaned J, Goicolea J, Alfonso F, *et al.* Propensity and mechanisms of restenosis in different coronary stent designs: complementary value of the analysis of the luminal gain-loss relationship. J Am Coll Cardiol 1999; 34:1490–7.

11. Pache J, Kastrati A, Mehilli J, *et al.* Intracoronary stenting and angiographic results: strut thickness effect on restenosis outcome (ISAR-STEREO-2) trial. J Am Coll Cardiol 2003; 41:1283–8.

12. Koning R, Eltchanioff H, Commeau P, *et al.* Stent placement compared with balloon angioplasty for small coronary arteries: in-hospital and 6-month clinical and angiographic results. Circulation 2001; 104:1604–8.

13. Doucet S, Schalij MJ, Vrolix MCM, *et al.* Stent placement to prevent restenosis after angioplasty in small coronary arteries. Circulation 2001; 104:2029–33.

14. Moer R, Myreng Y, Mølstad P, *et al.* Stenting in small coronary arteries (SISCA) trial. A randomized comparison etween balloon angioplasty and the heparin-coated beStent. J Am Coll Cardiol 2001; 38:1598–603.

15. Park SW, Lee CW, Hong MK, *et al.* Randomized comparison of coronary stenting with optimal balloon angioplasty for treatment of lesions in small coronary arteries. Eur Heart J 200; 21:1785–9.

16. Kastrati A, Schomig A, Dirschinger J, *et al.* A randomized trial comparing stenting with balloon angioplasty in small vessels in patients with symptomatic coronary artery disease. Circulation 2000; 102:2593–8.

17. Casella G, Prati F. Stenting small coronary arteries: The Multi-Link PIXEL Multicenter Italian Registry. J Invas Cardiol. 2003; 15:371–6.

18. Ardissino D, Cavallini C, Bramucci E, *et al.* Sirolimus-eluting vs uncoated stents for prevention of restenosis in small coronary arteriers. A randomized trial. JAMA 2004; 292:2727–34.

19. Schofer J, Schlüter M, Gershlick AH, *et al.* Sirolimus-eluting stents for treatment of patients with long atherosclerotic lesions in small coronary arteries: double-blind, randomized controlled trial (E-SIRIUS). Lancet 2003; 362:1093–99.

20. Schampaert E, Cohen EA, Schulter M, *et al.* The Canadian study of the sirolimus-eluting stent in the treatment of patients with long de novo lesions in the small native coronary arteries (C-SIRIUS). J Am Coll Cardiol 2004; 43:1110–15.

21. Lemos PA, Arampatzis CA, Saia F, *et al.* Treatment of very small vessels with 2.25-mm diameter sirolimus-eluting stents (from the RESEARCH registry). Am J Cardiol 2004; 93:633–6.

22. Stone GW, Ellis SG, Cox DA, *et al.* One-year clinical results with the slow-release polymer-based, paclitaxel-eluting TAXUS stent. The TAXUS-IV trial. Circulation 2004; 109:1942–7.

23. Ellis SG, Popma JJ, Lasala JM, *et al.* Relationship between angiographic late loss and target lesion revascularization after coronary stent implantation: analysis from the TAXUS-IV trial. J Am Coll Cardiol 2005; 45:1193–200.

24. Moses JW, Leon MB, Popma JJ, *et al.* Sirolimus-eluting stents versus standard stents in patients with stenosis in a native coronary artery. N Engl J Med 2003; 349:1314–23.

25. Umeda H, Iwase M, Kanda H, *et al.* Promising efficacy of primary gradual and prolonged balloon angioplasty in small coronary arteries: a randomized comparison with cutting balloon angioplasty and conventional balloon angioplasty. Am Heart J 2004; 147:e4.

26. Caputo R, Flately M, Ho KKL, Baim DS. Safety and effectiveness of stent implantation without predilation for small coronary arteries. Cathet Cardiovasc Intervent 2003; 59:455–8.

27. Popma JJ, Leon MB, Moses JW, *et al.* Quantitative assessment of angiographic restenosis after sirolimus-eluting stent implantation in native coronary arteries. Circulation 2004; 110:3773–80.

28. Grenadier E, Roguin A, Hertz I, *et al.* Stenting very small coronary narrowings (<2 mm) using the biocompatible phosphoryline-coated coronary stent. Cathet Cardiovasc Intervent 2002; 55:303–8.

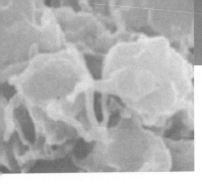

25

Percutaneous coronary intervention in saphenous vein graft disease

AZFAR G. ZAMAN AND JAGATH HERATH

KEY POINTS

- Long term outcome of CABG is limited by occlusive atherothrombotic disease of vein grafts in up to 50% of patients after ten years.

- Repeat surgical intervention carries a high risk of morbidity and mortality.

- PCI should be the preferred first route of revascularization in patients with previous CABG.

- Stent placement in vein grafts is associated with a high (up to 20%) risk of distal embolisation and consequent complications.

- Routine use of embolic protection devices significantly reduces procedural complications during vein graft PCI and where anatomy permits, their use is mandatory.

- Three types of embolic protection devices are available: distal occlusion, proximal occlusion and distal filter. The type to use is determined by lesion location in the vein graft.

- The routine use of glycoprotein IIb/IIIa inhibitors is not recommended for vein graft PCI. Some evidence suggests benefit in patients in whom a distal filter device is employed.

- The risk of restenosis with BMS is high (10–20%) and early data with DES show promising results in restenosis reduction.

- There is no benefit in using of PTFE coated stents over BMS.

- There is no evidence for the use of thrombectomy devices in vein graft PCI.

- For vein graft PCI both the radial and femoral access routes can be employed.

INTRODUCTION

Since first implantation of coronary grafts in 1967 the success of venous conduits in relieving myocardial ischaemia has been limited by their temporal attrition. Although internal mammary grafts have unsurpassed long term patency, utilisation is limited by scarcity. The use of gastroepiploic and radial arteries has been shown to be less than optimal.[1] Consequently, in spite of declining surgical revascularization rates worldwide, the use of venous grafts seems unlikely to diminish and treatment of symptomatic patients with degenerated venous grafts will remain a problem for interventional cardiologists.

Atherosclerotic disease in vein grafts can be either discrete (focal) or diffuse and degenerative. Most clinical trials forming the evidence base for percutaneous intervention in vein grafts report outcomes in patients with discrete disease. Initial trials demonstrated a high percentage of adverse events. The recognition that these were largely secondary to distal embolisation led to development of protection devices that have revolutionized percutaneous intervention in vein grafts with a significant reduction in periprocedural adverse events.

Vein graft disease progression and its timing

Three interlinked pathological processes – thrombosis, neointimal hyperplasia and atherosclerosis, which are temporally distinct, contribute to vein graft disease.[2,3] Awareness of the processes and their timing may help in optimising outcome from intervention.

Vein graft attrition occurring within a month of surgery is almost always due to graft thrombosis and the occlusion rate is 3 to 12% per month. Early thrombosis of vein grafts is caused by the combination of a prothrombotic state and technical factors present at the time of surgery.

Neointimal hyperplasia is defined as the accumulation of smooth muscle cells and extra cellular matrix in the intima and is the main pathological process that occurs one month to one year after graft implantation. It is similar to pathological changes that occur in native coronary arteries after balloon angioplasty.

Atherosclerosis is the main pathological process that contributes to vein graft occlusion one year and beyond after surgery.[2] The predisposing factors and the basic process of atheroma development are similar to those documented in native coronary arteries. However, there are a few distinct topographic, temporal, and histological differences in the pathology of vein graft disease.

The distinct morphological difference seen in vein grafts compared to native coronary arteries is that vein graft atheroma is diffuse, concentric, and friable with poorly developed or absent fibrous cap with little calcification. Intravascular ultrasound studies reveal the absence of focal compensatory enlargement ('Glagov's law') of diseased vein graft segments.[3,4] Late graft thrombosis triggers recurrent ischaemia and is frequently seen in old degenerating grafts with advanced atherosclerotic disease.[5]

REVASCULARISATION FOR VEIN GRAFT DISEASE

Redo surgery

Recurrence of anginal symptoms is seen in up to 20% of patients within one year following surgical revascularisation followed by 4% of patients annually during the next 5 years, 19% at 10 years and 31% at 12 years.[6]

There are limited data comparing percutaneous revascularisation to repeat surgery in patients with angina recurrence. Repeat surgery achieves complete revascularisation in 92% of patients compared to 38% in the percutaneous intervention group. However, in-hospital complications are more common in surgical patients: death (7.3 % vs. 0.3%), Q-wave MI (6.1% vs. 0.9%), and low output syndromes (24% vs. 9%). Both procedures result in equal survival rates at one and six years with equal relief of angina but repeat intervention and/or revascularisation is more frequent in the percutaneous group (64% vs. 8%) at six years.[7, 8]

Given the high morbidity and mortality of re-operation reduced symptomatic benefit as compared to first bypass surgery,[8,9] percutaneous revascularisation should be the preferred first route for post surgery angina recurrence.

Percutaneous coronary intervention

Lesion pathology explains the different outcomes in vein grafts when compared to native coronary arteries.

Balloon angioplasty for vein graft disease has moderate procedural success limited by high periprocedural complication rate, high incidence of restenosis (35%) and high repeat revascularisation rate.[10, 11] Clinical trials show BMS to be superior to balloon angioplasty in vein graft lesions. The use of stents is associated with a high procedural success, superior clinical outcome, and reduced TLR. However, as compared to native vessels the restenosis rate remains high[12, 13] coupled with higher periprocedural complications.

The high incidence of periprocedural complications is in the guise of myocardial necrosis resulting from distal embolisation. The major advance in vein graft intervention has been the advent of embolic protection devices for which extensive trial evidence exists for reducing complications from embolisation (*vide infra*).

The significant problems associated with vein graft intervention are:

1. distal embolisation;
2. no reflow; and
3. aggressive restenosis.

The use of DES in native coronary arteries has shown promising results with significant reduction in restenosis rates.[14, 15] Limited data is available on the long term efficacy of DES in patients with vein graft disease. Most studies confirm a high procedural success rate but there is conflicting data on how DES would affect the clinical outcome. Two nonrandomized trials have shown a trend towards a reduction in MACE at six to nine months follow up.[16, 17] The use of DES was associated with a lower restenosis rate (10% vs. 26.7%, P=0.03) and TVR (4.9% vs. 23.1%, P <0.01) at six to nine months. However, one study showed similar clinical outcome at 30 days, 60 days and 1 year.[18]

Diffuse SVG disease

The optimal treatment strategy for diffusely degenerative SVG (grafts >3-years-old, isolated lesion length >20 mm in length or diffusely diseased segment with multiple/sequential stenosis) is challenging and controversial.

Unlike focal graft lesions, diffusely degenerative graft disease with large ulcerated fragile plaques with associated thrombus is associated with a low procedural success, higher complication rates and low long term patency rate.[19]

Endoluminal reconstruction by stenting of diffuse lesions ('full metal jacket') is a possible option and clinical trials reveal a high procedural success for stenting of diffuse lesions. However, it has been associated with a high incidence of death (11.1%) or myocardial infarction (9.4%) and frequent need for repeat angioplasty.[20]

EMBOLIC PROTECTION DEVICES

Embolic protection devices are catheter-based devices used to capture atherothrombotic debris released during percutaneous vascular interventions and can be divided into three types:

1. distal occlusion;
2. proximal occlusion; and
3. distal filtration.

The first recorded use of these devices was during carotid stenting[21] and subsequent studies confirmed their efficacy in reducing the incidence of periprocedural embolic stroke and death. The high risk of periprocedural myocardial infarction and MACE during vein graft intervention led to exploration of embolic protection devices in this setting.

Distal occlusion devices

The distal occlusion devices have a large evidence base with early vein graft intervention studies using the GuardWire (Medtronic AVE, Santa Rosa, California). This is a temporary occlusion-aspiration system with a 2.8 F crossing profile. A guidewire with a central lumen and inflatable balloon is introduced beyond the lesion. The balloon (either 2.5–5 mm or 3–6 mm) is inflated (using saline/contrast solution) to occlude the vessel and thereby prevent antegrade flow. Following stent deployment over the central wire, any debris released is trapped by the inflated balloon and then aspirated through a 5 F monorail aspiration catheter. The balloon is then deflated and antegrade flow restored. The obvious downside of this device is the duration of ischaemia induced by balloon inflation. The advantage (over filter devices) is that the likelihood of debris passing around the device is minimised by the absolute occlusion thereby assuring complete debris removal.

An alternative device is the TriActiv system (Kensey Nash). In contrast to the GuardWire, this device utilises gas to fill the balloon and thus allows rapid inflation and deflation times. In addition there is an active flush and extraction system. In a randomised controlled trial, the TriActiv system was found to be non inferior to the GuardWire and Filter EZ systems.[22]

Distal filtration devices

The devices with most trial data are EZ-FilterWire (EPI, Boston Scientific), Spider and Microvena Trap (eV3, Minneapolis, Minnesota) and Angioguard (Cordis). The mechanism for all is similar. A non-occlusive filter within its own delivery sheath is delivered distal to the lesion and deployed. Once the sheath is removed the filter is released and assumes the shape of a windsock whose neck is composed of a nitinol loop fixed on its own wire. Following stent deployment, debris is caught in the filter which is then retrieved using a retrieval sheath passed over the wire. The FilterWire and Spider devices are 6 F compatible whilst the Angioguard requires a 7 F guiding catheter.

The major advantage with the filtration devices is flow preservation. One potential disadvantage is that the filter has pores of between 80 to 150 μm and, therefore, may allow debris smaller than 80μm to pass through. However, studies comparing to occlusive devices have failed to show a difference in MACE even though electron microscopy of material aspirated with the GuardWire reveal 50% of particles to be <100μm.[23]

Proximal occlusion devices

The Proxis (Velocimed, Maple Grove, Minnesota) is the only one of its kind licensed for use at the time of writing. Where the landing zone is inadequate, this type of device is the only one suitable for use. The Proxis is compatible with any guidewire. A sealing balloon is deployed proximal to the lesion and this occludes antegrade flow. Intervention is then performed in an environment of stasis created before the passage of any device whereas with the other products described above, prior stenosis dilation may be necessary before crossing with the device. The obvious advantage of the proximal occlusion device is that any and most importantly, all debris dislodged in the dilation process can be aspirated. The device is 7 F compatible with a maximum balloon size of 5mm. Predilation balloons and stents are delivered through the Proxis system, deployed and then debris aspirated before balloon deflation and restoration of antegrade flow.

This system also has the advantage of allowing interventions on multisequential lesions, whereas distal devices require multiple catheter exchanges for sequential lesions.

Preliminary data from a non-randomized trial of 40 patients, demonstrated successful deployment in 95%.[24] The reported MACE rate of 5% was much lower than that achieved with distal devices but data comparing the two are awaited.

A major limitation of this type of device is that they are contraindicated in ostial and proximal vein graft lesions.

Limitations of embolic protection devices

- The major limitation of distal devices is their requirement for a 'landing zone' distal to the lesion. Therefore, lesions within 30 mm of the graft to coronary anastomosis site cannot be safely protected with these devices and a proximal device is indicated.
- Most distal devices are bulky with large crossing profiles and poor torque. In order to cross the lesion, it may be necessary to predilate with consequent risk of embolisation.
- In the presence of subtotal occlusion and poor distal flow, it may be difficult to size the vein graft distal to the lesion. Undersizing the balloon or filter will lead to debris embolising around the occlusive site. Once again, a proximal occlusion device may be better suited under these circumstances.
- Embolisation secondary to incomplete apposition of inflated balloon or filter ring.
- Risk of retrieval device (for filter wires) snagging on stent struts.
- Proximal devices cannot be used in ostial or proximal vein graft lesions. They need a proximal 'landing zone' of 15 mm.

Clinical studies

The first such device evaluated in saphenous vein grafts with low thrombus burden was the GuardWire. A registry of 105 patients confirmed safety and reduction of MACE when compared to historical controls and led to the larger, randomized controlled, SAFER study.[25] This study excluded patients with acute myocardial infarction or severe left ventricular dysfunction but did include patients with a higher thrombus burden than that in the SAFE registry.

Use of the device confirmed a beneficial effect in reducing 30-day MACE (9.6% vs. 16.5%, P = 0.004) and incidence of no reflow (3% vs. 9%, P = 0.02).

The first registry evaluating FilterWire safety and efficacy excluded high risk patients with acute myocardial infarction or severe left ventricular dysfunction.[26] Confirmation of safety and efficacy led to direct comparison with the GuardWire (FIRE study) in patients with low thrombus burden and good pre procedural flow. Primary end-point analysis confirmed similar rates of successful deployment, angiographic and biomarker release and 30-day MACE.[23] Subgroup analysis revealed superiority of the FilterWire in smaller vessels and eccentric lesions.

The proximal occlusion device (Proxis) has been shown to be safe and effective. The first clinical trial with this device, involving 600 patients (PROXIMAL trial) confirmed the Proxis device to be at least as good as the distal devices. Although the trial design was complex, direct comparison with the distal devices revealed a non-significant reduction in MACE (6.2% vs 11.2%, P = 0.89).[27]

In conclusion, therefore, the role of embolic protection devices for vein graft intervention is firmly established. They represent a partial but incomplete solution to distal embolisation and their use during vein graft intervention should be mandatory. The use of a particular device will often be determined by the lesion location and in some grafts with multiple lesions it is possible that no device can be employed.

THROMBECTOMY DEVICES

The benefit of thrombectomy on clinical end points is unproven. In the X-Sizer AMI registry there was no difference in TIMI flow grade 3.[28] There may, however, be situations where the thrombus burden is so large as to preclude the use of embolic protection devices. In these rare instances the X-Sizer system (EndiCOR Medical, San Clemente, California) or the AngioJet device (Possis, Minneapolis, Minnesota) are available for use, although trial evidence of benefit is lacking.

GP IIB/IIIA RECEPTOR INHIBITORS IN VEIN GRAFT INTERVENTION

Even with appropriate use of embolic protection devices, acute complication rates after degenerative vein graft PCI may exceed 10%. This is most often secondary to 'no-reflow' resulting in Q or non Q-wave myocardial infarction. Adjunctive glycoprotein IIb/IIIa inhibitors have proven efficacy in patients with ACS undergoing PCI to native coronary arteries. Data supporting use in vein graft PCI, however, is lacking. Pooling results from several randomized trials[29–34] suggested worse 30-day outcomes. More recently, a differential effect of GP IIb/IIIa agents has been reported.[35] The authors reported on a pre specified subgroup analysis of the FIRE trial, where 651 patients undergoing vein graft PCI and stent insertion were randomized to the filter wire or distal occlusion embolic protection devices. Patients randomised to the distal occlusion device revealed a marked increase in MACE when assigned to GP IIb/IIIa inhibitors (16% vs. 6.3%; P=0.007). No difference was seen in patients in whom the filter device was used. Although the use of GP IIb/IIIa inhibitors was not randomly assigned, the results are nevertheless surprising given the central role of platelet aggregation in distal platelet embolisation. These findings underscore the recognition that pathophysiology of distal embolisation in vein graft PCI is multifactoral with involvement among others, of plaque embolisation and vasospasm. The difference between the two devices is most likely explained by the fact that the filter wire allows antegrade flow of small particulate matter and the reduced platelet aggregation and deposition with GP IIb/IIIa use translates to reduced MACE. During balloon occlusion use of these agents is unlikely to have a beneficial effect as embolic retrieval is facilitated by occlusion and aspiration of all particulate matter.

In conclusion, therefore, the use of filter wire devices may benefit from adjunctive therapy with GP IIb/IIIa inhibitors but use of occlusive embolic protection precludes GP IIb/IIIa therapy.

PTFE COVERED STENT

The aim of covered stents was to improve outcome in graft intervention through prevention of distal embolisation and reducing restenosis rate. This stent has a biocompatible PTFE membrane to 'seal' the lumen of the graft thus trapping embolic debris. In addition, the membrane would act as a mechanical barrier to prevent protrusion of proliferating tissue thereby inhibiting neointimal hyperplasia and restenosis.

However, three major randomised trials revealed no additional benefit in respect to restenosis and cumulative MACE when compared to BMS.[36–38] Use in vein graft interventions, therefore, cannot be recommended except in emergency situations to seal perforations.

SUMMARY

Long term outcome after surgical revascularization is limited by attrition of vein grafts such that up to 50% have significant disease at ten years with angina recurrence. Repeat surgical revascularization is associated with high morbidity and mortality and PCI offers a safer alternative for revascularization in the majority of patients with vein graft disease. Nevertheless, vein graft PCI with stent deployment also carries risk (up to 20%) of procedure related complications, largely as a result of distal embolisation. The advent of embolic protection devices has reduced such complications significantly and their use should be mandatory. Use of glycoprotein IIb/IIIa inhibitors in selected groups may also help in reducing procedure related complications. Drug-eluting stents hold the promise of further reduction in long term complications resulting from decreased restenosis rates. Saphenous vein graft PCI remains a challenge for the interventionist. A better understanding of the pathophysiology and progression of vein graft atheroma coupled to pharmacological and technological advances have tilted the balance in favour of the patient such that vein graft PCI should be considered the first route for revascularization in affected patients.

REFERENCES

1. Khot UN, Friedman DT, Pettersson G, *et al.* Radial artery bypass grafts having an increased occurrence of angiograghically severe stenosis and occlusion compared with

left internal mammary arteries and saphenous vein grafts. Circulation, 2004; 109: 2086–91.

2. Motwani JG, Topol EJ. Aortocoronary Saphenous Vein Graft Disease. Pathogenesis, Predisposition, and Prevention. Circulation 1998; 97:916–31.

3. Kalan JM, Roberts WC. Morphologic findings in saphenous veins used as coronary arterial bypass conduits for longer than 1 year: necropsy analysis of 53 patients, 123 saphenous veins, and 1865 five-millimeter segments of veins. Am Heart J. 1990; 119: 1164–84.

4. Nishioka T, Luo H, Berglund H, et al. Absence of Focal Compensatory Enlargement or Constriction in diseased human coronary saphenous vein bypass grafts: an intravascular ultrasound study. Circulation. 1996; 93:683–90.

5. Peykar S, Angillillo J, Bass TA, et al. Saphenous vein graft disease. Minerva Cardioangiol 2004; 52:379–90.

6. Weintraub WS, Jones EL, Craver JM, et al. Frequency of repeat coronary bypass or coronary angioplasty after coronary artery bypass surgery using saphenous venous grafts. Am J Cardiol. 1994; 73:103–12.

7. Stephan WJ, O'Keefe JH, Piehler JM, et al. Coronary angioplasty versus repeat coronary artery bypass grafting for patients with previous bypass surgery. J Am Coll Cardiol 1996; 28:1140–6.

8. Yau TM, Borger MA, Weisel RD, et al. The changing pattern of reoperative coronary surgery. J Thorac Cardiovasc Surg 2000; 120:156–63.

9. Schmuziger M, Christenson JT, Maurice J, et al. Reoperative myocardial revascularization: an analysis of 458 reoperations and 2645 single operations. Cardiovasc Surg 1994; 2:623–9.

10. Plokker HW, Meester BH and Serruys PW. The Dutch experience in percutaneous transluminal angioplasty of narrowed saphenous veins used for aortocoronary arterial bypass. Am J Cardiol 1991; 67:361–6.

11. de Feyter PJ, van Suylen RJ, de Jaegere PP, et al. Balloon angioplasty for the treatment of lesions in saphenous vein bypass grafts. J Am Coll Cardiol 1993; 21:1539–49.

12. Fenton SH, Fischman DL, Savage MP, et al. Long-term angiographic and clinical outcome after implantation of balloon-expandable stents in aortocoronary saphenous vein grafts. Am J Cardiol 1994; 74:1187–91.

13. Savage MP, Douglas JS, Fischman DL, et al. Stent placement compared with balloon angioplasty for obstructed coronary bypass grafts. Saphenous Vein de novo Trial Investigators. N Engl J Med 1997; 337:740–7.

14. Moses JW, Leon MB, Popma JJ, et al. Sirolimus-eluting stents versus standard stents is patients with stenosis in a native coronary artery. N Eng J Med 2003; 349:1315–23.

15. Colombo A, Drzewiecki J, Banning A, et al. Randomized study to assess the effectiveness of slow- and moderate-release polymer-based paclitaxel-eluting stents for coronary artery lesions. Circulation 2003; 108:788–94.

16. Lei GE, Iakovou I, Sangiorgi GM, *et al*. Treatment of saphenous vein graft lesions with drug-eluting stents. Immediate and midterm outcome. J Am Coll Cardiol 2005; 45: 989–94.

17. Lee MS, Shah AP, Aragon J, *et al*. Drug-eluting stenting is superior to bare metal stenting in saphenous vein grafts. Catheter Cardiovasc Interv. 2005 Dec; 66:507–11.

18. Chu WW, Rha SW, Kuchulakanti PK, *et al*. Efficacy of sirolimus-eluting stents compared with bare metal stents for saphenous vein graft intervention. Am J Cardiol. 2006; 97:34–7.

19. Ellis SG, Brener SJ, DeLuca S, *et al*. Late myocardial ischemic events after saphenous vein graft intervention-importance of initially "nonsignificant" vein graft lesions. Am J Cardiol 1997; 79:1460–4.

20. Choussat R, Black AJR, Bossi I, *et al*. Long-term clinical outcome after endoluminal reconstruction of diffusely degenerated saphenous vein grafts with less-shortening wallstents. J Am Coll Cardiol. 2000; 36:387–94.

21. Theron J, Courtheoux P, Alachkar F, *et al*. New triple coaxial catheter system for carotid angioplasty with cerebral protection. AJNR Am J Neuroradiol 1990; 11:869–74.

22. Carrozza JP, Mumma M, Breall JA, *et al*. Randomized evaluation of the TriActive balloon-protection flush and extraction system for the treatment of saphenous vein graft disease. J Am Coll Cardiol 2005; 46:1677–83.

23. Stone GW, Rogers C, Hermiller J, *et al*. Randomized Comparison of Distal Protection With a Filter-Based Catheter and a Balloon Occlusion and Aspiration System During Percutaneous Intervention of Diseased Saphenous Vein Aorto-Coronary Bypass Grafts. Circulation 2003; 108:548–53.

24. Sievert H, Wahr D, Schuler G, *et al*. Effectiveness and safety of the Proxis system in demonstrating retrograde coronary blood flow during proximal occlusion and in capturing embolic material. Am J Cardiol 2004; 94:1134–9.

25. Baim DS, Wahr D, George B, *et al*. Randomized Trial of a Distal Embolic Protection Device During Percutaneous Intervention of Saphenous Vein Aorto-Coronary Bypass Grafts. Circulation 2002; 105:1285–90.

26. Stone GW, Rogers C, Ramee S, *et al*. Distal filter protection during saphenous vein graft stenting: technical and clinical correlates of efficacy. J Am Coll Cardiol 2002; 40:1882–8.

27. White J. TCT 2005 Late-Breaking Trials Promise to Influence Practice Patterns.Journal of Interventional Cardiology 2006; 19(1):113–16.

28. Napodano M, Pasquetto G, Sacca S, *et al*. Intracoronary thrombectomy improves myocardial reperfusion in patients undergoing direct angioplasty for acute myocardial infarction. J Am Coll Cardiol 2003; 15;42(8):1395–402.

29. Use of a monoclonal antibody directed against the platelet glycoprotein IIb/IIIa receptor in high-risk coronary angioplasty. The EPIC Investigators. N Engl J Med 1994; 330:956–61.

30. Platelet glycopoten IIb/IIIa receptor blockade and low-dose heparin during percutaneous coronary revascularization. The EPILOG Investigators. N Engl J Med 1997; 336:1689–96.

31. Randomised placebo-controlled and balloon-angioplasty-controlled trial to assess safety of coronary stenting with use of platelet glycoprotein IIb/IIIa blockade. The EPISTENT

Investigators. Evaluation of platelet IIb/IIIa inhibitors for stenting. Lancet 1998; 352:87–92.

32. Randomised placebo-controlled trial of effect of eptifbatide on complications of percutaneous coronary interventions: IMPACT-II. Integrilin to minimize platelet aggregation and coronary thrombosis-II. Lancet 1997; 349:1422–8.

33. Inhibition of platelet glycoprotein IIb/IIIa with eptifbatide in patients with acute coronary syngrome. The PURSUIT Trial Investigators. Platelet glycoprotein IIb/IIIa in unstable angina: Receptor suppression using Integrilin therapy. N Engl J Med 1998; 339:436–43.

34. Jonas M, Stone GW, Mehran R, et al. Platelet glycoprotein IIb/IIIa receptor inhibition as adjunctive treatment during saphenous vein graft stenting: differential effects after randomization to occlusion or filter-based embolic protection. Eur Heart J. 2006; 27(8):920–8.

35. Laarman GJ, Kiemeneij F, Mueller R, et al. Feasibility, safety, and preliminary efficacy of a novel ePTFE-covered self-expanding stent in saphenous vein graft lesions: the Symbiot II trial. Catheter Cardiovasc Interv 2005; 64(3):361–8.

36. Mahmud E, Pezeshki B, Salami A, et al. Highlights of the 2004 Transcatheter Cardiovascular Therapeutics (TCT) annual meeting: Clinical implications. J Am Coll Cardiol 2005; 45:796–801.

37. Stankovic G, Colombo A, Presbitero P, et al. The Randomized Evaluation of polytetrafluoroethylene COVERed stent in Saphenous vein grafts (RECOVERS) Trial. Circulation 2003; 108:37.

38. Schachinger V, Hamm CW, Munzel T, et al. A randomized trial of Polytetrafluoroethylene-Membrane-Covered stents compared with conventional stents in aortocoronary saphenous vein grafts. J Am Coll Cardiol 2003; 42:1360–9.

Section Four

Non-Coronary
Intervention:
Peripheral Vascular
Intervention

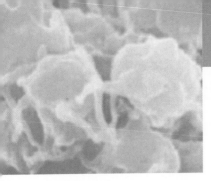

26

Carotid artery stenting

IQBAL MALIK, MD

KEY POINTS

- The time has now come to regard carotid artery stenting (CAS) as a realistic alternative to Carotid endarterectomy (CEA). Based on the availability of safe techniques, on trial evidence and the presence of a cohort of over 12 000 patients that have been treated successfully worldwide.

- Three major patient groups need to be considered for carotid intervention: symptomatic, asymptomatic and pre-cardiac surgery.

- Trials of CAS versus medical therapy are unlikely to be performed as CEA has been shown to be better than medical therapy in patients with significant ICA stenosis.

- Due to ease of access, the carotid duplex ultrasound scan has become the screening tool of choice.

- Use of adjunctive pharmacology has improved outcomes in coronary intervention, but not CAS as yet.

- Transcranial Doppler measurements suggest that without distal protection, the incidence of micro-embolisation is higher with CAS than CEA.

INTRODUCTION

Stroke is the third leading cause of death in the developed world.[1] Internal carotid artery (ICA) stenosis is a major cause of ischaemic stroke, with the risk being related to the degree of stenosis and the presence of recent symptoms.[2,3] Carotid endarterectomy (CEA) has become the preferred method of treatment for patients with asymptomatic or symptomatic high grade ICA stenosis, supplanting medical therapy alone. The time has now come to regard carotid artery stenting (CAS) as a realistic alternative to CEA. This statement is based on the availability of safe techniques, on trial evidence and the presence of a cohort of over 12 000 patients that have been treated successfully worldwide.[4]

HISTORY

Atherosclerosis of the carotid bifurcation was suggested as a risk factor for stroke over 50 years ago.[5] Surgery of this area was developed at a similar time by Eastcott in the UK, and Debakey in the US.[6,7] Following this, CEA became a popular procedure amongst vascular surgeons. In the USA alone, more than 100 000 CEA procedures were performed in 1985, well before the publication of randomised controlled trial data.[8] In the ensuing confusion about indications and outcomes, a number of trials began to clarify the correct role for CEA in both symptomatic and asymptomatic patients.[9,10–12] CEA remains the most common vascular operation in the US.

The report of first carotid angioplasty was published in 1983, with stenting becoming popular in the early 1990s.[13,14] By 1994, Roubin et al. were performing

TABLE 26.1 - TRIAL EVIDENCE FOR THE USE OF CEA IN SYMPTOMATIC AND ASYMPTOMATIC ICA STENOSIS. ALL END POINTS ARE 30-DAY DEATH AND STROKE RATES. CVA=STROKE

TRIAL	% STENOSIS	OPERATIVE RISK (CVA/death)	F/U PERIOD Ipsilateral CVA/death	MEDICAL Rx	CEA
Symptomatic					
NASCET		6.5%	2 yrs	13.1%	2.5%
N=659	>70% Angiographic				
NASCET	50–69%	–	5 yrs	22.2%	15.7%
N=858	Angiographic				
ECST	>70–99%	7%	3 yrs	16.8%	10.3%
N=778	Duplex				
Asymptomatic					
ACAS	>60%	–	5 yrs	11%	5.1%
N=1662	Angiographic				
ACST	>60%	–	5 yrs	11.8%	6.4%
	Angiographic				

CAS on a routine basis in the USA.[15] Distal protection devices (DPD) were developed in a primitive form in 1987.[16] It has really been the development of more usable DPD that has lead to the rapid growth of CAS in recent years.[4]

PATIENT SELECTION

Three major patient groups need to be considered for carotid intervention:

Symptomatic

Three trials have addressed the issue of the treatment of symptomatic ICA stenosis. The VA trial was terminated early due to publication of the results of the other two.[17] (Table 26.1).

The North American Symptomatic Carotid Endarterectomy Trial (NASCET) randomised 2885 patients with 30–99% ICA stenoses at angiography and recent stroke (CVA) or transient ischaemic attack (TIA) to medical therapy or CEA. In patients with 70–99% stenosis, operation reduced two-year ipsilateral CVA risk from 26% to 9% (relative risk reduction 65%) and combined major CVA and death rates from 13.1% to 2.5% (relative risk reduction 81%).[9] In those with 50–69% stenosis, five-year ipsilateral CVA risk was reduced from 22.2% to 15.7% (relative risk reduction 29%).[18] There was no benefit in patients with stenosis <50%, although this group still had an event rate of 15–19% at two years, suggesting medical therapy also needed to be improved.

The European Carotid Surgery Trial (ECST) randomised 3024 patients with symptomatic ICA stenosis in a similar manner, using duplex ultrasound criteria of >60% stenosis.[10,19] In patients with 70–99% stenosis, at three years, risk of ipsilateral CVA was reduced from 16.8% to 10.3% (relative risk reduction 39%). Risk of major stroke or death was reduced from 11% to 6% (relative risk reduction 45%). There was no benefit in patients with <70% duplex stenosis.

A meta-anaylsis of these and the VA trial suggested most benefit in men, those >75, and those treated within two weeks.[20] So, for symptomatic patients, a duplex stenosis of >70–75% (angiographic >50%) should be treated to improve prognosis. American guidelines suggest that the surgeon should have <6% peri-procedural CVA and death rates for the procedure to be useful.[21]

Asymptomatic

The value of CEA in asymptomatic ICA stenosis is less clear. Three small initial trials failed to show a benefit, but may have been underpowered to do so.[22-24] However, there are now two larger trials which have shown positive results[12,25] (Table 26.1).

The Asymptomatic Carotid Atherosclerosis Study (ACAS) studied 1662 patients under the age of 80 with >60% ultrasound stenosis, randomizing them to CEA or medical therapy.[25] At five years, the risk of ipsilateral CVA or death was reduced from 11% to 5.1% by CEA. The value of the procedure in women was not proven.

The Asymptomatic Carotid Surgery Trial (ACST) randomized 3120 patients, and again used >60% stenosis on ultrasound as the entry criterion, and showed that after five years, ipsilateral CVA or death rate was reduced from 11.8% to 6.4% by CEA.[12]

So, in asymptomatic patients, a stenosis of >60% could be treated, if the patient is male, <80- years-old, and has a good chance of living for five years. Since the benefits was mainly in those with >75% stenosis, this is a more robust cut-off to use, matching an angiographic stenosis of 50% by NASCET criteria (Fig. 26.3).

It should be recalled that the background event rate is <2% stroke risk per year, which would be reduced to 1% by the procedure. This compares well with the risk reductions offered by lipid lowering therapy, or comparing the benefit of Clopidogrel over Aspirin in patients with vascular disease.[26-27] American guidelines suggest that the surgeon should have a <3% peri-procedural CVA and death rate for asymptomatic patients for the procedure to be useful.[21]

Pre-cardiac surgery

Those patients with asymptomatic ICA stenoses facing CABG or valve surgery have elevated peri-operative CVA risk. Whether carotid intervention is beneficial in some or all is controversial, since CEA itself can carry a higher risk in the presence of severe cardiac disease.[28] A review of the limited data suggests that the hemodynamic consequences may not be relevant with a unilateral stenosis, but if the numerical addition of the stenoses of the ICA on both sides is >140%, then intervention on the more severe side is acceptable.[29] If brain imaging suggests an inadequate collateral supply to the hemisphere supplied by a tight carotid stenosis, then this unilateral stenosis may be worth treating. On the basis of the SAPPHIRE trial (see below), CAS would seem the more appropriate therapy in such cases.[30]

CAS versus CEA

Trials of CAS versus medical therapy are unlikely to be performed as CEA has been shown to be better than medical therapy in patients with significant ICA

TABLE 26.2 - INDICATION TO PERFORM CAS RATHER THAN CEA

CONDITION	DETAILS
High Medical Co-morbidity	Age >80
	Coronary disease (CAD) with acute myocardial infarction (AMI) <4 weeks ago
	Any severe CAD
	Congestive cardiac failure
	Dialysis dependant renal failure
	Chronic airways disease (FEV1 <1 L)
	Uncontrolled diabetes mellitus
Local surgical factors	Restenosis after Endarterectomy (CEA)
	Radiation induced Carotid stenosis
	Anatomically high ICA stenosis (above C2)
	Prior neck scarring or surgery
	Contralateral recurrent laryngeal nerve (RLN) injury
	Contralateral internal carotid artery occlusion

stenosis. Thus, on-going trials would need to confirm that CEA and CAS are equivalent if CAS is to become the mainstay of treatment for ICA stenosis. There are patients, however, who have been shown to be at elevated operative risk, and who might benefit from a percutaneous approach if risks were shown to be lower.[28,31-33] (Table 26.2).

CEA carries risks, including CVA, surgical haematoma, cranial nerve injury and risks related to anaesthesia.[34] These risks in real life are higher than those reported in the trials, both due to patient and indeed operator selection, since the best and largest volume operators often participate in these studies.[35] The same operator volume dependency has also been seen for CAS, with early cases having a higher complication rate than later ones, the so-called 'learning curve'.[36] Even in early experience of 528 cases of CAS from Roubin *et al.*, however, the safety of CAS became clear. Despite 83% of the symptomatic patients being ineligible for CEA by NASCET criteria due to co-morbidity, 30-day CVA and death rates were 7.4%, comparable to those for CEA in the NASCET trial.

There are now two published randomised trials of CAS against CEA. The Carotid and Vertebral Artery Transluminal Angioplasty Study (CAVATAS) randomised 504 patients with symptomatic ICA stenosis to balloon angioplasty (only 26% got a stent) or CEA. This showed that 30-day stroke and death rates were equivalent in both arms at 9%, but that hematomas and cranial nerve injuries were higher in the CEA arm (Fig. 26.1). Although it was argued that the peri-operative risk was too high in the CEA arm, these were experienced surgeons who had participated in previous trials, and in fact it was CAS, which was still a novel procedure, without the use of DPDs, that should have been disadvantaged.[37]

The Stenting and Angioplasty with Protection in Patients at High Risk for Endarterectomy (SAPPHIRE) study was the first trial to compare CEA with modern CAS utilising DPD.[30] All patients were considered high risk (Table 26.2). A total of 723 patients were enrolled with stenoses of >50% if symptomatic or

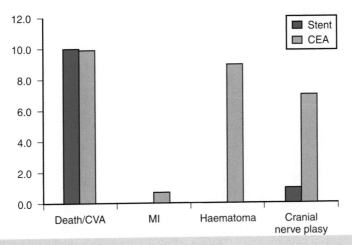

Figure 26.1:
30-day outcome of CAVATAS trial comparing CAS and CEA in symptomatic patients with ICA stenosis. There was no significant difference in death and stroke, or in myocardial infarction (MI) rates, but there were less cranial nerve palsies and haematomas with CAS (p=0.0015 and <0.0001 respectively).

>80% if asymptomatic. Of these, 307 were randomised to CAS versus CEA. However, 409 were considered unsuitable for CEA and were put in the CAS registry, whilst only seven patients were considered unsuitable for CAS, and were placed in the CEA registry. All CAS procedures were done with the Angioguard DPD and Precise stent (Cordis, Johnson and Johnson). The outcome of 30-day stroke and death rate was 3.1% for CAS versus 3.3% for CEA (p=ns). More interestingly, the rate in the stent registry was also only 3% (Fig. 26.2). Myocardial infarction was defined as rise of creatinine kinase twice the upper limit of normal. The combined endpoint of the study (death/CVA/MI) occurred in 5.8% of the CAS group versus 12.6% of the CEA group (p=0.047). The same trend was seen in asymptomatic and symptomatic patients, and was maintained at one year.

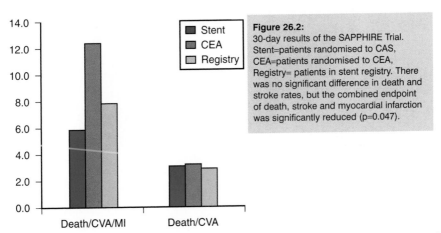

Figure 26.2:
30-day results of the SAPPHIRE Trial. Stent=patients randomised to CAS, CEA=patients randomised to CEA, Registry= patients in stent registry. There was no significant difference in death and stroke rates, but the combined endpoint of death, stroke and myocardial infarction was significantly reduced (p=0.047).

Thus, in higher risk patients with symptomatic or asymptomatic ICA stenosis, results of CAS are as good if not better than CEA. On this basis, CAS is a reasonable alternative strategy to be offered to such patients.

For lower risk patients, results of ongoing trials are awaited, but there appears no logical reason to assume CAS will not also be the treatment of choice in this larger cohort.[38–40,41]

Key investigations

Carotid duplex scanning Due to ease of access, the carotid duplex ultrasound scan has become the screening tool of choice. There is considerable skill involved in performing and interpreting the scan. There is a correlation between stenosis assessed at angiography and duplex measurement (Fig. 26.3). Attempts have been made to try to improve plaque characterisation, and these may develop further with the advent of virtual histology. There is some data to suggest that plaque morphology predicts outcome after intervention, although the jury is still out.[42,43]

Invasive angiography Selective angiography for assessing ICA stenosis carries a risk of TIA and CVA, and so is now rarely performed. Using arch aortography and digital subtraction, non-selective images can be obtained to allow measurement of stenosis.

MRA Access to magnetic resonance angiography (MRA) is limited in the UK, but can produce excellent images of the aortic arch, great vessels, and intra-cerebral vasculature. Decisions on treatment may be swayed by the presence

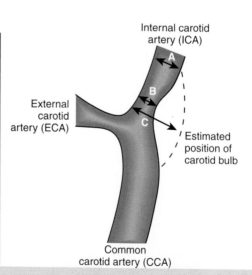

$$NASCET = \frac{A-B}{A} \quad ECST = \frac{C-B}{C}$$

NASCET (% stenosis)	ECST (% stenosis)
30	65
40	70
50	75
60	80
70	85
80	91
90	97

Figure 26.3:
Comparison of measurement of ICA stenosis using NASCET (angiographic) criteria or ECST (Duplex ultrasound) criteria.

or absence of intracerebral collaterals from the circle of Willis. However, pseudo-stenoses can result from movement artefact.

CT angiography With the advent of multi-slice CT, detailed imaging of the arch and great vessels can be achieved. In addition, the intracerebral circulation can be imaged. Although not yet validated against invasive angiography, which is seen as the gold standard, image quality is rapidly improving allowing accurate assessment of the stenosis, as well as plaque composition. The only drawback of CT is that brain imaging is not as detailed as with MRI.

TECHNIQUE FOR CAS

Planning and pre-treatment

Pre-operative medication The patient should be adequately hydrated as with all vascular catheterisation procedures. Aspirin and Clopidogrel need to be initiated at least 24 hours prior to the procedure. A loading dose of 300 mg of each is given if the patient is not on them regularly, with 75 mg daily thereafter. Anti-hypertensive medication is reviewed, and the beta-blocker stopped for the day of the procedure. The aim is to have a systolic pressure between 120–180 mmHg at the start of the procedure.

Use of adjunctive pharmacology has improved outcomes in PCI. Data in CAS suggests that use of DPDs gives greater benefit than use of glycoprotein IIb/IIIa agents.[44,45] There is a danger of haemorrhagic transformation if embolic CVA occurs with these agents on board. However, they may find a place *in addition* to DPDs to reduce platelet aggregation within the filter device. This needs to be tested in further trials.

Gaining a stable working platform The patient should be comfortable with a head cushion to maintain a stable position. There should be electrocardiographic and haemodynamic monitoring attached. An intravenous line should be available and functional.

A standard technique should be employed to gain familiarity with the approach (Table 26.3). Various catheter shapes are available to try to intubate the common carotid artery selectively, including Vitek, Berenstein and Sidewinder. Problems arise with a bovine origin of the left CCA or deep-seated origins of the great arteries (Fig. 26.4). Most commonly the procedure used by radiologist involves a long sheath as the conduit, whilst cardiologists prefer a 7 F or 8 F guide catheter. Care needs to be taken not to perforate a branch of the ECA with the stiff wire used to support placement of the guide catheter. The ability to store a roadmap of the lesion allows easy passage of the angioplasty wire or DPD.

Distal protection or not? Micro-embolisation is thought to be the major cause of peri-operative neurological complications during CAS.[46] Transcranial Doppler measurements suggest that without distal protection, the incidence of micro-embolisation is higher with CAS than CEA.[47] Thus prevention of distal embolisation would seem logical. This can be achieved with distal filter devices, distal occlusion devices, or proximal occlusion devices (Table 26.4). Most cardiologists are likely to prefer distal protection filters

Table 26.3 - SUMMARY OF TECHNIQUE TO PERFORM CAROTID ARTERY STENTING IN STANDARD CASES. MODIFIED FROM HOBSON *ET AL.*[55]

- Pre-treated with Aspirin and Clopidogrel
- Transfemoral 8 F sheath placed via Seldinger Technique
- 0.035" wire to reach aortic arch
- Aortogram to assess take-off of great vessels
- Heparin given to achieve ACT 250–300
- 5 F Vitek or other catheter to selectively cannulate innominate artery (IA) or left common carotid artery (CCA) (no wire)
- Imaging to visualise stenosis and origin of external carotid artery (ECA)
- 0.035" coated Terumo glide wire to advance catheter into ECA
- Exchange inside catheter for long 0.035" stiff Amplatser wire 3
- Place 8 F guide catheter (or sheath) into CCA 2 cm below bifurcation
- Remove stiff wire
- Cross lesion with distal protection device (DPD) on 0.014" wire and deploy device 2–3 cm above lesion in internal carotid artery (ICA)
- Predilate if needed with 3×20 mm balloon ESSENTIAL to give 600 micrograms of atropine prior to this
- Place self-expanding stent in position and release
- Post-dilate to achieve <20% residual stenosis
- Retrieve DPD
- Remove guide catheter/sheath and use closure device to seal femoral puncture
- Continue aspirin and Clopidogrel four weeks

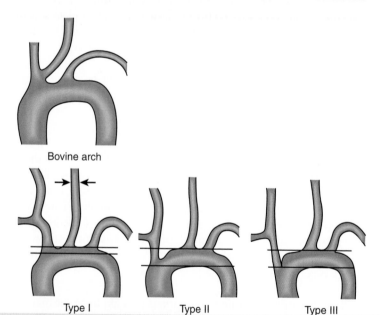

Bovine arch

Type I   Type II   Type III

Figure 26.4:
Difficult arch anatomy. When the left internal carotid artery (ICA) emerges from the innominate, a bovine anatomy is found. Type I arch has the origin of all the great vessel within one diameter of the ICA away from each other. Type II arch has the take-off of the innominate artery >1 ICA diameter away from the other great vessels but above the base of the arch. A type III arch has the origin of the innominate artery below the base of the arch.

TABLE 26.4 - EMBOLIC PROTECTION DEVICES USED FOR CAROTID ARTERY STENT (CAS) PROCEDURES WITH ADVANTAGE AND DISADVANTAGES LISTED. INTERNAL CAROTID ARTERY (ICA), EXTERNAL CAROTID ARTERY (ECA)

TECHNIQUE	ADVANTAGES	DISADVANTAGES
Balloon occlusion • Percusurge (Medtronic)	• Can be used in patients with low cardiac output • no embolic debris if used correctly	• Requires lesion to be crossed without protection to deliver device • Maximum vessel size 6 mm • Can lead to cerebral hypoperfusion • No flow of contrast, so imaging difficult • Risk of trauma to ICA with movement of the filter
Distal filter • Angioguard (Cordis) • Accunet (Guidant) • EZ-Filter (Boston) • Interceptor (Medtronic) • NeuroShield (Abbott) • Spider (EV-3)	• Maintain anterograde perfusion • Allow imaging whilst in use	• Requires lesion to be crossed without protection to deliver device • Filter may clog or get overloaded • Can be difficult to retrieve in tortuous vessels • Maximum size 8 mm • Risk of trauma to ICA with movement of the filter
Proximal occlusion • Parodi (Arteria) • MOMA (Invotec)	• Can be used in large vessels • No need to cross ICA lesion prior to protection	• Can lead to cerebral hypoperfusion • Large sheath size in femoral artery (10 F or 11 F) • Requires disease free ECA

due to familiarity. Large scale trials comparing outcomes with and without distal protection are lacking, but registry data suggests that some form of protection device should be used in most cases. Event rates (30-day stroke and death) in symptomatic patients having CAS in the pre-protection era were 6.7% versus 2.82% in the modern age (Wholey MH, ACC Scientific sessions presentation 2003). For asymptomatic patients, rates were 3.97% and 1.75% respectively.

Distal balloon occlusion requires crossing the ICA lesion with the device, inflation of a low pressure balloon to block the passage of debris distally during CAS, and removal of debris by aspiration prior to the end of the procedure. Because blood flow is interrupted, the patient may become restless due to cerebral hypoperfusion. Therefore, the CAS procedure must be completed within a few minutes.

Filter DPDs use 80–100 micron filters inserted via the guide catheter or sheath, and deployed beyond the ICA stenosis. The blood flow is maintained, and so the procedure is better tolerated. However, movement of the device can result in spasm or even dissection of the ICA, and if apposition is not perfect, some debris can still pass upwards to the brain. The device is re-captured after the CAS procedure and withdrawn through the stent.

The third device involves the proximal occlusion of the CCA and the external carotid artery (ECA). A large catheter with an extension arm for the ECA is advanced into the CCA. Occlusion balloons mounted on the catheter are inflated in the CCA and then the ECA. This creates a negative pressure in the ICA and should allow the collaterals in the circle of Willis to produce reverse flow, preventing distal embolisation into the ICA. The stent procedure is then performed and aspiration performed to clear debris from the ICA prior to device removal.

Balloon, stent and closure Once the DPD is in place, if the lesion is tight, with less than a 2 mm diameter, or looks calcified, the pre-dilatation with a 3 mm × 20 mm balloon is recommended. Direct stenting may be performed for less severe stenoses. It is vital to give atropine 600 micrograms prior to balloon inflation. Failure to do so will result is bradycardia and hypotension which can be difficult to manage and may be prolonged.

Which stent? The choice of stent depends on the characteristics of the lesion and the shape of the vessel. A closed cell design will improve lesion coverage if a lot of debris is expected, but will not be as flexible as an open cell design. A stainless steel stent (Carotid Wallstent, Boston) is likely to have more radial strength, but will not be as conformable as a nitinol stent (e.g. Precise stent, Cordis, or Acculink, Guidant). It is important to get familiar with a few stents and how they perform rather than use a large range. The role for tapered stents (designed to be smaller in the ICA section than the CCA section) is not clear (Acculink, Guidant). Self-expanding stents are used almost exclusively due to concerns about what might happen to a balloon expanded stent if carotid sinus massage was subsequently performed! It appears that stenting across the ECA origin does not matter clinically. Since many ICA stenoses extend into the carotid bifurcation, the norm is to stent into the CCA from the ICA.

Once the stent is in place, post-dilatation is usually required to allow the stenosis to be reduced to <20–30%. There appears to be no need to go for 0% as one might for the coronary, and high pressure, large balloon inflation may lead to unnecessary additional risk by causing more embolisation.

The DPD is then recovered, the guide catheter or sheath removed, and the femoral puncture site sealed with a closure device to allow the patient to sit up more rapidly.

Complications and management

General complications common to all percutaneous vascular procedures, such as femoral puncture complications, bradycardia, and hypotension are dealt with elsewhere. This section will focus on those related to CAS specifically.

Perforation of ECA If seen on angiography, then bleeding is occurring at a rate of at least 3 ml/minute.[48] Continued bleeding may cause substantial sub-glottic swelling and may necessitate intubation to protect the airway. If conservative management fails, there may be a need to embolise the branch of the ECA that is bleeding with a coil, glue or foam.[49]

Vessel rupture Although rare, high pressure balloon inflation in calcified lesions may cause ICA rupture. This is usually managed conservatively.[50]

Spasm Manipulation with the wire, and in particular distal filter devices, can result in spasm of the ICA. This usually resolves after removal of the device. The administration of 100–200 micrograms of Isosorbide Dinitrate will improve it if treatment is required.

Neurological The most dreaded complications are neurological. No DPD is 100% efficient in catching debris, and in addition, there is an incidence of late embolic stroke after the DPD is removed, in the first seven days post-procedure. This is presumably generated by detachment of a mobile piece of atheroma.[51] Late events are usually managed conservatively once bleeding has been excluded. Large CVAs occurring during the procedure should prompt intracerebral angiography to exclude acute occlusion due to embolism. The role of thrombolysis in this situation is not defined, and catheter and wire-based fragmentation of the debris may be warranted. Haemorrhagic stroke during the procedure will necessitate full reversal of anti-coagulants.

Either due to embolisation, or related to hypoperfusion, the patient can become restless and may have a seizure. Restlessness is resolved by improving perfusion by finishing the procedure and removing the distal or proximal protection device.

The hyperperfusion syndrome occurs in a small number of cases. Headache, fits or CVA may be the clinical manifestation. It is thought that increased cerebral perfusion after intervention (CEA and CAS) overwealms cerebral autoregulation. Intracerebral bleeding can be catastrophic. For this reason, bilateral procedures should be avoided and blood pressure control should be achieved prior to carotid intervention.[52]

The ideal training program

Consensus is slowly being reached on the ideal training program for becoming competent in CAS procedures.[53] Worldwide, interventional cardiologists, interventional radiologists and vascular surgeons are performing the procedures. An ideal pathway would include all the following:

1. Background information
   - knowledge of the causes of stroke;
   - causes of carotid artery disease;
   - understanding of the medical interventions available to reduce stroke risk;
   - evidence base for carotid intervention; and
   - interpretation of investigations (duplex, CTA, etc).

This may need a validated training program to ensure knowledge base is adequate.

2. Interventional skill
   - background in endovascular procedures;
   - able to perform balloon angioplasty; and
   - knowledge of management of complications.

This may be augmented by attending live-case meetings

3. Virtual simulator training in carotid procedures
   - able to practice procedures without risk to patients;

4. Proctorship when cases begun in home institution. ICSS suggests ten cases are proctored prior to solo operation. US guidelines suggest 25 cases, with half of these first operator.[39,53]

Perhaps more important still is that adequate clinical governance and review procedures are in place to allow practice to be monitored, and problems to be

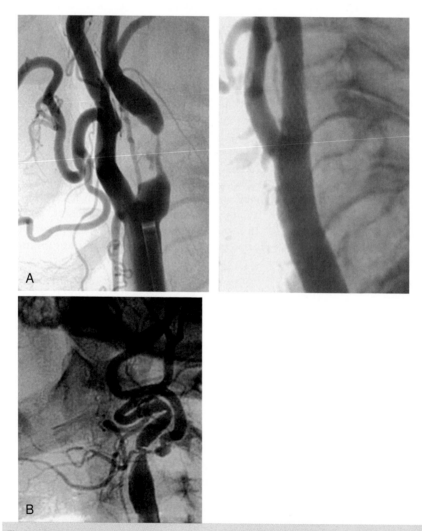

Figure 26.5:
Straightforward cases need to be performed initially: A, With greater experience, tortuous arteries, with multiple stenoses or bifurcation lesions will become possible B.

resolved without patient risk. Training of the staff in the interventional lab and recovery areas is vital to reducing patient risk.

CONCLUSIONS

CEA is not as invasive as CABG surgery, whilst CAS carries higher risks than PCI since the brain is more unforgiving than the myocardium. However, as with the coronary field, the move towards the development of less invasive treatments is unrelenting and with the appropriate training, many interventionalists will be able to perform CAS safely. As with coronary intervention, case selection in the early phase of the 'learning curve' will allow the program to develop. The more difficult lesion can still be referred for CEA until sufficient catheter skills have developed (Fig. 26.5).

It is important to pay attention to initial patient selection and appropriate investigation. This is best done in the context of a multi-disciplinary team (MDT). Selection of technique to be employed, choice of equipment, and meticulous pre-operative, peri-operative and post-operative care is vital to ensure that the procedure is performed at lowest possible risk. Careful liaison with the MDT allows clinical governance and audit to be transparent and honest.

The evidence base comparing CAS to CEA is enlarging, with both registry and trial data. There is a position of clinical equipoise in low-risk patients, but for high risk patients, if an intervention is planned, CAS makes a strong case to be the favoured treatment.

A review by NICE in the UK is awaited, but present guidelines on the management of stroke suggest that CAS is a rapidly evolving procedure and encourage those performing stenting to take part in the ICSS trial (http://www.nice.org.uk/page.aspx?o=218167).

REFERENCES

1. American Heart Association. Heart Disease and Stroke Statistics, 2003 update. 2003. Dallas Scientitic Sessions, Texas, USA, American Heart Association.

2. Barnett HJ, Gunton RW, Eliasziw M, Fleming L, Sharpe B, Gates P et al. Causes and severity of ischemic stroke in patients with internal carotid artery stenosis. JAMA 2000; 283(11):1429–36.

3. Inzitari D, Eliasziw M, Gates P, Sharpe BL, Chan RK, Meldrum HE et al. The causes and risk of stroke in patients with asymptomatic internal-carotid-artery stenosis. North American Symptomatic Carotid Endarterectomy Trial Collaborators. N Engl J Med 2000; 342(23):1693–700.

4. Wholey MH, Al Mubarek N, Wholey MH. Updated review of the global carotid artery stent registry. Catheter Cardiovasc Interv. 2003; 60(2):259–66.

5. Fischer CM, Gore I, Okabe N, White PD. Atherosclerosis of the carotid and vertebral arteries: extracranial and intracranial. J Neuropath Exp Neurol 1965; 24:455–76.

6. Eastcott HH, Pickering GW, Rob CG. Reconstruction of internal carotid artery in a patient with intermittent attacks of hemiplegia. Lancet 1954; 267(6846):994–6.

7. DeBakey ME. Successful carotid endarterectomy for cerebrovascular insufficiency. Nineteen-year follow-up. JAMA 1975; 233(10):1083–5.

8. Tu JV, Hannan EL, Anderson GM, Iron K, Wu K, Vranizan K *et al*. The fall and rise of carotid endarterectomy in the United States and Canada. N Engl J Med 1998; 339(20):1441–7.

9. Beneficial effect of carotid endarterectomy in symptomatic patients with high-grade carotid stenosis. North American Symptomatic Carotid Endarterectomy Trial Collaborators. N Engl J Med 1991; 325(7):445–53.

10. MRC European Carotid Surgery Trial: interim results for symptomatic patients with severe (70-99%) or with mild (0–29%) carotid stenosis. European Carotid Surgery Trialists' Collaborative Group. Lancet 1991; 337(8752):1235–43.

11. Endarterectomy for asymptomatic carotid artery stenosis. Executive Committee for the Asymptomatic Carotid Atherosclerosis Study. JAMA 1995; 273(18):1421–8.

12. Halliday A, Mansfield A, Marro J, Peto C, Peto R, Potter J *et al*. Prevention of disabling and fatal strokes by successful carotid endarterectomy in patients without recent neurological symptoms: randomised controlled trial. Lancet 2004; 363(9420):1491–502.

13. Bockenheimer SA, Mathias K. Percutaneous transluminal angioplasty in arteriosclerotic internal carotid artery stenosis. AJNR Am J Neuroradiol. 1983; 4(3):791–2.

14. Diethrich EB, Ndiaye M, Reid DB. Stenting in the carotid artery: initial experience in 110 patients. J Endovasc Surg 1996; 3(1):42–62.

15. Yadav JS, Roubin GS, Iyer S, Vitek J, King P, Jordan WD *et al*. Elective stenting of the extracranial carotid arteries. circ 1997; 95(2):376–81.

16. Theron J, Raymond J, Casasco A, Courtheoux F. Percutaneous angioplasty of atherosclerotic and postsurgical stenosis of carotid arteries. AJNR Am J Neuroradiol. 1987; 8(3):495–500.

17. Mayberg MR, Wilson SE, Yatsu F, Weiss DG, Messina L, Hershey LA *et al*. Carotid endarterectomy and prevention of cerebral ischemia in symptomatic carotid stenosis. Veterans Affairs Cooperative Studies Program 309 Trialist Group. JAMA 1991; 266(23):3289–94.

18. Barnett HJ, taylor DW, Eliasziw M, Fox AJ, Ferguson GG, Haynes RB *et al*. Benefit of carotid endarterectomy in patients with symptomatic moderate or severe stenosis. North American Symptomatic Carotid Endarterectomy Trial Collaborators. N Engl J Med 1998; 339(20):1415–25.

19. Randomised trial of endarterectomy for recently symptomatic carotid stenosis: final results of the MRC European Carotid Surgery Trial (ECST). Lancet 1998; 351(9113): 1379–87.

20. Rothwell PM, Eliasziw M, Gutnikov SA, Warlow CP, Barnett HJ. Endarterectomy for symptomatic carotid stenosis in relation to clinical subgroups and timing of surgery. Lancet 2004; 363(9413):915–24.

21. Goldstein LB, Adams R, Becker K, Furberg CD, Gorelick PB, Hademenos G *et al*. Primary prevention of ischemic stroke: A statement for healthcare professionals from the Stroke Council of the American Heart Association. circ 2001; 103(1):163–82.

22. Carotid surgery versus medical therapy in asymptomatic carotid stenosis. The CASANOVA Study Group. Stroke 1991; 22(10):1229–35.

23. Results of a randomized controlled trial of carotid endarterectomy for asymptomatic carotid stenosis. Mayo Asymptomatic Carotid Endarterectomy Study Group. Mayo Clin Proc. 1992; 67(6):513–18.

24. Hobson RW, Weiss DG, Fields WS, Goldstone J, Moore WS, Towne JB et al. Efficacy of carotid endarterectomy for asymptomatic carotid stenosis. The Veterans Affairs Cooperative Study Group. N Engl J Med 1993; 328(4):221–7.

25. Endarterectomy for asymptomatic carotid artery stenosis. Executive Committee for the Asymptomatic Carotid Atherosclerosis Study. JAMA 1995; 273(18):1421–8.

26. A randomised, blinded, trial of clopidogrel versus aspirin in patients at risk of ischaemic events (CAPRIE). CAPRIE Steering Committee [see comments]. Lancet 1996; 348(9038):1329–39.

27. LIPID study group. Prevention of cardiovascular events and death with Pravastatin in patients with coronary heart disease and a broad range of initial cholesterol levels. N Engl J Med. 1998; 339:1349–57.

28. Borger MA, Fremes SE, Weisel RD, Cohen G, Rao V, Lindsay TF et al. Coronary bypass and carotid endarterectomy: does a combined approach increase risk? A metaanalysis. Ann Thorac Surg. 1999; 68(1):14–20.

29. Naylor R, Cuffe RL, Rothwell PM, Loftus IM, Bell PR. A systematic review of outcome following synchronous carotid endarterectomy and coronary artery bypass: influence of surgical and patient variables. Eur J Vasc Endovasc Surg. 2003; 26(3):230–41.

30. Yadav JS, Wholey MH, Kuntz RE, Fayad P, Katzen BT, Mishkel GJ et al. Protected carotid-artery stenting versus endarterectomy in high-risk patients. N Engl J Med 2004; 351(15):1493–501.

31. McCarthy WJ, Wang R, Pearce WH, Flinn WR, Yao JS. Carotid endarterectomy with an occluded contralateral carotid artery. Am J Surg. 1993; 166(2):168–71.

32. Rothwell PM, Slattery J, Warlow CP. Clinical and angiographic predictors of stroke and death from carotid endarterectomy: systematic review. BMJ 1997; 315(7122): 1571–7.

33. Veith FJ, Amor M, Ohki T, Beebe HG, Bell PR, Bolia A et al. Current status of carotid bifurcation angioplasty and stenting based on a consensus of opinion leaders. J Vasc Surg. 2001; 33(2 Suppl):S111–S116.

34. Paciaroni M, Eliasziw M, Kappelle LJ, Finan JW, Ferguson GG, Barnett HJ. Medical complications associated with carotid endarterectomy. North American Symptomatic Carotid Endarterectomy Trial (NASCET). Stroke 1999; 30(9):1759–63.

35. Wennberg DE, Lucas FL, Birkmeyer JD, Bredenberg CE, Fisher ES. Variation in carotid endarterectomy mortality in the Medicare population: trial hospitals, volume, and patient characteristics. JAMA 1998; 279(16):1278–81.

36. Roubin GS, New G, Iyer SS, Vitek JJ, Al Mubarak N, Liu MW et al. Immediate and late clinical outcomes of carotid artery stenting in patients with symptomatic and asymptomatic carotid artery stenosis: a 5-year prospective analysis. circ 2001; 103(4):532–7.

37. Endovascular versus surgical treatment in patients with carotid stenosis in the Carotid and Vertebral Artery Transluminal Angioplasty Study (CAVATAS): a randomised trial. Lancet 2001; 357(9270):1729–37.

38. Hobson RW. CREST (Carotid Revascularization Endarterectomy versus Stent Trial): background, design, and current status. Semin Vasc Surg. 2000; 13(2):139–43.

39. Featherstone RL, Brown MM, Coward LJ. International carotid stenting study: protocol for a randomised clinical trial comparing carotid stenting with endarterectomy in symptomatic carotid artery stenosis. Cerebrovasc Dis. 2004; 18(1):69–74.

40. Ringleb PA, Kunze A, Allenberg JR, Hennerici MG, Jansen O, Maurer PC et al. The Stent-supported Percutaneous Angioplasty of the Carotid Artery versus Endarterectomy Trial. Cerebrovasc Dis. 2004; 18:66–8.

41. EVA-3S Investigators. Endarterectomy versus Angioplasty in patients with severe symptomatic carotid stenosis (EVA-3S) Trial. Cerebrovasc Dis. 2004; 18:62–5.

42. Biasi GM, Froio A, Diethrich EB, Deleo G, Galimberti S, Mingazzini P et al. Carotid plaque echolucency increases the risk of stroke in carotid stenting: the Imaging in Carotid Angioplasty and Risk of Stroke (ICAROS) study. circ 2004; 110(6):756–62.

43. Geroulakos G, Domjan J, Nicolaides A, Stevens J, Labropoulos N, Ramaswami G et al. Ultrasonic carotid artery plaque structure and the risk of cerebral infarction on computed tomography. J Vasc Surg. 1994; 20(2):263–6.

44. Levy EI, Hopkins LN. Editorial comment—Utility of abciximab during carotid stenting when distal protection is contraindicated. Stroke 2003; 34(11):2567.

45. Chan AW, Yadav JS, Bhatt DL, Bajzer CT, Gum PA, Roffi M et al. Comparison of the safety and efficacy of emboli prevention devices versus platelet glycoprotein IIb/IIIa inhibition during carotid stenting. Am J Cardiol. 2005; 95(6):791–5.

46. Ohki T, Marin ML, Lyon RT, Berdejo GL, Soundararajan K, Ohki M et al. Ex vivo human carotid artery bifurcation stenting: correlation of lesion characteristics with embolic potential. J Vasc Surg. 1998; 27(3):463–71.

47. Jordan WD, Jr., Voellinger DC, Doblar DD, Plyushcheva NP, Fisher WS, McDowell HA. Microemboli detected by transcranial Doppler monitoring in patients during carotid angioplasty versus carotid endarterectomy. Cardiovasc Surg. 1999; 7(1):33–8.

48. Berjljung L, Hjorth S, Svendler CA, Oden B. Angiography in acute gastrointestinal bleeding. Surg Gynecol Obstet. 1977; 145(4):501–3.

49. Ecker RD, Guidot CA, Hanel RA, Wehman JC, Sauvageau E, Guterman LR et al. Perforation of external carotid artery branch arteries during endoluminal carotid revascularization procedures: consequences and management. J Invasive Cardiol. 2005; 17(6):292–5.

50. Broadbent LP, Moran CJ, Cross DT, III, Derdeyn CP. Management of ruptures complicating angioplasty and stenting of supraaortic arteries: report of two cases and a review of the literature. AJNR Am J Neuroradiol. 2003; 24(10):2057–61.

51. Wholey MH, Wholey MH, Tan WA, Toursarkissian B, Bailey S, Eles G et al. Management of neurological complications of carotid artery stenting. J Endovasc Ther. 2001; 8(4):341–53.

52. Coutts SB, Hill MD, Hu WY. Hyperperfusion syndrome: toward a stricter definition. Neurosurgery 2003; 53(5):1053–8.

53. Rosenfield K, Babb JD, Cates CU, Cowley MJ, Feldman T, Gallagher A *et al.* Clinical competence statement on carotid stenting: training and credentialing for carotid stenting—multispecialty consensus recommendations: a report of the SCAI/SVMB/SVS Writing Committee to develop a clinical competence statement on carotid interventions. J Am Coll Cardiol. 2005; 45(1):165–74.

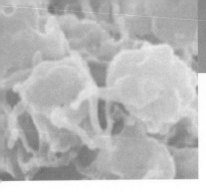

27

Percutaneous management of renal arterial disease

SRINIVASA P. POTLURI, MD, AND
STEPHEN RAMEE, MD

KEY POINTS

■ Renal artery stenting for severe atherosclerotic RAS improves renal function and blood pressure control; with the advent of less complicated and newer percutaneous techniques there is a potential for providing benefit to a broad spectrum of patients.

■ There is a need for considerable research to understand the pathophysiology of RAS and the benefit of treating percutaneously; there are several questions that need to be answered including the role of distal emboli protection devices during intervention to prevent worsening renal failure, DES in reducing restenosis in renal arteries, survival in patients after RAS intervention.

Renovascular disease has been increasingly recognized as a treatable cause of hypertension and ischemic renal insufficiency. The association between renal artery stenosis (RAS), coronary artery disease, hypertension, renal insufficiency, congestive heart failure and survival has been well studied. Surgical or percutaneous revascularization is effective in restoring patency, lowering blood pressure, stabilizing renal function, and preventing recurrent heart failure.[1–3] This chapter reviews the recent evidence concerning the clinical course of RAS and benefits of revascularization and proposes strategies for the management of such patients.

Renovascular disease affecting the main renal arteries is commonly caused by atherosclerotic disease and fibromuscular dysplasia (FMD), and much less commonly Takayasu's arteritis. Atheromatous disease is the most common cause of RAS and may be part of generalized atherosclerosis. Atherosclerotic stenosis usually occurs in the proximal 2 cm of renal arteries and in up to 80% of cases, it involves the renal ostia. FMD is the most common cause of RAS in children and young adults and affects women between 25 to 50 years in 90% of cases. The disease is frequently bilateral and may involve other arterial systems. In medial FMD, the internal elastic lamina is focally and variably thinned with thickened areas of collagen replacing the muscle producing the classic 'string of beads' appearance on angiography. Among patients who had serial angiography, it has been observed that 33% of cases progress, although there was no loss of renal function.[4] (Fig. 27.1B).

EPIDEMIOLOGY AND NATURAL HISTORY

RAS is frequently asymptomatic and its true prevalence and natural history is unknown. Autopsy studies reported RAS incidences of 4 to 53%. Increased age, severity of coronary artery disease, presence of congestive heart failure, presence of peripheral vascular disease, and female gender were each independently associated with the probability of having RAS.[5] The increasing frequency of RAS

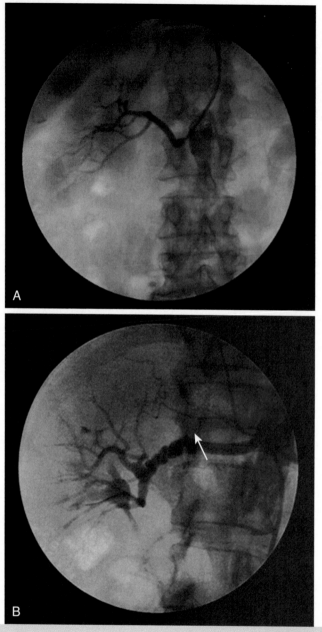

Figure 27.1:
Slide A: demonstrates the classic atherosclerotic renal artery stenosis and Slide B: Fibromuscular dysplasia.

TABLE 27.1 - PREVALENCE OF RENAL ARTERY STENOSIS

	NO. OF PATIENTS	STUDY GROUP	PREVALENCE OF RAS	COMMENTS
Sawicki et al.	5194	Autopsy	4.3%	73% had HTN
Olin et al.	395	PVD/AAA	33-39%	
Harding et al.	1302	Cardiac cath	11%	53% had HTN
Appel et al.	45	Dialysis	22%	All of them had HTN
Uzu et al.	297	Autopsy	12%	Patients died of MI
Crowley	14,152	Cardiac cath	6%	RAS progressed in 11%

AAA: abdominal aortic aneurysm, HTN: hypertension, MI: myocardial infarction, PVD: peripheral vascular disease.

with advancing age has been observed by many authors. Studies have shown that 22–59% patients with peripheral vascular disease have significant RAS. During cardiac catherterization the presence of RAS has been reported to be 6–11%, higher if the angiography was performed in patients with uncontrolled hypertension.[6] The prevalence of Angiographic RAS was seen in 36% of patients treated in hypertension clinics for severe hypertension. In patients with hypertension RAS probably account for between 0.2–5% and has been reported in 35–42% of patients with renovascular hypertension[7] Table 27.1.

Although there has been no prospective angiographic study to determine the progression of stenosis or deterioration of renal function, a number of investigators studied patients with known RAS. Various studies reported the progression of stenosis in 25 to 70% of patients. In an angiographic study of 85 patients with known atherosclerotic RAS, 44% had progression of disease and 16% progressed to complete occlusion after a mean follow up of 52 months.[4] The rate of progression to total occlusion occurred more frequently (39%) when there was a RAS more than 75%. Renal duplex studies showed that RAS progression was more in patients with greater than 60% RAS (18%, 28%, and 49% for renal arteries initially classified as normal, <60% stenosis, and >60% stenosis, respectively, P=0.03).[8] Advanced age, female sex, CAD, longer time between initial screening and follow-up were independently associated with the probability of progression of atherosclerotic RAS.

Mailloux et al. showed that, in 14% of patients starting dialysis RAS was the cause of their end stage renal disease (ESRD).[9] In another study of patients older than 50 years, RAS was seen in 22% of patients referred for renal replacement therapy.[10] The mere presence of RAS, even prior to developing ESRD, portends a poor prognosis. [9] Renovascular disease appears to be a risk factor for premature cardiac death. Conlon et al., followed 1235 cardiac catherterization patients, and their four-year unadjusted survival for patients with RAS was 65% compared with 86% for patients without significant RAS.[11]

PATHOPHYSIOLOGY

Hypertension

Unilateral RAS causes renin mediated form of hypertension and usually responds to angiotensin converting enzyme (ACE) inhibitor or angiotensin receptor blocker (ARB) therapy. In patients with bilateral or solitary functioning kidney stenosis the hypertension is volume dependent.[12] These patients do not respond as well to ACE inhibitor or ARB therapy, and functional renal insufficiency may occur when these drugs are administered. However, sodium restriction and diuresis will return the patient to the renin mediated form of hypertension, and restore sensitivity to ACE inhibitors and ARBs.

Ischemic nephropathy

It is difficult to completely understand the pathophysiology of ischemic nephropathy due to the lack of linear relationship between the degree of RAS and renal function, difficulty to ascertain the cause of nephropathy (RAS vs. parenchymal disease) and lack of consistent outcome after intervention (worsening renal function after intervention). Renal blood flow is three to fivefold greater than the perfusion of other metabolically active organs. This level of perfusion is necessary for driving the glomerular filtration rate (GFR). Renal blood flow and GFR are kept constant through wide variations in the systemic arterial blood pressure which is maintained by alteration in the tone of afferent and efferent arterioles. However, in patients with renal artery stenosis the perfusion pressure necessary to maintain the renal blood flow and GFR reaches a critical level below which point the patient develops nephropathy. This can be exacerbated by antihypertensive therapy.[13]

CLINICAL MANIFESTATIONS OF RENOVASCULAR DISEASE

There are several clinical features that may raise the suspicion of renovascular disease (Table 27.2.) RAS should be suspected in patients with atherosclerosis of other vascular territories. The diagnosis of renovascular disease should be strongly considered in patients with resistant hypertension which is defined as

---

TABLE 27.2 - CLINICAL FEATURES SUGGESTIVE OF RENOVASCULAR DISEASE

- Onset of hypertension before age 30 or after age 55
- Exacerbation of previously well controlled hypertension
- Absence of family history of hypertension
- Resistant hypertension
- Malignant hypertension or retinopathy
- Epigastric bruit (50 to 60%)
- Azotemia on initiation of ACE inhibitors (6 to 40%)
- Unexplained azotemia or hypokalemia (15%)
- Atherosclerosis elsewhere
- Atrophic or discrepant renal size of ultrasound (60 to 70%)
- Recurrent CHF or 'flash pulmonary edema' not related to CAD

ACE: angiotensin converting enzyme, CHF: congestive heart failure, CAD: coronary artery disease.

failure to normalize blood pressure to less than 140/90 mmHg following a trial consisting of at least three drugs with different mechanisms of action.[14] Accelerated or malignant hypertension has also been associated with a very high prevalence of RAS. An epigastric systolic bruit is audible in 50 to 60% of the patients with RAS; however, 10% of subjects with essential hypertension may also have an abdominal bruit.

DIAGNOSTIC EVALUATION OF RENOVASCULAR DISEASE

Improvements in the diagnostic tools, like duplex ultrasound, computed tomographic angiography, magnetic resonance angiography, have led to increased diagnosis of RAS. The ideal imaging test should identify the main renal arteries as well as accessory arteries, localize the site of stenosis, and provide insight into the functional significance. Angiogram the 'gold standard' for imaging is rarely necessary to make the diagnosis of RAS, as one of the noninvasive modalities can accurately assess the renal arteries (Fig. 27.2).

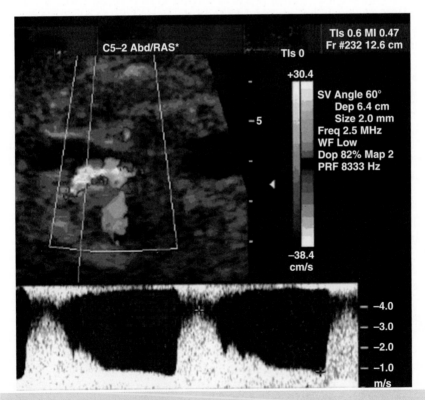

Figure 27.2:
Renal Doppler Ultrasound. Doppler ultrasound of right renal artery showing high velocities (arrow) in the proximal portion indicating severe ostial right renal artery stenosis (angiography showed severe stenosis as shown in the Fig. 27.1, slide A).

Laboratory testing

Renal vein renin is not a useful test to screen for RAS, as 15% of patients with essential hypertension have elevated levels and about 75% of patients with RAS have elevated levels. The renin levels may be depressed in the presence of bilateral RAS. Recently, elevated b-type natriuretic peptide is shown to be elevated in patients with RAS and predicts blood pressure response to intervention.[15]

Duplex ultrasonography

Renal ultrasound is an excellent test for detecting RAS and provides very useful information about the degree of stenosis, renal size, follow up after percutaneous or surgical intervention, and other associated renal abnormalities. It provides a good assessment of anatomical as well as hemodynamic nature of the disease. (Fig. 27.2). When compared to angiography it has a sensitivity of 84–98% and a specificity of 60–99% for the diagnosis of RAS.[16] Duplex ultrasound is also extremely useful in assessing the parenchymal renal resistive index (RI) (peak systolic velocity – peak end diastolic velocity/peak systolic velocity) which can assist in predicting the response to intervention. Greater than 90% of patients with RI greater than 0.8 demonstrated no improvement in hypertension and 80% had no improvement in renal function.[17] Major limitations exist with the use of duplex, including lack of reproducibility of results, and it is highly dependent on the operator skills and, therefore, there is a great variability in the reported sensitivity and specificity.

Computed tomographic angiography (CTA)

A spiral multislice computed tomography is used to render a three-dimensional reconstruction of the abdominal vasculature and has been reported to be highly sensitive and specific in the diagnosis of RAS.[18] However, it requires a large volume of contrast and limits its use in patients with renal insufficiency. With the advent of faster scanners, this technique is gaining in popularity.

Magnetic resonance angiography (MRA)

MRA provides visualization of the renal arteries and abdominal vessels with a non-nephrotoxic contrast agent. When compared to angiography the MRA has 90–100% sensitivity and 75–94% specificity. It also accurately identifies accessory renal arteries in 80% of cases. The sensitivity and specificity are low for the diagnosis of FMD.[19]

Captopril renography

Renal scintigraphy can detect differences in renal perfusion between each kidney and the sensitivity and specificity of the test greatly improves when an ACE inhibitor is added, especially in patients with unilateral renal stenosis. Overall, the accuracy of captopril renography in detecting RAS appears acceptable, with a sensitivity of 85–90% and the specificity of 90–98%. The presence of renal insufficiency or bilateral RAS may adversely affect the accuracy of the test. With the technologic improvement in the duplex ultrasonography, CTA and MRA, the captopril renography is now the secondary screening modality.[20]

Renal angiography

This is the 'gold standard' for the diagnosis of RAS. Since RAS is common in patients with coronary artery disease, some cardiologists perform a 'drive-by' abdominal aortogram during cardiac catheterization. If a patient meets the criteria for RAS intervention it is advisable to do the abdominal or renal angiography during the time of cardiac catheterization. This is still a controversial area and soon there will be guidelines for the management of these patients.[21] The technique of renal angiography will be detailed later.

MANAGEMENT OF RENAL ARTERY DISEASE

The treatment of RAS aims at preventing the clinical events such as hypertension and complications associated with it, renal insufficiency and preventing and diseases associated with progression of atherosclerosis. Medications with documented value at preventing clinical events including antihypertensives, hypolipidemic agents, antiplatelet agents, and renal artery revascularization all contribute to this primary goal.

Medications

Smoking cessation, diuretics, beta blockers, ACE inhibitors, Aspirin, and statins reduce mortality from coronary heart disease, congestive heart disease, and stroke in high-risk hypertensive patients. Most patients with RAS have hypertension and associated cardiovascular risk factors, and many have symptomatic atherosclerosis elsewhere. They should be provided with pharmacologic treatment according to current recommendations, described elsewhere in this book.

Use of ACE inhibitors can induce renal insufficiency in patients with bilateral or solitary functioning RAS. ACE inhibitor treatment should be stopped if the serum creatinine increases over 20%. The serum creatinine returns to normal after cessation of therapy.[22] Patients with RAS who are treated solely on medical therapy should be carefully followed for the progression of disease by monitoring renal function and serial duplex renal ultrasound. Unfortunately, unilateral renal artery occlusion and loss of an entire functioning kidney may not change the serum creatinine.

Revascularization

Since the introduction of stents in the last decade, surgical revascularization for RAS is rarely performed. There is still controversy regarding the benefit and appropriate indication for percutaneous transluminal angioplasty (PTA) or stent placement in patients with RAS. The indications for PTA or stent are presence of stenosis of at least 70% of unilateral or bilateral renal arteries and have either uncontrolled hypertension despite medical therapy, renal insufficiency not related to another clear-cut cause, or recurrent CHF not attributable to active ischemia.

RENAL ARTERY ANGIOGRAPHY AND INTERVENTION

Technique

Arterial Access: renal intervention can be performed through a femoral or brachial access depending on the anatomy and the operator's experience and preference. Femoral artery is the most used access by the cardiologists and in our institution. Brachial or radial artery access is preferred if intervention is planned when the renal arteries are oriented cranially. Femoral artery access is preferred if the renal arteries are oriented caudally or horizontally.

Diagnostic angiography can be performed non-selectively with a pigtail catheter placed at the level of L1–L2 lumbar vertebrae. We prefer a digital subtraction image with 15–20 cc of contrast per second for two seconds, in the anterior-posterior projection or 10 degree left anterior oblique projection. Selective diagnostic angiography through the brachial approach is performed with a multipurpose catheter and through the femoral approach several catheters can be used based on the orientation of the renal artery, including Judkins right coronary catheter, internal mammary artery catheter, Simmons catheter, or Cobra catheter. Hand injection of the contrast is performed to fill the artery, and ensuring 'reflux' of contrast into the aorta to visualize the ostium. Pressure gradients can be obtained across borderline stenoses to confirm the fuctional significance; ideally with a pressure wire (fractional flow reserve value of less than 0.8 is suggested to be significant). Systolic pressure gradient of >20 mmHg and a mean pressure gradient of 10 mmHg may be considered functionally significant.[23]

Renal artery intervention from the brachial approach is performed using a multipurpose guiding catheter or a long sheath. From the femoral approach we prefer using a 50 cm long Hockey stick or renal double curve guiding catheters, although, an internal mammary artery guiding catheter can be used as well. The size of the guiding catheter that is used should be based on the stent size that matches the renal artery size which is measured quantitatively. RAS often requires pre-dilation with a slightly smaller balloon. Stent should be placed cautiously so that it protrudes 1–2 mm into the aorta, the stent balloon is slightly withdrawn and balloon may be inflated to higher pressure to 'flare' the proximal stent at the renal artery ostium. Care should be taken while re-engaging the renal artery with the guiding catheter to prevent stent damage or displacement before performing the final angiogram. Renal FMD should be treated by balloon angioplasty alone using the same technique. Patient should be on Aspirin prior to the procedure and 3000–5000 IU Heparin should be given during the procedure. Aspirin with or without Clopidogrel should be continued for at least one month after the procedure. For further details on technique of renal intervention please refer to *Quick guide to peripheral vascular intervention*, Editor: White CJ (Physicians' Press, 2001)[24] (Fig. 27.3).

Follow up

Patients who undergo percutaneous revascularization should undergo periodic surveillance by duplex ultrasound imaging or CTA to detect progression of disease, restenosis, and loss of kidney volume. Imaging study should be obtained soon after renal artery intervention to assess the adequacy and again after 6 months, 12 months, and yearly thereafter, or whenever there is recurrence or worsening of hypertension.

CLINICAL RESULTS OF RENAL INTERVENTION

Angioplasty for FMD

Several small series published reports of PTA on FMD. Overall, the technical success is greater than 85%. (Table 27.3) Hypertension was cured in 22% to

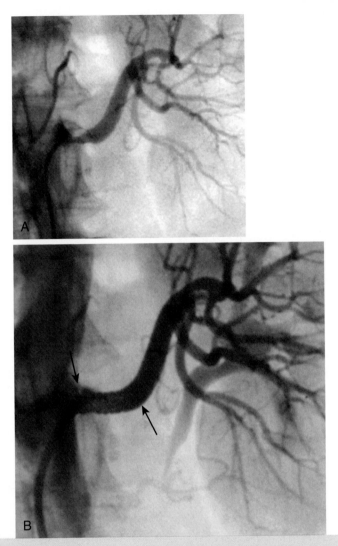

Figure 27.3:
Atherosclerotic renal artery stenting pre A and post procedure B (arrow shows stent location)

52%, improved in 22% to 74%, and failed to improve in 12% to 30%. The rate of restenosis following PTA ranges from 12% to 25% over follow up intervals of six months to two years.[25]

INTERVENTION FOR ATHEROSCLEROTIC RAS

Technical results

PTA for atherosclerotic RAS is now replaced by renal artery stenting; due to suboptimal results. The technical success PTA is 57% compared with greater than 90% for stenting and restenosis occurred in 48% of angioplasty compared to

TABLE 27.3 - RESULTS OF PTA ON FMD

	Year	Patients	Technical Success %	Follow-up mean months	HTN Benefit %
de Fraissinette *et al.*	2003	70	94	39	88
Birrer *et al.*	2002	27	100	10	74
Klow *et al.*	1998	49	98	9	70
Davidson *et al.*	1996	23	100	Not reported	74
Jensen *et al.*	1995	30	97	12	85
Bonelli *et al.*	1995	105	89	43	85
Tegtmeyer *et al.*	1991	66	100	39	98
Klinge *et al.*	1989	52	90	Not reported	93
Sos *et al.*	1983	31	87	16	92

HTN: hypertension, NR: not reported

14% with stenting. A study published from our institution evaluated the safety and efficacy of renal artery stenting in 100 consecutive patients. Our technical success was 99% and restenosis was 19%[3] (Table 27.4). Complications of percutaneous renal artery revascularization have been decreasing, a finding attributed to use of more flexible guiding catheters, lower profile premounted stents, and lower Heparin doses. In a series of 268 patients who underwent 320 procedures, the complication rate decreased from 16% in 1998 to 3% in 2001 and most are due to access site complications and rarely due to rupture of renal artery.[26] The restenosis rates after stenting depend on the diameter of the renal artery. In a recent study the rates of restenosis were 16% for ≤4 mm, 17% for 5 mm, 10% for 6 mm, and 0% for ≥7 mm diameter of the renal artery.[27]

Most of the further discussion pertains to the renal artery stenting and its effect on blood pressure and renal function. Results of the older PTA trials would not be discussed.

TABLE 27.4 - EFFECT OF RENAL ARTERY STENTING ON HYPERTENSION

	Year	Patients	Follow-up (months)	Technical success %	Restenosis %	Blood pressure benefit %*
Lederman *et al.*	1999	300	10	100	23	70
Dorros *et al.*	1998	163	48	99	NR	57
Blum *et al.*	1997	68	27	100	11	68
Bosclair *et al.*	1997	33	1-34	100	NR	67
Iannone *et al.*	1996	63	10	99	14	39
Henry *et al.*	1996	59	14	100	3#	76
Van de Ven *et al.*	1995	24	6	100	16	67
MacLeod *et al.*	1995	28	11	100	17	25
Hennequin *et al.*	1994	21	12-66	100	19	100
Wilms *et al.*	1991	11	7	100	29	70
Rees *et al.*	1991	28	2-18	96	39	65

* Benefit includes blood pressure cure and improvement.
# At follow up of 6 months
NR: not reported

Effect on blood pressure

The clinical effect of renal artery stenting on blood pressure is variable due to several reasons that are not well defined. In general, beneficial effect on blood pressure can be defined as, cure when the diastolic blood pressure <90 mm Hg and systolic blood pressure <140 mm Hg off antihypertensive medications, and improvement when the diastolic blood pressure <90 mm Hg and/or systolic blood pressure <140 mm Hg on the same or reduced number of medications or a reduction in diastolic blood pressure by at least 15 mm Hg on the same or reduced number of medications.[28] Most studies on renal artery stenting defined the benefit on blood pressure differently and overall, there was a cure of 20% (CI: 4, 37%) and a improvement of 49% (CI: 16, 83%)[29] (Table 27.4). The mortality in patients with RAS is caused primarily caused by cardiovascular disease and because even modest reduction in blood pressure are associated with greater reductions in the cardiovascular events, the efficacy of renal stenting should be assessed with regard to the overall benefit of stenting rather than cure of hypertension.

A distinct subgroup of patients, who present with recurrent pulmonary edema with hypertensive emergency and renal insufficiency, may represent severe bilateral RAS. They usually fail medical therapy and renal artery stenting provides effective resolution of hypertension and heart failure.

EFFECT ON RENAL FUNCTION

Effect of renal stenting on renal function may be defined as; improvement when the absolute value of estimated glomerular filtration rate (GFR) improves after the procedure and stabilization when the GFR remains same or the slope of decline is improved. In patients with normal renal function there was no significant change in the renal function. In patients with renal insufficiency there was improvement of function in 30% (CI: 22, 39%) and stabilization in 38% (CI: 25, 51%) of patients (Table 27.5). These results did not vary significantly across several studies of renal artery stenting.[29] The reasons for failure to improve or deterioration in renal function are not well known. Most reports suggest that treatment of severe bilateral RAS is the only condition with benefit on renal function.[30]

TABLE 27.5 - EFFECT OF RENAL ARTERY STENTING ON RENAL FUNCTION

	Patients	Age	Patients with RF	Follow-up (months)	Renal Function benefit %	
					Improve	Stable
Lederman *et al.*	300	70	111	10	19	54
Shannon *et al.*	21	63	21	9	43	29
White *et al.*	100	67	44	6	20	NR
Harden *et al.*	32	67	32	6	34	34
Bosclair *et al.*	33	63	17	1–34	41	35
Iannone *et al.*	63	70	29	10	36	45
Van de Ven *et al.*	24	67	0	6	36	64
Hennequin *et al.*	21	55	6	12–66	17	50
Rees *et al.*	28	66	14	2–18	36	36

NR: not reported

REFERENCES

1. Rimmer, J.M. and F.J. Gennari, Atherosclerotic renovascular disease and progressive renal failure. Ann Intern Med, 1993. 118(9): p. 712–19.

2. Khosla, S., et al., Effects of renal artery stent implantation in patients with renovascular hypertension presenting with unstable angina or congestive heart failure. Am J Cardiol, 1997. 80(3): p. 363–6.

3. White, C.J., et al., Renal artery stent placement: utility in lesions difficult to treat with balloon angioplasty. J Am Coll Cardiol, 1997. 30(6): p. 1445–50.

4. Schreiber, M.J., M.A. Pohl, and A.C. Novick, The natural history of atherosclerotic and fibrous renal artery disease. Urol Clin North Am, 1984. 11(3): p. 383–92.

5. Uzu, T., et al., Prevalence and predictors of renal artery stenosis in patients with myocardial infarction. Am J Kidney Dis, 1997. 29(5): p. 733–8.

6. Crowley, J.J., et al., Progression of renal artery stenosis in patients undergoing cardiac catheterization. Am Heart J, 1998. 136(5): p. 913–18.

7. van Jaarsveld, B.C., et al., The effect of balloon angioplasty on hypertension in atherosclerotic renal-artery stenosis. Dutch Renal Artery Stenosis Intervention Cooperative Study Group. N Engl J Med, 2000. 342(14): p. 1007–14.

8. Caps, M.T., et al., Prospective study of atherosclerotic disease progression in the renal artery. Circulation, 1998. 98(25): p. 2866–72.

9. Mailloux, L.U., et al., Renal vascular disease causing end-stage renal disease, incidence, clinical correlates, and outcomes: a 20-year clinical experience. Am J Kidney Dis, 1994. 24(4): p. 622–9.

10. Appel, R.G., et al., Renovascular disease in older patients beginning renal replacement therapy. Kidney Int, 1995. 48(1): p. 171–6.

11. Conlon, P.J., et al., Survival in renal vascular disease. J Am Soc Nephrol, 1998. 9(2): p. 252–6.

12. Wright, J.R., et al., A prospective study of the determinants of renal functional outcome and mortality in atherosclerotic renovascular disease. Am J Kidney Dis, 2002. 39(6): p. 1153–61.

13. Jacobson, H.R., Ischemic renal disease: an overlooked clinical entity? Kidney Int, 1988. 34(5): p. 729–43.

14. Chobanian, A.V., et al., The Seventh Report of the Joint National Committee on Prevention, Detection, Evaluation, and Treatment of High Blood Pressure: the JNC 7 report. Jama, 2003. 289(19): p. 2560–72.

15. Silva, J.A., et al., Elevated brain natriuretic peptide predicts blood pressure response after stent revascularization in patients with renal artery stenosis. Circulation, 2005. 111(3): p. 328–33.

16. Olin, J.W., et al., The utility of duplex ultrasound scanning of the renal arteries for diagnosing significant renal artery stenosis. Ann Intern Med, 1995. 122(11): p. 833–8.

17. Radermacher, J., *et al.*, Use of Doppler ultrasonography to predict the outcome of therapy for renal-artery stenosis. N Engl J Med, 2001. 344(6): p. 410–17.

18. Vasbinder, G.B., *et al.*, Accuracy of computed tomographic angiography and magnetic resonance angiography for diagnosing renal artery stenosis. Ann Intern Med, 2004. 141(9): p. 674–82; discussion 682.

19. Tan, K.T., *et al.*, Magnetic resonance angiography for the diagnosis of renal artery stenosis: a meta-analysis. Clin Radiol, 2002. 57(7): p. 617–24.

20. Nally, J.V., Jr., J.W. Olin, and G.K. Lammert, Advances in noninvasive screening for renovascular disease. Cleve Clin J Med, 1994. 61(5): p. 328–36.

21. White, C.J., Screening renal artery angiography at the time of cardiac catheterization. Catheter Cardiovasc Interv., 2003. 60(2): p. 295–6.

22. van de Ven, P.J., *et al.*, Angiotensin converting enzyme inhibitor-induced renal dysfunction in atherosclerotic renovascular disease. Kidney Int, 1998. 53(4): p. 986–93.

23. Subramanian, R., *et al.*, Renal fractional flow reserve: a hemodynamic evaluation of moderate renal artery stenoses. Catheter Cardiovasc Interv, 2005. 64(4): p. 480–6.

24. White, C.J., Ramee, S. R., Collins, T.C., Jenkins, J.S., Renal Artery Stent Placement, in Quick guide to peripheral vascular stenting, C.J. White, Editor. 2001, Physicians' Press.

25. Slovut, D.P. and J.W. Olin, Fibromuscular dysplasia. N Engl J Med, 2004. 350(18): p. 1862–71.

26. Zeller, T., *et al.*, Technological advances in the design of catheters and devices used in renal artery interventions: impact on complications. J Endovasc Ther, 2003. 10(5): p. 1006–14.

27. Zeller, T., *et al.*, Gold coating and restenosis after primary stenting of ostial renal artery stenosis. Catheter Cardiovasc Interv, 2003. 60(1): p. 1-6; discussion 7–8.

28. Rundback, J.H., *et al.*, Guidelines for the reporting of renal artery revascularization in clinical trials. American Heart Association. Circulation, 2002. 106(12): p. 1572–85.

29. Leertouwer, T.C., *et al.*, Stent placement for renal arterial stenosis: where do we stand? A meta-analysis. Radiology, 2000. 216(1): p. 78–85.

30. Harden, P.N., *et al.*, Effect of renal-artery stenting on progression of renovascular renal failure. Lancet, 1997. 349(9059): p. 1133–6.

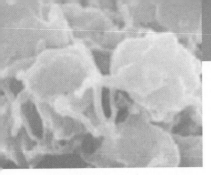

28

Percutaneous management of aortic and peripheral vascular disease

NORMAN SHAIA, MD, AND RICHARD R. HEUSER, MD

KEY POINTS

- From a technical standpoint, carotid stenting is less invasive and avoids the potential complications of a neck dissection that surgery involves.

- Currently, the decision to intervene with carotid disease is based primarily on two important clinical trials, NASCET and ACAS.

- A percutaneous approach to carotid revascularization appears to offer many advantages over CEA in select individuals.

- Secondary hypertension represents approximately 5% of the overall hypertensive population.

- Revascularization for atherosclerotic renal artery stenosis is primarily for the improvement of blood pressure control.

- Percutaneous revascularization of renal arterial stenosis has become an acceptable alternative to traditional surgical therapy.

- Aorto-iliac occlusive disease, like other types of peripheral arterial disease, may present with a wide range of symptomatology.

- Femoral arterial disease, like aorto-iliac pathology, can present with a wide variety of symptoms.

- Despite its theoretical advantage over PTA alone, there does not appear to be overwhelming data to support the use of stents in the femoral artery.

INTRODUCTION

Since the introduction of the first transluminal balloon therapy in the late 1970s, the field of PCI has exploded. Technological advances have included the widespread application of metallic stents in the mid-1990s and the recent utilization of DES in the 21st century. Adjunctive pharmacological therapy has further allowed the interventional cardiologist to succeed in high-risk coronary intervention. The practice of evidence-based medicine has fuelled the need for randomized controlled trials to access the safety and efficacy of coronary intervention. Numerous devices and drugs have been subjected to intense scrutiny, which has further advanced the field of percutaneous endovascular intervention.

With the success of percutaneous treatment in the coronary tree over the last decade, there has been a growing interest in its application to the peripheral arterial circulation. Despite its all too frequent association with coronary arterial disease, peripheral arterial pathology historically has been under-diagnosed and treated. However, with advances in peripheral device technology and the experience gained in coronary intervention, treatment of peripheral arterial disease is increasingly becoming an integral part of an interventionalist's practice.

Currently, a wide variety of balloons and stents are being utilized to treat aortic, iliac, femoral, renal, and carotid disease. The development of embolic protection devices has further allowed the advancement and application of these technologies. As a result, complication rates have decreased and have arguably allowed percutaneous therapy to become the preferred revascularization strategy. Randomized clinical trials continue to evolve and its results will ultimately dictate the superiority of a percutaneous rather than surgical approach. In this chapter, we will examine the current applications of percutaneous endovascular peripheral intervention and its potential to treat patients with severe disabling vascular disease.

CAROTID ANGIOPLASTY AND STENTING

Although it appears that the treatment of carotid disease has been a recent advance in peripheral intervention, elective carotid stenting first began over a decade ago. A multidisciplinary group, including Gary S. Roubin MD from the University of Alabama, began treating carotid lesions in 1994. This group was instrumental in introducing this technique to the field of interventional cardiology.

The rationale for a percutaneous vs. a surgical approach is multifactorial. From a technical standpoint, carotid stenting is less invasive and avoids the potential complications of a neck dissection that surgery involves. In addition, it does not require general anesthesia which can lead to various cardiovascular sequelae in high risk individuals. If complications do occur, symptoms are readily apparent because the patient is alert during the procedure. This allows the operator to identify the angiographic source of the patient's symptoms and provide immediate therapy. Finally, clinical and anatomical features which would typically preclude a surgical intervention may be ideal or even low risk for a percutaneous approach. It is for these reasons that a percutaneous revascularization strategy has gained momentum over the past few years. In this section, the indications, basic technique, and clinical trial data of carotid intervention will be reviewed.

Carotid revascularization, whether it be percutaneous or surgical, is indicated for the prevention of stroke. Carotid disease may lead to a cerebrovascular accident (CVA) through a variety of mechanisms. A stenosis may be a source of thrombo-embolism or if severe can cause ischemic-related neurological sequelae. The term 'TIA' or transient ischemic attack is utilized frequently in clinical practice and can be a 'wastebasket' term to explain a variety of symptoms. This is because neurological symptoms can be subtle and attributable to other neurovascular phenomena. However, a 'TIA' is often the reason for a referral to a neurologist and ultimately for an extensive cerebrovascular evaluation. If carotid disease is identified, the decision to intervene can be a difficult one.

Currently, the decision to intervene with carotid disease is based primarily on two important clinical trials, NASCET and ACAS. NASCET (North American Symptomatic Carotid Endarterectomy Trial) was a prospective, multi-center randomized trial which compared carotid endarterectomy (CEA) to best medical therapy.[36] In this relatively low risk symptomatic cohort, the two-year outcome for CEA with respect to freedom from ipsilateral stroke or death was 92%. This is in contrast with the medical management arm, who fared much worse with a 72% freedom from the above clinical endpoints. Although there were some shortcomings of this trial, it did provide significant insight on the treatment of carotid disease. The second pivotal trial was ACAS, the Asymptomatic Carotid Atherosclerotic Study.[36] Unlike the patient population in NASCET, these individuals were asymptomatic and found to have carotid disease based on duplex imaging. At five years, there was a statistically significant reduction in the incidence of ipsilateral stroke with CEA vs. medical management, 4.7% vs. 9.4% respectively.

The current recommendations for any type of carotid revascularization are primarily based upon the results of these two important trials. Simply stated, patients can be divided into two groups: symptomatic and asymptomatic. In symptomatic patients, CEA is advised for 60% lesions in females and 50% lesions in males. However, this is only if the peri-procedural stroke or death rate is 6% or less. In asymptomatic patients, CEA is recommended for 70% lesions in females and 60% lesions in males. Again, this must be accomplished with a complication rate of 3% or less. Therefore, in order for a percutaneous approach to be widely adapted, its safety and efficacy must be comparable to the above surgical results.

Indications for carotid angioplasty and stenting continue to evolve as more clinical trial data becomes available. Various medical, neurological, and angiographic risk factors for carotid surgical revascularization have been identified based on previous CEA trials. These are listed in Table 28.1.[38] Identification of these risk factors is crucial before proceeding with revascularization.

TABLE 28.1

Risk Factors for CEA
Medical
Angina pectoris
Recent MI (6 months)
Congestive heart failure
Severe hypertension (systolic >180)
Advanced PVD
Chronic obstructive lung disease
Age >70 years
Severe Obesity
Uncontrolled diabetes
Uncontrolled hypertension
Neurological
Progressive neurological deficit
Recently resolved (≥24 hrs.)
Generalized cerebral ischemia
Recent cerebral infarct (≥7 days)
Frequent TIA's not controlled by medications
Angiographic
Contralateral occlusion
Stenosis in region of siphon
Plaque extending 3 cm distally or 5 cm proximally into the CCA
High bifurcation at level of second cervical vertebra
Thrombus extending from an ulcerated lesion
Diffuse narrowing of entire distal ICA 2° to sub-totally occluded ICA

TABLE 28.2 - CONTRAINDICATIONS TO STENTING

- Severely tortuous, calcified and atheromatous aortic arch vessels that make access difficult.
- Pedunculated thrombus at the lesion site. This type of thrombus is best seen using 15 frame per second cine imaging.
- Severe renal impairment precluding safe use of contrast agents.
- Recent stroke (three weeks). These patients are best stabilized on antiplatelet and possibly anticoagulants prior to stenting.
- Patients unable to tolerate appropriate doses of antiplatelet agents.

In addition, based on early experience with carotid stenting, a number of contraindications have been recognized. These are summarized in Table 28.2.[38] With improvements in catheter-based technique and equipment, the above mentioned criteria will continue to evolve. Operator experience should also influence the types of patients considered appropriate for a percutaneous approach.

Although many of the above mentioned risk factors have been shown to increase both surgical and percutaneous complication rates, there are situations which overwhelmingly favor a percutaneous approach. These may include post-CEA restenosis, discrete stenosis in patients with prior neck radiation or radical dissection, discrete proximal or ostial common carotid lesions, and discrete lesions in the distal internal carotid or involving high bifurcations.[40] It is in these patients which percutaneous carotid intervention will hopefully find its niche and improve revascularization outcomes.

As with a majority of percutaneous cardiovascular procedures, a thorough non-invasive assessment is often performed. Aside from a detailed history and physical, adjunctive studies include carotid duplex, CT angiography, and magnetic resonance imaging/angiography (MRI/MRA). In patients with a previous history of TIA or CVA, collaboration with a neurologist is helpful for correlation of anatomical and clinical data. Once a decision has been made to pursue invasive testing, an extensive review of the risks and benefits of carotid angiography and/or stenting should be reviewed with the patient.

The technique of carotid angiography and/or stenting may vary somewhat among operators. Although details of various approaches are beyond the scope of this chapter, a basic review is warranted. The procedure can essentially be divided into six parts: (1) angiographic evaluation; (2) carotid sheath placement; (3) wire and embolic protection device (EPD) delivery; (4) pre-dilatation; (5) stent deployment; and (6) post-dilatation. The majority of diagnostic carotid procedures can be performed with one catheter, a 5 French Vitek. The catheter is shaped into a double curve with a tip, which allows for its upward orientation in the aortic arch. This allows for engagement of all brachiocephalic vessels and facilitates the advancement of a 0.038 glide wire for selective cannulation. The common carotid bifurcation is usually located at the level of C3 and C4, although there are numerous anatomical variations. Often a lateral and lateral oblique projection is ideal for separation of the internal and external carotid arteries.

Once the diagnostic study is completed and the location of the lesion has been identified, the Vitek catheter is advanced over the 0.038 glide wire into the ipslateral external carotid artery. A stiff 0.038 Amplatz wire is then exchanged for the glide wire and Vitek catheter is removed. Alternatively, a 0.014 Tad wire can also be utilized for this step. The stiffer wire provides adequate support for the insertion of a 7 French-90cm sheath, which is placed in the common carotid artery. The dilator and wire are removed and anticoagulation is administered prior to inserting the 0.014 wire/EPD into the internal carotid artery. Similar to coronary intervention, an activated clotting time (ACT) of 200–250 seconds is recommended. At this time, a 0.014 coronary guide wire/filter device is advanced across the area of interest. Various wires and embolic protection are available for carotid intervention. The selection of the appropriate system will depend on the type of lesion as well as the operator's familiarity with the equipment. The most commonly utilized filter wire at this time is the Accunet device (Cordis). The tip of the wire is usually placed at the base of the skull, and the filter is ideally deployed 2 cm distal to the stenosis.

Pre-dilatation is subsequently performed with a 4.0 mm balloon unless the stenosis is pre-occlusive or the artery is occluded. In these cases, a step-wise pre-dilatation strategy is advised with the initial placement of a 2 mm balloon. Short, repeat inflations are performed with careful monitoring of the heart rate, blood pressure, and patient symptomatology. Once adequate pre-dilation has been accomplished, the balloon is removed and a self-expanding stent is loaded onto the wire. Self-expanding stents are utilized much more frequently than balloon-expandable stents for a number of reasons. One, with balloon-expandable stents, the stent has to be differentially expanded to accommodate to the size of the common carotid artery, bifurcation, and internal carotid artery. Therefore, more than one balloon has to be delivered for optimal dilatation and stent expansion. Secondly, the balloon can rupture while deploying the stent and there may be difficulty in advancing the balloon-stent assembly through the guiding sheath. Finally, balloon-expandable stents tend to occlude the external carotid artery. There have been a few reports of external compression with the balloon expandable stents. For these reasons, self-expanding stents are recommended for carotid intervention in a majority of cases. The final step to successful carotid stenting is post-dilatation. A 5–6 mm balloon is utilized depending upon the size of the internal carotid artery. Once this has been performed, the retrieval sheath of the EPD is advanced over the filter, and the wire and filter are removed as one unit together. Final angiographic images are obtained through the common carotid sheath and the procedure is complete. A carotid angiogram both pre-intervention and post-intervention is demonstrated in Fig. 28.1.

Careful post-procedural monitoring of these patients is vital since they are prone to a number of possible complications. These include puncture-site bleeding issues, transient brady-arrhythmias, hypotension, and neurologic sequelae from thrombotic and athero-embolic material. Early recognition of these potential adverse outcomes of carotid revascularization is crucial. Vasopressor and vagolytic agents are often utilized for post-procedural hemodynamic alterations. These hemodynamic changes are often secondary to the mechanical pressure on the carotid baro-receptors. This effect can result in hypotension up to 24–48 hours after the procedure depending upon the sensitivity of the baro-receptors. Usually there are no long-term clinical ramifications if this is

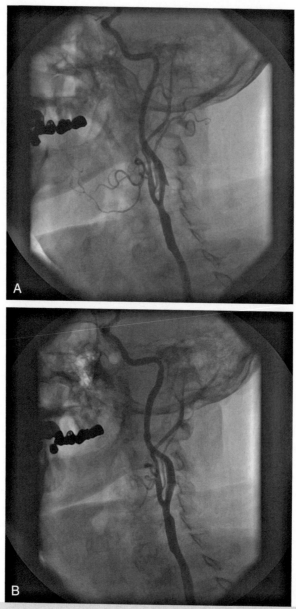

Figure 28.1:
A, A discrete internal carotid stenosis. B, Post carotid angioplasty and stenting.

treated in a prudent manner. Rarer complications such as carotid dissection, carotid perforation, and cerebral hemorrhage can obviously be fatal. The technical aspects of neurovascular rescue to treat these scenarios are beyond the scope of this chapter. However, as procedure-dedicated equipment continues to evolve and operator experience improves, it is anticipated that these complications will be infrequently encountered.

As alluded to above, the indications and technical aspects of a percutaneous approach to carotid revascularization have been evolving over the past decade. Just as NASCET and ACAS sought to establish the superiority of surgery over medical therapy for the treatment of carotid disease, percutaneous carotid intervention had to prove its safety and efficacy as well. Initially, the CAVATAS (Carotid and Vertebral Artery Transluminal Angioplasty Study) trial was conducted in Great Britain.[41] This was a prospective, randomized, controlled trial comparing CEA vs. carotid angioplasty in higher risk, symptomatic patients with high-grade carotid stenoses. Approximately two-thirds of the patients in the percutaneous arm were treated with carotid angioplasty without stenting. Despite sub-optimal equipment and operator experience in the percutaneous arm, both early and late outcomes were similar in the two groups. The 30-day incidence of major stroke and death was approximately 5% and the incidence for all strokes (disabling and non-disabling) was 11% in both arms.

The advent of EPD and improved stent design lead to the first randomized, prospective, multi-center trial for comparison of carotid stenting with protection vs. CEA. The SAPPHIRE (Stenting and Angioplasty with Protection in Patients at High Risk for Endarterectomy) trial was conducted in 2002 and randomized a total of 307 patients.[42] Eligible patients could be either asymptomatic with >80% stenoses by ultrasound or symptomatic with >50% stenosis and one high-risk factor (see Table 28.3). The primary endpoint was the incidence of MACE, including death, stroke, or MI within 30 days of the procedure. At 30 days, SAPPHIRE reported a composite endpoint of 5.8% and 12.6% for carotid stenting with embolic protection and CEA, respectively. In addition, complication rates were similar among the two groups of patients with respect to TIA and major bleeding. There was a statistically significant difference in cranial nerve injury, 0% in the stenting arm and 5.3% in the CEA arm. One-year results presented in 2003 demonstrated a MACE rate of 11.9% and 19.9% for carotid stenting and CEA respectively. SAPPHIRE was a landmark trial because it was the first randomized study to compare carotid stenting with distal embolic protection with carotid surgery in high-risk patients. Its results prove the hypothesis that among patients with severe carotid artery stenosis and coexisting conditions, carotid stenting is not inferior to carotid endarterectomy.

TABLE 28.3 - FDA-APPROVED AND INVESTIGATIONAL ENDOGRAFTS
Device
Ancure™
AneuRx™
Endologix™
Excluder™
Lifepath™
Quantum Lp™
Talent™
Vangaurd™
Zenith™

A percutaneous approach to carotid revascularization appears to offer many advantages over CEA in select individuals. As with all novel modalities in cardiovascular intervention, rigorous testing and clinical trial outcomes will be vital before it is widely accepted. However, initial clinical experience appears very promising at this time. Improvements in catheter, stent, and embolic protection design will likely lead to better outcomes with a reduction in complications. Obviously, formal training centers need to be established as well and incorporated in interventional cardiovascular programs. In parallel with the advancements made in coronary intervention, carotid stenting represents the natural progression to a successful, less-invasive technique for revascularization.

ABDOMINAL AORTIC ANEURSYMS AND ENDOLUMINAL TREATMENT

Abdominal aortic aneurysms (AAA) are atherosclerotic in origin in a majority of patients. Often times hypertension is present as well which contributes to the formation of an aneurysm. Because of the high morbidity and mortality associated with this vasculopathy, screening, monitoring, and aggressive treatment is vital.

Approximately 95% of AAAs are infra-renal in origin. Detection of an AAA during clinical examination has only moderate sensitivity at best. Therefore, if clinical suspicion is high, an abdominal ultrasound is warranted. If a patient is obese or if the ultrasound is suboptimal, other non-invasive studies such as MRI/MRA or CT can be performed with excellent sensitivity. Once the diagnosis is made, the decision whether to intervene is based upon the size and the rate of enlargement of the aneurysm. It is well accepted that a diameter of >5 cm is an indication for intervention. This size is based upon surveillance studies which have indicated that AAAs 5.5 cm and 6.5 cm have annual rupture rates of 11% and 26% respectively.[43] If an aneurysm is discovered measuring 3–4 cm, serial examinations with ultrasound are recommended every six months to monitor the rate of enlargement.

Historically, the treatment for AAAs has been surgical in nature. However, open surgical repair carries a considerable risk especially in patients with a host of cardiovascular and pulmonary co-morbidities. Consequently, many of these patients are turned down for open surgical repair. In a series of 109 patients who were refused AAA repair, death due to aneurysm rupture occurred in 36% of patients with AAA 5.5–5.9 cm and >50% in AAA 6.0–7.0 cm.[44] In patients with multiple risk factors for a poor surgical outcome, endoluminal grafting has gained substantial popularity in the last few years. The development of this technique to exclude the aneurysm by placement of an endoluminal graft began in 1991 by Parodi and collegues.[45] An illustration of a typical endoluminal graft is shown in Fig. 28.2. The procedure is performed under local anesthesia and involves the placement of a stent-anchored Dacron prosthetic graft in a retrograde femoral cannulation. A number of aortic endografts have been developed in the United States and are listed in Table 28.3.[46]

Various clinical and angiographic criteria are required for approval of an aortic endoluminal graft. Clinical criteria include the following: (1) the risks of an open repair are unacceptable; and (2) The risk of aneurysm rupture is high. These scenarios are listed in Table 4.[46] Anatomic criteria are also very important and

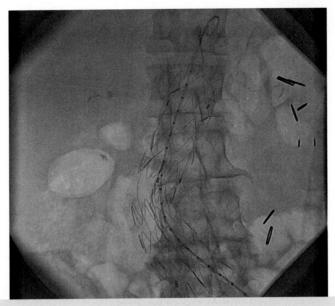

Figure 28.2:
A typical endoluminal graft.

must be evaluated carefully prior to proceeding with an endoluminal repair. These are listed in Table 28.5.[46] Once these criteria have been met, the decision to perform an endoluminal vs. surgical repair will depend on the expected peri-operative mortality and life-expectancy of the patient. If the peri-operative mortality is less than 5% and the life expectancy is >5 years, a conventional surgical approach is advised. On the other hand, if the perioperative mortality is >5% and the life expectancy is short secondary to other co-morbid conditions, an endoluminal repair should be considered.

Although a step-wise technical description of performing an endoluminal repair is beyond the scope of this chapter, one should be familiar with the potential adverse outcomes of these devices. Most importantly, the presence of an endoleak should be identified after endoluminal repair. An endoleak is defined as intraaneurysm flow around an endovascular graft. There are four types of endoleaks which are listed in Table 28.6.[46] Endoleaks can be diagnosed non-invasively with ultrasound, CT, and MRI, or invasively with angiography. Endoleaks can lead to rupture of an aneurysm because of their persistent pressure on the vessel wall. A variety of structural changes of the endograft can lead to the

TABLE 28.4 - RISK FACTORS FOR ANEURYSM RUPTURE

A. An aneurysmal diameter >5cm.

B. An aneurysmal diameter of 4–5 cm that has increased in size by 0.5 cm in the last six months.

C. An aneurysmal diameter that measures twice the size of the normal infrarenal aorta.

**TABLE 28.5 - ANATOMIC CONSIDERATIONS OF ENDOLUMINAL
GRAFT REPAIR**

- Length
- Shape
- Angulation of the infrarenal neck of the aneurysm
- Involvement of the common iliac arteries
- Size and tortuosity of the ileofemoral vessels

development of an endoleak. These include: suture breaks between the stent and
the graft, fracture of the hooks used to anchor the proximal end of the endograft
to the aortic wall, circular and longitudinal stent wire separation, separation of
the connection between wire loops, graft fatigue, device migration, component
separation, and endograft or vessel thrombosis.[47] The decision to intervene once
an endoleak has been discovered depends upon the type of endoleak as well as
the size of the aneurysm. Another potential adverse outcome is the development
of endotension. This refers to the expansion of the aneurysm in the absence of an
obvious endoleak. One of the leading causes of endotension is transmission of
pressure through a sealed or thrombosed endoleak.

Although numerous advancements have been made in the development of
endoluminal grafts, there has been variable results reported when compared to
traditional surgical repair. Up until recently, a variety of prospective, cohort,
controlled studies have been performed.[48,49,50] However, in the last year, early
results were released for two randomized trials comparing endoluminal and open
surgical repair. EVAR-1 (Endovascular Aneurysm Repair Trial 1) and DREAM
(Dutch Randomized Endovascular Aneurysm Management Trial) have both
reported lower operative mortality rates after endovascular repair as compared to
open repair.[51,52] In EVAR-1, the in-hospital mortality was 6% for open repair and
1.6% for endoluminal repair, while in DREAM, the in-hospital mortality was
4.6% and 1.2% for open repair and endoluminal repair, respectively. These trials
concluded that in patients who are candidates for both techniques, endovascular
repair is preferable to open repair. Further randomized data with long-term
follow up will be required.

The diagnosis and subsequent treatment of AAAs are vital because of the high
morbidity and mortality associated with it. Endovascular repair has made
dramatic advancements in the past few years with regard to device integrity and

TABLE 28.6 - TYPES OF ENDOLEAKS

- *Type I:* Flow into the aneurysm from proximal or distal end of the graft or
  between the segments of the graft. These leaks usually result from
  inappropriate sizing or inadequate deployment of the graft or from
  interposed thrombus.
- *Type II:* Retrograde flow into the aneurysm from patent lumbar or inferior
  mesenteric arteries.
- *Type III:* Flow into the aneurysm through tears or perforations in the graft
  material.
- *Type IV:* Flow into the aneurysm through the graft material by permeation.

durability. Early comparisons with the traditional open surgical repair have shown promise as an alternative treatment in a majority of patients. Long-term clinical results will ultimately dictate the popularity of this technique. Incorporating endoluminal repair procedures into training programs for interventional cardiologists is important for understanding how to diagnose and treat patients with AAAs/AAA repairs. As with all cardiovascular therapies, the goal is to continue to improve efficacy while striving for more non-invasive modalities to treat patients.

RENAL ANGIOPLASTY AND STENTING

Secondary hypertension represents approximately 5% of the overall hypertensive population. Atherosclerotic renal artery stenosis accounts for the majority of patients with secondary hypertension.[21] Although this appears to represent a small number of individuals, its prevalence is much higher among patients with co-existing coronary and peripheral arterial disease. Approximately 15–18% of patients undergoing cardiac catheterization for suspected coronary artery disease have been found to have reno-vascular stenosis.[22,23] Furthermore, the incidence increases even more in patients with aneurysmal or occlusive peripheral vascular disease.[24]

Renal arterial disease should be suspected in a number of clinical scenarios. These include an abdominal bruit, onset of hypertension >55 years of age, medically refractive hypertension, azotemia with ACE inhibitors, and the presence of an atrophic kidney. Often the combination of refractory hypertension and renal insufficiency represents the most common reason for further investigation of secondary hypertension. A non-invasive assessment may consist of a renal duplex scan, magnetic resonance angiography (MRA), computed tomographic angiography (CTA), and renal-captopril scan. Depending on the results of the above studies, a referral for invasive angiography may be warranted. A basic review of the indications, technical considerations, and clinical outcomes of renal arterial intervention will be discussed below.

Revascularization for atherosclerotic renal artery stenosis is primarily for the improvement of blood pressure control. Both immediate and long-term effects on hypertension have been demonstrated in various studies.[25,25] This has lead to a reduction in the number of anti-hypertensive agents required for optimal blood pressure control. This is beneficial in many regards including a smaller number of drug interactions and a limited exposure to pharmacological side effects. Secondly, renal arterial revascularization can potentially result in the preservation of renal function as well as a slowing in the progression of overt renal failure.[27] Even patients with end stage renal disease on hemo-dialysis who have stenotic renal arteries may experience a reversal in renal function.[28] Finally, patients with refractory congestive heart failure and angina may indirectly benefit.[29] Improved blood pressure control with afterload reduction may result in both improvements in systolic and diastolic performance.

If non-invasive imaging is suggestive of reno-vascular stenosis, a referral for diagnostic angiography is justified. Diagnostic renal angiography is most commonly performed from a femoral arterial access site. A variety of catheters are available for selective cannulation of the renal ostia. These include a Judkins' right configuration, an internal mammary, and a cobra catheter. A 6 French catheter is usually sufficient to engage the renal ostia without causing trauma to the aorta which may lead to potential cholesterol embolization. The renal ostia are usually located approximately 1–2 cm below the takeoff of the superior mesenteric artery. The left renal artery often has a higher origin than the right. In addition, multiple renal arteries can be present in up to 30% of patients. One of the most common anomalies include two separate arteries to the renal hilum. Atherosclerotic renal artery stenosis most often occurs at the ostium or proximal portion of the renal artery. This is in contrast to fibromuscular dysplasia which more commonly involves the distal segment of the artery.

Once imaging has been adequately performed, the decision to perform revascularization must be based on the degree of stenosis as well as the patient's presentation. The majority of percutaneous renal interventions can be safety and successfully performed from the original femoral arterial access site. In cases where the takeoff of the artery is located overly caudal, a brachial approach may be preferred. When retrograde femoral access is chosen, a 7 or 8 French arterial sheath is inserted. The original diagnostic catheter is kept in the renal ostium and a soft tip exchange length guidewire is utilized to cross the lesion and is placed in the distal vessel. At this time, the diagnostic catheter is exchanged for a renal angioplasty guiding catheter and anticoagulation is subsequently administered. Standard unfractionated Heparin is utilized with a goal activated clotting time (ACT) of 200–250 seconds. Bivalirudin, a direct thrombin inhibitor, may be substituted; however, clinical outcome data does not exist at this time for this indication. Pre-dilatation is performed next with a peripheral angioplasty balloon and sized accordingly to the measured diameter of the reference segment. Low-pressure inflations are recommended to avoid trauma and dissection of the vessel wall. After balloon deflation, the guiding catheter is advanced across the lesion over the balloon to allow safer delivery of the stent. If this is not performed, the stent edges may catch on plaque resulting in potential stent embolization.

After adequate pre-dilatation, a balloon-expandable stent is advanced over the wire and positioned at the lesion site. Once a satisfactory position has been obtained, the guiding catheter is withdrawn slightly, uncovering the stent. Optimization of the location of the stent is then obtained with low-volume contrast injections. If an ostial lesion is present, it is ideal to have approximately one millimeter of stent protrude into the aorta. This is to ensure complete coverage of the ostium of the artery. The stent is subsequently deployed at an appropriate pressure and the balloon is withdrawn into the guiding catheter after deflation. Additional contrast injections are performed to assess for adequate stent expansion. If this is not the case, post-dilatation may be performed with higher pressure or a larger balloon may be required.

Percutaneous renal revascularization has been shown to be an acceptable therapy for renovascular stenosis. Balloon angioplasty alone can achieve adequate short-term angiographic results; however, the incidence of restenosis is unacceptably high in many instances.[30] This is especially true for aorto-ostial lesions which are prone to vascular recoil. For this reason, endovascular stents are frequently utilized despite optimal immediate results with balloon angioplasty alone. Similar to coronary arterial stents, renal arterial stents are able to scaffold the arterial wall and prevent elastic recoil. Early clinical results demonstrate superior angiographic and hemodynamic outcomes with stenting vs. balloon angioplasty alone.[31,32] Primary success rates have been reported between 95–100% while restenosis rates vary widely between 1.6–39%.[33,34] As mentioned earlier, one of the primary indications for renal arterial revascularization is improvement in blood pressure control. Various studies have reported promising results. White *et al.* reported a statistically significant improvement in blood pressure control with a reduction in the number of anti-hypertensive medications from 2.6 +/– 1.0 to 2.0 +/– 0.9 (p<0.001).[35] In patients who underwent follow-up angiography, a restenosis rate of 18.8% was demonstrated. The only procedural variable which was associated with angiographic restenosis was the immediate post-stent minimum lumen diameter (MLD). Other studies have demonstrated benefit for unstable angina as well as congestive heart failure symptoms.[32] However, there has not been a clear benefit in improvement in creatinine clearance. Their still remains debate as to whether revascularization can result in normalization of renal function in patients with chronic renal insufficiency. It does appear that the rate of progression to renal failure can be slowed with revascularization. Additional multi-center, randomized trials will be needed to address some of these issues.

Percutaneous revascularization of renal arterial stenosis has become an acceptable alternative to traditional surgical therapy. Renal artery stenting has resulted in improved long-term patency and control of hypertension in many patients. Its effect on slowing the progression of renal failure and potentially reversing end-stage renal disease has been encourgaging in select patients. However, as alluded to above, more clinical data will be necessary to clearly define its benefit in these scenarios. Currently, in patients with medically refractive hypertension, renal artery stenting appears to be the treatment of choice.

AORTO-ILIAC ANGIOPLASTY AND STENTING

Aorto-iliac occlusive disease, like other types of peripheral arterial disease, may present with a wide range of symptomatology. Depending upon numerous co-existing factors, patients may be asymptomatic, have mild claudication or limb-threatening ischemia. The presence of collateral vessels, lesion severity, and the location of the stenosis will influence the clinical presentation.

As with all types of peripheral arterial pathology, an initial assessment includes a thorough history and physical. However, a classic claudication description is often not present in a majority of patients. Symptoms may overlap with other conditions such as degenerative disc disease or neuropathic pain syndromes. Therefore, a careful review of co-morbidities should be performed and prompt further investigation if clinical suspicion is high. Non-invasive studies such as measurement of the ankle-brachial index (ABI), segmental and exercise ABI's, and duplex ultrasound can be extremely beneficial. These tests can not only detect the presence of peripheral arterial disease, but the location as well. Once a complete non-invasive assessment has been performed, a referral for aorto-iliac angiography may be warranted.

Vascular access for aorto-iliac angiography is usually obtained from the ipslateral femoral artery. However, a contralateral retrograde femoral approach may be necessary if a contra-indication exists for ipslateral access. Likewise, in rare instances, an upper extremity arterial cannulation may be required. In any case, a standard Seldinger technique is employed, with the initial placement of a 6 French vascular sheath. A 0.035 Wholey wire or hydrophilic glide wire is utilized for crossing aorto-iliac disease, with subsequent placement of a pigtail catheter in the abdominal aorta. Diagnostic angiography is performed with visualization of occlusive disease and distal runoff of the lower extremities. An antero-posterior (AP) projection is usually standard, however, caudal angulation may be beneficial in some aorto-iliac disease. A roadmap is obtained in preparation for possible aorto-iliac intervention.

Early experience with intervention of aorto-iliac disease involved PTA only in a majority of cases. An example of a stenotic lesion in the iliac artery is shown in Fig. 28.3. Ideal characteristics of iliac lesions for PTA included a stenotic, noncalcified, discrete (<3 cm) lesion with >2 patent run-off vessels.[1] In contrast, relative contraindications for a percutaneous approach involved total occlusions, long lesions (>5cm), bilateral disease and the presence of an aneurysm. If the above criteria were met for a lesion, accurate assessment of vessel size and length was subsequently made with quantitative angiography or IVUS. Pre-treatment with Aspirin and intra-procedural Heparin was the standard pharmacological regimen utilized. After balloon dilation, a pressure gradient was obtained. In the case of a >5 mmHg pressure gradient or a residual stenosis of >30%, stenting or repeat higher-pressure balloon inflation would be performed.

In the case of aorto-iliac stenting, two types of stents exist: balloon-expandable and self-expanding. Advantages of balloon-expandable stents include a greater radial force and easier precision for optimal placement. In contrast, self-expanding stents are more longitudinally flexible and lower profile, allowing for easier delivery. This is especially useful when performing an intervention from the contra-lateral access site. In addition, self-expanding stents are more suited for longer lesions as they allow for more normal vessel tapering.

Similar to coronary intervention, the long-term patency of iliac vessel angioplasty is dependent upon both clinical and anatomical variables.[2] Favorable criteria include non-diabetic, male patients with discrete non-occlusive stenoses with good distal run-off. In contrast, restenosis tends to be higher in diabetic, female patients with diffuse and lengthy occlusive lesions with poor distal run-off.

Prior to the routine placement of iliac stents as a preferred strategy for revascularization, early clinical trials examined the efficacy of PTA vs. medical and surgical therapy.[3] Patient enrollment criteria in these early trials included lifestyle-limiting or progressive claudication, ischemic pain at rest, non-healing ischemic ulcerations and gangrene. After randomized clinical trial data established the superiority of iliac PTA over medical therapy, investigators began to compare this percutaneous approach with traditional surgical therapy.[3] Wilson *et al.* conducted a randomized trial comparing PTA vs. bypass surgery for 157 iliac lesions.[4] No significant differences were found for the clinical endpoints of death, amputations, or loss of patency at three years. In addition, measurement of the ABI at three years demonstrated no difference in the two treatment arms.

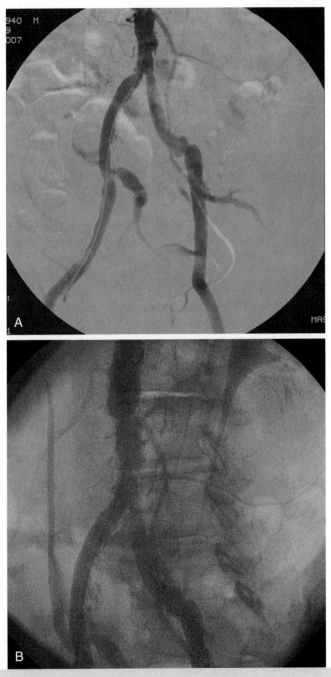

Figure 28.3:
A, A stenotic lesion in the common iliac artery. B, Post common iliac artery stenting

In parallel with the advancements made in coronary intervention, the availability of stents dramatically affected the results of iliac intervention. Bosch *et al.* published a meta-analysis of over 2000 patients undergoing PTA and stent placement for aorto-iliac occlusive disease.[5] Compared with PTA only, iliac stenting had a higher procedural success rate and a 43% reduction in late (four year) failures. Other randomized trials have studied PTA with provisional stenting (stent placement for unsatisfactory balloon angioplasty results) vs. primary iliac stenting.[6,7,8] Results have demonstrated that there is a significantly improved technical success rate as well as reduction in the pressure gradient with primary stenting. In addition, if provisional stenting was implemented in the PTA arm, the outcomes were similar to the primary stenting arm. Again indicating the overall improved clinical and angiographic outcome with iliac stenting. Additional clinical trials have yielded similar results. Richter *et al.* demonstrated a four-year patency rate of 92% and 74% for iliac stenting and PTA, respectively.[9]

With improved stent design and deliverability, as well as improved pharmacological adjunctive therapy, percutaneous therapy of aorto-iliac disease has become standard of care in the majority of settings. Clinical trials have clearly demonstrated its superiority over medical management and its non-inferiority to a surgical approach. This has allowed for an acceptable alternative to the management of occlusive aorto-iliac disease.

FEMORAL ARTERY ANGIOPLASTY AND STENTING

Femoral arterial disease, like aorto-iliac pathology, can present with a wide variety of symptoms. Often times, patients may be asymptomatic especially with the development of an adequate collateral circulation. If symptoms of intermittent claudication develop, the progression to critical limb ischemia is approximately 5% per year.[10] The risk of revascularization, whether it be surgical or percutaneous, is 11% at five years and 14% at ten years in these patients.[11] Therefore, as with all types of peripheral arterial disease, lifestyle modification should be implemented first. Only in the presence of ischemic rest pain, disabling claudication, or ischemic tissue loss should revascularization be considered as a first option.

Prior to the availability of endovascular treatment, surgical bypass was the primary means of revascularization. Historically, patency rates of above the knee femoropopliteal bypass were 80% at one year and approximately 50% at five years.[12] Because of the need for less invasive means to treat these patients, percutaneous therapies for femoral arterial stenotic and occlusive disease began to emerge in the early to mid-1990s. Early experience with PTA of femoral arterial disease demonstrated patency rates comparable to traditional surgical revascularization.[13,14]

Similar to aorto-iliac disease, ideal characteristics for PTA of femoral disease included a stenotic, short, and non-calcified lesion. In parallel with coronary intervention, long and chronically occluded lesions had poor short and long term patency rates.[15,16] A chronic total occlusion in the SFA is shown in Fig. 28.4. Initially, 'debulking' modalities such as rotational and directional atherectomy were employed. Unfortunately, these strategies did not prove to be beneficial.[17,18]

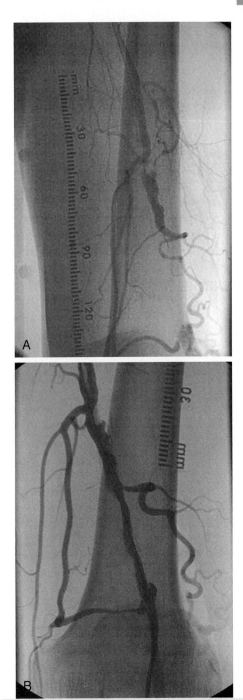

Figure 28.4:
A, In stent restenosis of the left renal artery. B, Post renal artery angioplasty.

The advent of stenting for femoral disease was thought to eliminate some of the shortcomings of PTA alone. Initial indications for stenting included the presence of a significant residual stenosis (>30%) after PTA, an arterial dissection, and the incidence of restenosis. The types of stents available for utilization in the femoral artery included a self-expanding and a balloon expandable stent. Advantages and disadvantages of each of these were mentioned previously.

Vascular access for femoral arterial intervention depends primarily upon the location of the lesion. The most common approaches include: (1) an antegrade puncture of the ipslateral common femoral artery; (2) a retrograde puncture of the contralateral common femoral artery; and (3) a retrograde puncture of the ipslateral popliteal artery. If intervention is to be performed in the mid to lower femoral artery, an ipslateral puncture is often the preferred approach. This access site not only allows for close proximity to the lesion of interest, but also allows for easier guidewire and catheter manipulation. In contrast, if the lesion is higher in the femoral tree or there is an existing contraindication for ipslateral access, a contralateral puncture may be employed. However, one may encounter difficulty with guidewire and catheter manipulaton around the aortic bifurcation. In addition, deliverability of balloons and stents may present a problem. This is especially true with longer and bulkier devices. Finally, if the above techniques prove to be unsuitable, an ipslateral popliteal approach may be required. In this case, smaller sheaths are utilized which may limit the number and types of devices that can be delivered.

The technique of performing the intervention is similar in priniciple to that described with aorto-iliac intervention. Hydrophillic glide wires may be utilized for crossing calcified and chronically occluded lesions. Once a lesion has been transversed, exchange for a more supportive wire will allow one to guide the placement of a balloon or stent. Anticoagulation regimens are similar to other peripheral arterial intervention, with administration of Aspirin and intra-procedural Heparin. Intravascular ultrasound can be a useful tool for both vessel sizing and for optimization of stent apposition. The later is vital for minimizing the risk of early thrombosis as well as for late in-stent restenosis.

Despite its theoretical advantage over PTA alone, there does not appear to be overwhelming data to support the use of stents in the femoral artery. Thus far, little randomized clinical data exists to support the routine practice of stenting over PTA. A small study was conducted which randomized 51 patients to PTA vs. stenting in the femoral artery.[19] At one year of follow up, no statistically significant difference was found with regard to patency between the two arms. Other observational data to date yield similar results.[20] Obviously, larger randomized clinical trials are needed to justify the routine utilization of stents in the femoral artery.

Immediate complications of femoral artery intervention mainly include groin access issues. Pseudoaneurysm, arterio-venous fistula, and groin hematoma are all potential complications, especially with the use of larger sheaths. Early thrombosis and distal thrombo-embolization are rare, but serious sequelae of peripheral intervention. Late complications include restenosis and reocclusion, which occur more often in longer and complicated lesions.

With the improvements in technology that has emerged in coronary intervention, there has been parallel advancements in peripheral therapies. Novel devices, such as the Fox Hollow atherectomy device, has shown some initial success in treating de novo and in-stent restenotic lesions. Thermo-cooling catheters, namely the Polar-catheter (Boston Scientific) have also shown some initial promise in the femoral and even popliteal arterial circulation. As with all new devices, randomized data will be needed to justify the costs of these techniques. However, there has been encouraging results with these devices in a number of individuals. Currently, percutaneous femoral arterial intervention provides an alternative therapy for revascularization in many patients. The optimal endovascular strategy, both from a pharmacologic and mechanical standpoint, will continue to evolve with further operator experience and clinical trial results.

CONCLUSIONS

The diagnosis and treatment of peripheral vascular disease is an essential part of a cardiovascular specialist's practice. In the last decade, a number of advancements have been made in the endovascular treatment of peripheral arterial disease. This has allowed for an alternative therapy for many patients who may not be ideal candidates for a surgical intervention. Many of the techniques of coronary intervention have been applied to the treatment of carotid, renal, aortic, iliac, and femoral disease. The new generation of interventional cardiologists must be exposed to these techniques and be prepared to offer them to their patients. With continued clinical research and operator experience, the goal of treating a wide array of peripheral disease in a non-invasive manner may be reached in the near future.

REFERENCES

1. Heuser RR. Peripheral Vascular Stenting for Cardiologists. Martin Duntz Ltd. 1999; Chapter 5: Page 47.

2. Johnston KW. Balloon Angioplasty: Predictive factors for long term success, Semin Vasc Surg 1989; 3: 117–122.

3. Whyman MR, Kerracher EMG, Gillespie IN et al. Randomized Controlled Trial of Percutaneous Transluminal Angioplasy for Intermittant Claudiaction. Eur J Vasc Surg 1996; 12: 167–172.

4. Wilson SE, Wolf GL, Cross AP. Percutaneous transluminal angioplasty versus operation for peripheral arteriosclerosis: report of a prospective randomized trial in a selected group of patients. J Vasc Surg 1989; 9: 1–9.

5. Bosch JL, Hunink MGM. Meta-analysis of the results of percutaneous transluminal angioplasty and stent placement for aortoiliac occlusive disease. Radiology 1997; 204: 87–96.

6. Henry M, Amor M, Thevenof G *et al.* Palmaz stent placement in iliac and femoropoplitieal arteries: primary and secondary patency in 310 patients with 2–4 year follow up. Radiology 1995; 197: 167–174.

7. Vorwerk D, Gunther RW, Schumann K, Wendt G. Aortic and iliac stenosis: follow-up results of stent placement after insufficient balloon angioplasty in 118 cases. Radiology 1996; 198: 45–48.

8. Tetteroo E, Haaring C, Van der Graaf Y *et al.* Intraarterial pressure gradients after randomized angioplasty or stenting of iliac artery lesions. Dutch Iliac Stent Trial Study Group. Cardiovasc Intervent Radiol 1996; 19: 411–417.

9. Richter GM, Noeldige G, Roeren T *et al.* First long-term results of a randomized mulitcenter trial: iliac balloon-expandable stent placement versus regular percutaneous transluminal angioplasty. In: Lierman D (ed.) State of the Art and Future Developments. Morin Heights, Canada: Polyscience, 1995; 30–35.

10. Hertzer NR. The natural history of peripheral vascular disease. Implications for its management. Circulation 1991; 83 (Suppl): 112–119.

11. Cox GS, Hertzer NR, Young JR *et al.* Nonoperative treatment of superficial femoral artery disease: long-term follow-up. J Vasc Surg 1993; 17: 172–181.

12. Michaels JA. Choice of material for above-knee femoropopliteal bypass graft. Br J Surg 1989; 76: 7–14.

13. Holm J, Arfridsson B, Jivegard L *et al.* Chronic lower limb ischemia. A prospective randomized controlled study comparing the 1-year results of vascular surgery and percutaneous transluminal angioplasty (PTA). Eur J Vasc Surg 1991; 5: 517–522.

14. Yucel EK. Femoropopliteal angioplasty: Can we predict success with duplex sonography? AJR AM J Roentgenol 1994; 162: 184–186.

15. Matsi PJ, Manninen HI, Soder HK *et al.* Percutaneous transluminal angioplasty in femoral artery occlusions: primary and long-term results in 107 claudicant patients using femoral and popliteal catherization techniques. Clin Radiol 1995; 50: 237–244.

16. Capek P, McLean GK, Berkowitz HD. Femoropopliteal angioplasty. Factors influencing long-term success. Circulation 1991; 83 (Suppl): I 700–I80.

17. Belli AM, Murphy GJ, Bolia A. Recanalization using a low speed rotational device (ROTACS) in total occlusions of the femoropopliteal artery. Clin Radiol 1994; 49: 304–306.

18. Vroegindeweij D, Tielbeck AV, Buth J *et al.* Directional atherectomy versus balloon angioplasty in segmental femoropopliteal artery disease: two-year follow-up with color-flow Doppler scanning. J Vasc Surg 1995; 21: 255–268.

19. Vroegindeweij D, Vos LD, Tielbeek AV *et al.* Balloon angioplasty combined with primary stenting versus balloon angioplasty alone in femoropopliteal obstructions: a comparative randomized study. Cardiovasc Intervent Radiol 1997; 20: 420–425.

20. Do-dai-Do, Triller J, Walpoth BH *et al.* A comparison study of self-expandable stents versus balloon angioplasty alone in femoropopliteal artery occlusions. Cadiovasc Intervent Radiol 1992; 15: 301–312.

21. Simon N, Franklin Ss, Bleifer KH, Maxwell MH. Clinical characteristics of renovascular HTN. JAMA 1972; 220: 1209–1218.

22. Olin JW, Melia M, Young JR *et al.* Prevalence of atherosclerosis renal artery stenosis in patients with atherosclerosis elsewhere. Am J Med 1990; 88: 46N–51N.

23. Harding MB, Smith LR, Hinmelstein SI *et al.* Renal artery stenosis: prevalence and associated risk factors in patients undergoing routine cardiac catherization. J Am Soc Nephrol 1992; 2: 1608–1616.

24. Valentine RJ, Clagett GP, Miller GL *et al.* The coronary risk of unsuspected renal artery stenosis. J Vasc Surg 1993; 18: 433–440.

25. Derkx F, Schalekamp M. Renal artery stenosis and HTN. Lancet 1994; 344: 237–239.

26. Losinno F, Zuccala A, Busato F, Zucchelli P. Renal artery angioplasty for renovascular HTN and preservation of renal function: long-term angiographic and clinical F/V. Am J Radiol 1994; 162: 853–857.

27. Harden PN, Macleod MJ, Rodiger RSC *et al.* Effect of renal artery stenting on progression of renovascular renal failure. Lancet 1997; 349: 1133–1136.

28. Novick AC, Pohl MA, Schreiber M *et al.* Revascuarization for preservation of renal function in patients with atherosclerotic renovascular disease. J Urol 1983; 129: 907–912.

29. Khosla S, White CJ, Collins TJ *et al.* Effects of renal artery stent implantation in patients with renovascular HTN. Presenting with USA or CHF. Am J Cardiol 1997; 80: 363–366.

30. Weibull H, Bergquist D, Jonsson K *et al.* Long-term results after percutaneous transluminal angioplasty of atherosclerotic renal artery stenosis: The importance of intensive follow-up. Eur J Vasc Surg 1991; 5: 291–301.

31. Isles CG, Robertson S, Hill D. Management of renovascular disease: A review of renal artery stenting in ten studies: QJ Med 1999; 92: 159–167.

32. Khosla S, White CJ, Collins TJ *et al.* Effects of renal artery stenting implantation in patients with renovascular HTN presenting with USA or CHF. Am J Cardiol 1997; 80: 363–366.

33. Van de Ven PJG, Kaatee R, Beutler JJ *et al.* Arterial stenting and balloon angioplasty in ostial atherosclerotic renovascular disease: A randomized trial. Lancet 1999; 353: 282–286.

34. Dorros G, Jaff M, Jain A *et al.* Follow-up of primary Palmaz-Schatz stent placement for atherosclerotic renal artery stenosis. Am J Cardiol 1995; 75: 105i–1055.

35. White CJ, Ramee SR, Collins TJ *et al.* Renal artery stent placement: utility in difficult lesions for balloon angioplasty. J A Cell Cardiol 1997; 30: 1445–1450.

36. North American Symptomatic Carotid Endarterectomy Trial Collaborators. Beneficial effect of carotid endarterectomy in symptomatic patients with high grade carotid stenosis. New Eng J Med 1991; 325: 445–453.

37. Executive Committee for the Asymptomatic Carotid Atherosclerotic Study. Endarterectomy for asymptomatic carotid artery stenosis. JAMA 1995; 274: 1421–1428.

38. Heuser RR, Periperal Vascular Stenting for Cardiologists. Martin Dunitz Ltd. 1999; Chapter 7, Page 71.

39. Heuser RR, Periperal Vascular Stenting for Cardiologists. Martin Dunitz Ltd. 1999; Chapter 7, Page 73.

40. Heuser RR, Periperal Vascular Stenting for Cardiologists. Martin Dunitz Ltd. 1999; Chapter 7, Page 77.

41. CAVATAS Investigators. Endovascular versus surgical treatment in patients with carotid stenosis in the Carotid and Vertebral Artery transluminal Angioplasty study (CAVATAS): a randomized study. Lancet 2001; 357: 1729–1737.

42. SAPPHIRE (Stenting and Angioplasty with Protection in Patients of High Risk for Endarterectomy) Investigators. NEJM 2001; 351: 1493–1501.

43. The UK Small Aneurysm Trial Participants. Mortality results for randomized controlled trial of early elective surgery or ultrasonographic surveillance for small abdominal aortic aneurysms. The UK Small Aneurysm Trial Participants. Lancet 1998; 352: 1649–1655.

44. Conway KP; Byrne J, Townsend M *et al*. Prognosis of patients turned down for conventional abdominal aortic aneurysm repair in the endovascular and sonographic era: Szilagy; revisited? J Vasc Surg 2001; 33: 762–757.

45. Parodi JC, Palmaz JC, Barone HD. Transfemoral intraluminal graft implantation for abdominal aortic aneurysms. Ann Vasc Surg 1991; 5: 491–499.

46. Kamineni R, Heuser RR. A review of endoluminal treatment. Journal of Interventional Cardiology 2004; 17: 437–445.

47. Beebe HG. Late failures of devices used for endovascular treatment of abdominal aortic aneurysm: What have we learned and what is the task for the future? New York: Thieme Medical Publishers, 2001.

48. Zarins CK, White RA, Schwarten D *et al*. Aneurx Stnet graft versus open surgical repair of abdominal aortic aneurysms: Multicenter prospective clinical trial. J Vasc Surg 1999; 29: 292–305.

49. May J, White GH, Waugh R *et al*. Improved survival of endoluminal repair with second-generation prostheses compared with open repair in the treatment of abdominal aortic aneurysms: A 5-year concurrent comparison using life table method. J Vasc Surg 2001; 33: 21–6.

50. Cohnert TV, Oelert G, Wahlers T *et al*. Matched-pair analysis of conventional versus endoluminal AAA treatment outcomes during the initial phase of an aortic endografting program. J Endovasc Ther 2000; 7: 94–100.

51. EVAR-1 Comparison of endovascular aneurysm repair with open repair in patients with abdominal aortic aneurysm (EVAR trial 1), 30-day operative mortality results: randomized controlled trial. Lancet. 2004 Sep 4; 364(9437): 843–848.

52. DREAM Investigators. A Randomized Trial Comparing Conventional and Endovascular Repair of Abdominal Aortic Aneurysms. N Engl J Med 2004; 351: 1607–1618.

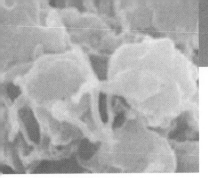

29

Coarctation of the aorta

TONY NICHOLSON, MD, FRCR

KEY POINTS

- Coarctation of the aorta has an interesting pathophysiology based on the developing cardiovascular system in utero.

- Recognition of coarctation of the aorta is important if late complications and early death are to be avoided.

- The literature and experience would suggest that balloon angioplasty, possibly aided by stenting, offers a safe effective treatment.

- We do not, as yet, have long term follow up data to prove that balloon angioplasty also alters the natural history of the condition.

Coarctation of the aorta is a congenital narrowing of the aorta in the region of the aortic isthmus which may present in the neonate or remain undetected well into adult life. About 80% of patients are male. 50% of patients have bicuspid aortic valve and it is common in Turner's syndrome.

In utero, conditions that reduce blood flow in the aortic arch and increase right to left flow through the ductus arteriosus, such as aortic stenosis and other left heart obstructive lesions predispose to coarctation. Conversely, where pulmonary artery and right to left ductal flow is reduced, such as in tetralogy of Fallot and pulmonary atresia, coarctation is very rare.

CLINICAL CONSIDERATIONS

The site of the aortic obstruction influences the age of presentation. If the coarctation is proximal to the ductus arteriosus, the distal aorta will be well perfused by the duct in utero, and collaterals will not develop. Closure of the duct in the neonatal period will then precipitate left ventricular hypertension and heart failure. If the coarctation is at or beyond the insertion of the duct, collaterals will have developed, and closure of the duct may produce no symptoms. These patients present incidentally or, more commonly, with hypertension as adults.

If undiagnosed the natural history is variable. Of those who survive infancy, 25% die before the age of 20 years, 50% by 32, and 90% by 58 years.[1] The commonest causes of death are cardiac failure, aortic rupture, infective endocarditis, and intracerebral haemorrhage from associated cerebral aneurysm rupture.[1]

Hypertension, as measured in the arms, is common and will result in varying degrees of left ventricular hypertrophy. The femoral pulses are usually delayed and weakened compared with the carotid and arm pulses and there is a characteristic murmur. Rarely patients present in middle age and beyond, usually with hypertension and ischaemic heart disease. At this stage the coarctation may have completely occluded and the murmur may no longer be heard.

The coarctation site is usually asymmetric, containing some duct tissue with a posterior shelf which may be preceded by some tapering of the aortic lumen. The degree of stenosis is variable. Adjacent tortuosity of the aorta may develop, particularly in adults. There are associated abnormalities which are now recognized as part of an aortic syndrome such as tubular hypoplasia in the arch both proximal and/or distal to the origin of the left subclavian artery. This is more commonly seen in young children and rarely in adults. Bicuspid aortic valve and the association with cystic medial degeneration may lead to dilatation of the ascending aorta and carries an increased risk of dissection and rupture aggravated by hypertension.[2]

When present post-stenotic dilatation is more diffuse than one would expect and in most cases is due to abnormal structure of the elastic tissue in the media. The normal cranial migration of the left subclavian artery which develops from the seventh intersegmental artery may be impaired. Its origin will then be abnormally low and may be involved in the coarctation.

The coarctation is usually short but longer lesions rarely occur. The aetiology and morphology of interrupted aortic arch is quite distinct from that of coarctation.

One of the striking features in adults and older children is the collateral circulation around the obstruction (Fig. 29.1). This is usually in proportion to the degree of stenosis and is generally used as an indicator of its severity. The main collateral routes are the internal mammary arteries with retrograde flow to the aorta below the coarctation through the 3rd–9th intercostal arteries, the inferior epigastric arteries, plus scapular and various mediastinal arteries. This results in enlargement of both subclavian arteries. Rib notching usually takes several years to develop; it is caused by pressure erosion of the inferior aspects of the adjacent ribs, and requires both enlargement and tortuosity of the intercostal arteries. This is the reason why rib notching is rare in young children, even in severe coarctation. The typical rib notching of coarctation is bilateral but asymmetric, and is best seen on the inferior aspects of the posterior thirds of the upper ribs, sparing the first two because these arise from the costocervical trunk proximal to

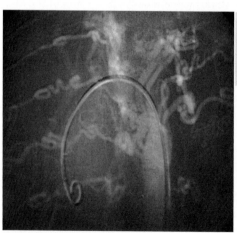

Figure 29.1:
Angiography in a patient with hypertension and radio-femoral delay demonstrates the extensive internal mammary and intercostal artery collateral circulation.

the usual site of coarctation and do not form part of the collateral circulation. If the left subclavian artery is stenosed or occluded there will be no rib notching on the left side. If there is an anomalous origin of the right subclavian artery from below the level of the coarctation there will be no rib notching on the right side.

IMAGING

In adults and older children the PA chest radiograph is almost always abnormal. Chest x-ray features include cardiomegally particularly in older adults, a prominent ascending aorta (especially with a bicuspid aortic valve) and various aortic knuckle abnormalities. There may be a 'three sign' due to enlargement of the left subclavian artery above the coarctation, the narrowed segment, and then localized post stenotic dilatation of the aorta below. Occasionally this post stenotic dilatation gives the impression of a low aortic knuckle. The whole area of the aortic knuckle may appear small and flat. On a lateral film the enlarged internal mammary artery may be seen behind the sternum.

True coarctation should not be confused with pseudocoarctation that results from an elongation of the distal aortic arch which, because it is fixed at the arterial ligament, then bulges backwards above and below this point. Increasing aortic tortuosity may develop with age but there is usually no significant haemodynamic obstruction. On the chest radiograph a double prominence of the aortic knuckle may be seen and may be thought to be a mediastinal mass. CT or MRI will demonstrate the true anatomy.

The clinical signs together with a chest x-ray are usually enough to make the diagnosis. Echocardiography may be difficult in adults and older children but in infants it may be useful in identifying the area of stenosis and identifying associated congenital cardiac defects. Using continuous wave Doppler measurements of flow velocities above and below the coarctation and a modified Bernoulli equation it is possible to assess the degree of stenosis.

MRI is now the imaging modality of choice in both infantile and adult coarctation (Fig. 29.2). It has considerable advantages as it is noninvasive and

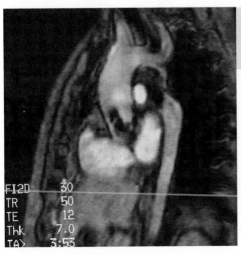

Figure 29.2:
Gradient echo T2 weighted MRI scan of the thorax reveals a tight coarctation beyond the origin of the left subclavian artery.

also is useful for post-treatment follow up. T1-weighted spin-echo sequences will show the whole of the aorta, the major branches, and the larger collaterals. Cine phase contrast imaging can be used to estimate the gradient across the coarctation. Gadolinium-enhanced 3D MRA gives the best anatomical images.

Multislice CT can also provide exquisite images but is rarely used because of the radiation implications. Angiography, previously the imaging procedure of choice, is now rarely required unless cardiac catheterization is necessary for the investigation of associated cardiac abnormalities. The coarctation can usually be crossed from the femoral arterial route but this may be impossible and require brachial artery catheterization. Asymmetry of the lesion may require the acquisition of multiple views.

TREATMENT

Previously the most common treatment for significant coarctation was surgery. Short lesions that can be mobilized are resected with end-to-end anastomosis and this will give the best long-term result. Failing this, the most usual procedure is repair by subclavian patch. Synthetic graft material is unsuitable in children because of the lack of growth.

Percutaneous transluminal angioplasty for the treatment of aortic coarctation in adults and children is well established.[3–10] The technique compares favorably with surgical repair with respect to blood pressure control, reduction of the coarctation gradient, and complication rates in the short term.[3–14] It has been proposed that stenting may offer superior long-term outcomes (Fig. 29.3).[15–17] However, the use of metallic stents in the treatment of aortic coarctation has only

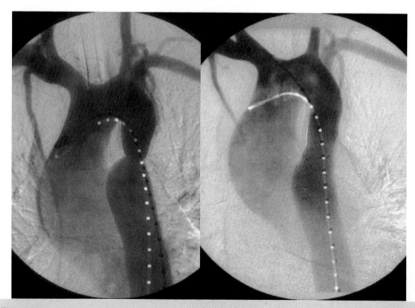

Figure 29.3:
Tight coarctation with a gradient of 50 mm Hg and the result after stenting with abolition of the gradient (courtesy of Dr Peter Gaines).

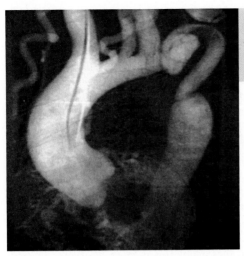

Figure 29.4:
Post surgical repair of a coarctation there is the development of a pseudoaneurysm and Restenosis. However, extreme tortuosity precluded endovascular repair.

been reported in patients with recurrence following surgical repair,[15] or in small series.[16–17] Long-term follow-up of primary stent use is not available. Medium- and long-term follow-up of angioplasty in children, adolescents and adults has been published.[8–10] Not all coarctations are suitable for endovascular repair, extreme tortuosity at the coarctation site being a contraindication (Fig. 29.4).

TECHNIQUE

PTA or stenting is performed in an angiography suite under either general anesthesia or neuroleptanalgesia depending on patient preference. Practitioners should have a stent graft of suitable size available and be experienced with their use in case of rupture. The availability of stent grafts means that thoracic surgical stand by is no longer required.

The technique is modified from other PTA procedures. The common femoral artery is punctured and an introducer sheath inserted. A shaped catheter is then advanced to the level of the coarctation and, using a steerable wire, the coarctation is crossed. The wire and catheter are then advanced into the ascending aorta. The steerable wire is removed and replaced with a 260 cm long Amplatz wire (Cook, Letchworth, Herts, UK). The catheter is withdrawn and replaced by a 5 Fr marker pigtail catheter. Heparin (5000 IU) is then given intravenously. Simultaneous pressures are measured in the ascending aorta and at the femoral level via the sheath. An angiogram is performed using the pigtail catheter and, using the calibration markers, the diameter of the aorta immediately below the left subclavian artery is measured. A balloon catheter with diameter 2 mm less than this measurement is used for dilatation (usually 18–24 mm). Stents are sized 1 mm larger than the aortic measurement.

With the Amplatz wire in place an appropriate sheath is inserted into the femoral artery and the PTA catheter advanced over the Amplatz wire to the coarctation site and inflated using dilute contrast. Waisting of the balloon confirms its position within the area of the coarctation and full inflation is then performed to abolish the waist. A single appropriately sized balloon is far preferable to 'kissing balloons' which will not produce 360 degree dilatation. After deflation and withdrawal through the sheath, simultaneous pressures are again measured and, if these show a systolic gradient of less than 10 mmHg, check angiography should be performed to make sure there are no complications at the PTA site. If the systolic gradient remains above 10 mm then a stent can be used to abolish any recoil.

RESULTS AND COMPLICATIONS

The literature would suggest that PTA has a lower morbidity and mortality then surgery.[3–10] Overall surgical mortality is 2.6–3.1% while only one death has been reported with PTA and that was eight months following the procedure secondary to aortic dissection away from the coarctation site.[4] Post surgical paraplegia has been reported in most surgical series but not yet reported post endovascular treatment. Localized dissections and pseudoaneurysms are reported in 0–10% of PTA series but their long term significance is unknown. Most are treated by stent graft if they become complicated.

Restenosis rates of 39–46% have been reported in children.[18,19] However the accepted restenosis rate in adults is much lower at 14%.[3–6,10] One study did demonstrate a 69% restenosis rate over nine years but used predominately 'kissing balloons' instead of appropriately sized single balloons.[17] Most studies do demonstrate a sustained fall in systolic blood pressure and antihypertensive requirement.

REFERENCES

1. Campbell M. Natural history of coarcation of the aorta. Br Heart J 1970; 32: 633–640.

2. Lindsay J. Coarctation of the aorta, bicuspid aortic valve and abnormal ascending aortic wall. Am J Cardiol 1988; 61: 182–184.

3. Fawzy ME, Sivanandam V, Galal O. One to ten year follow up of balloon angioplasty of native coarctation of the aorta in adolescents and adults. J Am Coll Cardiol 1997; 30: 1542–1546.

4. Schrader R, Bussmann WD, Jacobi V, Kadel C. Long-term effects of balloon coarctation angioplasty on arterial blood pressure in adolescent and adult patients. Cathet Cardiovasc Diagn 1995; 36: 220–225.

5. Tyagi S, Arora R, Kaul UA, Sethi KK, Gambhir DS, Khalilullah M. Balloon angioplasty of native coarctation of the aorta in adolescents and young adults. Am Heart J 1992; 123: 674–680.

6. Biswas PK, Mitra K, De. S. Follow-up results of balloon angioplasty for native coarctation of aorta. Indian Heart J 1996; 48: 673–676.

7. Phadke K, Dyet JF, Aber CP, Hartley W. Balloon angioplasty of adult aortic coarctation. Br Heart J 1993; 69: 36–40.

8. Lababida Z. Percutaneous balloon coarctation angioplasty: Long term results. J Intervent Cardiol 1992; 5: 57–62.

9. Ledesma Velasco M, Ramirez Reyes H, Aldana Perez T, Acosta Valdez JL, Munayer Calderon J, Carpio Hernandez JC, Verdin Vasquez R. Percutaneous transluminal angioplasty in aortic coarctation in adolescents and adults: Mid term results. Arch Inst Cardiol Mex 1992; 62: 339–343.

10. Paddon AJ, Nicholson AA, Ettles DF *et al.* Long term follow up of perctaneous balloon angioplasty in adult coarctation. Cardiovascular & Interventional Radiology 2000; 23: 364–367.

11. Bobby JJ, Emami JM, Farmer RDT, Newman CGH. Operative survival and 40 year follow up of surgical repair of aortic coarctation. Br Heart J 1991; 65: 271–276.

12. Kirklin JW, Barratt-Boyes BG (eds) (1986) Cardiac Surgery. Churchill Livingstone, London, chapt 34, pp 1263–1327.

13. Sabiston DC, Spencer FC (eds) (1990) Surgery of the Chest. WB Saunders, Philadelphia, chapt 33, pp 1126–1221.

14. Knyshov GV, Sitar LL, Glagola MD, Atamanyuk MY. Aortic aneurysm at the site of repair of coarctation of the aorta: A review of 48 patients. Ann Thorac Surg 1996; 61: 935–939.

15. Ebeid MR, Prieto LR, Latson LA. Use of balloon expandable stents for coarctation of the aorta: Initial results and intermediate term follow-up. J Am Coll Cardiol 1997; 30: 3847–1852.

16. Bulbul ZR, Bruckheimer E, Love JC, Fahey JT, Hellenbrand WE. Implantation of balloon-expandable stents for coarctation of aorta: Implantation data and short-term results. Cathet Cardiovasc Diagn 1996; 39: 36–42.

17. Macdonald S, Thomas SM, Cleveland TJ, Gaines PA. Angioplasty or stenting in adult coarctation of the aorta? A retrospective single center analysis over a decade. Cardiovascular & Interventional Radiology 2003; 26(4): 357–64.

18. Sharma S, Bhagwat AR, Loya YS. Percutaneous balloon angioplasty for native coarctation of the aorta: Early and intermediate term results. J Assoc Physicians India 1991; 39: 610–613.

19. Rao PS, Galal O, Smith PA, Wilson AD. Five to nine year follow up of balloon angioplasty of native aortic coarctation in infants and children. J Am Coll Cardiol 1997; 27: 462–470.

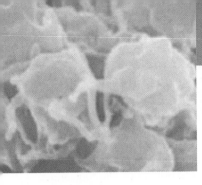

30

Percutaneous vascular intervention in the venous system

ARUN SEBASTIAN, MRCP, FRCR AND
DUNCAN F. ETTLES MD, FRCP (ED) FRCR

KEY POINTS

- While many of the techniques described in this chapter are common to other cardiovascular interventions, the venous system poses certain unique challenges.

- The operator must possess a good knowledge of variant anatomy and recognise the important differences between the nature and behaviour of venous, as opposed to arterial lesions.

- Careful attention to technique is required within these low flow vessels to avoid thrombotic occlusion and damage to relatively thin walled vessels.

- Restenosis rates following venous angioplasty tend to be higher and repeated interventions may be required to maintain patency in dialysis fistulas and native veins.

- Level 1 evidence is lacking with regard to most of the procedures and further research is needed to strengthen the evidence base.

INTRODUCTION

Percutaneous intervention in the venous system has been relatively slow to develop in comparison to coronary and peripheral arterial intervention. There are several reasons for this, including the relatively low incidence of clinically significant venous disease, incompletely understood pathophysiology and a perception that technical and clinical success rates are much more limited in the venous circulation compared to the arteries. Many clinicians remain ill-informed about the scope of interventional procedures available. Nevertheless, more aggressive management of malignant disease, the need for vascular access in renal disease and renewed interest in pulmonary embolic disease have led to a rapid increase in the burden of cases presenting to the interventional radiologist. There are very few randomised studies of interventional procedures in venous disease and the evidence base is derived largely from retrospective analyses and case series. However, the potential for improved quality of life and relief of disabling symptoms makes endovascular treatment of venous disease both challenging and rewarding.

ENDOVASCULAR TREATMENT OF SUPERIOR VENA CAVAL OBSTRUCTION AND SUBCLAVIAN VEIN THROMBOSIS

The clinical syndrome of superior vena caval obstruction (SVCO) most commonly occurs as a result of mediastinal malignancy but has a number of other aetiologies including radiotherapy, chemotherapy and caval stenosis or occlusion due to central lines and cardiac pacemakers. The resulting constellation of symptoms includes facial and arm swelling, headaches, dysphagia and mental impairment. In malignant SVCO, conventional treatment includes the use of steroids and radiotherapy but reponse is often slow and only partial. The use of endovascular stents allows rapid and effective relief of caval obstruction which allows a dramatic improvement in quality of life for these patients, many of whom have a poor prognosis.[1]

Diagnosis of SVCO is clinical and most often will be confirmed by contrast enhanced CT of the mediastinum. The decision to intervene is based on severity of symptoms. Preliminary venography, usually from bilateral arm injections, confirms the diagnosis and allows treatment to be planned. In order to relieve SVCO, it is necessary to re-establish patency between the distal SVC and one of the brachiocephalic veins only, as good collaterals exist across the midline. Where SVCO is due to malignancy, the stent is usually placed in the brachiocepahlic vein least involved by the tumour mass. The obstruction can be crossed either from the arm or via a femoral approach using a multipurpose or cobra type catheter. In the presence of a large thrombus burden, preliminary thrombolysis or thrombus aspiration may be necessary. However, in patients with malignant SVCO, lysis carries a high risk and a preliminary CT of the brain is needed to exclude metastatic disease. Predilatation of the SVC is rarely needed and a 12 to 16 mm diameter stent of sufficient length to exclude the encased portion of the vein is deployed (Fig. 30.1). Self expanding stents (Wallstent or Smart stent) are preferred and may be post-dilated if necessary to establish a lumen of at least 10mm.[1,2] Procedural success rates are high with few serious reported complications. Patients are warned that they may experience some chest discomfort for a few days following treatment and are also advised to expect a large diuresis as the upper limbs and torso decompress. Objective follow-up of implanted central venous stents is difficult and often inappropriate in patients with advanced malignancy. However, several clinical studies confirm excellent symptomatic relief, such that most patients experience no recurrence of their symptoms prior to death.

Subclavian and axillary vein thrombosis is usually secondary to indwelling catheters or devices and malignant infiltration. Primary or idiopathic thrombosis of the subclavian vein may occur and is known as Paget-Schroetter syndrome. It occurs in otherwise healthy subjects and is thought to be caused by repeated trauma to the subclavian vein between the clavicle, first rib and surrounding muscles and ligamentous tissue. It is often seen in bodybuilders and heavy goods vehicle drivers. The subclavian vein eventually becomes stenotic and fibrosed with a resulting episode of acute thrombosis. Careful questioning can often elicit a history of similar episodes in the preceding months. Often, conservative management, by simple elevation, is sufficient to relieve arm swelling but better results are obtained by combining this with the use of anticoagulation. Interventional treatment including the use of thrombolysis, angioplasty, stenting and rib resection has been shown to reduce post-phlebitic symptoms and recurrent presentations. Catheter directed thrombolysis rapidly clears thrombus and typically demonstrates high grade stenosis where the subclavian vein crosses the clavicle. Opinion differs as to whether angioplasty and stenting alone or in combination with rib resection offers the best long term outcome. Despite a high initial success rate, recurrent stenosis is common in the subclavian vein.

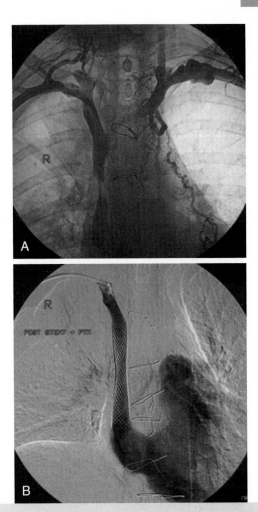

Figure 30.1:
A, Severe stenosis of the superior vena cava causing SVCO syndrome B, A 12mm diameter Wallstent has been deployed in the SVC using a right antecubital approach, with an excellent result.

Stents offer a better immediate luminal gain, but are prone to fracture because of continued mechanical stresses and should probably be avoided in young patients. Because venous collateralisation around the shoulder is good, some authorities recommend a conservative approach in all but the severely symptomatic and disabled patients.[3,4]

INFERIOR VENA CAVA FILTERS

Accurate estimates of morbidity and mortality due to pulmonary embolic disease are very difficult to obtain. Embolic disease is still under-recognised and often only considered after other investigations have proved inconclusive. Estimates of mortality have suggested a figure of up to 35% over 12 months in patients following untreated pulmonary emboli. There is a growing body of evidence to show that caval filtration reduces the incidence of early fatal repeat emboli and that IVC filters have a very low long term morbidity, despite fears of potential device related complications.[5,6]

The commonest indications for caval filter placement include those patients with proven pulmonary emboli who have contraindications to anticoagulation therapy. In patients where repeated episodes of pulmonary embolism occur despite effective anticoagulation, IVC filter insertion is also indicated. The increasing use of IVC filters has led to a wider range of indications including prophylaxis for patients with pelvic trauma, prophylaxis prior to pelvic surgery and in patients with known iliocaval thrombus (Fig. 30.2).

A wide range of devices is available to the interventionist, including stainless steel and nitinol types. All can be delivered through 8 F or smaller introducer sheaths. Most designs allow placement through either the transfemoral or transjugular approach, and the Simon nitinol filter can also be placed from the antecubital fossa. This latter approach can be very useful in the dyspnoeic patient who is unable to lie flat during filter insertion. Caval filters may be permanent (i.e. Birds Nest Filter) or retrievable (Gunther Tulip filter) in type. Retrievable or temporary filters offer an attractive solution in younger patients requiring prophylaxis. These filters can be removed at up to several weeks after implantation or alternatively, repositioned within the cava at suitable intervals to avoid incorporation into the wall of the cava. In the authors' unit, temporary filters have been used for prophylaxis in the late stages of pregnancy and successfully removed after delivery.

Filter placement is a generally straightforward and well tolerated procedure. Cannulation of a suitable access vein is followed by preliminary venography to demonstrate venous anatomy and exclude the presence of caval thrombus. Occasionally, caval anomalies such as left-sided or double IVC will be encountered and placement of two filters has been described. Once the level of the renal veins and position of the iliac confluence is established, the filter is deployed in the infrarenal portion of the IVC. When preliminary imaging shows extensive caval thrombus, a jugular approach is used. Occasionally, suprarenal filter placement is indicated which can be technically difficult if the intrahepatic portion of the IVC is short. In these cases, one of the more compact filters, such as the Gunther Tulip, is preferred to avoid the risk of prolapse into the right atrium. In the management of subacute massive pulmonary embolism, IVC filter placement can follow preliminary pulmonary angiography and mechanical clot disruption or intrapulmonary thrombolysis. The endovascular management of pulmonary embolism is, however, outwith the scope of this chapter.

Device related complications are rare but include device fracture and occasionally fatal migration. Modern designs are much less prone to migration but some authorities recommend surveillance by plain abdominal radiography. Perforation of the IVC wall is well recognised but clinically unimportant (Fig.30.3). Occlusion of the IVC following filter insertion has been reported but may relate to filter type. In the author's unit we found a less than 5% incidence using the Birds Nest filter.[7] Recurrent pulmonary emboli occur with an incidence of between 2 and 5% after filter implanation. This may be due to failure of thrombus trapping, collateral venous pathways or thrombus propagation on the superior aspect of the implanted device. Unless contraindicated, anticoagulation

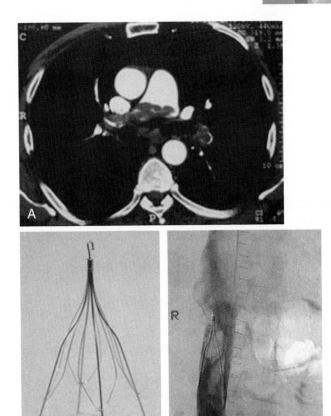

Figure 30.2:
A, CT pulmonary angiogram showing massive emboli at the bifurcation of the pulmonary trunk B, The Gunther retrievable Tulip filter C, Large thrombi can be seen trapped within the filter which was therefore left in situ.

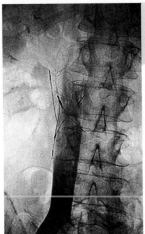

Figure 30.3:
A Bird's Nest permanent IVC filter. Note superior prolapse of filter wires which is of no clinical significance.

should be continued for at least six months after filter insertion to minimise the risks of recurrent emboli and DVT.

Retrievable filters are removed using a jugular approach and a specially adapted snare set. Check venography is performed to ensure that no trapped thrombi are present. If this is shown to be the case, then the filter is left in situ and regarded as a permanent device. Even after short implantation periods, some temporary filters become incorporated into the cava and in these circumstances, forcible removal should not be attempted. Maldeployment of temporary devices or subsequent tilting within the cava may also make retrieval impractical in a small number of cases.

INTERVENTION IN DIALYSIS FISTULAS

There is an ever increasing number of patients with chronic renal failure requiring regular haemodialysis, which is usually achieved through a fistula. The most common fistula -related problem is outflow vessel stenosis which leads in turn to thrombosis and occlusion. Haemodialysis fistulas are created communications between the native artery and vein in an extremity and this may be a native arteriovenous fistula or a prosthetic arteriovenous graft. Haemodialysis failure and occlusion is most commonly the result of progressive narrowing of the outflow vein in native fistulas and the venous anastomosis in prosthetic grafts.

Clinical examination may raise suspicion of fistula stenosis which may be palpable beneath the skin. Arterial inflow stenosis can cause vacuum phenomenon during dialysis and stenosis at the site of cannulation can make routine needling difficult. Venous stenoses remote from the fistula result in a congested fistula with loss of thrill and increased compression times after dialysis. Screening for stenoses is often undertaken by Doppler ultrasound to detect falling flow rates and impending failure. Such programmes are worthwhile as prospective angioplasty of venous stenoses that narrow the lumen by more than 50% improves fistula function and prolongs access survival.[8,9]

Percutaneous transluminal angioplasty can be used to manage more than 80% of arterial and venous stenoses in the stenoses in both native fistulas and grafts (Fig. 30.4). Fistulography is initially performed to delineate the arterial and venous anatomy and to evaluate the subclavian veins and SVC for evidence of central venous stenosis. Access for intervention is usually achieved by direct fistula puncture but transarterial and retrograde venous approaches are sometimes necessary. In keeping with venous stenoses at other sites, high inflation pressures (10–20 atmospheres) are commonly required to abolish the lesions. Balloon dilatation of these lesions is often very painful and the fibrous nature of venous stenoses increases the risk of vessel laceration and rupture. Suitably sized bare and covered self-expanding stents should be available for bailout should this occur. PTA of graft-related stenoses yields primary success rates ranging from 94 to 98% with secondary patency of 85 and 82% in the forearm and upper arm respectively. For native forearm fistulas, rates range from 91 to 95%.

The role of stents in the management of venous stenosis of dialysis access is unclear. As mentioned above, stent placement is used for treatment of outflow vein rupture after balloon angioplasty, when attempts to tamponade bleeding by prolonged balloon inflation fail and for treatment of stenosis recoil. Future access

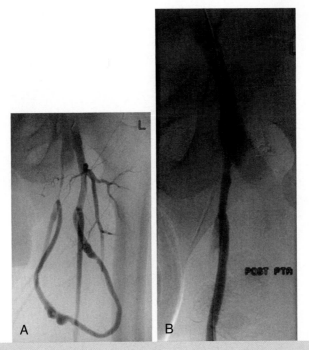

Figure 30.4:
A, Severe stenosis (arrowed) affecting the venous outflow of a loop thigh dialysis graft B, Successful result following balloon angioplasty.

sites must be anticipated before placing a stent. Primary stent placement is recommended due to poor results after simple balloon dilatation of central venous stenosis (Fig. 30.5). Continued patency of venous stents require aggressive reintervention and the cumulative patency rate is around 70% per year.

Dialysis fistula thrombosis usually relates to outflow lesions and results in loss of access in 80–85% if not corrected rapidly. Therapeutic options for fistula thrombosis include surgical thrombectomy, thrombolysis, thromboaspiration and mechanical dissolution. Pharmaco-mechanical methods involve low or high dose local infusion of the thrombolytic agent before detaching or crushing the thrombus with a balloon. Purely mechanical methods include clot extraction or disruption methods using devices such as Trerotola catheter and Sharaffuddin balloon. Technical success rates for pharmaco-mechanical and mechanical methods are between 89 and 95% with secondary patency rates in the region of 75% at one year.[8,9,10] Subclinical pulmonary emboli as a result of these procedures are common but seem to be rarely of clinical significance.

VENOUS ACCESS

The use of central venous access (CVA) catheters has increased dramatically over the last decade for administration of chemotherapy, antibiotics, total parenteral nutrition and as temporary access for haemodialysis. Numerous catheter types are available and the choice depends on the indication for access and its intended duration. Short-term catheters are usually placed without imaging unless there is

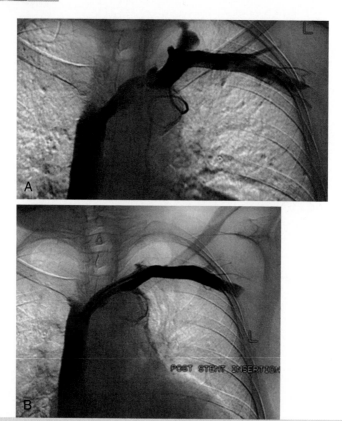

Figure 30.5:
A, Severe stenosis of the left brachiocephalic vein with resulting in impaired function of forearm dialysis fistula B, A Smart stent has been used to abolish the venous stenosis and restore rapid central venous flow.

abnormal venous anatomy. Long-term venous access is through central venous catheters, peripherally inserted central catheters (PICC) and ports. Central venous catheters have a subcutaneous tunnelled route between the skin and the site of venous puncture. A Dacron cuff at the proximal end of the subcutaneous tract allows in growth of fibrous tissue to provide mechanical stability and a barrier to infection. PICC lines are usually placed via a superficial arm vein without imaging, but if this is not possible, access using deeper veins and fluoroscopic control is undertaken. Ports have a subcutaneous reservoir connected to the central venous catheter. Although these have traditionally been placed surgically, the smaller port systems placed radiologically are preferred by many patients. An ideal location for the reservoir is the anteromedial aspect of the second rib.

When multiple, possibly incompatible, substances need to administered simultaneously, multi lumen catheters are preferred. When continuous access or high flow rates are required, tunnelled lines are preferred, while ports are more suited for intermittent access, as the skin will act as an antimicrobial barrier between treatment periods.

Ease of access makes the subclavian vein a favourite puncture site, but carries the risks of thrombosis and stenosis which may preclude future use of this limb for graft or fistula access. For this reason, in dialysis patients, the internal jugular vein is the preferred site of access. The superficial and vertical course of the internal jugular allows easy cannulation access. The inferior vena cava (IVC) is another alternative and can be approached via transfemoral, translumbar and transhepatic routes. Collateral veins can be used for venous access in patients with central venous occlusion.

The subclavian and internal jugular veins are easily punctured under ultrasound guidance with the patient placed in the Trendeleburg position to aid puncture and reduce the risk of air embolism.[11] Fluoroscopy is used to position a guidewire and peelaway sheath and the catheter is cut to size prior to insertion so that its tip lies at the cavo-atrial junction. Catheter malposition (Fig 30.6), arterial puncture, the risk of pneumothorax have all been minimised by ultrasound guidance and during the translumbar approach, ureteral injury is avoided by advancing the needle close to the vertebral body. The frequency of catheter related infections varies between 10 and 30% or 1.4 per 1000 catheter days. About 7% of all patients who have central catheters require catheter removal as a result of infection, with a higher incidence of infection in multilumen catheters. Catheter-related thrombosis can occur in up to 10% of patients from peri-catheter fibrin sheath, peri-catheter or intra-catheter thrombus. Contrast injection may help identify the problem and a loop snare can be used to strip the fibrin sheath from the catheter while catheter thrombosis can be treated by thrombolysis.[12,13,14] Central venous stenoses occur especially in patients on haemodialysis, due to direct vessel trauma and high flow rates. Management often necessitates the use of self-expanding stents as balloon angioplasty is often insufficient.

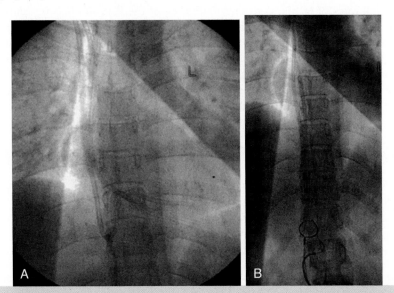

Figure 30.6:
A, Dialysis lines inserted without imaging have been malpositioned in the right ventricle. A pigtail catheter introduced from the groin is used for the repositioning procedure. B, The additional use of an Amplatz snare inserted from the left femoral vein was needed to successfully reposition the lines within the IVC.

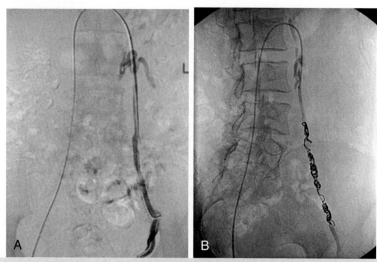

Figure 30.7:
A, Symptomatic left sided varicocele. The left testicular vein is cannulated from a right femoral venous approach B, Complete occlusion is achieved by deployment of fibered coils.

OTHER VENOUS INTERVENTIONS

The creation of transjugular intrahepatic porto-systemic shunts (TIPS) for the management of variceal bleeding and intractable ascites was described over 20 years ago but became clinically feasible with the introduction of metallic stents. TIPS procedures are now routinely undertaken in most radiology departments with high rates of technical success.[15] Stenting of the IVC and hepatic veins for Budd Chiari syndrome are well established techniques and embolisation procedures for symptomatic varicoceles have largely replaced conventional surgical treatment[16] (Fig. 30.7). There has been a recent renewal of interest in thrombolytic procedures for iliofemoral deep venous thrombosis[17] and, on the other side of the coin, significant developments in endovenous laser ablation.

REFERENCES

1. Nicholson AA, Ettles DF, Arnold A, Greenstone M, Dyet JF: Treatment of malignant superior vena cava obstruction: metal stents or radiation therapy. J Vasc Intervent Radiol 1997; 8:781–8.

2. Crow MTI, Davies CH, Gaines PA: Percutaneous management of superior vena cava occlusions. Cardiovasc Intervent Radiol 1995; 18:367–72.

3. Meier GH, Pollak JS, Rosenblatt M, *et al*. Initial experience with venous stents in exertional axillary-subclavian vein thrombosis. J Vasc Surg 1996; 24:974–83.

4. Lee MC, Grassi CJ, Belkin M, *et al*. Early operative intervention after thrombolyitc therapy for primary subclavian vein thrombosis: An effective treatment approach. J Vasc Surg 1998; 27:1101–8.

5.   Walsh DB, Birkmeyer JD, Barrett JA, *et al*. Use of inferior vena cava filters in the medicare population, Ann Vasc Surg 1995; 9:483–7.

6.   Decousus H, Leizorovicz A, Parent F, *et al*. A clinical trial of vena caval filters in the prevention of pulmonary embolism in patients with proximal deep vein thrombosis. N Engl J Med 1998; 338:409–15.

7.   Nicholson A, Ettles DF, Paddon AJ, Dyet JF: Long term follow-up of the Bird's Nest IVC Filter. Clinical Radiology 1999; 54:759–64.

8.   Turmel-Rodrigues L, Pengloan J, Baudin S, *et al*. Treatment of stenosis and thrombosis in haemodialysis fistulas and grafts by interventional radiology. Nephrol Dial Transplant 2000; 15:2029–36.

9.   Hunter DW, Castaneda-Zuniga WR, Coleman CC, *et al*. Failing arteriovenous dialysis fistulas: evaluation and treatment. Radiology 1984; 152:631–5.

10. Valji K: Transcatheter treatment of thrombosed hemodialysis access grafts: Am J Roentgenol 1995; 164:823–9.

11. Gordon AC, Saliken JC, Johns D, *et al*. US-guided puncture of the internal jugular vein: complications and anatomic considerations. J Vasc Intervent Radiol 1998; 9:333–8.

12. Haskal ZJ, Leen VH, Thomas-Hawkins C, *et al*. Transvenous removal of fibrin sheaths from tunneled hemodialysis catheters. J Vasc Intervent Radiol 1996; 7:513–17.

13. Kidney DD, Nguyen DT, Deutsch LS. Radiologic evaluation and management of malfunctioning long-term central vein catheters. Am J Roentgenol 1998; 171:1251–7.

14. Rockall AG, Harris A, Wetton CW, *et al*. Stripping of failing haemodialysis catheters using the Ampltaz gooseneck snare. Clin Radiol 1997; 52:616–20.

15. Richter GM, Noeldge G, Palmaz JC, *et al*. Transjugular intrahepatic portocaval stent shunt: Preliminary clinical results. Radiology 1990; 174:1027–30.

16. Zuckerman AM, Michell SE, Venbrux AC, *et al*. Percutaneous varicocele occlusion: Long term follow-up. J Vasc Intervent Radiol 1994; 5:315–19.

17. Semba CP, Dake MD: Iliofemoral deep venous thrombosis: Aggressive therapy using catheter-directed thrombolysis. Radiology 1994; 191:487–94.

Section Five

Non-Coronary
Intervention:
Non-Vascular
Intervention

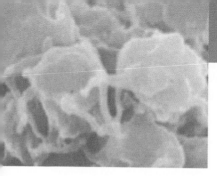

31

Percutaneous balloon mitral valvuloplasty and mitral valve repair

BERNARD D. PRENDERGAST, ROGER J.C. HALL, AND ALEC VAHANIAN

KEY POINTS

- Approximately 250 mitral valvuloplasty procedures are carried out annually in the UK.

- The procedure requires experience in trans-septal puncture.

- It is ideal in non-calcified and non-regurgitant valves.

- Expert echocardiographic assessment is required before and after the procedure.

- Results are similar to surgery in the long-term.

- There is very large experience of the procedure in countries with high incidence of rheumatic fever.

- The presence of left atrial thrombus is a contraindication to the procedure.

PERCUTANEOUS MITRAL VALVULOPLASTY

INTRODUCTION

Despite the decline of rheumatic fever, mitral stenosis remains a common and important problem. The incidence of rheumatic heart disease in immigrants and ethnic minority groups is not inconsiderable and acute rheumatic fever is still a common problem in the developing world. In the West, rheumatic heart disease in the elderly represents a medico-historical remnant of widespread streptococcal infection during the first half of the twentieth century. Although degenerative valve disease now predominates in this age group, rheumatic mitral stenosis is by no means unusual. Older patients with mitral stenosis tend to fall into two categories: those who have restenosis after a previously successful surgical or percutaneous mitral valvotomy, and those with more slowly progressive rheumatic disease which has only become symptomatic in later life, these latter subjects illustrating selective survival in that the more seriously afflicted died at a young age.

Since the first publication on the implementation of the technique of percutaneous balloon mitral valvuloplasty by Inoue in 1984, numerous reports have confirmed its safety and efficacy. The technique has now virtually replaced surgical commissurotomy for the treatment of mitral stenosis and indications for the technique in developed countries have now been extended to include younger patients in challenging clinical situations and older patients with more severe disease.

PATHOPHYSIOLOGY

The frequency of mitral stenosis parallels the incidence of acute rheumatic fever: the current prevalence, though clearly decreasing, is unknown. Rheumatic mitral valve disease is characterised by fusion of one or both commissures. The valve leaflets may be thickened, fibrous and calcified, causing reduced mobility, and the chordae tendinae may shorten and thicken, before fusing to form secondary subvalvular stenosis.

The normal mitral valve orifice is 4 cm^2, but in severe mitral stenosis this may be reduced to less than 1 cm.^{2} Pulmonary hypertension and increased pulmonary vascular resistance are frequent associated findings. These abnormalities usually become haemodynamically significant in the fourth and fifth decades, although initial presentation at the age of 70 or above is not uncommon. In mild–moderate disease the cardiac output may remain normal but is unable to increase with exercise, leading to exertional dyspnoea. With more severe degrees of stenosis, cardiac output becomes subnormal, even at rest. Symptoms may also be precipitated during tachycardia, when the abbreviation of diastole is associated with impaired left ventricular filling, and by the onset of atrial fibrillation when cardiac output may fall by 20–25% due to the loss of atrial transport and an associated sudden increase in heart rate.

The mechanism of balloon mitral valvuloplasty is splitting of the fused commissures and the procedure is only likely to work when there is significant fusion. The results of valvuloplasty are inversely related to the degree of leaflet thickening, calcification and mobility, and, in particular, the extent of subvalvular disease. In general, marked thickening and calcification of the subvalvular apparatus makes the valve less amenable to valvuloplasty.

PATIENT SELECTION

Patient selection is fundamental in predicting the immediate outcome of balloon mitral valvuloplasty. The procedure may have its most significant impact in the developing world where mitral stenosis is common, particularly in young patients, and cardiac surgical resources are sparse. In western populations, patients with mitral stenosis may have moderately mobile and pliable valves, but generally are far older and have much more valvular thickening and calcification. Despite the lack of scientific evidence in this group of patients, a consensus regarding the place of balloon valvuloplasty is emerging which is consistent with common sense and a knowledge of the pathology of mitral stenosis. In practice, the choice of percutaneous balloon valvuloplasty will depend on the following factors: the patient's clinical condition, anatomical aspects and the experience of the practitioners concerned.

Clinical considerations

Clinical evaluation focuses on functional disability and the risks of the procedure in comparison with mitral valve replacement. Traditionally, surgical treatment of mitral stenosis has been withheld until symptoms become quite severe because of the very definite risk and inconvenience of surgery. In such markedly symptomatic patients the indication for balloon valvuloplasty is clear. However, now that the mitral valve can be dilated with excellent symptomatic results, a risk of major complications <1% and only a couple of days in hospital, it is also reasonable to consider the procedure in mildly symptomatic patients in the hope that early intervention may postpone the onset of atrial fibrillation and pulmonary vascular disease and allow the patient normal or near normal exercise tolerance. Truly asymptomatic patients are not usually candidates for mitral valvuloplasty, except in the following circumstances: a need for major non-cardiac surgery, to allow pregnancy, and possibly in patients with an increased risk of embolism (e.g. previous embolic event, heavy left atrial spontaneous echo contrast), recurrent atrial arrhythmias or evidence of pulmonary hypertension at rest or with exercise.

Percutaneous valvuloplasty is the only interventional alternative when mitral valve replacement is contraindicated. It may also be preferable to surgery, at least as a first attempt, in patients with mitral stenosis who have undergone previous surgical mitral commissurotomy or aortic valve replacement. Although a good immediate outcome is frequently achieved, overall event-free survival is inferior in patients undergoing balloon valvuloplasty following previous valve surgery compared with those in whom balloon valvuloplasty is the primary procedure. However, the immediate outcome and long-term follow-up results are excellent in carefully selected patients with suitable valves and valvuloplasty is a valuable treatment option in this group.

The procedure may also be preferable to valve replacement in patients with impaired left ventricular function since the subvalvular apparatus is spared and the insult of cardiopulmonary bypass is avoided. In cases of co-existent mitral stenosis and moderate aortic valve disease, balloon valvuloplasty can be performed as an interim measure, and may postpone the need for eventual double valve replacement. Concomitant mitral/aortic and mitral/tricuspid valvuloplasty have also been reported in exceptional clinical circumstances.

In western populations, many patients with mitral stenosis have concomitant non-cardiac disease which may increase the risk of surgery and balloon mitral valvuloplasty represents an attractive therapeutic option in this setting. This situation is particularly common in frail elderly patients, where balloon dilatation usually results in a moderate but significant improvement in valve function, associated with a clinically useful symptomatic result, although subsequent functional deterioration is frequent. The procedural mortality is 3% in the elderly, which is considerably less than the risks of mitral valve replacement in this group. In centres with greater experience, complication rates may be even lower.

Several series indicate that balloon valvuloplasty is a safe and efficacious treatment in pregnant patients with mitral stenosis to improve the mother's haemodynamic status; it is also well tolerated by the foetus. The risks of exposing the foetus to radiation may be minimised by adequate lead screening of the abdomen and successful outcomes using transoesophageal echocardiographic guidance alone, i.e. dispensing with radiation, have also been described. It must be borne in mind, however, that the procedure always carries a risk of complications, albeit small, so that it should be limited to pregnant women who remain symptomatic despite appropriate medical treatment, and undertaken by highly experienced operators.

Anatomical aspects

The evaluation of candidates for the procedure requires a precise assessment of valve morphology and function for advance planning of balloon dilatation and subsequent follow-up. Subsequent to clinical examination, two-dimensional colour Doppler echocardiography is currently the best and most widely used non-invasive technique for assessing the suitability of the mitral valve for balloon dilatation, allowing evaluation of the anatomical characteristics of the valve and subvalvular apparatus, and the size of the valve annulus (Table 31.1).

In rheumatic mitral stenosis the valve leaflets are characteristically thickened (and often calcified) at echocardiography with evidence of commissural fusion. The degree of commissural fusion is usually best assessed using transthoracic echocardiography in the parasternal short axis view. Cusp mobility is reduced and bowing of the leaflets occurs in diastole. Associated features such as left atrial enlargement and/or thrombus, pulmonary hypertension and mitral regurgitation may also be apparent. Transthoracic imaging is satisfactory in most patients, but the valve is better defined by transoesophageal imaging. The aims of echocardiographic assessment prior to balloon valvuloplasty are to identify features predictive of a poor outcome, such as extensive valvular calcification, marked thickening and scarring of the subvalvular apparatus and the presence of associated mitral regurgitation. In addition, it is important to exclude the presence of left atrial thrombus, which increases the risk of systemic thromboembolism during or following the procedure. Since transoesophageal echocardiography allows more accurate assessment of the degree of leaflet involvement and subvalvular disease and is better at visualising left atrial and appendage thrombus, it is now considered mandatory in all patients prior to balloon valvuloplasty. The presence of thrombus within the left atrium (either floating or localised), particularly on the inter-atrial septum, is a contraindication to balloon valvuloplasty. A number of small series have reported that the procedure is feasible in patients with thrombus restricted to the left atrial appendage, but this remains controversial. Unless there is a need for urgent intervention or anticoagulation is contraindicated for other reasons, the patient can be treated with oral anticoagulants for at least 1 month, after which a follow-up transoesophageal echocardiographic examination often shows disappearance of the thrombus. Spontaneous echo contrast, an echocardiographic marker of

TABLE 31.1 - ECHOCARDIOGRAPHIC ASSESSMENT PRIOR TO BALLOON MITRAL VALVULOPLASTY
Degree of mitral stenosis
Commissural fusion
Valvular calcification
Subvalvular involvement
Associated mitral regurgitation
Left atrial thrombus
Atrial septal anatomy

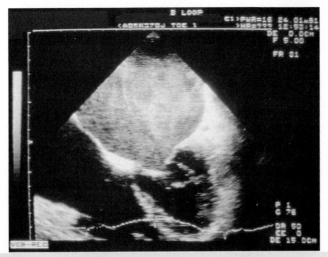

Figure 31.1:
Transoesophageal echocardiogram (horizontal plane, four-chamber view) taken from a patient with severe rheumatic mitral stenosis. Note calcification of the anterior leaflet and spontaneous echo contrast within a grossly dilated left atrium, indicative of stagnant blood flow.

blood stasis within the left atrium, is a frequent finding in mitral stenosis and does not prohibit balloon valvuloplasty (Figures 31.1 & 31.2).

The valve area can be assessed using a combination of planimetry of the valve orifice in early diastole and measurement of the pressure half-time (the time interval for the velocity of flow across the valve to fall from its peak value to the

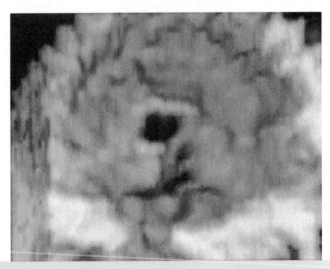

Figure 31.2:
Three-dimensional echocardiographic reconstruction of a severely stenosed mitral valve viewed from the ventricular aspect in late diastole.

peak value divided by the square root of 2, normal <100 ms) from which valve area can be calculated as follows:

$$\text{Mitral valve area (cm}^2\text{)} = \frac{220}{\text{pressure half-time (ms)}}$$

Generally speaking, it is not advisable to define an arbitrary threshold valve area above which balloon valvuloplasty should not be performed, since overall assessment should also take account of functional disability and the presence of pulmonary hypertension. In practice, however, it is unusual to undertake the procedure in patients with a valve area greater than 1.5 cm^2 (or 1 cm^2/m^2 body surface area if the patient is unusually large).

Coexistent mitral regurgitation can be quantified using Doppler techniques. Severe regurgitation (Sellers grade 3 or 4) contraindicates balloon valvuloplasty whereas mild regurgitation (Sellers grade 1) is acceptable. Patients with moderate mitral regurgitation (Sellers grade 2) present a dilemma and an overall decision should be made in the light of other clinical and echocardiographic variables. In cases where mitral stenosis is combined with severe aortic stenosis, the need for surgery is obvious. Tricuspid regurgitation is usually present to some degree and measurement of the velocity of the jet allows estimation of the pulmonary artery pressure. Reports in relatively small numbers of patients have suggested that balloon valvuloplasty can be performed safely and effectively in patients with severe pulmonary hypertension, though long term outcome may be inferior in this group.

Clinician experience

In addition to these patient-related parameters, the experience of the medical team is important in reaching a management decision. Several series have confirmed that major complications are significantly fewer in centres undertaking a relatively large caseload. Inevitably, complications are more frequent when the operator has only a small throughput, since the procedure is technically demanding. In general terms, balloon valvuloplasty should only be performed by groups who are experienced in trans-septal catheterisation and who carry out an adequate number of procedures to maintain the technical skills required. These considerations are highly relevant in western countries where mitral stenosis is relatively infrequent. Specialist experience is of particular importance in cases with minimal symptoms, cardiothoracic deformity or during pregnancy.

PATIENT PREPARATION

Patient preparation is essentially similar to that for routine left/right heart catheterisation. Informed consent should be obtained and the patient made aware of the small risks of systemic thromboembolism and severe mitral regurgitation requiring urgent surgery. Where appropriate, anticoagulant medication should be terminated 48 hours prior to valvuloplasty (with a target INR of < 1.2 on the day of the procedure), and then recommenced the following day (assuming there are no vascular complications and the indication for anticoagulation persists). All other medication is continued. A recent transthoracic and transoesophageal echocardiogram should be available to confirm valve suitability and exclude the presence of left atrial thrombus (see above). In practice, these are often performed during the 24 hours prior to the procedure.

On the day of valvuloplasty, the patient is fasted for 4–6 hours before the procedure and one or both groins are prepared for vascular access. A light sedative (e.g. diazepam 5 mg) may be helpful in anxious patients. Vascular sheaths may be removed immediately or 3–4 hours later when the anticoagulant effects of heparin have elapsed. Generally, the patient can be discharged the day after a successful procedure providing there have been no complications. A further echocardiogram is performed before discharge (a transthoracic study is usually sufficient) to exclude significant mitral regurgitation or residual left-to-right shunt and to provide a baseline assessment of residual stenosis, which assists future follow-up.

TECHNIQUE

Although a variety of techniques are available, mitral valvuloplasty is most widely undertaken using the Inoue balloon in view if its relative simplicity of use and lower risk of complications. Specific advantages of the Inoue balloon include a lower risk of left ventricular perforation, easier manoeuvrability, its slender profile (creating a smaller defect in the inter-atrial septum), its self-positioning characteristics, short inflation-deflation cycle, and capacity to permit gradually increasing successive balloon inflation sizes, which allow the operator to terminate the procedure when commissural splitting is achieved or when there is an increase in the severity of mitral regurgitation.

Trans-septal catheterisation of the left atrium is required preceded by routine right heart catheterisation via the femoral vein. Right atrial angiography with late filling and filming of the left atrium to guide trans-septal puncture, and use of a retrograde pigtail catheter positioned in the ascending aorta to delineate the position of the aortic valve and posterior aortic sinus (thereby reducing the risk of inadvertent aortic puncture) may be of assistance for low volume operators or those early in their experience of the procedure. Trans-septal puncture is performed using a Brockenbrough needle and satisfactory left atrial positioning is confirmed by dye injection through the puncture needle or direct measurement of left atrial pressure or oxygen saturation. If satisfactory, the trans-septal catheter (either a Mullins or Brockenbrough catheter) is advanced into the left atrium, heparin (3000–10000 IU according to operator preference) is administered, and mitral valve area (if required) may be derived by measurement of the trans-valve pressure gradient and cardiac output.

The Inoue, single balloon technique makes use of a double loop guidewire, a 14 F dilator and the Inoue balloon catheter (Fig. 31.3). The size of Inoue balloon is selected according to the patients size (usually height or body surface area – Table 31.2) and the balloon prepared by successive inflation and deflation with contrast to extrude excess air. Balloon diameter at peak inflation is then verified using graduated calipers. The double loop guidewire is inserted into the left atrium through the trans-septal catheter, which is then removed. The 14 F dilator is introduced over this guidewire and advanced to dilate both the femoral vein and the atrial septal puncture site. It is then removed and the Inoue balloon

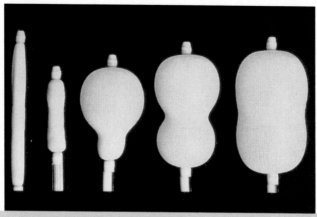

Figure 31.3:
The Inoue balloon at various stages of inflation. Note the initial selective inflation of the distal balloon which allows optimal positioning across the stenosed mitral valve.

catheter is inserted over the guidewire and placed in the left atrium. Following partial inflation of the distal balloon to assist flotation and avoid entanglement in the sub-valve apparatus, the balloon catheter is then manipulated across the mitral valve aided by a pre-shaped stylet. In cases where gross left atrial dilatation or puncture unduly low in the inter-atrial septum make this difficult, the catheter may be looped within the left atrium with the assistance of the guidewire, thereby allowing more direct access to the valve orifice. Once across the valve, the distal balloon is then inflated, moved back and forth inside the left ventricle to ensure that it is mobile and not entangled between the mitral valve chordae, and then pulled back against the mitral valve until resistance is felt and immediately fully inflated. It is then deflated at once (recommended maximal occlusion time 5 seconds) and the catheter allowed to retreat into the left atrium. The degree of success may then be estimated, either by measurement of the pressure gradient or immediate echocardiographic assessment, and serial inflations using stepwise increases in balloon diameter undertaken until a satisfactory result is obtained (see below). In routine practice, transthoracic echocardiography is a key monitoring tool throughout the procedure. However, "real time" three-dimensional imaging provides additional information regarding valve morphology and intracardiac echocardiography is useful in guiding technical

TABLE 31.2 - INOUE BALLOON SELECTION	
HEIGHT (CM)	**BALLOON SIZE (DIAMETER IN CM)**
<150	24
>150	26
>165	28
>180	30

aspects of the procedure – both are now used in several specialist centres. When intra-procedural echocardiography is unavailable, mitral regurgitation is monitored between inflations by assessment of the left atrial v-wave and left ventriculography. Before terminating the procedure, a final left ventricular angiogram is usually performed to compare the degree of mitral regurgitation with that in the baseline study (Figures 31.4 & 31.5).

The older double balloon technique is rarely used nowadays and requires a Brockenbrough needle, a Mullins catheter and sheath, and a dilator. Trans-septal puncture is performed as described above, the Mullins sheath advanced over the dilator into the left atrium and heparin given. A 7 F floating balloon catheter is passed through the sheath antegradely across the mitral valve and valve area determined. Once the left ventricle has been catheterised, the sheath is advanced over the floating balloon catheter, which is subsequently withdrawn. One or two

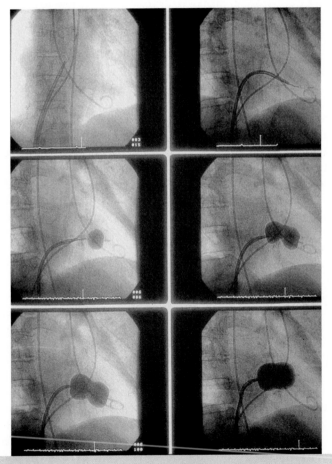

Figure 31.4:
Percutaneous balloon mitral valvuloplasty using the Inoue balloon. Note 'wasting' of the stenosed mitral valve prior to full inflation.

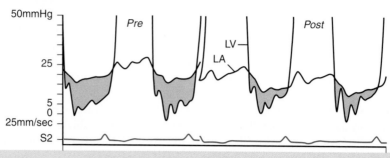

Figure 31.5:
Reduction in the gradient between left atrium (LA) and left ventricle (LV) (hatched) before and after balloon valvuloplasty.

precurved long exchange guidewires are then positioned at the left ventricular apex, or alternatively they are manipulated across the aortic valve into the ascending aorta. The sheath is removed and the dilating balloon catheters are advanced over the wires and positioned across the stenotic mitral valve. Occasionally, pre-dilatation of the atrial septum using a 6 mm balloon may be necessary. A variety of dilating balloon combinations may be used: a 20 mm and 15 mm balloon, two 20 mm balloons, a Trefoil 3x10 mm and a 19 mm balloon or a Trefoil 3x12 mm and a 19 mm balloon. Alternatively, a single balloon catheter such as Trefoil 3x15mm or a Bifoil 2x19mm have been used. After 1–2 inflations (each no longer than 20 seconds to avoid prolonged hypotension and syncope), the balloon dilating catheters are removed, leaving the wire(s) in place, and the floating balloon catheter and Mullins sheath are replaced to allow calculation of mitral valve area. If a satisfactory result has been obtained, the floating balloon, Mullins sheath and wires are removed and mitral regurgitation assessed by left ventriculography. This technically demanding approach has recently been simplified by the availability of the multi-track system allowing use of Monorail balloons on a single guidewire, though its application remains infrequent.

There is controversy as to which of these antegrade techniques provides superior immediate and long-term results. Compared with the Inoue balloon, the multiple balloon technique usually results in a larger mitral valve area and a lesser degree of mitral regurgitation after valvuloplasty, particularly in patients with anatomically favourable valves. However, these differences in immediate outcome are subtle, with no significant differences in survival, adverse clinical events or restenosis at long-term clinical follow-up. As indicated, the Inoue technique is now the default technique at most major centres since it is easier to perform and has a lower risk of complications, particularly left ventricular perforation.

A third, rarely used approach is a retrograde technique utilizing arterial access alone (thereby avoiding the need for trans-septal puncture and creation of a left-to-right atrial shunt with the inherent risk of a residual atrial septal defect). However, although this clearly reduces the hazards associated with trans-septal catheterisation (and may be indispensable in the rare event when this is contraindicated or impossible), the risks of chordal rupture, peripheral arterial damage and significant bleeding are increased.

A final more recent development is the application of a percutaneous metallic valvulotome, which can be autoclaved after each procedure to allow repeated use in many patients, thereby overcoming the prohibitive costs of the Inoue balloon which limit its use in developing nations. Further potential advantages include a greater increase in valve area in comparison with the Inoue balloon, and selective commissural splitting, especially in calcified valves with a reduction in leaflet trauma. Experiences in more than 1000 patients, predominantly in developing nations, have been promising though minimal randomised data are available to provide a comparison with more established techniques leading to its poor overall uptake.

OUTCOME

Initial results

Technical failure rates range from 1–15% and usually occur in the early stage of the operator's experience. Successful balloon mitral valvuloplasty converts severe mitral stenosis to a mild-moderate narrowing, usually providing an increase in valve area of over 100% (average final area 2cm^2), which results in an immediate decrease in left atrial pressure, pulmonary arterial pressure and pulmonary vascular resistance. These physiological changes are associated with a parallel improvement in the patient's clinical state, often by two or more New York Heart Association classes. These results are well maintained and encouraging long term follow-up results up to 15 years following the procedure have been reported.

After the procedure, the most accurate evaluation of valve area is provided by echocardiography allowing calculation of final valve area by means of planimetry, the pressure half-time or the continuity equation. Assessment may be undertaken immediately following the procedure since elastic recoil is insignificant. Two definitions of an optimal initial result are in current use: a final valve area > 1 cm^2/m^2 body surface area or complete opening of at least one commissure (both without significant increase in mitral regurgitation, ie. >Sellers grade 2/4).

Predictors of outcome

Initial reports stressed the predictive value of echocardiographic anatomical assessment using semi-quantitative scores to predict immediate outcome. Of these, the best known is that originally developed by Wilkins *et al.* at the Massachusetts General Hospital. Leaflet rigidity, leaflet thickening, valvular calcification, and subvalvular disease are each scored on a scale from 0 to 4 yielding a maximum total echocardiographic score of 16. A higher score represents a heavily calcified, thickened and immobile valve with extensive thickening and calcification of the subvalvular apparatus. Among the four components of the score, valve leaflet thickening and subvalvular disease provide the best correlates for the increase in mitral valve area produced by balloon valvuloplasty. Patients with lower echocardiographic scores have a higher likelihood of a good outcome with minimal complications and a haemodynamic and clinical improvement that persists at long-term follow-up. Furthermore, in long-term follow-up studies, patients with echocardiographic scores <8 display a higher rate of survival and freedom from combined events (death, mitral valve replacement, repeat valvuloplasty and symptoms in New York Heart Association class III or IV). Conversely, patients with higher scores have a relatively poor outcome. In particular, rigid thickened valves, extensive subvalvular fibrosis and valve calcification herald a suboptimal result.

However, these echocardiographic scores do not predict immediate or long-term outcome of balloon mitral valvuloplasty with complete reliability. Limitations of echocardiographic classification include the difficulties of reproducibility, underestimation of lesion severity, and the fact that the use of scores takes no account of localised changes in specific portions of the valve apparatus, particularly in the commissural area. Reflecting these limitations, more recent publications have been less enthusiastic, reporting a poor correlation between echocardiographic scores and the initial increase in valve area. Furthermore, anatomical prediction of the development of severe mitral regurgitation following the procedure is even less reliable. It is now generally accepted that other factors influence outcome, including the age, sex and size of the patient, the presence of mitral valve calcification, pre-existent mitral regurgitation, atrial fibrillation, left atrial dilatation or pulmonary hypertension, tricuspid regurgitation, a small initial valve area, balloon size and a history of previous surgical commissurotomy. These parameters should therefore also be taken into consideration (Table 31.3)

Outcome following mitral balloon valvuloplasty in elderly patients is generally inferior compared with the younger population, particularly since other adverse factors such as valve calcification and atrial fibrillation are frequently present. Nevertheless, the procedure has an established useful role in carefully selected patients. Independent predictors of success in the elderly include a lower echocardiographic score, lower New York Heart Association functional class and a larger mitral valve area prior to valvuloplasty. A low echocardiographic score, particularly the absence of valve calcification, is the strongest predictor of event-free survival in this group.

Patients with heavily calcified valves, either on fluoroscopy or echocardiography, have a worse immediate outcome, as reflected in a smaller increase in valve area

---

TABLE 31.3 - FACTORS PREDICTING OUTCOME AFTER BALLOON MITRAL VALVULOPLASTY

- Age and sex
- Body size
- Valve anatomy
- Mitral valve calcification
- Pre existent mitral regurgitation
- Previous surgical commissurotomy
- Small initial valve area
- Left atrial size
- Sinus rhythm
- Pulmonary aterial pressure
- Balloon size

Complications 31

after balloon valvuloplasty and inferior long-term, event-free survival. These outcomes correlate closely with the degree of calcification. Similar findings have also been reported in long-term follow-up studies after surgical commissurotomy. Further studies are needed to refine the indications for balloon valvuloplasty in this frequently encountered, heterogeneous group of patients. Current strategy recommends surgery in patients with massive or bi-commissural calcification, whereas balloon valvuloplasty can be attempted as an initial therapeutic approach in patients with mild or unicommissural calcification, particularly when other clinical factors are favourable. Traumatic mitral regurgitation requiring surgery is a more frequent complication of balloon valvuloplasty in this group. Patients with valve calcification who undergo uncomplicated balloon dilatation require careful appraisal and follow up – those with poor early results or subsequent clinical deterioration should be considered for surgery.

Patients in atrial fibrillation often have other factors associated with an inferior result, i.e. advanced age, unsuitable valve anatomy and a history of previous surgical commissurotomy. Nevertheless, it seems that atrial fibrillation itself predicts a poor outcome after balloon valvuloplasty, i.e. a smaller initial increase in mitral valve area after valvuloplasty and inferior event-free survival.

Restenosis

The incidence of restenosis following successful balloon valvuloplasty is usually low (approximately 40% over 7 years). Repeat balloon valvuloplasty has been successfully performed for restenosis in several series of patients and may represent an attractive treatment option in cases of symptomatic restenosis occurring several years following the initial procedure, providing that the predominant mechanism of restenosis is commissural refusion and that overall valve anatomy remains suitable.

COMPLICATIONS

Reported mortality of balloon valvuloplasty averages 0.5% in experienced hands. Although this is considerably less than the risk associated with mitral valve replacement, a fairer comparison would be with closed mitral commissurotomy, which has a very similar risk. The main causes of death are left ventricular perforation or the poor initial condition of the patient. Important complications of balloon valvuloplasty are cardiac perforation leading to tamponade, embolic stroke due to displacement of thrombus from the left atrium, severe damage to the valve leading to severe regurgitation, and residual atrial septal defect (Table 31.4).

The rate of haemopericardium varies from 0.5–12%, and usually results from trans-septal catheterisation or, more rarely, from apex perforation, either by the guidewires or the balloon itself. This complication has become relatively infrequent since the widespread use of the Inoue balloon.

Embolism is encountered in 0.5–5% of cases but is seldom the cause of permanent incapacity. It may be due to fibrino-thrombotic material (despite the absence of detectable thrombus prior to the procedure), gas, or, on rare occasions, calcium. The risk of thromboembolism can be minimised by careful scanning of the left atrium using transoesophageal echocardiography before the dilatation.

409

TABLE 31.4 - COMPLICATIONS FOLLOWING BALLOON MITRAL VALVULOPLASTY

- Cardiac perforation
- Systemic embolism
- Mitral regurgitation
- Residual atrial septal defect
- Vascular damage
- Arrhythmias

Mild mitral regurgitation is relatively common and usually seems to occur via the commissures that have been split by balloon dilatation. Severe mitral regurgitation results from a tear in a valve cusp and is unusual, with rates ranging from 2–10%. Effective balloon dilating area normalised for body surface area (EBDA/BSA) and valve calcification are the only established predictors of increased mitral regurgitation following balloon valvuloplasty. Echocardiographic scores to predict the likelihood of significant mitral regurgitation complicating the procedure (evaluating uneven distribution of thickness in the anterior and posterior leaflets and the degree of commissural and subvalvular disease) have been proposed, consistent with the longstanding clinical impression that mitral regurgitation occurs most often in patients with unfavourable anatomy, especially in those with extensive subvalvular disease. Moderate–severe regurgitation may be well tolerated initially, but surgery is often necessary, usually on a scheduled basis. Valve replacement is needed in most cases because of the severity of the underlying valve disease, but conservative surgery, combining suture of the valve tear and commissurotomy may be possible in cases with less severe valve deformity if appropriate surgical expertise is available. Particularly encouraging results using this approach have been reported by Acar in Paris (Fig. 31.6).

The frequency of residual atrial septal defect varies from 10–20%, as assessed by oximetry, and from 40–80% by colour flow Doppler. The associated shunts are nearly always small and without clinical consequence. Some data suggest that the incidence of significant left-to-right atrial shunting is higher in patients with anatomically unsuitable valves. The vast majority (45–80%) close spontaneously. Persistence is related to size (> 5mm diameter), unsatisfactory relief of valve obstruction such that left atrial pressure remains high, or to the development of restenosis.

Other complications, including arrhythmias and vascular damage, are rare.

Urgent surgery (i.e. within 24 hours) is rarely needed (<1%) for complications of balloon mitral valvuloplasty. It may occasionally be required for massive haemopericardium or less frequently for severe mitral regurgitation which is poorly tolerated. Overall, the procedure is of low risk when performed by experienced operators on properly selected patients.

COMPARISONS WITH SURGICAL COMMISSUROTOMY

Balloon valvuloplasty may achieve an increase in mitral valve area comparable with that obtained using the well established surgical techniques of open and

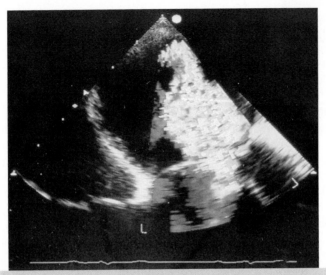

Figure 31.6:
Transoesophageal echocardiogram (horizontal plane, four plane chamber view) demonstrating severe mitral regurgitation secondary to a tear in the anterior leaflet complicating balloon valvuloplasty. This patient developed acute pulmonary oedema and required urgent mitral valve replacement.

closed mitral commissurotomy. Furthermore, the technique overcomes the need for thoracotomy, general anaesthesia and cardiopulmonary bypass, and requires a short hospital stay and brief convalescence. Most patients return to normal activities within a day or two of the procedure. Such advantages are meaningless, however, unless the dilatation procedure and conventional surgery have comparable safety and efficacy.

Interpretation of long-term follow-up studies of patients undergoing balloon mitral valvuloplasty and their comparison with surgical series are confounded by heterogeneity in the patient populations studied. In patients with optimal mitral valve morphology, surgical commissurotomy has favourable long-term haemodynamic and symptomatic results. However, as observed following balloon valvuloplasty, elderly patients and those with calcified valves or atrial fibrillation do less well.

Several randomised studies from developing countries have compared the techniques of balloon valvuloplasty and surgical commissurotomy. The two methods appear to be comparable in safety and give similar immediate and mid-term clinical and haemodynamic improvement. However, a valid comparison remains difficult since (i) these series are few and concern relatively small numbers of patients; (ii) the duration of follow-up after balloon valvuloplasty is still insufficient, given that deteriorating valve function following surgical commissurotomy is most commonly seen after a period of 8–10 years; and (iii) the patients in these series were nearly always young with favourable mitral valve morphology.

Although long-term follow-up studies will continue to define the precise role of balloon valvuloplasty, these initial randomised controlled trials comparing the technique with surgical commissurotomy are encouraging and support the percutaneous approach for the treatment of patients with rheumatic mitral stenosis who have suitable valve anatomy. Given its practical advantages, balloon valvuloplasty should be considered in all patients with mitral stenosis who are symptomatic despite medical treatment.

PERCUTANEOUS MITRAL VALVE REPAIR

The progressive refinement of surgical techniques of mitral valve repair and their adoption into routine surgical practice have had a major impact on the management of mitral regurgitation worldwide. Indeed, current guidelines for surgical intervention encourage earlier referral if repair is feasible and surgery is now undertaken in many asymptomatic subjects with exceedingly low mortality. However, not all patients are suitable candidates for surgery and, encouraged by their successes elsewhere, interventional cardiologists have developed two main techniques for the percutaneous repair of mitral regurgitation over the past five years: edge-to-edge repair and prosthetic ring annuloplasty.

The edge-to-edge technique is akin to the Alfieri surgical procedure, requiring the placement of a stitch to oppose the mid portion of both mitral leaflets and thereby creation of a double mitral valve orifice. The percutaneous procedure is challenging requiring a trans-septal approach and transoesophageal echocardiographic guidance and has been performed in less than 100 patients worldwide. However, initial results of a feasibility study have been encouraging and a head-to-head randomised comparison with surgery is now underway in the USA. Potential limitations include the inability to address co-existent annular dilatation (restricting its use to repair of localised prolapse of the medial portions of either leaflet) and the possibility of leaflet or chordal trauma. These constraints together with the procedure's technical demands may ultimately limit its application.

Alternative approaches are being addressed in animal models and first patient series. Percutaneous prosthetic ring annuloplasty aims to reproduce the effects of surgical ring placement by the delivery of a constraining device within the coronary sinus. Experience derived from electrophysiological procedures suggests easier performance than the edge-to-edge technique and outcome in animal models and early clinical feasibility studies has been favourable. However, procedural challenges remain including the inconsistent relation of the coronary sinus to the posterior mitral annulus, incomplete annular coverage, the inability to anchor the device in both fibrous trigones, potential damage to the adjacent circumflex coronary artery and problems related to annular calcification. Further refinements of the procedure to overcome these issues are being explored and early non randomised clinical trials are ongoing. Ultimately a combination of the edge-to-edge and annuloplasty techniques may prove useful though further assessment is awaited.

Overall, it seems unlikely that percutaneous mitral valve repair will be able to match the excellent results of surgical repair in the foreseeable future. Exploration of these evolving techniques against established surgical procedures whilst ensuring patient safety and interest therefore presents an ethical dilemma. In the first instance, experience will remain limited to those patients in whom surgery is contraindicated or presents excessive risk. Thereafter, careful clinical trial design and assessment of efficacy are critical and a recent position statement endorsed by the American College of Cardiology and the American Heart Association has addressed these difficult regulatory issues.

CONCLUSIONS

Balloon valvuloplasty is now firmly established as the procedure of choice for the treatment of patients with rheumatic mitral stenosis whose valves are anatomically suitable for balloon dilatation, and in patients where surgery is contraindicated or presents too high a risk. The best results are obtained when the valve shows definite commissural fusion, is pliable, has little or no disease of the subvalvular apparatus and is not heavily calcified. Despite these ideal criteria, good palliation may also be obtained by dilating quite heavily calcified valves in the elderly and patients who are unfit for surgery. The procedure results in a significant decrease in the mitral gradient and an increase in mitral valve area in the majority of patients with minimal mortality and morbidity. These haemodynamic changes are usually associated with a marked immediate clinical improvement which persists at medium and long-term follow-up. Although immediate and long-term results are comparable with long established surgical procedures, it is important to consider percutaneous and surgical approaches as complementary techniques in the management of patients with mitral stenosis, each applicable at the appropriate stage of the disease. Techniques for percutaneous mitral valve repair are currently in their infancy. Although preclinical models and preliminary experience in humans have been encouraging, experience to date is concentrated in a handful of specialist centres worldwide and whilst conclusions remain speculative, further developments are awaited with interest.

FURTHER READING

Block PC, Bonhoeffer P. Percutaneous approaches to valvular heart disease. Curr Cardiol Rep 2005; 7:108–13.

Cheng TO. Long-term results of percutaneous balloon mitral valvuloplasty with the Inoue balloon catheter in elderly patients. Am J Cardiol 2002; 90:686–7.

Feldman T. Core curriculum for interventional cardiology: percutaneous valvuloplasty. Catheter Cardiovasc Interv 2003; 60:48–56.

Guerios EE, Bueno R, Nercolini D et al. Mitral stenosis and percutaneous mitral valvuloplasty (part 1). J Invasive Cardiol 2005; 17:382–6.

Guerios EE, Bueno R, Nercolini D et al. Mitral stenosis and percutaneous mitral valvuloplasty (part 2). J Invasive Cardiol 2005; 17:440–4.

Inoue K, Okawi T, Nakamura T et al. Clinical application of transvenous mitral commissurotomy by a new balloon catheter. J Thorac Cardiovasc Surg 1984; 87:394–402.

Iung B, Cormier B, Ducimetière P et al. Immediate results of percutaneous mitral commissurotomy. A predictive model on a series of 1514 patients. Circulation 1996; 94:2124–30.

Iung B, Garbarz E, Michaud P et al. Late results of percutaneous mitral commissurotomy in a series of 1024 patients: analysis of late clinical deterioration: frequency, anatomical findings, and predictive factors. Circulation 1999; 99:3272–8.

Iung B, Garbarz E, Michaud P et al. Immediate and mid-term results of repeat percutaneous mitral commissurotomy for restenosis following earlier percutaneous mitral commissurotomy. Eur Heart J 2000; 21:1683–90.

Iung B, Vahanian A. The long-term outcome of balloon valvuloplasty for mitral stenosis. Curr Cardiol Rep 2002; 4:118–24.

Iung B, Nicoud-Houel A, Fondard O et al. Temporal trends in percutaneous mitral commissurotomy over a 15 year period. Eur Heart J 2004; 25:701–8.

Lau KW, Hung JS, Ding ZP et al. Controversies in balloon mitral valvuloplasty: the when (timing for intervention), what (choice of valve), and how (choice of technique). Cathet Cardiovasc Diagn 1995; 35:91–100.

Mack MJ. Percutaneous mitral valve repair: a fertile field of innovative treatment strategies. Circulation 2006; 113:2269–71.

Palacios IF. Farewell to surgical mitral commissurotomy for many patients. Circulation 1998; 97:223–6.

Prendergast BD, Shaw TRD, Vahanian A et al. Percutaneous balloon mitral valvuloplasty: contemporary indications and the role of emergent technology. Heart 2002; 87:401–404.

Presbitero P, Prever SB, Brusca A. Interventional cardiology in pregnancy. Eur Heart J 1996; 17:182–8.

Sutaria N, Shaw TRD, Prendergast BD et al. Transoesophageal echocardiographic assessment of mitral valve commissural morphology predicts outcome following balloon mitral valvotomy. Heart 2006; 92:52–7.

Tawn Z, Himbert D, Brochet E et al. Percutaneous valve procedures: present and future. Int J Cardiovasc Intervent 2005; 7:14–20.

Vahanian A, Palacios I. Percutaneous approaches to valvular heart disease. Circulation 2004; 109:1572–9.

Vahanian A, Acar C. Percutaneous valve procedures: what is the future? Curr Opin Cardiol 2005; 20:100–6.

Vassiliades TA, Block PC, Cohn LH et al. The clinical development of percutaneous heart valve technology: a position statement of the Society of Thoracic Surgeons, the American Association for Thoracic Surgery, and the Society for Cardiovascular Angiography and Interventions. J Am Coll Cardiol 2005; 45:1554–60.

Wilkins GT, Weyman AE, Abascal VM et al. Percutaneous balloon dilatation of the mitral valve: an analysis of echocardiographic variables related to outcome and the mechanism of dilatation. Br Heart J 1988; 60:299–308.

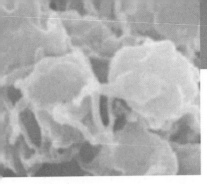

32

Aortic valve intervention

DAVID HILDICK-SMITH

KEY POINTS

■ The practice of percutaneous aortic valve intervention is entering an exciting phase in its history.

■ Widely-applicable percutaneous valve implantation is on the horizon, and this promises to be the most important development in cardiology since the introduction of the coronary stent.

■ Balloon aortic valvuloplasty is re-emerging as a technique of importance following gradual loss of enthusiasm over the preceding 15 years.

PATHOPHYSIOLOGY OF BALLOON DILATATION

Fracture of calcific nodules, separation of fused commissures and stretching of the annulus are the main mechanisms whereby valve dilatation occurs.[1] Calcific nodules may fracture (though fortunately rarely embolise) relieving leaflet restriction. Fused commissures, seen most commonly in rheumatic aortic valve disease, may be separated. Direct annular dilatation may occur, though early recoil can be brisk. Recently, it has been established from macroscopic specimens excised at valve replacement that patients who develop adult calcific aortic stenosis have a much higher incidence of aortic valve abnormalities than was previously thought, at around 50%, the majority of which are biscuspid.[2]

HISTORY OF BALLOON AORTIC VALVULOPLASTY

This procedure was first described in contemporary terms in 1984[3] in a series of 23 children. Immediate haemodynamic were good, with reduction in transvalvular gradient from ~110mmHg to ~30mmHg and acceptable morbidity and mortality. Balloon aortic valvuloplasty quickly became established as the treatment of choice for children and young adults with symptomatic congenital pure aortic stenosis.

For adults, however, calcification and valvular rigidity militated against such good results. The first few cases were reported in 1986[4,5] and were quickly followed by a larger cohort.[6] Although the immediate results were encouraging, with gradient reduction from ~75mmHg to ~30mmHg, complications were not infrequent. However, the population chiefly comprised patients who were either not fit for, or had refused, surgical intervention, and as a result the Mansfield Balloon Aortic Valvuloplasty Registry was set up in 1986 to see if good results could be obtained across a broader cross-section of patients, operators and centres. 490 patients were enrolled. Acute treatment was effective, with increase in aortic valve area from 0.5cm^2 to 0.8cm^2 and a reduction in transvalvar gradient from ~60mmHg to ~30mmHg. The major complication rate, however, for the procedure was 22%, including procedural death (5%), early post-procedure death (3%), embolic phenomena (2%), tamponade (1%), and severe aortic regurgitation (1%). Vascular injury due to the large calibre of arterial sheath also accounted for an 11% morbidity.

The next large study was the NHLBI Aortic Valvuloplasty Registry.[7] Encompassing over 600 patients from multiple American centres, this Registry also demonstrated good initial haemodynamic results (valve area increased from ~0.5cm^2 to ~0.8cm^2; transvalvar gradient decreased from ~60mmHg to ~30mmHg), with a 15% 30-day mortality, and a 30% incidence of vascular complications or need for transfusion.

Follow up, however, gave disappointing results. The first studies suggested that the chance of continued clinical improvement after one year was <50%, but later studies were to prove even more discouraging, and in the last large published study of this procedure as a stand-alone treatment, Lieberman et al. reported a 'dismal' event-free survival rate of 40%, 19% and 6% at 1, 2 and 3 years respectively.[8] No other major series has been published since, and it is notable that a bibliographic search for relevant literature on aortic valvuloplasty demonstrates a publication peak between 1986 and 1989, followed by a gradual decline over the ensuing 15 years.

INDICATIONS

Indications for balloon aortic valvuloplasty in mature adults are, therefore, few, and are listed in Table 32.1.

One of the common indications for balloon aortic valvuloplasty in contemporary practice is as a bridge to aortic valve surgery. Patients with decompensated aortic stenosis who are in a critical condition and are not fit for surgery may have their chances of a successful operation increased if they have a bridging balloon valvuloplasty.[9] Clinical features which may suggest a possible role for a percutaneous bridging procedure are persisting hypotension, pulmonary oedema, renal dysfunction or poor left ventricular function despite optimal medical therapy. In these cases balloon valvuloplasty may be undertaken at an acceptable risk.

Balloon valvuloplasty forms an integral part of percutaneous aortic valve implantation. Patients who are undergoing a percutaneous valve implant will have a balloon valvuloplasty as an integral part of the procedure. This establishes how restrictive the valve is, and whether any implant difficulties are likely to be encountered, for example, if calcification is extensive.

TABLE 32.1 - INDICATIONS FOR AORTIC VALVULOPLASTY IN PATIENTS WITH SEVERE AORTIC STENOSIS
As a bridge to aortic valve replacement
As a precursor to percutaneous aortic valve implantation
Palliation of symptoms in patients unfit for surgery
Palliation prior to non-cardiac surgery
Palliation during pregnancy

Patients who are unfit for surgery due to co-morbidities and frailty may elect to undergo balloon aortic valvuloplasty in the face of disabling symptoms, aware of the risks and the likely relatively temporary nature of the symptomatic relief they may obtain.

The procedure

Patient selection is usually made on the basis of history, examination and echocardiography. As with mitral stenosis, greater degrees of calcification are felt to be associated with less good outcomes. More than Grade II aortic regurgitation is a contraindication to the procedure, and impaired left ventricular function is a predictor of poor medium-term outcome (though may equally be the primary reason for balloon valvuloplasty). Concomitant coronary disease is also a predictor of adverse outcome.

Preparation

All patients need to be carefully consented for the procedure. Patients should have a coronary angiogram to establish the extent of any coronary disease, either before or at the time of the intended valvuloplasty. This establishes the degree of risk more clearly, and adds important surgical information if the patient might transfer to theatre in the event of serious complications. For patients in extremis an intra-aortic balloon pump can be particularly helpful.

RETROGRADE APPROACH

The commonest approach to the aortic valve is via the retrograde approach. This has the advantage of directness, but the disadvantage of large bore arterial access. A 6 F venous sheath is sited from the right femoral vein, and a temporary pacing wire advanced to the right ventricular apex. This is not in expectation of complete heart block, though this can occur, but rather to stabilise the heart by rapid pacing during balloon inflation. A 12 F or 14 F arterial sheath is placed via the right femoral artery. This requires stepwise dilatations, with liberal use of fluoroscopy at the groin ensuring uncomplicated passage of the sheath. Intravenous Heparin 70iu/kg is given.

An aortogram is done in standard left anterior oblique projection to confirm that aortic regurgitation is less than moderate. The aortic valve is crossed with a straight wire on Amplatz or Feldman catheters as preferred and left ventricular versus systemic pressures are measured (using the sheath access port) to estimate the transvalvular gradient. A superstiff exchange guidewire is then taken and the distal end is pigtail-curved so that it will coil in the left ventricle minimising risk of perforation.

Balloon sizing is according to the annular dimensions of the aortic valve. In practice, this usually means that a 20 mm balloon is initially taken for women, 23 mm for men. Prior to introducing the balloon across the valve, a short burst of right ventricular pacing is tested at 210 bpm. Cardiac output is usually grossly reduced with this; systemic pressure may fall to 40 mmHg or below. Once pacing is terminated, normal rhythm and systemic pressures return. This technique is extremely effective for stabilising the balloon in the aortic valve orifice, and it is remarkable that serious sustained arrhythmias are rarely provoked.

Dilatation occurs in a stepwise fashion. Once the balloon has been de-aired in the descending aorta and introduced through the aortic valve orifice, pressure may fall significantly as the balloon now obstructs a significant part of the outflow orifice. Right ventricular pacing is started and the balloon is quickly inflated with 1:9 saline:contrast mix under fluoroscopy. The relatively low contrast content ensures rapid inflation/deflation cycles. For the first inflation, waisting of the middle of the balloon is the aim, to ensure correct positioning of the apparatus (Fig. 32.1). The patient, who has the procedure under local anaesthesia with mild sedation only, should be warned that they may feel dizzy for a few seconds. Active deflation of the balloon by hand is then undertaken. After a gentle first and a more robust second inflation of the balloon to achieve full dilatation (Fig. 32.2), the balloon is removed and a pigtail catheter introduced into the left ventricle to allow measurement of the simultaneous transvalve gradient. A third inflation may be made if the haemodynamic result is inadequate. Hand inflation of the balloon is more than adequate for this. The goal of valvuloplasty should be a 50% decrease in transvalvar gradient and a 100% increase in valve area, with a final aortic valve area of at least 1.0 cm^2. A final aortogram is done to check the degree of aortic regurgitation. Given the rather agricultural nature of the procedure, it is surprising that severe aortic regurgitation is not more common, with an incidence of ~2%.

Post-procedure, haemostasis is the most important issue given the calibre of arterial sheath used. Perclose or Prostar techniques have been advocated and may

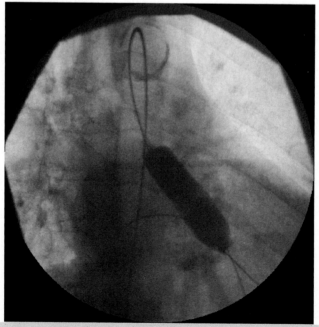

Figure 32.1:
Initial balloon inflation.

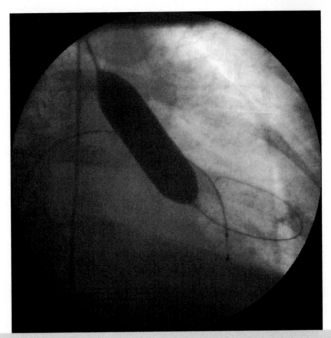

Figure 32.2:
Fully expanded balloon.

offer advantages, otherwise the sheath needs to be removed under controlled hypotension. This can successfully be achieved post valvuloplasty with an infusion of glyceryle trinitrate at low dose, aiming for a systolic pressure of 100–110 mmHg. Firm manual pressure for a minimum of 30 minutes or a femoral clamp can be applied. With the most recent balloons (e.g. BALT) the introducing sheath is now 10 F rather than 12F/14 F and, therefore, the arterial access site can be closed if preferred with an 8 F Angioseal. If manual compression is used, strict bedrest for six hours is mandatory as the moribidity and mortality from associated vascular complications is significant, and a rebleed on mobilisation can prove disastrous.

ANTEGRADE APPROACH

In this lesser used technique, the large bore introducing sheath is inserted into the femoral vein. This route greatly reduces the risk of important vascular complications, but complicates the procedure in every other respect.

Firstly, a transseptal puncture must be made, bearing in mind that the interatrial septum may lie more vertical than usual. Once in the left atrium, however, it is not simply a case of advancing the wire and balloon around the bends. Fluoroscopically the heart appears smooth, but the trabeculations, chordae and papillary muscles constitute a major hazard for the unwary and considerable care must be taken to negotiate these. If the guidewire passes between chordae, the deflated balloon, which remains bulky, may cause disruption of the mitral valve apparatus on withdrawal.

Once in the left atrium with the Mullins sheath, intravenous Heparin 70iu/kg is given. An inflated Swan-Ganz catheter is the best device for crossing into the left ventricle through the mitral valve orifice. In the left ventricle, the balloon is orientated towards the aortic valve, and the 0.025" wire advanced. The deflated balloon follows and the wire is then exchanged, if necessary via a multipurpose catheter, for a stiffer 0.035" exchange wire. The interatrial septum is dilated either with a tailor-made dilator (for example, from the Inoue system), or with an 8 mm angioplasty balloon. Again, it is important to dilate the inter-atrial septum adequately to prevent possible balloon entrapment during retrieval. Finally the 20 mm or 23 mm Z-Med or BALT balloon is advanced over the wire and sequential dilatations are made as for the retrograde approach. (Fig. 32.3 A–D) Some operators have described successful use of the Inoue balloon for this procedure. A pigtail in the aorta allows for accurate haemodynamic monitoring of the results. Post-procedure care is much less of a problem, as the 14 F sheath is venous. Simple manual compression followed by two hours bedrest is more than adequate.

COMPLICATIONS

There is no doubt that percutaneous balloon aortic valvuloplasty for adults with calcific aortic stenosis is a procedure which carries significant risk of complications. Unsurprisingly, complications are more frequent when the pre-morbid condition of the patient is worse. For patients in cardiogenic shock at the time of the procedure, in-hospital mortality approaches 50%, and two-year survival is 30%.[10]

The range of complications is shown in Table 32.2. Although per-procedural death is uncommon, 30-day mortality is ~10% across the series, with a high incidence of vascular complications. Embolic events are surprisingly uncommon, though when they occur they may be serious (Fig. 32.4).

Percutaneous aortic valve replacement

The percutaneous approach to valve replacement has been in development for over a decade in animal models. The first human implant was the Bonhoeffer pulmonary valve in 2000,[11] and this was closely followed by the Cribier aortic valve in 2002.[12] While the first was a triumph of engineering in the relatively rarified world of congenital valvular heart disease, the second caused ripples of excitement throughout the Cardiology world. Aortic stenosis is an extremely common condition, and many patients are not even considered for surgical correction. If percutaneous aortic valve replacement were to prove possible, this would open up a whole new set of possibilities for many currently untreated patients.

Antegrade approach

The antegrade approach is theoretically advantageous as it avoids very large bore arterial access, and, therefore, minimizes the risk of vascular injury. However, this approach is more technically demanding than the retrograde approach, and would significantly limit the number of interventionists able to underake the procedure, and, therefore, the companies have been keen to develop the trans-femoral arterial route by preference.

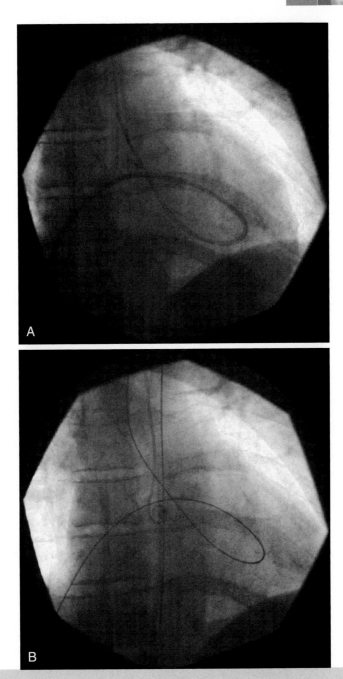

Figure 32.3:
A–D, An inflated Swan-Ganz catheter is the best device for crossing into the left ventricle through the mitral valve orifice. In the left ventricle, the balloon is orientated towards the aortic valve, and the wire advanced. The deflated balloon follows and the wire is then exchanged, if necessary via a multipurpose catheter, for a stiffer 0.035" exchange wire.

Continued

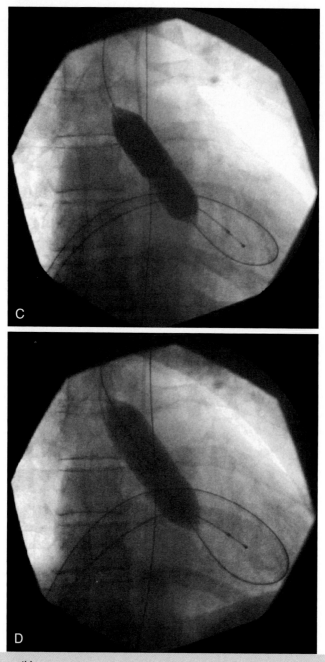

Figure 32.3, cont'd.

TABLE 32.2 - MORBIDITY AND MORTALITY ASSOCIATED WITH PERCUTANEOUS BALLOON AORTIC VALVULOPLASTY

STUDY	NO. PATIENTS	PROCEDURAL DEATH	30-DAY MORTALITY	VASCULAR COMPLICATIONS	EMBOLIC EVENTS
NHLBI	674	3%	14%	30%	5%
Letac	218	0.5%	5%	13%	2%
McKay	492	5%	8%	11%	2%

5 F femoral arterial access is made and aortograms taken in right and left anterior oblique projections. A pacing wire is advanced to the right ventricular apex from the left femoral vein for pace-stabilisation. Following transseptal puncture, heparinisation and introduction of an 8 F Mullins sheath into the left atrium, a Swan-Ganz catheter is advanced to the aorta as for the balloon valvuloplasty procedure, and the guidewire exchanged for a 260 cm 0.035" wire. Because the aortic valve prosthesis is bulky, the guidewire has to be snared and exteriorised at the right femoral artery to create an arteriovenous loop with enough inherent strength to allow the percutaneous valve to track. The interatrial septum is predilated as for balloon valvuloplasty and a 23 mm balloon inflation of the valve is made. Following this the 14 F venous sheath is removed and replaced by a 22 F venous sheath. The percutaneous valve itself is a radioopaque tubular slotted stainless steel expandable stent, 14 mm in length with an integrated trileaflet tissue valve made of three equal sections of bovine or equine pericardium, firmly sutured to the stent frame. This is crimped onto the delivery balloon with a dedicated tool, and introduced into the 22 F sheath. The whole apparatus is then advanced across the interatrial septum, into and round the left ventricular cavity and across the aortic valve. It is important not to allow the guidewire to lose its intraventricular loop during this process, otherwise the anterior leaflet of the mitral valve may be held open, which, particularly in patients with poor cardiac reserve, can lead to haemodynamic collapse. Using valvular calcification as a marker, the stent valve is positioned at the mid-point of the aortic valve and checked against the aortograms. Transoesophageal echocardiography is also frequently used, but interventionists generally find procedural fluoroscopy to be more useful than echocardiography for allowing accurate placement of the device. During rapid pacing the balloon is quickly inflated and deflated by hand with a saline/contrast mix under acquisition, ensuring full expansion of the valve stent within the aortic valve annulus. The deflated balloon is then removed.

The 260 cm guidewire is withdrawn from the right femoral vein until its distal end is in the left ventricle. A 6 F pigtail catheter is advanced over this guidewire into the left ventricle and simultaneous pressure measurements are made through this and a pigtail catheter in the aorta. Gorlin formula measurements of the aortic valve area can be made, with the aid of the Swan Ganz catheter re-positioned in the pulmonary artery. Left ventriculography and aortography is done to assess mitral or aortic regurgitation. At the end of the procedure, the venous and arterial introducers are removed and manual compression applied on the venous entry sites and right femoral artery site. Six hours post-procedure bedrest is required.

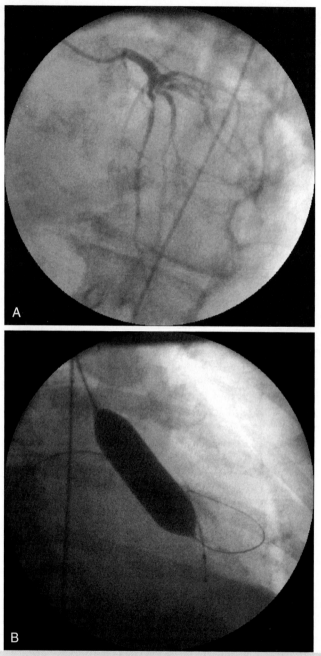

Figure 32.4:
A–D, Percutaneous balloon aortic valvuloplasty has a high incidence of vascular complications. Embolic events are surprisingly uncommon, though when they occur they may be serious.

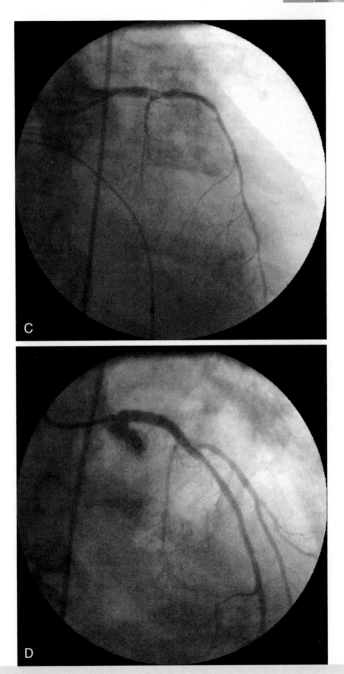

Figure 32.4, cont'd.

RETROGRADE APPROACH

As with balloon valvuloplasty, the retrograde approach has the attraction of being a more direct route, but requires very large bore arterial sheath insertion, which inevitably risks serious vascular complications. This approach has been pioneered in Rouen and Vancouver simultaneously.

The technique is broadly similar to the retrograde balloon aortic valvuloplasty approach, though direct femoral arterial access and repair needs to be made as the delivery sheath is 22 F. As with the antegrade approach, a preliminary balloon dilatation of the valve is undertaken. Once the 14 F sheath has been replaced with a 22F sheath, the valve stent is crimped onto the delivery balloon (the opposite way round to the antegrade approach!) and delivered to the valve traversing the arch.

This approach is very much 'under development' at the time of writing, and it remains to be seen whether sophistication and miniaturisation of equipment make the technically more straightforward retrograde approach a realistic prospect for valve replacement. The retrograde approach would undoubtedly open the technique up to a broader range of interventionists.

RESULTS, COMPLICATIONS, DEVELOPMENTS

As with any technique involving a wholly new treatment concept, percutaneous aortic valve implantation will not have a smooth passage into the interventional armamentarium. Early results have naturally been punctuated by failures as well as successes, and optimal techniques will take time to develop.

Cribier recently presented data from the first 29 implants involved in the pilot, I-REVIVE and RECAST studies. Peri-procedural MACE rates were significant, but as of April 2005, 14 patients were alive, three of whom had survived for more than one year following percutaneous aortic valve implantation. Webb has presented 13 retrograde cases done in Vancouver under general anaesthesia with transoesophageal echocardiographic control. Results were encouraging, with three technical failures and one procedural death.

Percutaneous valve technologies are evolving very rapidly. Recently, a 26 mm aortic valve prosthesis has been introduced. This might address the issues of valve migration and paravalvular leaks in selected patients. Femoral closure systems, preplaced through 6 F sheaths, may allow percutaneous closure of the large bore arterial access site at low risk of complications. For the intracoronary stent, many painful generations of crimped stents had to be endured before the development of the low-profile, pre-mounted third generation stent systems which we now take for granted. The same will surely happen with percutaneous aortic valve technologies.

REFERENCES

1. Safian RD, Mandell VS, Thurer RE, Hutchins GM, Schnitt SJ, Grossman W, et al. Postmortem and intraoperative balloon valvuloplasty of calcific aortic stenosis in elderly patients: mechanisms of successful dilation. J Am Coll Cardiol 1987; 9(3):655–60.

2. Roberts WC, Ko JM. Frequency by decades of unicuspid, bicuspid, and tricuspid aortic valves in adults having isolated aortic valve replacement for aortic stenosis, with or without associated aortic regurgitation. Circulation 2005; 111(7):920–5.

3. Lababidi Z, Wu JR, Walls JT. Percutaneous balloon aortic valvuloplasty: results in 23 patients. Am J Cardiol 1984; 53(1):194–7.

4. Cribier A, Savin T, Saoudi N, Rocha P, Berland J, Letac B. Percutaneous transluminal valvuloplasty of acquired aortic stenosis in elderly patients: an alternative to valve replacement? Lancet 1986; 1(8472):63–7.

5. McKay RG, Safian RD, Lock JE, Mandell VS, Thurer RL, Schnitt SJ, et al. Balloon dilatation of calcific aortic stenosis in elderly patients: postmortem, intraoperative, and percutaneous valvuloplasty studies. Circulation 1986; 74(1):119–25.

6. Cribier A, Savin T, Berland J, Rocha P, Mechmeche R, Saoudi N, et al. Percutaneous transluminal balloon valvuloplasty of adult aortic stenosis: report of 92 cases. J Am Coll Cardiol 1987; 9(2):381–6.

7. NHLBI Balloon Valvuloplasty Registry. Percutaneous balloon aortic valvuloplasty. Acute and 30-day follow-up results in 674 patients from the NHLBI Balloon Valvuloplasty Registry. Circulation 1991; 84(6): 2383–97.

8. Lieberman EB, Bashore TM, Hermiller JB, Wilson JS, Pieper KS, Keeler GP, et al. Balloon aortic valvuloplasty in adults: failure of procedure to improve long-term survival. J Am Coll Cardiol 1995; 26(6):1522–8.

9. Kitamura H, Doi T, Okabayashi H, Shimada I, Hanyu M, Saitoh Y. Percutaneous transluminal balloon aortic valvuloplasty with a small balloon as a bridge to surgery for severe aortic stenosis in an 83-year-old patient. Jpn J Thorac Cardiovasc Surg 2003; 51(10):562–4.

10. Moreno PR, Jang IK, Newell JB, Block PC, Palacios IF. The role of percutaneous aortic balloon valvuloplasty in patients with cardiogenic shock and critical aortic stenosis. J Am Coll Cardiol 1994; 23(5):1071–5.

11. Bonhoeffer P, Boudjemline Y, Saliba Z, Merckx J, Aggoun Y, Bonnet D, et al. Percutaneous replacement of pulmonary valve in a right-ventricle to pulmonary-artery prosthetic conduit with valve dysfunction. Lancet 2000; 356(9239):1403–5.

12. Cribier A, Eltchaninoff H, Bash A, Borenstein N, Tron C, Bauer F, et al. Percutaneous transcatheter implantation of an aortic valve prosthesis for calcific aortic stenosis: first human case description. Circulation 2002; 106(24):3006–8.

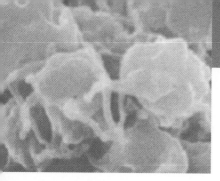

33

Pulmonary valvoplasty

J. D. R. THOMSON AND SHAKEEL A. QURESHI

KEY POINTS

▪ There are significant advantages to trans-catheter intervention compared with the surgical approach such that balloon valvoplasty is accepted as the treatment of choice for pulmonary stenosis.

▪ Patients with severe valvar obstruction require intervention but the timing of therapy in lesser degrees of obstruction is more controversial.

▪ Although by the standards of congenital cardiac catheter interventions, pulmonary valvoplasty is relatively straightforward, complications do occur and are inversely related to the age of the patient.

▪ Not only do most deaths and major complications occur when the procedure is performed in the first month of life, the neonatal group of patients are by far the most technically demanding and are frequently dependent on ductal patency to maintain pulmonary blood flow prior to transcatheter therapy requiring careful assessment of the viability of the right heart before treatment.

▪ In adult patients with pulmonary stenosis the response to balloon valvoplasty is similar to children, particularly with regard to the gradual resolution of secondary infundibular hypertrophy and longer term maintenance of gradient reduction.

▪ Patients with relatively large right ventricular outflow tracts may require the simultaneous deployment of multiple balloons for the successful relief of the stenosis.

▪ Residual gradients after immediately balloon valvoplasty often relate to infundibular stenosis, which usually resolves with time.

BACKGROUND

Although Rubio-Alvarez *et al.* described a technique for the relief of pulmonary valve stenosis using a combination of a balloon-tipped catheter and a guidewire in 1953,[1] the first successful clinical application was 21 years later, when an inflated angiographic balloon was withdrawn from the pulmonary artery into the right ventricle rupturing the valve.[2] It was the introduction of the static balloon technique in 1982 by Kan and colleagues and the demonstration by the same group that valvoplasty resulted in a significant reduction in right ventricular obstruction that led to widespread dissemination of the technique.[3,4] Prior to this, treatment for pulmonary stenosis was surgical, initially 'blind' pulmonary valvotomy using inflow occlusion, followed in later years by open valvotomy on cardiopulmonary bypass.[5,6]

The procedural, medium and long term results of balloon pulmonary valvoplasty have been robustly reported and are excellent.[7–18] There are no randomised trials of surgery and transcatheter treatment, but in the small number of comparative studies between balloon valvoplasty and surgery, transcatheter treatment has compared favourably in terms of the initial reduction of the gradient and the incidence of important complications with the additional benefit of avoiding cardiopulmonary bypass and its associated risks.[18,19] Although surgery may provide marginally more effective longer term gradient reduction,[18] pulmonary incompetence is less severe after balloon valvoplasty and there is increasing evidence of the need for pulmonary valve replacement in a proportion of patients after surgery.[20,21]

Balloon pulmonary valvoplasty is now firmly established as the treatment of choice for patients of all ages with pulmonary stenosis. Surgery for isolated pulmonary stenosis is rarely performed in the current era, the exception being those patients with severe stenosis due to valvar dysplasia unresponsive to balloon dilation. In these cases, surgical valvotomy is generally inadequate and a valvectomy is usually required.

CLINICAL ANATOMY

An understanding of the clinical anatomy of the right ventricular outflow tract is important for successful percutaneous valvoplasty. In contrast to the aortic valve, the pulmonary valve exists within a free standing muscular infundibulum unsupported by the ventricular septum or fibrous structures of the heart. Unlike the aortic valve, the pulmonary valve leaflets arise in part from both the muscular infundibulum and the arterial wall. The semilunar valve attachments of the pulmonary valve leaflets are not circumferential in the manner of a 'clover leaf', rather a more complex arrangement with longitudinal valvar extension such that the valve resembles a 'crown' with the line of attachment of the valve leaflets moving from proximal infundibular wall (muscle) to distal arterial wall.[22]

Obstructive pulmonary valve abnormalities fall into two categories. In the majority of cases, the primary abnormality is the fusion of the zone of apposition between valve leaflets. In these cases, the base of the valve does not attach in the same way as a normal pulmonary valve and frequently has a shallow line of apposition between leaflets. In extreme cases, fusion of the leaflets means that the valvar orifice is the size of a pin hole or there is no opening at all as in membranous atresia of the pulmonary valve. Successful balloon valvoplasty results from tearing of the fused areas of apposition between valve leaflets and this process occurs in the longitudinal as well as the transverse plane.

A small proportion of abnormal pulmonary valves are dysplastic with severe thickening of the valve tissue, often with myxomatous degeneration but little or any fusion along the zones of apposition.[23] In these cases, stenosis of the right ventricular outflow tract is a result of mechanical obstruction caused by the size and immobility of the valve. Pulmonary valvoplasty in patients with genuinely dysplastic valve tissue is often fruitless.

Secondary changes due to pulmonary valvar stenosis also occur. Most frequently infundibular obstruction occurs as a result of right ventricular hypertrophy, which often resolves after successful treatment of the primary valve stenosis. Ventricular fibrosis is often seen in longstanding cases of significant right ventricular obstruction and subendocardial right ventricular ischaemia and infarction are a relatively frequent finding in post mortem specimens.[24]

NATURAL HISTORY

Pulmonary stenosis is the commonest lesion with a prevalence of between 7 and 12% in live born congenital heart disease populations.[25,26]

The majority of patients with pulmonary valve abnormalities have mild pulmonary valve stenosis, which almost without exception follows a benign clinical course.[27] However, there are longitudinal data showing progression of pulmonary stenosis over time, particularly in those patients with at least moderate valvar obstruction.[28] In patients with mild pulmonary stenosis, progression of valvar obstruction can occur but rarely to the degree that treatment is required. It is also important to note that progression of stenosis is not invariable and the degree of obstruction will often remain unchanged and indeed in some instances will improve or even spontaneously resolve.[29] This is often attributed to growth of the stenotic pulmonary valve orifice.

Although valvar pulmonary stenosis is usually compatible with a normal life span, there is clear evidence of progressive damage to the right ventricular myocardium as a result of fibrosis and ischaemia in some patients with significant right ventricular outflow tract obstruction.[24] Untreated, significant pulmonary valve stenosis in adults often leads to a 'stiff' right ventricle, which, with time, may become a problem in its own right.

Infants with critical pulmonary stenosis

These patients are an important subgroup and often present with desaturation in early life due to right-to-left shunting at atrial level related to severe right ventricular outflow tract obstruction. These babies may be dependent on ductal patency to maintain adequate pulmonary blood flow and can present in extremis following closure of the arterial duct, which then requires urgent resuscitation and treatment of the underlying valve problem. In some cases a degree of right ventricular hypoplasia can occur (Fig. 33.1) and careful evaluation of the viability of the right heart prior to treatment is always required.[16]

PATIENT SELECTION AND TIMING OF INTERVENTION

Timing of intervention is a controversial issue in pulmonary stenosis. Clinical signs, symptoms, electrocardiographic changes and echocardiography all play a part in deciding when to intervene. Symptoms associated with pulmonary stenosis increase in frequency with age. Dyspnoea, fatigue and exercise intolerance are most commonly reported and are caused by inadequate cardiac output in the face of exertion. In extreme cases, in older patients, angina and sudden death (usually occurring in association with exercise) can occur. Symptoms are rare in patients without important pulmonary stenosis and, therefore, are almost always an indication for intervention.

Echocardiography and Doppler-derived transvalvar gradients are increasingly used to select patients for intervention (Fig. 33.2). In the current era, it is unusual for the decision for intervention not to have been taken by the time a patient

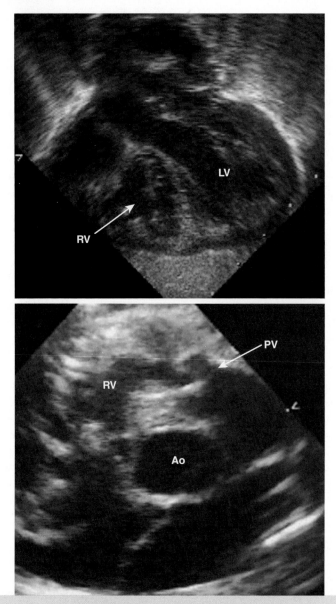

Figure 33.1:
Echocardiogram.
Critical PS in an infant with hypoplasia of the right ventricle. Four chamber view (apex to the bottom). A small but viable right ventricular cavity with considerable ventricular hypertrophy. Parasternal short axis view. Stenosed pulmonary valve with right ventricular hypoplasia and hypertrophy.
LV = Left ventricle, RV = Right ventricle, Ao = Aorta, PV = Pulmonary valve

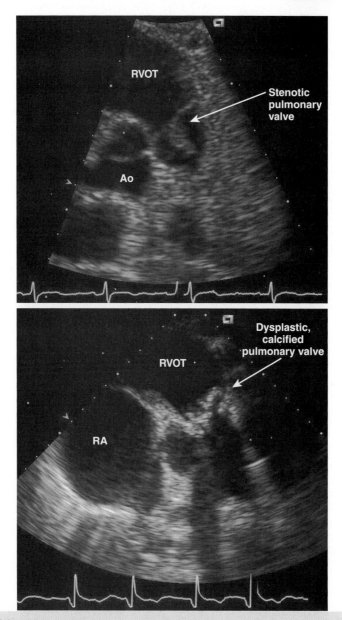

Figure 33.2:
Echocardiography.
Parasternal short axis view. Stenosed but non dysplastic pulmonary valve. Parasternal short axis view.
Dysplastic and calcified pulmonary valve in an adult. Parasternal short axis view. Colour Doppler across
a stenosed pulmonary valve. Continuous wave Doppler recording from the suprasternal notch. Peak to
peak gradient of 78 mmHg across a stenosed pulmonary valve. RVOT = Right ventricular outflow tract,
RA = Right atrium, Ao = Aortic valve

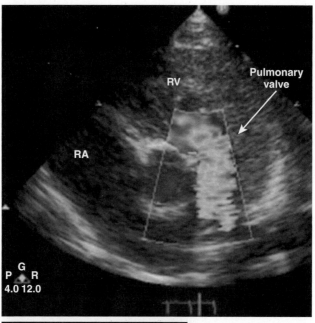

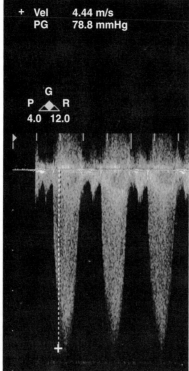

Figure 33.2, cont'd.

comes to cardiac catheterisation and as such invasive gradients are rarely used as triage tool. Most clinicians would advocate balloon pulmonary valvopasty in patients with Doppler gradients in excess of 4 m per second (equating to a peak-to-peak pressure drop of >64 mmHg), particularly if there is electrocardiographic or echocardiographic evidence of right ventricular hypertrophy.[30] Similarly there is general consensus that patients with mild pulmonary stenosis (Doppler gradient equating to a peak pressure gradient of less than 30 mmHg) do not require treatment and should be followed on an intermittent basis to monitor for progression.[27] Those patients in between (Doppler gradients between 30 and 64 mmHg) are more controversial. Many cardiologists treat these patients conservatively but there are those who argue that there are potentially deleterious long term effects on the right ventricle related to this degree of obstruction and this along with a propensity to progression of obstruction in these patients justifies intervention.[31]

There is good evidence of the effectiveness of balloon pulmonary valvoplasty for valvar stenosis in all age groups from neonates through to late adulthood.[7-18,34] In contrast to aortic valvoplasty, balloon dilation of the pulmonary valve appears effective even in adults with cusp calcification. Despite the availability of suitable equipment there is little published data on the treatment of premature and low birth weight infants with pulmonary stenosis and the exact role of the procedure in this group remains undefined with very high re-intervention rates reported in one small series (10 patients).[32]

Despite the different anatomical substrates, predicting the success of percutaneous pulmonary valvoplasty based on the pre-procedural appearance of the valve is unreliable.[8] Occasionally, surprisingly good results can be obtained in valves that appear severely dysplastic and conversely, the occasional valve with apparent isolated appositional fusion can be frustratingly resistant to balloon dilation. Thus, most interventional paediatric cardiologists would attempt balloon valvoplasty in patients fulfilling their unit criteria for intervention regardless of echocardiographic appearances of the valve.

BALLOON VALVOPLASTY

Procedure

Technically balloon pulmonary valvoplasty is relatively straightforward in infants, children and older patients. The procedure can be performed in patients under sedation but many operators prefer general anaesthesia as the temporary cessation of pulmonary blood flow is often associated with discomfort. Many operators do not routinely use anticoagulants in patients undergoing pulmonary valvoplasty, although it is the practice in some units. All patients undergoing valvoplasty procedures in our catheterisation laboratory receive prophylactic intravenous antibiotics. Initially a diagnostic right heart study is performed. Pressure measurements throughout the right heart are taken (Fig. 33.3). It is generally good practice to establish femoral arterial access to allow direct comparison of the right-sided and systemic pressures, although there are situations, particularly in smaller babies where arterial access may be undesirable. High quality angiography is a pre-requisite of successful valvoplasty and a majority of units performing this form of intervention utilise biplane fluoroscopic systems.

A right ventricular angiogram, usually obtained in the right anterior oblique (approximately 30 degrees RAO) and lateral projections, best defines the anatomy and the dimensions of the right ventricular outflow tract (Fig. 33.4). Modern fluoroscopic equipment allows for accurate measurements of the pulmonary valve annulus at the hinge points. It is generally best assessed on the lateral angiogram (Fig. 33.4).

Following the initial diagnostic study, an end-hole catheter (such as a multipurpose or Judkins right coronary catheter) is passed through the obstructed valve (this occasionally requires the aid of a hydrophilic guide wire) and a stable position in the distal left pulmonary artery is obtained. An exchange length guide-wire appropriate to the lumen of the intended balloon

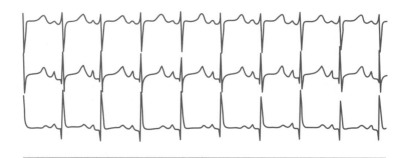

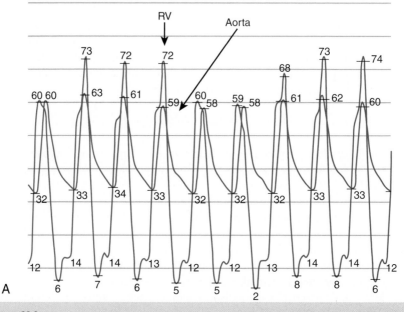

Figure 33.3:
Haemodynamics. A, Sequential right ventricular and aortic pressure measurements before pulmonary valvoplasty. B, Sequential right ventricular and aortic pressure measurements after pulmonary valvoplasty.

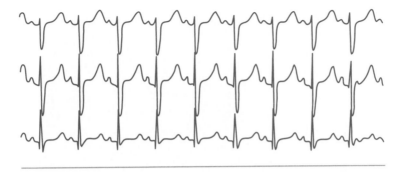

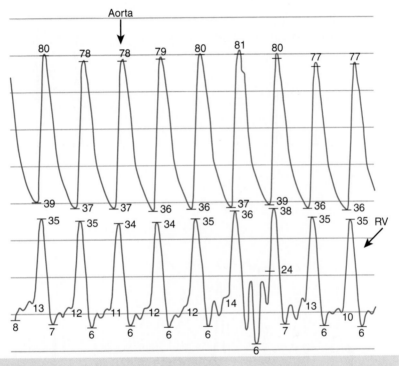

Figure 33.3, cont'd.

catheter is positioned and the guide catheter removed. Wire position is important in the execution of a successful valvoplasty and the majority of technically ineffective procedures have their origins in either a poorly supportive guidewire or inadequate wire position. A stiff exchange length guidewire positioned in the left pulmonary artery provides both the optimum line for passage of a balloon and its secure inflation but this is not an absolute pre-requisite for a successful valvoplasty. Care should be taken when using a floppy-tipped wire to ensure that the flexible distal portion is well beyond the pulmonary valve annulus otherwise the balloon will not be adequately supported and will be difficult to pass across the valve.

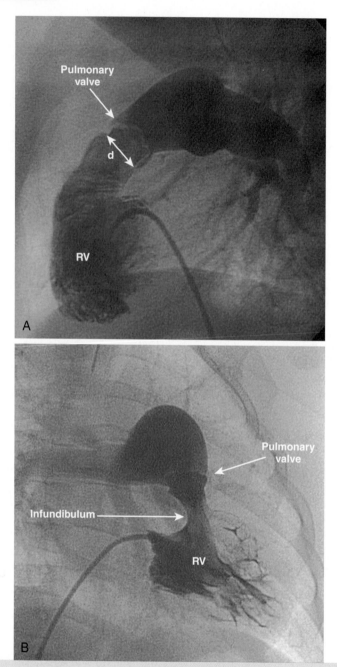

Figure 33.4:
A, Angiogram, lateral projection, d = pulmonary annular diameter. B, Angiogram, right anterior oblique projection (30°). C, Angiogram, lateral projection showing infundibular narrowing. RV = Right ventricle.

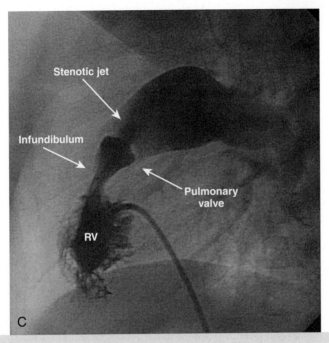

Figure 33.4, cont'd.

After establishing a good wire position, an appropriately sized balloon (see below) is advanced over the wire across the stenosed valve. Modern low profile balloons generally do not require de-airing prior to the insertion into the patient although with some larger balloons it is often advisable. Once the balloon is in the correct position, it is steadily inflated with dilute contrast (25% strength diluted with saline) using a pressure monitoring inflation device. Generally a waist is observed which disappears rapidly if the selected balloon is of the correct size and in the correct position (Fig. 33.5). It is our practice and belief that after successful abolition of the waist, there is little to be gained by further routine dilation, although some operators will routinely re-inflate on multiple occasions.

Following the valvoplasty manoeuvre, the balloon is removed and the pressure measurements repeated. Although some operators will repeat a right ventricular angiogram, it is our practice not to do this routinely. There are a number of reasons why the right ventricular pressure may remain significantly elevated (more than 50% systemic pressure). The balloon may be undersized relative to the right ventricular outflow tract and this is, of course, an indication for dilation with a larger balloon. More commonly there is a degree of pre-procedural reactive infundibular hyperplasia leading to muscular obstruction which will not respond to balloon dilation of any kind. This form of muscular overgrowth is a response to valvar stenosis and gradually resolves in the months following a successful valvoplasty.[12,13] In some cases, there may be a residual gradient relating to valvar dysplasia. In practice, the best definition of a dysplastic pulmonary valve is one which fails to respond to balloon dilation. In our

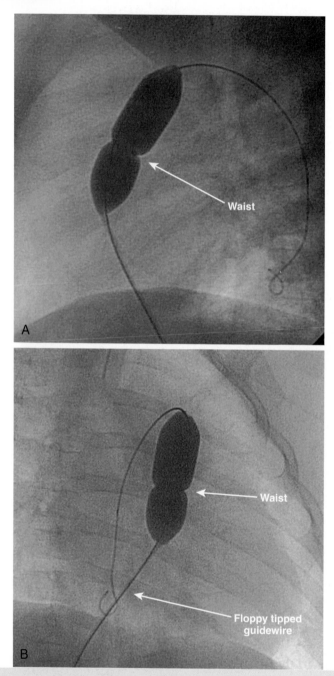

Figure 33.5:
A, Balloon inflation, lateral projection. Waist at site of pulmonary annulus. B, Balloon inflation, RAO projection (30 degrees) C, Resolution of waist, lateral projection.

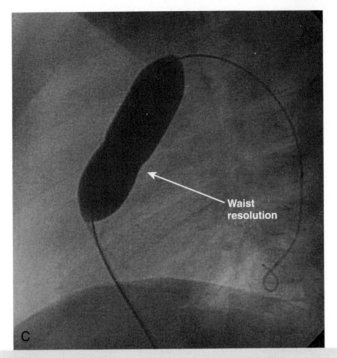

Waist resolution

Figure 33.5, cont'd.

experience, repeated dilations with progressively larger balloons are unlikely to improve the outcome, although there are anecdotal reports to the contrary.[15] Therefore, unless the balloon is undersized relative to the pulmonary valve annulus, in most instances the correct path of action with a suboptimal result is to terminate the procedure and observe the patient carefully over the coming months. Often a gradual reduction in the gradient is seen on echocardiography during the follow up period.

There are reports of the use of propanolol following balloon valvoplasty to reduce the effects of infundibular stenosis, although there is no clear evidence of a beneficial effect.[33]

TECHNICAL VARIATIONS

Dual balloon technique (Fig. 33.6): Although improved balloon technology (see below) has resulted in the production of larger diameter balloons, which are clinically effective, many operators feel there are still advantages to the dual balloon technique for dilation of larger pulmonary valves (>20 mm).[34,35] The technique requires bilateral femoral venous access. Two balloons with a combined diameter 50–60% greater than the annular measurements are inserted such that they 'kiss' when straddling the pulmonary valve.[36] When inflated, the balloons adopt an elliptical profile such that the right ventricle is vented during peak inflation. Although the procedure is safe and efficacious, and there are occasions, particularly in adult patients where such an approach

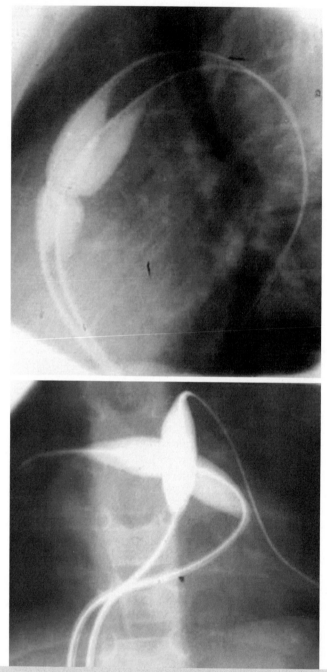

Figure 33.6:
Dual balloon technique. Lateral projection. RAO (30°) projection.

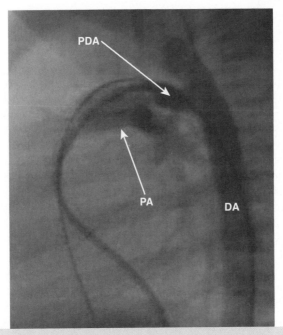

Figure 33.7:
Guidewire positioned across the ductus arteriosus in a neonate with critical PS. PA = Pulmonary artery,
PDA = Ductus arteriosus, DA = Descending aorta.

may be required, there is little firm data showing improved outcome compared with the single balloon technique and generally the marginal benefits are outweighed by the technical requirements (e.g. bilateral femoral vein access) and the need for multiple assistants.[8]

Neonates (less than one month of age): Balloon valvoplasty is technically more demanding in the neonate. Anatomically the right ventricular outflow tract can be more challenging to cross and may require the use of end-hole catheters of different shapes (Cobra or Judkins right coronary catheters are often the most useful) and small floppy tipped guidewires (0.014 or 0.018"). In addition tricuspid regurgitation and right ventricular hypertrophy add further challenges to the operator. It is important to maintain babies on a prostaglandin infusion if they have duct-dependent pulmonary stenosis.

Floppy tipped wires often have a long floppy distal segment and so in very small hearts obtaining a stable wire position can be difficult. If a persistent ductus arteriosus can be crossed with a floppy guidewire, this provides an excellent and stable pathway for the guidewire and the subsequent passage of the balloon (Fig. 33.7). After crossing the ductus arteriosus, some operators will snare the wire in the descending aorta in order to create an arterio-venous circuit for maximum stability.

These neonates can be haemodynamically fragile and in particular can react adversely to the cessation of pulmonary blood flow during balloon inflation.

Balloon valvoplasty in these patients should only be undertaken by operators experienced in the treatment of patients of this age group. In particular, the procedure requires an experienced anaesthetist.

BALLOONS

It was not until the early 1990s that the first commercially available non compliant valvoplasty balloons were constructed with the needs of the paediatric population specifically in mind (Fig. 33.8). Contemporary valvoplasty balloons are available with inflated balloon diameters ranging from 4–25 mm. Balloons are available with such low profile shafts that they can be inserted through a 3 F sheath for use in the smallest of infants. Inflation/deflation times are excellent due to modern coaxial technology, but valvoplasty balloons should only be inflated with radiographic contrast diluted with saline, as there are anecdotal reports of failure of deflation, in cases in whom dextrose solutions were used. Pre-inflation is only required in larger balloons in order to remove air bubbles which can potentially destabilise the inflated balloon position.

The majority of balloon valvoplasty procedures do not require high inflation pressures (generally valoplasty balloons operate at rated burst pressures of 3–6 atmospheres), however, high pressure balloons (burst pressures >10 atmospheres) are available and may be required in patients with severely dysplastic pulmonary valves.

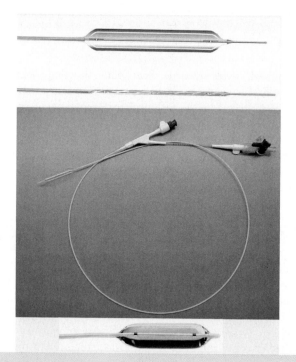

Figure 33.8:
Tyshak balloons.
Top panel shows Tyshak Mini, middle panel shows Tyshak II and lower panel shows the original Tyshak balloon – all are low profile balloons.

From the published data, a balloon to pulmonary annular diameter ratio of 1.2–1.4 appears to be optimal for effective gradient reduction.[8] Balloon to annular diameters in excess of 1.5 appear to result in right ventricular outflow tract damage in experimental animal models and may cause more pulmonary regurgitation (see below).[37]

COMPLICATIONS

The largest published series of pulmonary valvoplasty procedures (822 attempted procedures at 26 centres) reported major complications (death, tamponade, procedural tricuspid valve damage) in 0.6% of cases.[7] Minor complications such as femoral venous thromboses and tears, bleeds associated with access sites, femoral arterial thromboses, arrhythmia requiring treatment during the procedure, transient atrioventricular block and probable perforation of the right ventricular outflow tract (without apparent clinical sequelae) with guide wires are consistently reported in studies with an incidence of approximately 2–3%.

Complications are significantly more frequent in patients under one month of age. In the VACA series, the early mortality for this group was 3.5% (no reported deaths in older patients) with other complications occurring 2–3 times more frequently than in older patients.[7] Subsequent studies have consistently shown a mortality risk of 3–4% for this group of patients, related to both procedural complications and right heart hypoplasia.[11,16]

LONG TERM RESULTS

There are a number of studies reporting long term results after balloon pulmonary valvoplasty (Table 33.1). The requirement for re-intervention for residual or recurrent stenosis is reported in 0–16% of patients. Although most series contain relatively small numbers of patients and are, therefore statistically underpowered for the identification of risk factors for a suboptimal outcome, the VACA registry investigators reported long term follow-up data in a proportion of the original cohort (533 patients from the original 822) with a mean follow up time of 8.7 years. Twenty-three percent of patients had a suboptimal outcome defined as either the need for reintervention or a Doppler derived gradient of >36 mmHg.[8] From this data, adjusted risk factors for a suboptimal outcome were ascertained (Table 33.2). Patient age, presence of Noonan's syndrome (associated with valve

TABLE 33.1 - LONG TERM RESULTS AFTER PULMONARY BALLOON VALVOPLASTY

AUTHOR	YEAR	AGE GROUP	NUMBER	FU YEARS	SUBOPTIMAL OUTCOME/ REINTERVENTION RATE
McCrindle[8]	1994	All ages	533	8.7	23%Φ
Fawzy[10]	2001	Adults	87	8	6%*
Masura[15]	1993	Children	34	5.2	8.8%Φ
Peterson[18]	2003	Children	108	5.4	14.1%*
Jarrar[13]	1999	All ages	62	6.4	9.6%Φ
Rao[9]	1998	All ages	85	7	16%*
Chen[14]	1996	Adolescent/adults	53	6.9	0%

* = reintervention

Φ = either suboptimal result or reintervention

TABLE 33.2 - RISK FACTORS FOR SUBOPTIMAL OUTCOME

Small pulmonary valve hinge point
Higher immediate residual gradient

dysplasia), pre-balloon haemodynamic characteristics and the use of simultaneous balloons were not identified as risk factors for residual stenosis or restenosis.

As has been discussed previously, establishing the cause of a suboptimal outcome is not always easy. In many cases, late after the procedure, when infundibular obstruction has resolved, the cause will be residual stenosis related to valvar dysplasia unlikely to respond to further valvoplasty. There is, however, clear evidence that valvar obstruction may recur, although the mechanisms are poorly understood.[13] In this situation repeat valvoplasty is indicated and is usually effective.

For historical reasons, longer follow up data is available in surgical cohorts after treatment for pulmonary stenosis. These data show that surgically induced pulmonary incompetence in this setting is not benign and that pulmonary valve replacement is often required.[20, 21] Balloon pulmonary valvoplasty results in less pulmonary incompetence and currently progressive right ventricular dilation following transcatheter intervention has not been a problem, although clearly follow up times are shorter and, therefore, vigilance is required. It is for this reason that many operators feel it prudent to minimise the balloon to pulmonary valve annular diameter required to achieve acceptable gradient reduction at the same time minimising pulmonary incompetence.

REFERENCES

1. Rubio-Alvarez V, Limon-Larson R, Soni J. Valvulotomias intracardiacas por medio de un cateter. Arch Inst Cardiolo Mex 1953; 23:183–92.

2. Semb BK, Tjonneland S, Stake G, Aabyholm G. "Balloon valvulotomy" of congenital pulmonary valve stenosis with tricuspid valve insufficiency. Cardiovasc Radiol. 1979 Nov; 2(4):239–41.

3. Kan JS, White RI, Mitchell SE, Gardner TJ. Percutaneous balloon valvulopasty: a new method for treating congenital pulmonary stenosis. N Eng J Med 1982; 307:540–2.

4. Kan JS, White RI, Mitchell SE, Anderson JH, Gardner TJ. Percutaneous transluminal alloon valvuloplasty for pulmonary valve stenosis. Circulation 1984; 69:554–60.

5. Sellors T. Surgery of pulmonary stenosis: a case in which pulmonary valve was successfully divided. Lancet 1948; 1:988.

6. Sade RM, Crawford NC, Hohn AR. Inflow occlusion for semilunar valve stenosis. Ann Thorac Surg 1982; 33:570–5.

7. Stanger P, Cassidy SC, Girod DA, Kan JS, Lababidi Z, Shapiro SR. Balloon pulmonary valvuloplasty: results of the Valvuloplasty and Angioplasty of Congenital Anomalies Registry. Am J Cardiol. 1990 Mar 15; 65(11):775–83.

8. McCrindle BW. Independent predictors of long-term results after balloon pulmonary valvuloplasty. Valvuloplasty and Angioplasty of Congenital Anomalies (VACA) Registry Investigators. Circulation. 1994 Apr; 89(4):1751–9.

9. Rao PS, Galal O, Patnana M, Buck SH, Wilson AD. Results of three to 10 year follow up of balloon dilatation of the pulmonary valve. Heart. 1998 Dec; 80(6):591–5.

10. Fawzy ME, Awad M, Galal O, Shoukri M, Hegazy H, Dunn B, Mimish L, Al Halees Z. Long-term results of pulmonary balloon valvulotomy in adult patients. J Heart Valve Dis. 2001 Nov; 10(6):812–8.

11. Gournay V, Piechaud JF, Delogu A, Sidi D, Kachaner J. Balloon valvotomy for critical stenosis or atresia of pulmonary valve in newborns. J Am Coll Cardiol. 1995 Dec; 26(7):1725–31.

12. Fawzy ME, Galal O, Dunn B, Shaikh A, Sriram R, Duran CM. Regression of infundibular pulmonary stenosis after successful balloon pulmonary valvuloplasty in adults. Cathet Cardiovasc Diagn. 1990 Oct; 21(2):77–81.

13. Jarrar M, Betbout F, Farhat MB, Maatouk F, Gamra H, Addad F, Hammami S, Hamda KB. Long-term invasive and noninvasive results of percutaneous balloon pulmonary valvuloplasty in children, adolescents, and adults. Am Heart J. 1999 Nov; 138(5 Pt 1): 950–4.

14. Chen CR, Cheng TO, Huang T, Zhou YL, Chen JY, Huang YG, Li HJ. Percutaneous balloon valvuloplasty for pulmonic stenosis in adolescents and adults. N Engl J Med. 1996 Jul 4; 335(1):21–5.

15. Masura J, Burch M, Deanfield JE, Sullivan ID. Five year follow up after balloon pulmonary valvulplasty. J Am Coll Cardiol. 1993; 21(1):132–6.

16. Tabatabaei H, Boutin C, Nykanen DG, Freedom RM, Benson LN. Morphologic and haemodynamic consequences after percutaneous balloon valvotomy for neonatal pulmonary stenosis: Medium term follow up. J Am Coll Cardiol 1996; 27:473–8.

17. McCrindle BW, Kan JS. Long term results after balloon pulmonary valvoplasty. Circulation 1991; 83:1915–22.

18. Peterson C, Schilthuis JJ, Dodge-Khatami A, Hitchcock JF, Meijboom EJ, Bennink GB. Comparative long-term results of surgery versus balloon valvuloplasty for pulmonary valve stenosis in infants and children. Ann Thorac Surg. 2003 Oct; 76(4):1078–82.

19. O'Connor BK, Beekman RH, Lindauer A, Rocchini A. Intermediate-term outcome after pulmonary balloon valvuloplasty: comparison with a matched surgical control group. J Am Coll Cardiol. 1992 Jul; 20(1):169–73.

20. Roos-Hesselink JW, Meijboom FJ, Spitaels SEC, vanDomburg RT, vanRijen EHM, Utens EM, Bogers AJ, and Simoons ML. Long-term outcome after surgery for pulmonary stenosis (a longitudinal study of 22–33 years) Eur Heart J. 2006 Feb; 27(4):482–8.

21. Earing MG, Connolly HM, Dearani JA, Ammash NM, Grogan M, Warnes CA. Long-term follow-up of patients after surgical treatment for isolated pulmonary valve stenosis. Mayo Clin Proc. 2005 Jul; 80(7):871–6.

22. Stamm C, Anderson RH, Ho SY. Clinical anatomy of the normal pulmonary root compared with that in isolated pulmonary valvar stenosis. J Am Coll Cardiol 1998; 31:1420–5.

23. Robertson M, Benson LN, Smallhorn JS, Musewe N, Freedom RM, Moes CA, Burrows P, Johnston AE, Burrows FA, Rowe RD. The morphology of the right ventricular outflow tract after percutaneous pulmonary valvotomy: long term follow up. Br Heart J. 1987 Sep; 58(3):239–44.

24. Franciosi RA, Blanc WA. Myocardial infarcts in infants and children. A necropsy study in congenital heart disease. J Pediatr 1968; 73:309–19.

25. Abrahams DG, Wood P. Pulmonary stenosis with normal aortic root. Br Heart J. 1951; 13:519.

26. Nadas AS, Fyler DC. Pediatric cardiology. 3rd ed. Philadelphia: WB Saunders, 1972.

27. Hayes CJ, Gersony WM, Driscoll DJ, Keane JF, Kidd L, O'Fallon WM, Pieroni DR, Wolfe RR, Weidman WH. Second natural history study of congenital heart defects. Results of treatment of patients with pulmonary valvar stenosis. Circulation 1993 Feb; 87(2 Suppl):I28–37.

28. Lange PE, Onnasch DGW, Heintzen PH. Valvular pulmonary stenosis: natural history and right ventricular function. In: Doyle EF et al. eds. Pediatric cardiology. New York: Springer-Verlag, 1986.

29. Kirk CR, Wilkinson JL, Qureshi SA. Regression of pulmonary valve stenosis due to a dysplastic valve presenting in the neonatal period. European Heart Journal 1988; 9: 1027–9.

30. Gibbs JL. Interventional catheterisation. Opening up I: The ventricular outflow tracts and great arteries. Heart 2000; 83:111–15.

31. Rao PS. Indications for balloon pulmonary valvuloplasty. Am Heart J. 1988; 116:1661–2.

32. Simpson JM, Moore P, Teitel DF. Cardiac catheterization of low birth weight infants. Am J Cardiol 2001 Jun 15; 87(12):1372–7.

33. Buheitel G, Hofbeck M, Leipold G, Singer H. Incidence and treatment of reactive infundibular obstruction after balloon dilatation of critical pulmonary valve stenoses. Z Kardiol. 1999; 88(5):347–52.

34. Radtke W, Keane JF, Fellows KE, Lang P, Lock JE Percutaneous balloon valvotomy of congenital pulmonary stenosis using oversized balloons. J Am Coll Cardiol. 1986 Oct; 8(4):909–15.

35. Al Kasab S, Ribeiro P, Al Zaibag M. Use of a double balloon technique for percutaneous balloon pulmonary valvotomy in adults. Br Heart J. 1987 Aug; 58(2):136–41.

36. Rao PS. Influence of balloon size on short term and long term results of balloon pulmonary valvuloplasty. Tex Heart Inst J. 1987; 14:56–61.

37. Ring JC, Kulik TJ, Burke BA, Lock JE. Morphologic changes induced by dilation of the pulmonary valve annulus with overlarge balloons in newborn lambs. Am J Cardiol. 1984; 55:210–14.

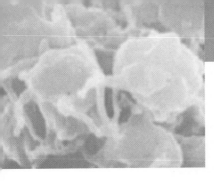

34

Percutaneous closure of patent foramen ovale, atrial septal defects and the left atrial appendage

STEPHAN WINDECKER, MD AND
BERNHARD MEIER, MD FESC FACC

KEY POINTS

- Patent foramen ovale (PFO) represents the most common persistent congenital heart anomaly.

- Atrial septal dysmorphogenesis has recently been correlated with heterozygous mutations of the cardiac homeodomain transcription factor *NKX2-5* in mice.

- Several studies established a strong association between the presence of PFO and cryptogenic stroke.

- Diagnosis of PFO requires either non-invasive imaging modalities, i.e. transthoracic or transesophageal echocardiography or invasive right heart catheterization with catheter passage of the defect.

- Patients with both PFO and ASA represent a high-risk group for recurrent paradoxical embolism and may particularly benefit from percutaneous PFO closure.

- Patients with more than one cerebrovascular event at baseline and those with complete occlusion of PFO have a significantly lower risk for recurrent stroke/TIA after device closure than with medical treatment.

- Atrial fibrillation is responsible for 16% of all ischemic strokes with about two-thirds (10% of all ischemic strokes) being cardioembolic related to left atrial thrombi.

- Strokes related to left atrial appendage (LAA) thrombus embolism are larger and more disabling compared to strokes of other etiology presumably related to the relatively large thrombus size nested within the LAA cavity.

PERCUTANEOUS CLOSURE OF INTERATRIAL SEPTAL DEFECTS

Anatomy

The atrial septum is formed by two overlapping embryological structures, the left-sided partially fibrous septum primum, and the right-sided muscular septum secundum. The foramen ovale is an opening in the atrial septum secundum, with the septum primum serving as a one-way slit allowing right-to-left shunt during in utero development (Fig. 34.1). The postnatal establishment of the pulmonary circulation with subsequent increase in left atrial pressure results in functional closure of the foramen ovale by pressing the septum primum against the septum secundum. This is generally followed by anatomical closure in the ensuing months. However, autopsy studies revealed that fusion of the two septae fails to occur in approximately 1 out of 4 people.1 Patent foramen ovale represents the most common persistent congenital abnormality. The prevalence of PFO declines

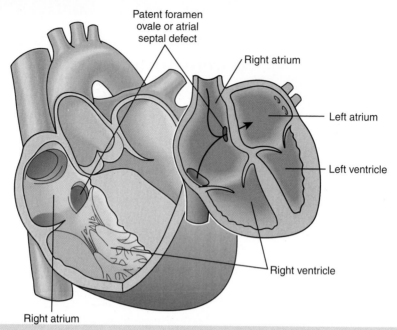

Patent foramen
ovale or atrial
septal defect

Right atrium

Left atrium

Left ventricle

Right ventricle

Right atrium

Figure 34.1:
Interatrial septal anatomy of patent foramen ovale and atrial septal defect.

in older age groups from 34% during the first three decades, to 24% for the 4th to 8th decade, and to 20% in the 9th decade and beyond. Together with the tendency of an increasing PFO size with age from a mean of 3.4 mm in the first decade to 5.8 mm in the 10th decade of life, this suggests that smaller PFOs may spontaneously close even late in life. There is no gender preference, but in females a family trait has been reported.

Atrial septal aneurysm (ASA) is a congenital abnormality of the atrial septum characterized by a redundant, amuscular membrane in the region of the fossa ovalis, corresponding to a sector of the central part of the septum primum. The prevalence of ASA in the general population varies from 1% in autopsy series to 2% in transesophageal echocardiographic studies.[2] ASA is rarely an isolated abnormality but associated with PFO in 50–85% of cases.

Atrial septal dysmorphogenesis, evident as increased frequency of PFO and atrial septal aneurysm (ASA) has recently been correlated with heterozygous mutations of the cardiac homeodomain transcription factor *NKX2-5* in mice. This observation provides first evidence that the incidence of PFO may be related to genetic factors, and that the PFO represents an index of septal dysmorphogenesis encompassing other defects such as ASA and atrial septal defects.[3]

Atrial septal defects (ASD) are 2–3 times as common in females as in males. Most cases result from spontaneous mutations, while a minority are inherited. Anatomically, ASDs are classified into four types according to their location relative to the fossa ovalis, their embryogenesis, and their size. Ostium secundum type defects are located in the region of the fossa ovalis. They are by far the most frequent ASDs (about 70%) and may be singular or multiple. Ostium primum defects are located in the lower part of the interatrial septum, anteriorly to the fossa ovalis, and may be associated with mitral or tricuspid regurgitation or a ventricular septal defect. Sinus venosus defects are located posteriorly to the fossa ovalis, in the most superior and posterior part of the interatrial septum. They are often associated with anomalous drainage of right pulmonary veins into the right atrium and with a biatrial connection of the superior vena cava (SVC). Finally, the rare coronary sinus defects, located at the site of the coronary sinus ostium, are often associated with an unroofed coronary sinus and a left atrial connection of a persistent left SVC.

Pathophysiology and clinical presentation Beside its physiologic role in the fetal circulation, the pathophysiological aspects of PFO have been increasingly appreciated giving rise to disease manifestations such as: (1) paradoxical embolism; (2) orthostatic desaturation in the setting of the platypnea-orthodeoxia syndrome; (3) refractory hypoxemia due to right-to-left shunt in patients with right ventricular infarction; or severe pulmonary disease; (4) decompression illness in divers; and (5) migraine headaches with aura.[4]

The mechanism for right-to-left shunting via PFO in patients with paradoxical embolism, right ventricular infarction, or severe pulmonary disease is related to a transient (phase after Valsalva maneuver during coughing, defecation, etc.) or permanent pressure gradient (decreased right ventricular compliance following right ventricular infarction or increased pulmonary artery pressure in case of severe pulmonary disease). In contrast, the mechanism for right-to-left shunting with the platypnea-orthodeoxia syndrome remains unknown as the right-sided pressures are typically normal and without measurable changes when assuming an upright posture during cardiac catheterization. Hypothetical explanations for right-to-left shunting in the upright position have been related to redistribution of blood flow, unequal compliance between diseased right and left heart chambers, subtle changes in pulmonary vascular resistance, and right ventricular output, or mechanical distortion of the fossa ovalis and the atria.

No etiology is found in up to 20–40% of strokes in young adults, hence they are called cryptogenic. Several case-control studies using contrast echocardiography established a strong association between the presence of PFO and cryptogenic stroke in adults aged <55 years, whereas the relationship remains less well defined in older age groups (Table 34.1).[5] Morphologic risk

TABLE 34.1 - ASSOCIATION OF PATENT FORAMEN OVALE AND ATRIAL SEPTAL ANEURYSM WITH STROKE IN YOUNG ADULTS (<55 YEARS)			
ODDS RATIO (95% CI)			
	PFO	ASA	PFO + ASA
Stroke vs non-stroke controls	3 (2–4)	6 (3–15)	16 (3–86)
Cryptogenic stroke vs known cause	6 (4–10)	7 (2–31)	17 (2–133)
Cryptogenic stoke vs non-stroke controls	5 (3–8)	19 (3–150)	24 (3–185)

Adapted from: Overell JR et al. Neurology 2000; 55:1172-9[5]

characteristics for paradoxical embolism include larger PFO size, greater degree of right-to-left shunt, association of ASA, or a prominent Eustachian valve.

The major pathophysiological consequences of an ASD are related to the shunting of blood from one atrium to the other, with the direction and amount of shunting determined by the relative compliance of the ventricles and the size of the defect. Because left atrial pressure exceeds right atrial pressure through most of the cardiac cycle, interatrial shunting is mostly left to right. This may lead to volume overload of the right heart with increased pulmonary blood flow and dilatation of the right ventricle and pulmonary arteries. Eventually, as the right ventricle fails, the left-right shunt diminishes and may even revert. The development of irreversible severe hypertensive pulmonary vascular disease (Eisenmenger's syndrome), which has a striking female preponderance, is rare in adult ASD patients, but may occur in 5–10% of untreated patients. In adults, a small ASD (Qp:Qs <1.5) usually causes no symptoms, with the exception of paradoxical embolism. It does not require closure for hemodynamic reasons. Conversely, a sizeable ASD is commonly associated with a significant shunt, with substantial hemodynamic consequences. Nonetheless, even patients with large ASDs usually report no symptoms until the 3rd or 4th decade, at which time fatigue and dyspnea on exertion may develop. In addition, the incidence of supraventricular arrhythmias, notably atrial fibrillation, increases with age and may precipitate heart failure and an increase in thromboembolic risk.

While a few patients with untreated large ASD have survived into their 8th and 9th decade of life, most patients with significant shunt die of right ventricular failure or arrhythmia in their 30s or 40s. Thus, in patients with a significant left-to-right shunt (Qp:Qs> 1.5), closure of the defect is recommended for prognostic reasons.[6, 7]

Diagnostic evaluation PFO cannot be detected on clinical grounds, but requires either non-invasive imaging modalities, i.e. transthoracic or transesophageal echocardiography or invasive right heart catheterization with catheter passage of the defect. An indirect proof of PFO can be derived with transcranial contrast Doppler ultrasound. In experienced hands the sensitivity and specificity of transcranial contrast Doppler ultrasound approaches that of transesophageal echocardiography, and the quantification of right-to-left shunt using provocative maneuvers may be more easily accomplished.[8] Multiplane transesophageal contrast echocardiography with Valsalva maneuver remains the most sensitive and specific method for the noninvasive detection of PFO (Fig. 34.2). It allows for sizing of the separation between septum primum and secundum, enables the definition of anatomic boundaries, the association with ASA, and the demonstration of a right-to-left shunt by either color flow mapping or contrast bubble injection. In addition, it allows for reliable exclusion of other potential cardiac sources of embolism. The shunt may be semi-quantitatively assessed by the amount of bubbles crossing from the right to the left atrium after intravenous injection of agitated saline.

The criteria for distinction between a floppy atrial septum and ASA vary between autopsy, transthoracic, and transesophageal echocardiography studies. ASA is generally diagnosed if the diameter of the base of the aneurysm

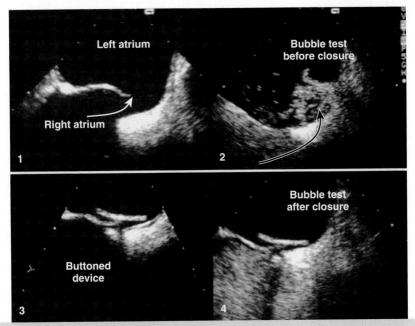

Figure 34.2:
Contrast transesophageal echocardiography for diagnosis of patent foramen ovale. The left upper picture: (1) indicates the slit-like defect with separation of septum primum and secundum acting as a one-way valve. The physiological effect of patent foramen ovale is shown in the right upper picture; (2) demonstrating a right-to-left shunt with transit of intravenously injected contrast bubbles from the right to the left atrium. The left lower picture; (3) shows the result following closure of patent foramen ovale with a Sideris Buttoned device. The right lower picture (4) indicates complete closure of patent foramen ovale without transit of contrast bubbles from the left to the right atrium.

exceeds 15 mm, and the excursion of the interatrial septum 10–15 mm in total amplitude.

The confirmation of paradoxical emboli through a PFO is a diagnostic challenge. The documentation of a thrombus crossing the PFO is rarely possible (Fig. 34.3). The diagnosis of paradoxical embolism is essentially done by exclusion, based on three presumptive criteria: (1) the presence of a right-to-left shunt; (2) the absence of a left-sided thrombo-embolic source, and; (3) the detection of venous thrombosis, thrombus in the right heart, or pulmonary embolism. In contrast, the diagnosis of orthostatic desaturation related to PFO in the setting of the platypnea-orthodeoxia syndrome can be definitely established by arterial blood gas analysis demonstrating desaturation in the upright position or by tilt-table contrast transesophageal echocardiography.

An ASD can be suspected clinically based on history and physical examination. However, the symptomatology (dyspnea, fatigue, and palpitations) is nonspecific, and the abnormalities on physical examination are subtle (soft ejection-type systolic murmur from the relative pulmonary stenosis, characteristic wide and fixed splitting of the 2nd heart sound, right ventricular impulse palpable in patients with large ASDs). Thus, they may go undetected for decades. The ECG may show right-axis deviation and incomplete right bundle branch block.

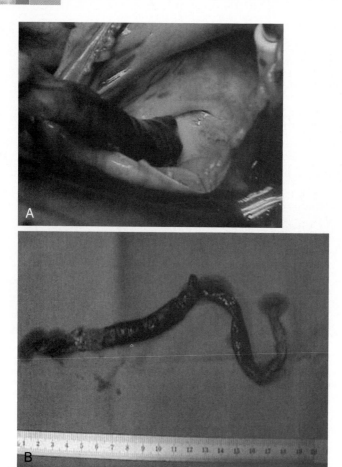

Figure 34.3:
A, Large thrombus as viewed from the right atrium lodged in the patent foramen ovale in a patient presenting with acute onset of shortness of breath and pulmonary embolism. Proven paradoxical embolism. B, Thrombus following emergency surgical resection.

Left-axis deviation occurs with ostium primum defects. Chest radiography may show prominent pulmonary arteries, and cardiomegaly from atrial and ventricular enlargement. Most ostium primum and secundum ASDs are readily diagnosed by transthoracic echocardiography, with direct visualization of the defect. Transesophageal echocardiography is useful for precise anatomical characterization, especially if percutaneous closure is intended, since it allows for determination of the septal rim separating the defect from neighboring cardiac structures. In addition, it is essential to identify multiple ASDs, sinus venous or coronary sinus defects, and anomalous pulmonary venous drainage.

Treatment Initial techniques of percutaneous ASD closure were documented by King *et al.* in the 1970s, Rashkind in the 1980s, and Sideris in the 1990s.

After Bridges *et al.*[9] first proposed that percutaneous PFO closure would reduce the incidence of recurrent stroke, this procedure has been shown feasible and safe using a variety of devices in numerous studies. In these studies, the success rate varied from 98 to 100% with complication rates between 0 and 10%. Complete PFO closure was achieved in 51 to 100% of patients, and the reported yearly recurrence rate varied between 0 and 3.4%. In our own experience, device implantation was successful in 98% of 80 cases, with an actuarial annual risk of recurrence of 2.5% for TIA, 0% for stroke, and 0.9% for peripheral emboli (combined end point 3.4%) over five years of follow up. We found that a post-procedural transseptal right-to-left shunt was a predictor of recurrent paradoxical embolism with a relative risk of 4 (95% CI 1–18, p=0.03).[10] The presence of ASA had no impact on the prognosis after percutaneous PFO closure. Since patients with both PFO and ASA are thought to represent a high-risk group for recurrent paradoxical embolism, this patient population may particularly benefit from percutaneous PFO closure.[11]

In contrast to the earlier devices initially developed for closure of secundum ASDs, dedicated PFO closure devices have a lower risk of embolization and a higher closure potential (complete closure in >95% of patients) (Fig. 34.4 and Table 34.2). Figure 34.5 A–F illustrates an example of percutaneous PFO closure using the Amplatzer PFO Occluder. After venous access is gained following local anesthesia via the right femoral vein, the PFO is crossed using a Multipurpose catheter. The Multipurpose catheter is then exchanged for a device-specific delivery system. Its tip is placed into the left atrium. The left-sided disk is then deployed and gently pulled back against the atrial septum under fluoroscopic guidance in a left anterior oblique projection. To deploy the right atrial disc, tension is maintained on the delivery cable while the delivery sheath is further withdrawn. A right atrial contrast angiography by a hand injection through the sidearm of the delivery sheath serves to delineate the atrial septum. The so-called Pacman sign refers to the aspect of the device on fluoroscopy that should be achieved before release (Fig. 34.6). Transesophageal or preferably intracardiac echocardiography can also be used to ascertain correct device position. Finally, the device is released from the delivery cable and hemostasis is achieved by manual compression of the femoral vein. Antibiotics during the intervention are commonplace, and prevention against endocarditis is recommended for a few months until the device is fully covered by tissue. Potential complications arising from percutaneous device closure of PFO include device embolization, air embolism, tamponade, retroperitoneal hematoma (inadvertent femoral artery puncture during venous access), and thrombus formation on the occluder device. Follow-up treatment for antithrombotic protection until full device endothelialization includes acetylsalicylic acid (80–300 mg per day) for a few months, with the addition of Clopidogrel (75 mg per day). The incidence of thrombus formation on ASD or PFO closure devices was reportedly low (<7%) in a large prospective study, with most thrombi resolving quickly with anticoagulation therapy.[12] There was, however, a significantly different propensity for thrombosis among the devices. At 3–6 months after device closure, a transesophageal echocardiographic examination is repeated to assess for a residual shunt following endothelial overgrowth and exclude thrombosis of the device.

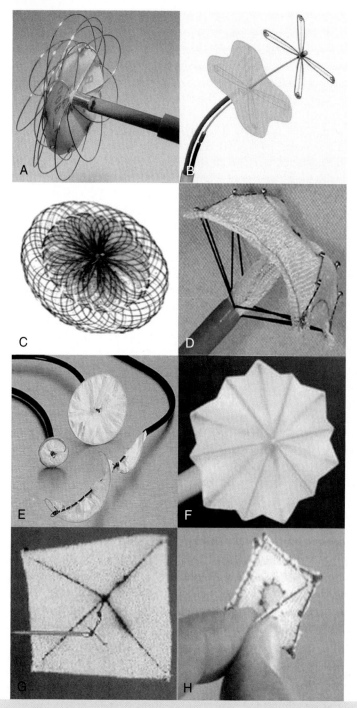

Figure 34.4:
Currently available devices. A, SolySafe. B, Premere. C, Amplatzer PFO Occluder. D, STARFlex.
E, Helex Septal Occluder. F, Transseptal device. G, Buttoned device. H, Angel Wings device.

TABLE 34.2 - CURRENTLY AVAILABLE PERCUTANEOUS PFO CLOSURE DEVICES. THE ASDOS AND DAS (ANGEL-WINGS OCCLUDER) ARE NO LONGER AVAILABLE FOR PERCUTANEOUS TRANSSEPTAL OCCLUSION PROCEDURES

	AMPLATZER PFO OCCLUDER	STARFLEX SEPTAL OCCLUDER	PFO STAR	SIDERIS BUTTONED OCCLUDER	SEPTAL HELEX OCCLUDER	PFO PREMERE CLOSURE SYSTEM
Manufacturer	AGA Medical Corporation	Nitinol Medical Technologies, Inc.	Applied Biometrics, Inc.	Custom Medical Devices	W.L. Gore & Associates Inc.	St. Jude Medical
Design	two self-expandable, round Nitinol discs interconnected by a thin flexible waist	Double umbrella with eight flexible metal arms covered with Dacron patches connected by a single post	two square components with four-arm, stainless steel wire cross covered with Dacron patches	two square components with wire skeleton and polyurethane cover, a counterocclucer, a counteroccluder and a button loop occluder	Two opposing discs formed by a single nitinol wire with a patch of polytetrafluoroethylene	Two square components with flexible nitinol wires cross covered with Dacron patch
PFO dedicated	Yes	No	Yes	No	No	Yes
Centering	non-centering	self-centering with help of microsprings	non-centering	non-centering	Non-centering	Non-centering
Fixation	passive countertension	passive countertension	passive countertension	sutured counterbutton	Passive and active with locking mechanism	Passive and active with locking mechanism
Device size	right atrial disc 25, 35 mm	23, 33, 40 mm	umbrella size 22, 26, 30 mm	umbrella size 15–50 mm	Diameter 15, 20, 25 mm	Diameter 15, 20, 25 mm
Delivery Sheath	8–9F	10–11F	10–13F	11–13F	9F	11F
Advantages	fully retrievable fully repositionable easy delivery		Small profile device	inexpensive	Small profile Fully retrievable Fully repositionable Retention suture	Fully retrievable Low surface profile of left atrial anchor Retention suture
Disadvantages	– bulky right atrial disc	– not easily repositionable	– not easily repositionable – high incidence of air embolism mediated through sheath	– complex multistep implantation procedure – not easily repositionable – spontaneous unbuttoning with device embolization	Potential for wire fracture	Too small for large floppy atrial septum

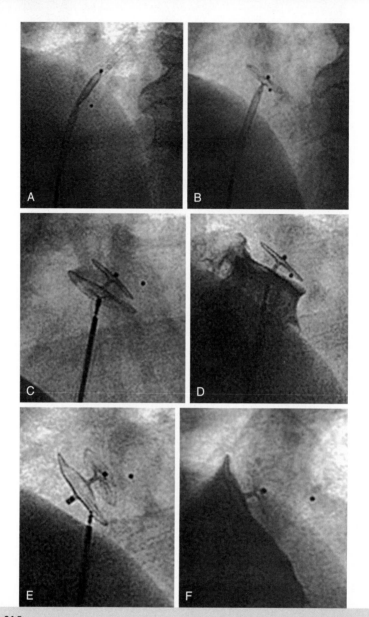

Figure 34.5:
A–F: Percutaneous PFO closure using the Amplatzer PFO Occluder (left cranial oblique view).
A, The constrained Amplatzer PFO Occluder is advanced within the Amplatzer delivery sheath, which is positioned across the PFO in the left atrium. B, The left atrial disc is deployed by withdrawing the delivery sheath and then gently pulled against the interatrial septum. C, Further retention of the delivery sheath under tension of the left atrial disc against the interatrial septum allows for release of the right atrial disc. The device has reassumed its double disc shape connected by a thin waist, passing across the PFO. D, A right atrial contrast injection by hand through the delivery sheath opacifies the right side of the interatrial septum, confirming a correct position of the device. Note the nearly horizontal orientation of the Amplatzer PFO Occluder and the indentation of the septum by the lower part of the disc. This results from the tension of the delivery cable upon the device. E, Release of the device from its delivery cable by counter-clockwise rotation. The device assumes the more perpendicular position of the interatrial septum. F, Control right atrial angiography by hand injection through the sheath delineating the right atrial septum and correct device position. The left atrial septum can be visualized during the levo-phase. Obtained with permission from Windecker S, Meier B. ACC Current Journal Review May/June 2002; 97–101; published by Elsevier Science, Inc.

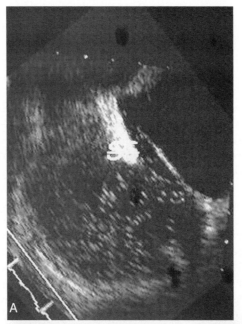

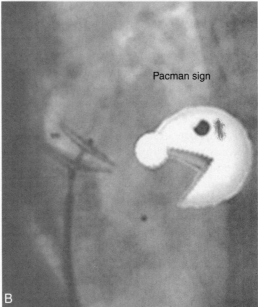

Pacman sign

Figure 34.6:
Echocardiographic and angiographic landmarks for adequate placement of a percutaneously inserted double-umbrella closure device. A, The echocardiographic appearance of the thick septum secundum (SS), which is sandwiched by the Amplatzer PFO occluder. B, Shows the correct position of an Amplatzer PFO Occluder as seen during right atrial contrast dye injection while still attached to the delivery cable in a left anterior oblique projection with cranial tilt. The two disks form two lines almost parallel in the inferior part, where the membranous part of the septum primum barely divides them. In the superior part the two disks are gaping at a certain angle as they embrace the wedge–like septum secundum. The insert shows the arcade figure 'Pacman' gobbling up a dot and providing the name Pacman sign in anology.

If the PFO proves completely closed, anti-thrombotic medication can be discontinued. In case of persistence of a small shunt, we recommend the continuation of acetylsalicylic acid and a further transesophageal echocardiogram after 1–2 years. Small residual shunts may close late. In case of persistence of a large residual shunt, implantation of a second device can be considered, which results in complete closure in most cases.

Comparison between medical therapy and percutaneous PFO closure for secondary prevention of stroke/TIAs has been reported in a case-control study[13] and in a meta-analysis of observational studies.[14] In our experience based on an analysis of patients with cryptogenic stroke and PFO referred to our university hospital-based stroke center, percutaneous PFO closure proved at least as effective as medical treatment. In patients with more than one cerebrovascular event at baseline and those with complete occlusion of PFO, there was a significantly lower risk for recurrent stroke/TIA after device closure than with medical treatment (Fig. 34.7A–B). In a recent systematic review of the relative benefits of percutaneous PFO closure compared with medical treatment, Khairy et al.[14] also reported a protective effect of percutaneous PFO closure compared with medical treatment on stroke/TIA recurrence (annual incidence 2% vs. 5%; relative risk 0.4, 95% CI 0.2–0.6, p<0.0001). At one year follow up, 1 of every 23 patients undergoing percutaneous PFO closure was prevented from recurrent stroke/TIA compared with medical treatment. Several ongoing, randomized trials compare percutaneous PFO closure with medical treatment in patients with cryptogenic stroke and PFO. Until the outcomes of these trials are known, there are no data to conclusively support PFO closure for paradoxical embolism.

Percutaneous ASD closure is quite similar to percutaneous PFO closure, as described above, with the exception that most centers use transesophageal or intracardiac echocardiographic guidance, and that balloon sizing of the defect is recommended in order to choose the appropriate device size. The almost invariably employed Amplatzer ASD occluder is selected about 1–5 mm larger than the ASD diameter as assessed during balloon sizing of the defect. If a balloon cannot be stabilized in the ASD, the device is oversized by 5–10 mm, assuming a nonrobust rim. Partial anomalous pulmonary venous drainage should have been excluded using preprocedural transesophageal echocardiography. Most small to moderate ostium secundum ASDs (<25 mm) can be closed percutaneously. Some operators exclude patients without a rim of tissue of at least 5 mm from the margins of the defect to the adjacent mitral and tricuspid valves, SVC, right upper pulmonary vein, and coronary sinus. Both the incidence of compete closure (98%) and the periprocedural complications appear similar to contemporary surgical closure.

PERCUTANEOUS CLOSURE OF THE LEFT ATRIAL APPENDAGE

Atrial fibrillation

Atrial fibrillation is the most common sustained cardiac arrhythmia and is a strong, independent risk factor for stroke and mortality. The incidence of the arrhythmia increases with age and affects approximately 5% of people at age 70 years and 10% of people >80 years of age. Atrial fibrillation is responsible for 16% of all ischemic strokes with about two-thirds (10% of all ischemic strokes)

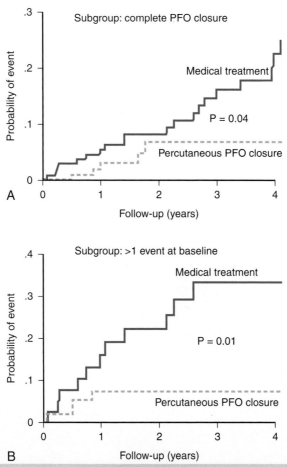

Figure 34.7:
A Probability of recurrent stroke or transient ischemic attack stratified for medical treatment (continuous line) and percutaneous patent foramen ovale (PFO) closure (dashed line) in the subgroup of patients with complete PFO occlusion. B Probability of recurrent stroke or transient ischemic attack stratified for medical treatment (continuous line) and percutaneous patent foramen ovale (PFO) closure (dashed line) in the subgroup of patients with more than one cerebrovascular event at baseline. Obtained with permission from Windecker S *et al*. J Am Coll Cardiol 2004; 44:750–8 published by Elsevier Science, Inc.[13]

being cardioembolic related to left atrial thrombi.[15] Strokes related to atrial fibrillation are particularly large and disabling, presumably due to the relatively large thrombi size. While rhythm control does not appear to reduce the risk of stroke, oral anticoagulation with Vitamin K antagonists constitutes the mainstay of therapy by reducing the stroke risk by 65% compared with placebo and 45% compared with Aspirin.[16] However, there is marked underuse of Vitamin K antagonist therapy in patients with atrial fibrillation related to the narrow therapeutic window, variability in pharmacokinetics, contraindications and fear of bleeding complications (0.5% annual risk of cerebral hemorrhage).

Left atrial appendage

The trabeculated left atrial appendage (LAA) is a remnant of the embryonic left atrium, whereas the smooth walled left atrial cavity is formed by the outgrowth of the pulmonary veins. The LAA is lined by endothelium and contains pectinate muscles, which run largely parallel to each other and give rise to the trabeculated surface.[17] The LAA lies anterolaterally in the left atrioventricular sulcus and is in close contact with the pulmonary artery superiorly and the left ventricular free wall inferiorly. The anatomy of the LAA is rather complex with a windsocklike configuration consisting of multiple lobes and a narrow junction, which is connected to the left atrium (Figs. 34.8 and 34.9).[18] The size of the LAA varies considerably with an orifice measuring 5–27 mm in diameter and a LAA length measuring 16–51 mm. The LAA has been considered a decompression chamber at times of increased atrial at pressure due to its high distensibility, the anatomical location high in the left atrium and the ability to secrete ANF.

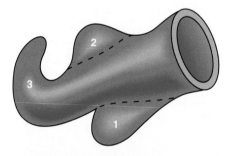

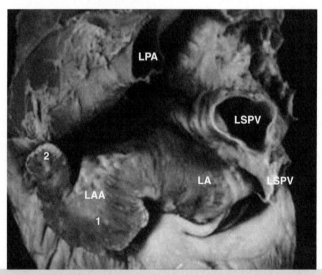

Figure 34.8:
LAA, left atrial appendage; LIPV, left inferior pulmonary vein; LPA, left pulmonary artery; LSVP, left superior pulmonary vein schematic diagram of LAA with typical windsock-like appearance and multiple lobes (1–3) anatomic specimen of LAA with two lobes as viewed from the outside Figure obtained with permission from Veinot JP *et al.* Anatomy of the normal left atrial appendage. Circulation 1997;96:3112-3115, figure 2.[18]

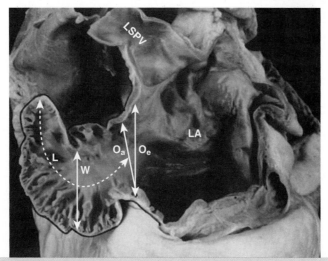

Figure 34.9:
LAA, left atrial appendage; Oe, echocardiographic orifice; Oa, anatomic orifice; L, length; W, width; LA, left atrium; LSVP, left superior pulmonary vein Anatomic specimen of LAA as viewed when opened from the left atrium (LA). Note the landmarks for anatomic and echocardiographic measurements of the LAA. Figure obtained with permission from Veinot JP *et al*. Anatomy of the normal left atrial appendage. Circulation 1997;96:3112-3115, figure 1.[18]

Atrial fibrillation not only affects remodelling of the left atrium but also of the LAA. Thus, LAA casts of patients with atrial fibrillation have been found more voluminous with larger orifices and fewer branches compared with patients in normal sinus rhythm. In addition, appendage Doppler flow velocities and LAA ejection fraction have been observed in patients with atrial fibrillation. These pathological changes result in stasis and predispose to thrombus formation within the LAA cavity (Fig. 34.10). Of note, transesophageal echocardiographic studies revealed that >90% of all thrombi related to atrial fibrillation originate from the LAA.[19] Unfortunately, strokes related to LAA thrombus embolism are larger and more disabling compared to strokes of other etiology presumably related to the relatively large thrombus size nested within the LAA cavity.

Percutaneous obliteration of the left atrial appendage

The pivotal observation that the vast majority (90%) of thrombi related to stroke in patients with atrial fibrillation originated from the LAA, stirred the therapeutic interest to obliterate the LAA as a means of stroke prophylaxis in patients with atrial fibrillation.[19] Indeed, it has become common practice to remove the LAA at the time of mitral valve surgery, and it is also routine part of the surgical MAZE procedure in patients with atrial fibrillation. Currently, a randomized clinical trial examines the potential of surgical LAA amputation to reduce stroke risk in patients at high risk for the development of atrial fibrillation undergoing heart surgery.[20]

Recently, a dedicated device for LAA obliteration via the percutaneous route was introduced. The Percutaneous Left Atrial Appendage Occluder (PLAATO™) system consists of the implant (Fig. 34.11) made of a nitinol metal cage with

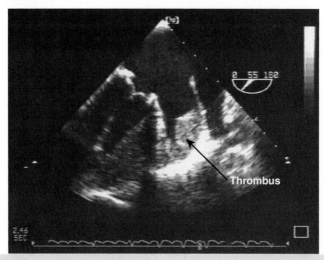

Figure 34.10:
LAA, left atrial appendage Transesophageal echocardiography of LAA revealing a thrombus attached to LAA wall in a patient with atrial fibrillation.

multiple outwardly bent anchors covered by a polytetrafluoroethylene (PTFE) membrane, and the delivery catheter, which houses the restrained implant.[21]

The implantation procedure is commenced by femoral venous puncture followed by transseptal access to the left atrium using routine technique. The transseptal sheath is exchanged for the delivery catheter, which either directly or guided by a diagnostic catheter is used to perform an angiogram of the LAA to determine the implant size. Following placement of the delivery catheter within the LAA, the implant is positioned by withdrawal of the catheter from the LAA.

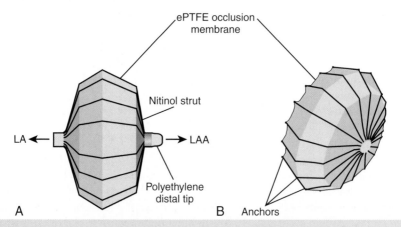

Figure 34.11:
LA, left atrium; LAA, left atrial appendage; ePTFE, expanded polytetrafluoroethylene PLAATO implant consisting of a nitinol metal cage with outward bent anchors and covered with ePTFE. Figure obtained with permission from Nakai T *et al*. Percutaneous Left Atral Appendage Occlusion (PLAATO) for preventing cardioembolism. Circulation 2002; 105:2217–2222, figure 1.[21]

The implant position is checked by a series of criteria including effective occlusion of the LAA by the device, a residual compression (>10%) of the device and a wiggling manoevre.[22] Device embolization is prevented by careful assessment of the above release criteria, oversizing the implant relative to the measured parameters by 20–40% and the anchors on the implant surface. In case of unsatisfactory results the device is fully retrievable and can be collapsed in the delivery sheath for another placement attempt. Animal studies revealed complete LAA occlusion, no evidence for thrombi on the implant surface and complete healing three months after device implantation (Figs. 34.12 A–B and 34.13).

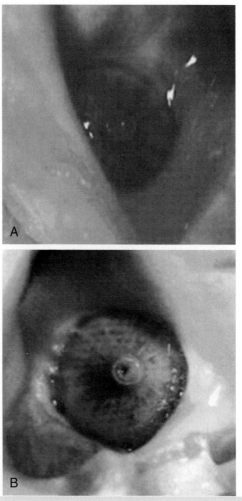

Figure 34.12:
A and B: A 1 month B 3 months. LAA, left atrial appendage; PLAATO, percutaneous left atrial appendage occlusion device. Anatomic specimen of LAA with device one and three months after PLAATO implantation in dogs. Note the snug fit of the implant and the endothelialization of the device surface. Figure obtained with permission from Nakai T *et al*. Percutaneous Left Atral Appendage Occlusion (PLAATO) for preventing cardioembolism. Circulation 2002;105:2217–2222, figure 4.[21]

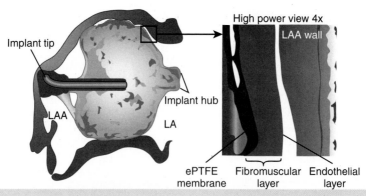

Figure 34.13:
LAA, left atrial appendage; PLAATO, percutaneous left atrial appendage occlusion device Light
microscopic specimen 3 months after PLAATO implantation in a dog. Note the device apposition
against the LAA endocardial surface without evidence of residual gaps. Figure obtained with permission
from Nakai T *et al.* Percutaneous Left Atral Appendage Occlusion (PLAATO) for preventing
cardioembolism. Circulation 2002;105:2217–2222, figure 5.[21]

The clinical performance of the device has been investigated in a recent study of
87 patients with atrial fibrillation and at least one high risk feature for embolic
stroke and a contraindication for treatment with Vitamin K antagonists. Patients
received Aspirin indefinitely and Clopidogrel for a duration of six months. The
procedure was successful in 86 (99%) patients and complicated by hemopericardium
in 6 (8%) patients. During follow up two deaths, one minor stroke, two transient
ischemic attacks and three gastrointestinal bleeds were observed.

The ease of use of the Amplatzer device for closure of PFO and atrial septal
defects led to the investigation of the Amplatzer technique for percutaneous
obliteration of the LAA. Percutaneous LAA obliteration using the Amplatz technique
has been reported in 16 patients with atrial fibrillation at high risk for stroke and
with a contraindication for therapy with Vitamin K antagonist.[23] The procedure was
successful in 15 (94%) patients and complicated by device embolization in one
patient. During follow up of five patient years no device related complications or
embolic events noted. In addition, the LAA was occluded in all successfully treated
patients without evidence of thrombosis at the atrial side of the device.

Thus, percutaneous LAA obliteration has been shown feasible in patients with
atrial fibrillation using the LAA dedicated PLAATO device and the Amplatzer
Septal Occluder. The incidence of complications appears acceptable in this
population at high risk of stroke and contraindications for Vitamin K antagonist
therapy. Future studies will further elaborate on the mid and long-term safety of
percutaneous LAA obliteration. Furthermore, the therapeutic efficacy of
percutaneous LAA obliteration compared to medical treatment with Vitamin K
antagonists or the novel ximelagatran to prevent thromboembolism.

REFERENCES

1. Hagen PT, Scholz DG, Edwards WD. Incidence and size of patent foramen ovale during the first
    10 decades of life: an autopsy study of 965 normal hearts. Mayo Clin Proc 1984; 59:17–20.

2. Agmon Y, Khandheira BK, Meissner I, *et al*. Frequency of atrial septal aneurysms in patients with cerebral ischemic events. Circulation 1999; 99:1942–1944.

3. Biben C, Weber R, Kesteven S, *et al*. Cardiac septal and valvular dysmorphogenesis in mice heterozygous for mutations in the homeobox gene Nkx2-5 [In Process Citation]. Circ Res 2000; 87:888–95.

4. Meier B, Lock JE. Contemporary management of patent foramen ovale. Circulation 2003; 107:5–9.

5. Overell JR, Bone I, Lees KR. Interatrial septal abnormalities and stroke: a meta-analysis of case-control studies [In Process Citation]. Neurology 2000; 55:1172–9.

6. Campbell M. Natural history of atrial septal defect. Br Heart J 1970; 32:820–6.

7. Konstantinides S, Geibel A, Olschewski M, *et al*. A comparison of surgical and medical therapy for atrial septal defect in adults. N Engl J Med 1995; 333:469–73.

8. Di Tullio M, Sacco RL, Venketasubramanian N, Sherman D, Mohr JP, Homma S. Comparison of diagnostic techniques for the detection of a patent foramen ovale in stroke patients. Stroke 1993; 24:1020–4.

9. Bridges ND, Hellenbrand W, Latson L, Filiano J, Newburger JW, Lock JE. Transcatheter closure of patent foramen ovale after presumed paradoxical embolism. Circulation 1992; 86:1902–8.

10. Windecker S, Wahl A, Chatterjee T, *et al*. Percutaneous closure of patent foramen ovale in patients with paradoxical embolism: long-term risk of recurrent thromboembolic events [see comments]. Circulation 2000; 101:893–8.

11. Wahl A, Krumsdorf U, Meier B, *et al*. Transcatheter treatment of atrial septal aneurysm associated with patent foramen ovale for prevention of recurrent paradoxical embolism in high-risk patients. J Am Coll Cardiol 2005; 45:377–80.

12. Krumsdorf U, Ostermayer S, Billinger K, *et al*. Incidence and clinical course of thrombus formation on atrial septal defect and patient foramen ovale closure devices in 1,000 consecutive patients. J Am Coll Cardiol 2004; 43:302–9.

13. Windecker S, Wahl A, Nedeltchev K, *et al*. Comparison of medical treatment with percutaneous closure of patent foramen ovale in patients with cryptogenic stroke. J Am Coll Cardiol 2004; 44:750–8.

14. Khairy P, O'Donnell CP, Landzberg MJ. Transcatheter closure versus medical therapy of patent foramen ovale and presumed paradoxical thromboemboli: a systematic review. Ann Intern Med 2003; 139:753–60.

15. Hart RG, Halperin JL. Atrial fibrillation and stroke: concepts and controversies. Stroke 2001; 32:803–8.

16. Hart RG, Halperin JL, Pearce LA, *et al*. Lessons from the Stroke Prevention in Atrial Fibrillation trials. Ann Intern Med 2003; 138:831–8.

17. Al-Saady NM, Obel OA, Camm AJ. Left atrial appendage: structure, function, and role in thromboembolism. Heart 1999; 82:547–54.

18. Veinot JP, Harrity PJ, Gentile F, *et al.* Anatomy of the normal left atrial appendage: a quantitative study of age-related changes in 500 autopsy hearts: implications for echocardiographic examination. Circulation 1997; 96:3112–15.

19. Blackshear JL, Odell JA. Appendage obliteration to reduce stroke in cardiac surgical patients with atrial fibrillation. Ann Thorac Surg 1996; 61:755–9.

20. Crystal E, Lamy A, Connolly SJ, *et al.* Left Atrial Appendage Occlusion Study (LAAOS): a randomized clinical trial of left atrial appendage occlusion during routine coronary artery bypass graft surgery for long-term stroke prevention. Am Heart J 2003; 145:174–8.

21. Nakai T, Lesh MD, Gerstenfeld EP, Virmani R, Jones R, Lee RJ. Percutaneous left atrial appendage occlusion (PLAATO) for preventing cardioembolism: first experience in canine model. Circulation 2002; 105:2217–22.

22. Sievert H, Lesh MD, Trepels T, *et al.* Percutaneous left atrial appendage transcatheter occlusion to prevent stroke in high-risk patients with atrial fibrillation: early clinical experience. Circulation 2002; 105:1887–9.

23. Meier B, Palacios IF, Windecker S, *et al.* Transcatheter Left Atrial Appendage Occlusion With Amplatzer Devices to Obviate Anticoagulation in Patients With Atrial Fibrillation. Catheter Cardiovasc Interv 2003; in press.

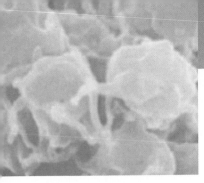

35

Septal ablation for HCM

AMY L. SEIDEL, MD, SAMIR R. KAPADIA, MD,
HARRY M. LEVER, MD AND E. MURAT TUZCU, MD

KEY POINTS

- PTSMA is a less invasive alternative to surgical myectomy for the treatment of LVOT obstruction in HCM patients who have drug refractory symptoms.

- PTSMA involves instillation of ethanol into a specific septal perforating branch of the LAD to create a localized myocardial infarction in the basal portion of the interventricular septum.

- Following PTSMA, LVOT gradients are significantly reduced and patients experience long term improvements in NYHA functional class, exercise capacity and quality of life.

- PTSMA appears to be safe and the incidence of CHB requiring permanent pacemaker implantation has decreased significantly with the institution of MCE and slight modifications in the procedure since its debut in 1995.

- PTSMA is not appropriate for all forms of LVOT obstruction which makes appropriate selection of patients of paramount importance.

- Long-term follow up and randomized studies are needed for optimum utilization of the percutaneous technique.

INTRODUCTION

Hypertrophic cardiomyopathy (HCM), an autosomal dominant disease that occurs in approximately 0.2% of the general population, results from mutations involving genes that encode for proteins of the cardiac sarcomere.[1,2] The various mutations result in a marked degree of clinical heterogeneity which includes differences in left ventricular anatomy, clinical symptomatology, prognosis, and ultimately treatment. Left ventricular outflow tract (LVOT) obstruction is one possible manifestation of HCM and is defined by the presence of an LVOT gradient at rest or with provocative maneuvers designed to decrease preload, decrease afterload, or increase cardiac contractility. In previous years, it was felt that this occurred in approximately 25% of the HCM population. However, recent data and expert opinion suggests that LVOT obstruction is more common and occurs in up to 70% of these patients.[3]

When LVOT obstruction is present it is often associated with mitral regurgitation (MR) as a result of systolic anterior motion (SAM) of the anterior mitral valve leaflet. The combination of outflow tract obstruction and MR can result in congestive heart failure. Once symptoms develop, negative inotropic agents that reduce the degree of LVOT obstruction should be instituted. These include beta-blockers, non-dihydropyridine calcium channel blockers, and the antiarrhythmic disopyramide.[1,2,4] In spite of maximal pharmacologic therapy, approximately 15% of patients will develop debilitating heart failure and should be considered for a mechanical intervention designed to relieve outflow tract obstruction.[5]

The current gold standard is surgical myectomy, which involves excision of approximately 5 grams of muscle from the basal anterior portion of the interventricular septum to just beyond the distal margins of the mitral valve leaflets.[1,2,4] Removal of the hypertrophied tissue decreases the degree of outflow tract obstruction and frequently improves the severity of MR secondary to SAM. Mortality is between 0–3% and patients experience long lasting symptomatic improvement that often includes an enhanced exercise capacity.[1,2,5–8] It is important to note, however, that these results come from a small number of North American and European medical centers where surgeons have extensive experience with myectomy. This highlights the fact that there is limited accessibility to this modality of treatment. In addition, elderly patients and those with multiple co-morbidities are not always considered optimal surgical candidates because of increased surgical risk. For these reasons, a less invasive non-surgical technique, percutaneous transluminal septal myocardial ablation (PTSMA), was developed for the relief of outflow tract obstruction in HCM.

PERCUTANEOUS TRANSLUMINAL SEPTAL MYOCARDIAL ABLATION

PTSMA for the treatment of LVOT obstruction in HCM was initially performed in 1995.[2,9–10] Ethanol is infused into a septal perforating branch of the LAD coronary artery to create a localized transmural myocardial infarction at the base of the interventricular septum. This leads to necrosis and thinning of the hypertrophied myocardium and subsequently, a decrease in the LVOT gradient. Several observational studies have shown that both resting and provokable gradients are reduced by more than 50%, with the majority being reduced by 90% or more.[9,11–18] These reductions are apparent immediately following the procedure and frequently remain stable and often improve over various periods of follow-up (Figs. 35.1 and 35.2). Many studies have also demonstrated significant improvements in patients' quality of life. This includes improvements in exercise capacity, a reduction in New York Heart Association (NYHA) functional class, and the ability to discontinue multiple medications previously used for the treatment of their disease.[11–12,14–16,18–20]

Two studies have compared PTSMA with surgical myectomy.[19,20] While each study is limited by its retrospective nature and inability to control for multiple procedural and patient variables, important information can be gleaned from each. Both techniques appear to effectively reduce resting LVOT gradients and NYHA symptomatology (Tables 35.1 and 35.2). However, the decrease in LVOT gradient following myectomy is more immediate and initially, more complete than that seen following PTSMA (Table 35.1). Within a years time, the reduction in LVOT gradients following each procedure do not differ significantly (Table 35.2), which demonstrates the gradual reduction in LVOT gradient that typically occurs over time following PTSMA. It is important to realize that even though the

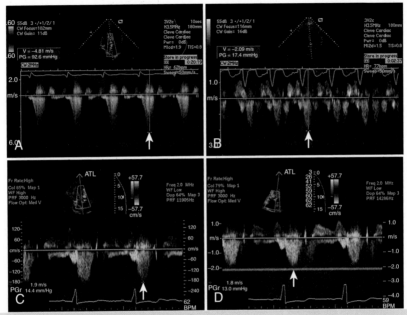

Figure 35.1:
This is a series of transthoracic echocardiogram continuous wave Doppler measurements through the left ventricular outflow tract in a patient prior to and at various time points following PTSMA. Velocity scales differ for each image and arrows are used to indicate peak instantaneous velocity across the LVOT. A, This image was taken prior to PTSMA and demonstrates a peak instantaneous velocity of 4.81 m/s which is equivalent to a peak LVOT gradient of 92.6 mmHg. B, Immediately following PTSMA, peak instantaneous velocity has decreased to 2.09 m/s, equivalent to a peak LVOT gradient of 17.4 mmHg. C, 7 months following PTSMA, peak instantaneous velocity is 1.9 m/s, equivalent to a peak LVOT gradient of 14.4 mmHg. D, 1 year following PTSMA, peak instantaneous velocity is 1.8m/s, equivalent to a peak LVOT gradient of 13 mmHg.

reductions in resting LVOT gradients upon follow up are comparable over time, a significant degree of provokable LVOT obstruction has been seen in patients having undergone PTSMA three months following the procedure.[19] These factors, in addition to the higher incidence of permanent pacemaker implantation following PTSMA (Tables 35.1 and 35.2), are all important considerations when selecting the most appropriate therapy for patients (see below).

TECHNICAL ASPECTS OF THE PROCEDURE

Due to the risk of complete heart block (CHB), a temporary pacemaker wire should be placed in the right ventricular apex. Stable and reliable pacing thresholds are essential and some operators will utilize screw-in leads for this purpose. Baseline intraventricular pressure measurements are obtained and coronary angiography is performed in the usual fashion. Particular care is warranted to obtain multiple views of the proximal and mid-LAD so that the origin and course of septal perforating branches can be seen. Throughout the case, simultaneous pressures can be recorded from the left ventricle with an end hole pigtail catheter positioned away from the LVOT, and from the aorta,

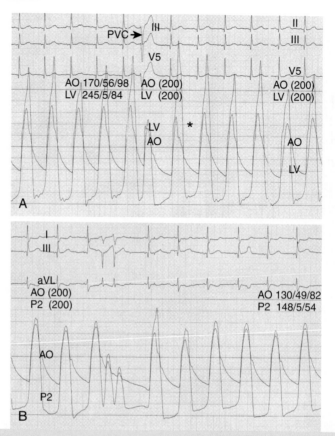

Figure 35.2:
These are simultaneous hemodynamic tracings from the left ventricle and aorta in a patient prior to and immediately following PTSMA. A, This tracing was recorded prior to PTSMA and demonstrates the hemodynamic features characteristic of dynamic LVOT obstruction. Note that there is a great degree of variability in the LVOT gradient. It is between 50–100 mmHg at rest and significantly increases in response to provocation (PVC). The Brockenbrough-Braunwald-Morrow sign (*), which refers to a decrease in the pulse pressure in the beat following a PVC is pathoneumonic of dynamic LVOT obstruction and nicely demonstrated in this tracing. B, Immediately following PTSMA, the resting gradient has decreased to approximately 10 mmHg. The provokable gradient, following a series of 2 PVCs, is now approximately 40 mmHg which is significantly less than that prior to the procedure.

through a left coronary guide catheter. The guide catheter may vary depending on the patient's anatomy, however, we prefer one with an XB curve. Once the guide is advanced to the left main trunk, Heparin is administered to achieve an ACT of more than 250s. A 0.014" flexible guide wire followed by an over the wire angioplasty balloon is initially advanced into the largest and most proximal septal perforating branch (Fig. 35.3). The balloon is then positioned in the proximal portion of the artery and techniques to identify it as an appropriate target for ablation are performed. During the early days of PTSMA, operators did this by assessing the impact that temporary balloon occlusion had on the LVOT gradient. The most proximal septal branch that caused an acute and significant reduction in the gradient, typically >50%, was selected if unwanted areas of the

TABLE 35.1 - OUTCOMES OF PTSMA VS. SURGICAL MYECTOMY AT THE CLEVELAND CLINIC FOUNDATION

PROCEDURE	AGE (YRS)	RESTING GRADIENT (mmHg)		NYHA CLASS		PPM (%)	MORTALITY (%)
		Pre	Imm	Post	Pre	Post	
PTSMA (N=25)	63+/-14	64+/-39	28+/-29[a]	24+/-19[b]	3.5+/-0.5	1.9+/-0.7	24[c]	0
Myectomy (N=26)	48+/-13	62+/-43	7+/-7	11+/-6	3.3+/-0.5	1.5+/-0.7	7.7	0

[a] p <0.001 vs. myectomy, [b] p <.01 vs. myectomy, [c] p <.05 vs. myectomy

PTSMA = percutaneous transluminal septal myocardial ablation, NYHA = New York Heart Association Functional Class,

PPM = permanent pacemaker, Pre = prior to the procedure, Post = three months following the procedure.

Modified from Qin JX, et al. J Am Coll Cardiology, 2001.

TABLE 35.2 - OUTCOMES OF PTSMA PATIENTS AT BAYLOR COLLEGE OF MEDICINE VS. AGE AND GRADIENT MATCHED MYECTOMY PATIENTS AT THE MAYO CLINIC

PROCEDURE	AGE (YRS)	Δ GRADIENT (mmHg)	NYHA III/IV (%)		PPM (%)	MORTALITY (%)	METS	
			Pre	Post			Pre	Post
PTSMA (N=41)	49+/-17	42+/-19	90	0	22[a]	2	5.9+/-1.4	7.5+/-1.9
Myectomy (N=41)	49+/-16	41+/-19	78	2	2	0	5.3+/-1.7	6.5+/-1.5

[a] p <.05 vs. myectomy, PTSMA = percutaneous transluminal septal myocardial ablation, NYHA III/IV = New York Heart Association Functional Class III/IV, PPM = permanent pacemaker, METs = metabolic equivalents, Pre = prior to the procedure, Post = one year following the procedure. Modified from Nagueh SF, et al. J Am Coll Cardiol, 2001.

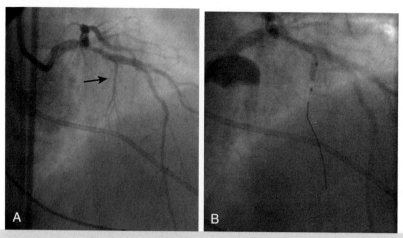

Figure 35.3:
A, This is an RAO cranial view that demonstrates the first major septal perforating branch of the LAD coronary artery (arrow). B, This is the same view showing a flexible guide wire within the branch and a balloon over the wire, inflated in the branch's most proximal portion.

myocardium were not at risk.[13] More recently, myocardial contrast echocardiography (MCE) has been employed in addition to this, to aide in the selection of the most appropriate target branches. The guidewire is removed and while the balloon is inflated, 1 to 2 ml of an echocardiographic contrast agent is injected into the balloon's central lumen and transthoracic echo images are obtained.[15,21,22] The contrast will define the myocardial territory supplied by that artery and delineate the area of planned infarction. The branch is chosen if the area of SAM-septal contact is opacified at the area of maximal flow acceleration and remote regions of the left and right ventricle are spared (Fig. 35.4).[15,22] MCE is now standard practice in most laboratories because precise localization of target arteries has many benefits. When compared to routine probatory balloon occlusion, ablations utilizing MCE have resulted in smaller infarcts, greater reductions in LVOT gradients, faster atrioventricular (AV) nodal recovery times, more significant reductions in NYHA functional class, and reduced incidences of recurrent LVOT obstruction.[15]

Once a vessel is determined to be appropriate for ablation, the operator must consider the amount of alcohol to infuse. There is a higher incidence of CHB and permanent pacemaker implantation when large volumes are used.[2, 22] Typically, 1–2 ml of alcohol is adequate per artery, however, anatomical considerations regarding the size of the region to be infarcted, the speed of contrast washout, and the desired degree of gradient reduction must be taken into consideration.[8,22] Alcohol is then infused into the central lumen of the balloon at a rate of 1 ml per 60–120 seconds, after repeat angiography upon balloon occlusion has demonstrated no reflux of dye in the LAD (Fig. 35.5). The balloon should remain inflated for at least five minutes.[22] Patients will frequently experience chest discomfort during this time. However, this is transient and typically responds to intravenous analgesic agents.

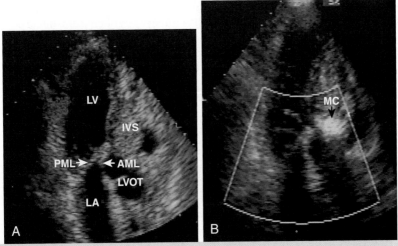

Figure 35.4:
A, This is an apical three chamber transthoracic echocardiogram image that demonstrates LVOT obstruction due to anterior mitral valve leaflet to ventricular septal contact (arrow). Note that the mechanism of contact is systolic anterior motion of the anterior mitral valve leaflet B, This is the same image taken immediately after myocardial contrast was instilled into the central lumen of the balloon. LV = left ventricle, LA = left atrium, LVOT = left ventricular outflow tract, IVS = interventricular septum, AML = anterior mitral valve leaflet, PML = posterior mitral valve leaflet, MC = myocardial contrast.

Once ethanol infusion is complete, angiography is performed to confirm obstruction of the targeted artery and gradient measurements are repeated (Fig. 35.5). It is then necessary to determine if additional septal branches should be ablated. Practice patterns differ in this respect because when to end the procedure remains a point of disagreement. Some operators continue to ablate

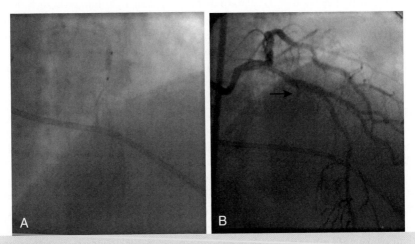

Figure 35.5:
A, This is an RAO cranial view showing contrast being injected into the central lumen of the balloon while the balloon is inflated in the proximal portion of the septal perforator. B, This is an RAO cranial view demonstrating obstruction of the septal perforator following alcohol injection (arrow).

additional branches until the LVOT gradient is at a particular value, typically less than 50% of its baseline or less than 20 mmHg.[4,16] Others stop the procedure when they are satisfied that the anatomic location of the alcohol bathed territory involves the desired area.

Following completion of the procedure, the temporary pacemaker wire is left in place because CHB can occur transiently or permanently in up to 50% of patients.[23] While some late occurrences have been reported, it typically occurs during or within the first 72 hours of the procedure.[14–17,23] Therefore, if the patient remains free of any concerning AV conduction abnormalities by this time, the temporary wire can be removed. Monitoring should occur in an intensive care unit for the first 48 hours, and telemetry continued for the duration of the patient's stay. Cardiac biomarkers should be cycled and will follow a pattern similar to that seen following an acute myocardial infarction. A transthoracic echocardiogram that includes LVOT gradient measurements should be obtained prior to the patient's discharge.

Complications

Complications inherent to any PCI are possible during PTSMA. However, some are more frequent than others and result from the intentional creation of a myocardial infarction in the interventricular septum.

Conduction disturbances are most common. Upon entry into the muscular portion of the interventricular septum, the right bundle branch is a discrete cord-like structure that is located deep within its mid-portion and does not begin to branch until is reaches the level of the papillary muscles. This is unlike the left bundle branch, which enters the muscular portion of the interventricular septum as multiple branches in a sheet like array that are located much closer to the septum's endocardial surface throughout its anterior, mid- and inferior portions (Fig. 35.6).[24] The trans-mural infarction created by alcohol ablation typically involves the mid-portion of the septum that contains the right bundle branch (RBB). Thus, the incidence of right bundle branch block is high and exceeds 60%.[25] It is important to know that individual septal perfusion patterns do vary and it is possible that the targeted artery or arteries also supply the myocardial region containing the more sub-endocardial left bundle. In this situation, CHB can occur. While incidences of CHB vary from study to study, permanent pacemaker implantation following PTSMA has been reported as high as 30% and pre-existing left bundle branch block (LBB) is a major risk factor for its development.[24] Fortunately, with the use of MCE, slower alcohol infusion rates, and smaller volumes of alcohol, the incidence of CHB has decreased to less than 10%.[12,15, 24,26]

While not frequently reported, myocardial infarction, most commonly involving the LAD territory, can occur at sites beyond the septal region.[26] Dissection can be the culprit, however, this not unique to PTSMA. What is unique is abrupt closure of the LAD distal to the targeted branch if spill-over of alcohol occurs during its infusion.[11, 26] This highlights the need to confirm precise balloon positioning in the proximal portion of the branch and exclude reflux of dye into the LAD prior to alcohol infusion (Fig. 35.5). Other potential infarct locations,

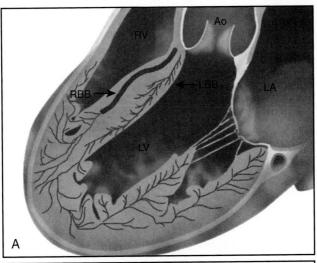

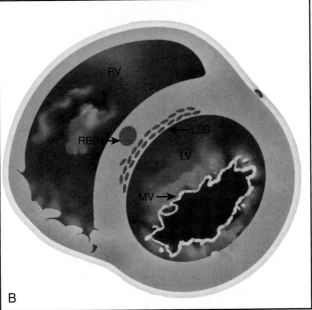

Figure 35.6:
This figure demonstrates the location and anatomy of the left and right bundle branches within the interventricular septum. A, This parasternal long axis cartoon of the heart shows that the right bundle branch begins as a cord like structure, deep within the mid-portion of the interventricular septum and does not begin to branch until it reaches the level of the papillary muscles (RBB). The left bundle branch is a sheet like structure with multiple branches as soon as it exits into the muscular portion of the interventricular septum (LBB). Note its proximity to the endocardial surface of the left ventricle. B, This cartoon demonstrates the same bundle branch anatomy at the level of the mitral valve in a short axis view. LV = left ventricle, RV = right ventricle, LA = left atrium, Ao = aorta, MV = mitral valve.

while less common, are areas of the left ventricular free wall and rarely regions of the right ventricle.[26]

The risk of sudden death following PTSMA remains unclear. There is concern that the resultant scar tissue may serve as substrate for the development of lethal ventricular arrhythmias in a group of patients already prone to their occurrence.[1,2,4, 25] The results of programmed electrical stimulation in a group of patients before and after PTSMA are mixed and there are two case reports demonstrating monomorphic ventricular tachycardia 1–2 weeks following the procedure.[13,27–28] Thus, there is currently not enough information available to suggest that PTSMA increases the risk of sudden death. However, a longer duration of follow up is needed to assess the true potential for this complication and its risk in relation to that of myectomy.

Mortality following PTSMA has been reported between 1–4% with incidences between 0–2% at more experienced centers.[2]

PATIENT SELECTION

Mechanical intervention for LVOT obstruction should be considered when a patient develops drug refractory NYHA functional class III or IV heart failure associated with a resting or provokable LVOT gradient of 50 mmHg or more.[4] In addition, the basal septum should be ≥18mm in thickness.[4] Once these criteria have been met, multiple anatomic and patient related characteristics must be considered to determine if PTSMA is appropriate.

For ablation to be effective, the mechanism of LVOT obstruction must be SAM of the anterior mitral valve leaflet, with leaflet to ventricular septal contact.[2] In addition, one must exclude structural abnormalities that contribute to symptoms and might lead to an incomplete result if not surgically corrected. This includes abnormalities of the mitral valve, atypical patterns or excessive degrees of septal hypertrophy, and severe coronary artery disease amenable to coronary artery bypass surgery.[2,4,29] It is also important to keep in mind that while PTSMA does result in an immediate significant lowering of the resting LVOT gradient, the reduction is not as pronounced as that seen following myectomy.[20,26] In addition, provokable gradients, while significantly reduced from baseline, often remain elevated upon follow up. There have also been reports of an increase in the LVOT gradient above the immediate post procedure level prior to hospital discharge following PTSMA.[10] While these gradients typically decrease after several months of follow up and patients ultimately experience a significant improvement in their symptoms, this may take several months. Therefore, in addition to the patient's expectations, one must consider the degree of his/her illness and need for complete and immediate symptomatic relief.

Once it has been determined that PTSMA would be a reasonable alternative to myectomy from an anatomical and symptom related standpoint; age and surgical risk must be considered. While PTSMA appears to be a safe and effective technique, until long-term follow up and randomized controlled studies are available, it is most useful in patients with high surgical risk or those without access to a high volume surgical center with documented excellent outcome measures, including a surgical mortality of ≤2%.

REFERENCES

1. Maron BJ. Hypertrophic Cardiomyopathy: A Systematic Review. *JAMA* 2002; 287(10):1308–1320.

2. Maron BJ, Mckenna WJ, Danielson GK, *et al.* American College of Cardiology/European Society of Cardiology Clinical Expert Consensus Document on Hypertrophic Cardiomyopathy. J Am Coll Cardiol 2003; 42(9):1687–1713.

3. Maron MS, Olivotto I, Zenovich AG, Udelson JE, Link MS, Pandian NG, *et al.* Clinical Aspects of Hypertrophic Cardiomyopathy [abstract]. *J Am Coll Cardiol* 2005; 45(3):161. Abstract 818–813.

4. Kimmelstiel CD, Maron BJ. Role of Percutaneous Septal Ablation in Hypertrophic Obstructive Cardiomyopathy. Circulation 2004; 109:452–455.

5. Cohn LH, Trehan H, Collins JJ. Long-Term Follow-Up of Patients Undergoing Myotomy/Myectomy for Obstructive Hypertrophic Cardiomyopathy. Am J Cardiol 1992; 70:657–660.

6. Woo A, Williams WG, Choi R, Wigle ED, Rozenblyum E, Fedwick K, *et al.* Clinical and Echocardiographic Determinants of Long-Term Survival after Surgical Myectomy in Obstructive Hypertrophic Cardiomyopathy. Circulation 2005; 111:2033–2041.

7. Ommen SR, Maron BJ, Olivotto I, Maron MS, Cecchi F, Betocchi S, *et al.* Long-Term Effects of Surgical Septal Myectomy on Survival in Patients with Obstructive Hypertrophic Cardiomyopathy. J Am Coll Cardiol 2005; 46(3):470–476.

8. Ten Berg JM, Suttorp MJ, Knaepen PJ, Ernst SMPG, Vermeulen FEE, Jaarsma W. Hypertrophic Obstructive Cardiomyopathy: Initial Results and Long-Term Follow-Up after Morrow Septal Myectomy. Circulation 1994; 90(4):1781–1785.

9. Sigwart U. Nonsurgical Myocardial Reduction for Hypertrophic Obstructive Cardiomyopathy. Lancet 1995; 346:211–214.

10. Abbas A, Brewington S, Dixon S, Grines C, O'Neill W. Alcohol Septal Ablation for Hypertrophic Obstructive Cardiomyopathy. J Inter Cardiol 2005; 18(3):155–162.

11. Knight C, Kurbaan AS, Seggewiss H, *et al.* Nonsurgical Septal Reduction for Hypertrophic Obstructive Cardiomyopathy: Outcome in the First Series of Patients. Circulation 1997; 95(8):2075–2081.

12. Seggewiss H, Faber L, Gleichmann U. Percutaneous Transluminal Septal Ablation in Hypertrophic Obstructive Cardiomyopathy. J Thorac Cardiovasc Surg 1999; 47:94–100.

13. Gietzen FH, Leuner CJ, Raute-Kreinsen U, *et al.* Acute and Long-Term Results after Transcoronary Ablation of Septal Hypertrophy (TASH). Eur Heart J 1999; 20(18):1342–1354.

14. Lakkis NM, Nagueh SF, Kleiman NS, *et al.* Echocardiography Guided Ethanol Septal Reduction for Hypertrophic Obstructive Cardiomyopathy. Circulation 1998; 98:1750–1755.

15. Faber L, Seggewiss H, Gleichmann U. Percutaneous Transluminal Septal Myocardial Ablation in Hypertrophic Obstructive Cardiomyopathy: Results with Respect to Intraprocedural Myocardial Contrast Echocardiography. Circulation 1999; 98:2415–2421.

16. Lakkis NM, Nagueh SF, Dunn JK, Killip D, Spencer WH. Nonsurgical Septal Reduction Therapy for Hypertrophic Obstructive Cardiomyopathy: One Year Follow-up. J Am Coll Cardiol 2000; 36(3):852–855.

17. Mazur W, Nagueh SF, Lakkis NM, et al. Regression of Left Ventricular Hypertrophy after Septal Reduction Therapy for Hypertrophic Obstructive Cardiomyopathy. Circulation 2001; 103:1492–1496.

18. Faber L, Meissner A, Ziemssen P, and Seggewiss H. Percutaneous Transluminal Septal Myocardial Ablation for Hypertrophic Obstructive Cardiomyopathy: Long Term Follow-up of the First Series of 25 Patients. Heart 2000; 83:326–331.

19. Qin JX, Shiota T, Lever HM, Kapadia SR, Stiges M, Rubin DN, et al. Outcome of Patients with Hypertrophic Obstructive Cardiomyopathy after Percutaneous Transluminal Septal Myocardial Ablation and Septal Myectomy Surgery. J Am Coll Cardiol 2001; 38(7):1994–2000.

20. Nagueh SF, Ommen SR, Lakkis NM, Killip D, Zoghbi WA, Schaff HV, et al. Comparison of Ethanol Septal Reduction Therapy with Surgical Myectomy for the Treatment of Hypertrophic Obstructive Cardiomyopathy. J Am Coll Cardiol 2001; 38(6):1701–1706.

21. Nagueh SF, Lakkis NM, HE Z et al. Role of Myocardial Contrast Echocardiography During Nonsurgical Septal Reduction Therapy for Hypertrophic Obstructive Cardiomyopathy. J Am Coll Cardiol 1998; 32:225–229.

22. Sigwart U, Asher CR, Lever HM. Catheter-Based Treatment for Patients with Hypertrophic Obstructive Cardiomyopathy. In: Topol EJ, ed. Textbook of Interventional Cardiology. 4th ed. Philia, PA: Saunders; 2003:987–995.

23. Chang Su Min, Nagueh SF, Spencer WH, and Lakkis NM. Complete Heart Block: Determinants and Clinical Impact in Patients with Hypertrophic Obstructive Cardiomyopathy Undergoing Nonsurgical Septal Reduction Therapy. J Am Coll Cardiol 2003; 42(2):296–300.

24. Talreja DR, Nishimura RA, Edwards WD et al. Alcohol Septal Ablation Versus Surgical Septal Myectomy. JACC 2004; 44(12):2329–2332.

25. Qin JX, Shiota T, Lever HM, Asher CR, Popovic ZB, Greenberg NL, et al. Conduction System Abnormalities in Patients with Obstructive Hypertrophic Cardiomyopathy Following Septal Reduction Interventions. Am J Cardiol 2004; 93:171–175.

26. Wigle ED, Schwartz L, Woo A, Rakowski H. To Ablate or Operate? J Am Coll Cardiol 2001; 38(6):1707–1710.

27. McGregor JB, Rahman A, Rosanio S, Ware D, Birnbaum Y, Saeed M. Monomorphic Ventricular Tachycardia: A Late Complication of Percutaneous Alcohol Septal Ablation for Hypertrophic Cardiomyopathy. Am J Med Sci 2004; 328(3):185–188.

28. Boltwood CM, Chien W, Ports T. Ventricular Tachycardia Complicating Alcohol Septal Ablation [Letters to the editor]. N Engl J Med 2004; 351(18); 1914–1915.

29. Faber L, Welge D, Ziemssen P, Seggewiss H, Fassbender D, Horskotte D, et al. Septal Ablation for Symptomatic Hypertrophic Obstructive Cardiomyopathy: An Analysis of Patients with Dissatisfactory Intervention Results [abstract]. J Am Coll Cardiol 2003; 41(6) suppl 1:145. Abstract 1014–63.

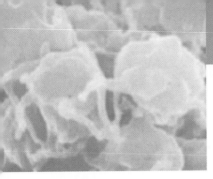

36

Percutaneous balloon pericardiotomy

JOHN L. CAPLIN

KEY POINTS

- PBP is effective in recurrent (usually malignant) pericardial effusion.

- It is performed in a cardiac catheterisation laboratory by an experienced operator.

- Cardiac and pulmonary injury are avoided by fluoroscopic guidance.

- Pleural effusion is common but usually transient.

- PBP is useful in critically ill patients with advanced malignancy.

INTRODUCTION

Most recurrent pericardial effusions are due to malignant disease, but it is unusual, which is perhaps surprising, as cardiac metastases are relatively common. Patients with recurrent effusions often spend a long time in hospital for treatment of their underlying condition, and effective pericardial drainage, in addition to relieving symptoms, can reduce hospital stays in a group of patients who particularly value the quality of life and the remaining time spent at home. Sclerosant therapies have been shown to be ineffective in the management of recurrent malignant pericardial effusions, and the choices facing the physician managing these patients include open pericardiectomy, surgical subxiphisternal pericardial window, and video-assisted thoracoscopic surgery to create a pericardial window. The development of percutaneous balloon pericardiotomy (PBP) has allowed the interventional cardiologist to contribute to the management of these patients.[1] The procedure has been shown to be a safe and effective procedure with a low recurrence rate.[2,3]

PATIENT SELECTION

Patients with recurrent pericardial effusions irrespective of the aetiology may be considered. In patients with definite malignant effusions who have not had previous pericardiocentesis, a decision can be made to perform PBP if the effusion is felt likely to recur.[4] Echocardiography is the most important pre-procedure investigation. There must be at least 1 cm of fluid inferior to the heart when viewed subxiphisternally. In addition if the effusion is loculated then the procedure is unlikely to succeed. If the patient has clinical signs of tamponade, but the procedure cannot be carried out promptly, pericardiocentesis with the removal of a few hundred millilitres of fluid will relieve the symptoms and allow PBP to be performed electively. If pericardiocentesis is performed a sheath should be left in the pericardial space for future access. Percutaneous balloon pericardiotomy has also be used successfully in non-malignant pericardial effusions in children,[5] and following Fontan revision in children.[6]

PROCEDURE

The procedure should be performed in a cardiac catheterisation laboratory with access to X-ray screening, haemodynamic monitoring and resuscitation equipment.[7] The patient is placed on the operating table with a back wedge to bring the patient's chest to about 30 degrees from horizontal. Subxiphisternal echocardiography is performed to confirm that there is adequate fluid inferior to the heart and the depth from the skin to the effusion is measured so that an adequate needle length can be selected. The balloon dilatation stretches both the pericardium and the diaphragm and is painful. Intravenous sedation with a small dose of a short-acting benzodiazepine, and pain prevention with narcotic analgesia is recommended. Continuous electrocardiographic monitoring is required and saturation monitoring is suggested in view of the sedation. The subxiphisternal region is prepared and a small skin incision is made about 2 cm below the subxiphisternal notch. The pericardium is punctured in the normal manner, directing the needle towards the left shoulder. A 0.035" J-tipped guidewire is inserted through the needle and a 4 to 6 F angiographic sheath inserted into the percardial sac. Five to ten millilitres of contrast may be injected into the pericardial sac to confirm the position of the sheath, that the effusion is not loculated, and that there is adequate pericardial fluid inferior to the heart for the procedure. A 0.038" soft-tipped stiff shaft Amplatz wire is then inserted into the pericardial space. The tip of the wire is positioned in the superior part of the pericardial sac if possible (Fig. 36.1). A 20 mm diameter 3 cm long dilating balloon is prepared in the usual way by suction using a syringe containing contrast diluted to half-strength with saline. The track is then pre-dilated using a 10 F dilator and the balloon catheter is advanced over the guidewire. The aim is to centre the balloon across the parietal pericardium and diaphragm (Fig. 36.1). The balloon catheter is then connected via a three-way tap to an indeflator. The balloon is initially filled by hand injection using half-strength contrast. The distal part of the balloon fills first (Fig. 36.2), and the balloon catheter shaft should be pulled back whilst simultaneously filling the balloon until a 'dog-bone' shape is noted (Fig. 36.3). The indeflator is then used to fill the balloon to a pressure of approximately 3 atmospheres. The aim is to abolish, if possible, the indentation caused by the diaphragm and pericardium (Fig. 36.4). It may be necessary to increase the pressure in the balloon or to perform more then one inflation to open a hole. The balloon may not fill completely if the proximal part of the balloon is within the skin or superficial tissues. If this occurs, gentle traction of the skin downwards is sometimes necessary. The main problem is that the balloon prolapses into the pericardial sac when the indeflator is used. In order to prevent this the balloon should be partially filled within the pericardial sac and then pulled back and fully inflated (Fig. 36.2).

Once the dilatation is completed the balloon catheter is withdrawn over the wire and replaced with a 6 F pigtail catheter. As much pericardial fluid as possible should be drained off at this stage as this probably limits the size of any pleural effusions. The catheter is then sewn in place and left on free drainage. There have

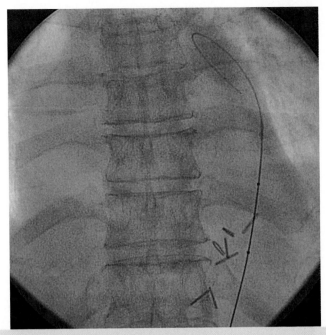

Figure 36.1:
The soft-tipped stiff shaft Amplatz wire is in the superior part of the pericardial sac. The two markers indicate the proximal and distal ends of the balloon.

been reports of the use of double balloons,[3,8] Inoue balloon catheters,[9] and the apical approach.

POST PROCEDURE MANAGEMENT AND FOLLOW UP

The patient should be monitored on the ward after return from the catheter laboratory. The volume of pericardial drainage should be noted every six hours. Once the volume is negligible (<75 millilitres in 24 hours), echocardiography should be performed, and provided the effusion is absent or very small the catheter should be withdrawn. If there is persistent fluid the pigtail catheter should be gently flushed with 5–10 millilitres of heparinised saline and manipulated around to enter the residual fluid. Once the catheter is removed the patient should be monitored for a further 24 hours, a departmental chest radiograph obtained and echocardiography performed. If there is no large pleural effusion and the pericardial sac is dry; the patient can be discharged home. It is suggested that the patient be reviewed in clinic after one month with a repeat chest radiograph and echocardiogram to check for complications or recurrent effusion.

Complications

● Pleural effusions: The development of left pleural effusions occurs in most successful PBP procedures. Most are small and temporary, but between 10 and

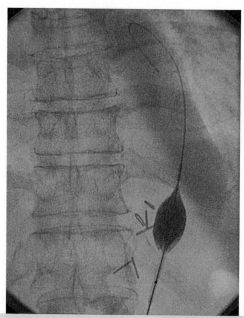

Figure 36.2:
The distal part of the balloon in the pericardial sac is filled and the balloon shaft is pulled back.

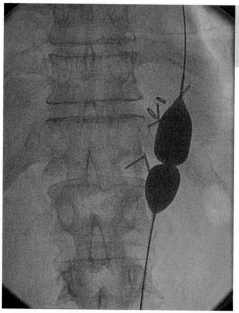

Figure 36.3:
The balloon is across the parietal pericardium and diaphragm at the level of the 'dog-bone' constriction.

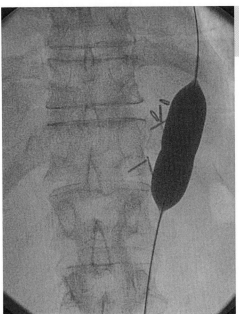

Figure 36.4:
The balloon is fully inflated with an aim of eliminating the waist.

15% of patients develop effusions large enough to require pleural drainage.[2] The highest risk is in patients with a pre-existing effusion. In patients with borderline pulmonary function who would be severely compromised by a large pleural effusion, close monitoring of the size of any pleural effusion is important.

- Cardiac or pulmonary injury: Pericardiocentesis is a potentially hazardous procedure. Before echocardiography was widely available there was significant morbidity and mortality due to myocardial or pulmonary injury. Echocardiography has substantially reduced these risks, but only operators experienced in pericardiocentesis should perform PBP.

- Balloon rupture: Rupture of the balloon is not uncommon: not surprisingly it is related to the use of high pressure and large balloons and the presence of an inelastic pericardium. Generally there are no other complications and the catheter is removed over a guidewire. If dislodgment of the balloon or catheter fracture occur, then the fragments may be removed using a snare inserted through a second pericardial catheter.[10]

- Fever: Pyrexia was noted frequently in initial reports, but sepsis was rare. Initially it was recommended that patients receive prophylactic antibiotics,[7] although this is no longer current practice.

RESULTS OF THE MULTICENTRE PBP REGISTRY

Data were collected from 130 patients in the years 1987–94.[2] The mean age was 59 years (range 25–78). There was an equal sex distribution. Malignant disease was present in 85%; the majority was from lung or breast primaries. Of the non-malignant aetiologies 4 of 20 were HIV-related. Tamponade was present in 69%, and prior pericardiocentesis had been performed in 58%.

The overall success rate of the procedure, defined as an uncomplicated procedure without the need for surgical pericardial window, and no recurrent effusion over an average follow up of five months, was 85%. Five patients required surgery for pericardial bleeding. Thirteen patients had recurrent effusion usually within three months, and 12 of these had surgery; however, six of the surgical patients had further recurrences.

There were minor complications in 13% of patients with fever as the most frequent complication; however, no patients had septicaemia. About one in six patients required thoracocentesis, and this was more common in patients with pre-existing pleural effusions. Survival in the majority of patients was consistent with the diagnosis of disseminated malignancy. The success rate in this registry was better than that reported for surgical procedures such as pericardiectomy, pleuropericardial window and subxiphisternal pericardiotomy, and much better than pericardiocentesis alone and sclersosant therapy.[11]

A recently reported study of 50 patients treated with a double-balloon technique for large malignancy-related effusions showed an overall success rate of 88% with fever in 28% and pneumothorax in 6%.[3]

CONCLUSIONS

Percutaneous balloon pericardiotomy is a safe and effective treatment of pericardial effusions, especially when due to disseminated malignant disease. It can reduce the duration of hospitalisation, and is less invasive and more effective than surgical therapy. In experienced hands the risks of the procedure are low, and it should be available in cardiac units which serve specialist cancer centres.

REFERENCES

1. Palacios IF, Tuzcu EM, Ziskind AA et al. Percutaneous balloon pericardial window for patients with malignant pericardial effusion and tamponade. Cathet Cardiovas Diagn 1991; 22:244–9.

2. Ziskind AA, Lemmon C, Rodriguez S et al. Final report of the percutaneous balloon pericardiotomy registry for the treatment of effusive pericardial disease. Circulation 1994; 1–121.

3. Wang HJ, Hsu KL, Chiang FT et al. Technical and prognostic outcomes of double-balloon pericardiotomy for large maligancy-related pericardial effusions. Chest 2003; 123(5):1775.

4. Jalisi FM, Morise AP, Haque R et al. Primary percutaneous balloon pericardiotomy. W V Med J 2004; 100(3):102–5.

5. Thanopoulous BD, Georgakopoulous D, Tsaousis GS et al. Percutaneous balloon pericardiotomy for the treatment of large, nonmalignant pericardial effusions in children: immediate and medium-term results. Cathet Cardiovasc Diagn 1997; 40(1):97–100.

6. Forbes TJ, Horenstein SM, Vincent JA. Balloon pericardiotomy for recurrent pericardial effusions following Fontan revision. Pediatr Cardiol. 2001; 22(6):27–9.

7. Ziskind AA, Palacios IF. Percutaneous balloon pericardiotomy for patients with pericardial effusion and tamponade. In: Topol EJ (ed.) Textbook of interventional cardiology, 3rd edn. Philadelphia: WB Saunders, 1999, pp. 869–77.

8. Hsu KL, Tsai CH, Chiang FT *et al.* Percutaneous balloon pericardiotomy for patients with recurrent pericardial effusion: using a novel double-balloon technique with one long and one short balloon. Am J Cardiol. 1997; 80(12):1635–7.

9. Chow WH, Chow TC, Yip AS, Cheung KL. Inoue balloon pericardiotomy for patients with recurrent pericardial effusion. Angiology 1996; 47:57–60.

10. Block PC, Wilson MA. Hemi-balloon dislodgement during percutaneous balloon pericardial window procedure: removal using a second pericardial catheter. Cathet Cardiovasc Diagn 1993; 29:289–91.

11. Vaitkus PT, Herrmann HC, LeWinter MM. Treatment of malignant pericardial effusion. JAMA 1994; 272:59–64.

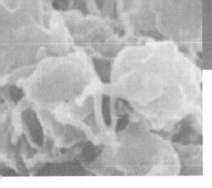

37

Foreign body retrieval

EVER D. GRECH AND DAVID R. RAMSDALE

KEY POINTS

- With the widespread use of intravascular catheters for diagnostic use and therapeutic purposes, the iatrogenic embolisation of materials employed for catheterisation has increased and is probably more prevalent than previously recognised.

- Many intravascular foreign bodies can be successfully removed using a variety of devices such as loop-snares, retrieval baskets or grasping forceps.

- The requirement for pacemaker/ICD electrode extraction will continue to increase as device implantations escalate. Adequate training and experience in lead extraction techniques is necessary.

- Intra-coronary stent deployment failure is a problem that has received little attention in the medical literature and is associated with significant morbidity and mortality. It can be avoided by prudent interventional techniques. Retrieving detached stents may be difficult and should only be performed by experienced operators.

- Operators should have a wide selection of retrieval devices and equipment, and be familiar in their use.

INTRODUCTION

The volume and complexity of percutaneous diagnostic and therapeutic techniques involving the heart and circulation has increased worldwide. These procedures are carried out not only by the cardiologist, but also by radiologists, anaesthetists, surgeons and physicians. Procedures commonly involve insertion of temporary or permanent pacing electrodes and central venous lines or catheters. Moreover, subcutaneously implanted long-term intravenous cannulae, such as Hickman lines, have proved useful for treating various conditions. Catheter-based coronary diagnostic and interventional procedures have also become widely practised.

Unfortunately, hand-in-hand with this rise in vascular intervention has come an increase in the incidence of lost or embolised foreign bodies in the venous and arterial circulations. It is, therefore, necessary for practising interventional cardiologists to become familiar with retrieval equipment and the techniques for their percutaneous removal. This not only circumvents the need for major thoracic or open heart surgery, but may also avoid potentially life-threatening complications. For the adult cardiologist, the commonest sites for retrieval of lost components are the great veins and right heart including the pulmonary arteries, and the coronary arterial tree. This chapter reviews the various types of retained components and the different methods for their successful retrieval.

DEVICES

A variety of transcatheter devices for retrieval of components are available. These include the following:

Loop-snare retrieval systems

The loop-snare device is often the first choice in view of its safety and ease of use. Two examples of loop-snare systems are shown in Fig. 37.1. The Welter retrieval loop catheter consists of a wire snare and is operated from a proximal handle. Its design permits orientation of the loop at right angles to its shaft, enabling access to free-floating foreign bodies. Other examples are the Curry loop snare (see Fig. 37.1) and the Amplatz goose neck snare, which has a nitinol 90 degree snare-loop to shaft orientation and remains co-axial to the vessel lumen (Fig. 37.2).

Retrieval baskets

Examples of retrieval baskets include the Dotter retrieval catheter (Fig. 37.1, bottom), the minibasket and the Dormia stone catcher. These consist of an outer sheath enclosing movable parallel metal wires, which can be opened or closed by sliding a cone in and out of the coronary catheter. To deploy these devices, the

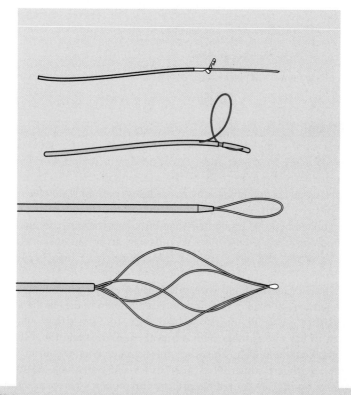

Figure 37.1:
Four examples of transcatheter retrieval devices. From top to bottom: Grasping forceps, Welter retrieval loop, the Curry loop snare, the Dotter retrieval basket.

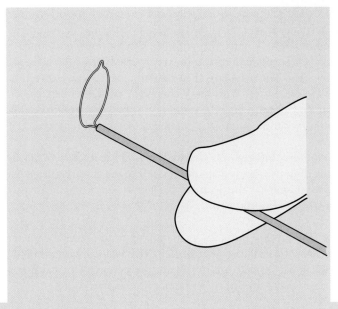

Figure 37.2:
The Amplatz goose neck snare.

basket is placed beyond the fragment and then opened. It is then withdrawn, allowing entrapment of the foreign body, at which time the basket is pulled shut and removed as a single unit. Retrieval basket devices are particularly useful in retrieving objects in the great veins or intracardiac chambers. In the arterial circulation, they are only useful if the object extends into the aorta.

Bioptome/grasping forceps
Different types of jaw forceps are available and an example is the Cook retrieval grasping forceps (Fig. 37.1, top). The grasping jaws are operated from a proximal handle, and care is needed when used to retrieve foreign bodies in less resilient vascular areas.

Miscellaneous techniques
Handmade wire snares A simple, handmade snare may be fashioned using single or twin guidewires. The snare is created by doubling over an exchange-length wire at its midsection and inserting it down a 4 F probing catheter. Alternatively, a snare may be created by looping the distal 5 cm of a standard-length wire, or tying together the flexible ends of two 0.014" wires. The probing catheter is then passed through the guide catheter and positioned just proximal to the retained fragment. The loop is front-loaded through the probing catheter and gently passed over the object. Ideally, the loop should have a moderate bend to help encompass the fragment. Once the object is trapped, the wire ends are pulled firmly to secure the object against the catheter tip. The whole assembly is then withdrawn until it passes through the

femoral sheath. If the snare device cannot be steered into a tortuous or acutely angled coronary artery, twin 0.014" guidewires may be used. The wires are advanced separately into the coronary artery and positioned beside the fragment. The proximal wire ends are inserted into a torquer and clamped firmly together. The torquer is then rotated in a clockwise direction to form a helix of the two wires. With the Y-connector partially open, the double helix is propagated distally into the coronary artery, ensnaring the object, which can then be withdrawn into the guiding catheter and removed.

Balloon catheters Inflated or deflated balloon catheters may be used to physically drag fragments from the vessel into the guide catheter. The inflated-balloon technique has the potential for significant mechanical vascular injury and must be used cautiously.

Pigtail ventriculography catheter A pigtail ventriculography catheter has been used to snare a catheter fragment in the venous system[1] and a broken guidewire in a coronary artery.[2] Again the potential for causing vessel wall damage demands caution when attempting this procedure.

SITES OF RETAINED COMPONENTS

Retained components can only be removed percutaneously if they are radio-opaque. High-resolution fluoroscopy is required, preferably digital with magnification options to enable accurate definition of the object. Full haemodynamic monitoring is essential. Systemic Heparin (10 000–15 000 units) should be administered if not already given beforehand, to avoid thrombus formation on the retrieval device or the retained fragment.

Right heart

For retrieval of central venous or right heart objects, the preferred technique is to use the right femoral vein for access. Under local anaesthetic, an 8 F haemostatic sheath is inserted into the right femoral vein using a Seldinger technique. A long sheath is then advanced over a 0.035 mm diameter long guidewire into the appropriate part of the great veins or right heart chamber. On removing the guidewire, the retrieval device is inserted to grip or ensnare the free end of the foreign body. Once captured, the device is withdrawn into the long sheath and the long sheath, retrieval device and foreign body are removed intact from the vein. A second venous sheath may sometimes be useful for insertion of another catheter such as a pig-tail, Judkins or Cournand which can be used to help unfold loops of catheters in order to present a free end for the retrieval device. Alternatively, a grasping forceps or snare device can be used. At the end of the procedure, haemostasis can be achieved by simple direct pressure when larger objects, knots or loops have been removed. Protamine sulphate can be given to reverse Heparin anticoagulation.

Pacemaker electrodes The transvenous extraction and/or repositioning of chronically implanted permanent pacemaker electrodes presents special difficulties due to scar-tissue adhesion at the lead tip, which may extend along the length of the lead. If a lead has failed, the usual practice is to cap it at the connector terminal so that it is sealed, leaving it buried under the patient's skin. However, removal is essential if the lead becomes infected, the patient develops septicaemia or there is a free-floating lead in the vascular system.

In some instances, removal of an adherent electrode can be achieved by continuous traction on the lead until it comes away from the myocardium. However, this is generally unsatisfactory because of the risk of myocardial avulsion. Until recently, the alternative and more complex option has been thoracotomy. However, a purpose-made lead extraction system enables removal to be performed reasonably safely without the need for surgery. The system uses a countertraction technique and hence lessens the risk of myocardial avulsion (Fig. 37.3A).

Lead extraction can be performed via the superior approach, when the lead is extracted through the implant vein (the subclavian, cephalic or jugular vein). Alternatively, the femoral approach is used if the lead is inaccessible or if the superior approach is difficult or unsuccessful.

Using the superior approach, surgical cutdown to the pacemaker generator is performed and it is removed. The terminal connector of the pacing lead is cut off cleanly using the clippers supplied. The two main tools used are the special locking stylet and the dilator sheath set. The locking stylet, which stiffens the

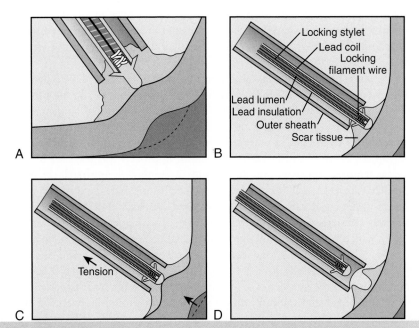

Figure 37.3:
A Pacing lead tension applied with contertraction within the sheath. B The stylet is locked inside the lead coil. If the lead has not been freed by the time the sheaths reach the heart, the outer is advanced to the myocardium. C Firm traction is placed on the locking stylet, whilst the sheath provides countertraction, preventing invagination of the heart and confining the force within the circumference of the sheath. D When the lead tip is freed from the scar tissue, it is removed through the sheath. The outer sheath can even be used as an introducer for a new lead.

lead, is passed down the lumen of the lead to its tip. It consists of a loop handle at the proximal end and an expandable wire coil at the distal end. The size of the locking stylet is selected beforehand using gauge pins. By rotating the loop handle anti-clockwise several times, the fine-wire filament unwinds inside the coil, wedging the stylet shaft tightly into the coil at the lead tip and locking it there. A system of two telescoping dilator sheaths is advanced over the protruding lead end and manipulated along its length via the subclavian vein and on into the heart, thus disrupting the scar tissue along the lead. If the lead has not been freed by the time the sheaths reach the myocardium, the outer sheath is advanced onto the myocardium (Fig. 37.3B). With firm traction on the lead via the locking stylet and countertraction on the sheath supporting the myocardial wall, the lead can be freed and pulled through the sheath (Figs. 37.3C and D). If required, a new lead can now be inserted through the outer sheath. Lead removal using this system may not be possible if there is excessive scar tissue along the length of the lead or if the locking stylet will not pass through a damaged lead. It may, therefore, be necessary to use the femoral approach if the lead has retracted into the venous system and cannot be reached with the superior approach.

The femoral system comprises a long sheath with a tip-deflecting guidewire threaded through a Dotter retrieval basket. A long sheath system is inserted via the femoral vein using routine Seldinger technique and advanced up to the right atrium. A tip-deflecting wire is lassoed around the lead and is pulled down onto the Dotter basket. A longer sheath is then advanced over the lead in a similar manner to the superior approach, thus removing the lead from the scar tissue and myocardium. The femoral system with the lead attached is then removed from the body.

In the largest published series using the above technique, Byrd *et al.* performed 3540 lead extractions in 2338 patients over a period of 28 months. The indications for extraction were infection (27%), non-functional or incompatible leads (25%), removal of Accufix or Encor atrial J-leads following their re-call by Teletronics due to the risk of potential fracture and protrusion of their J-retention wires (46%), or other causes (2%). A superior approach was used for 84.4% of leads, a femoral approach in 4.3% and a combined approach in 11.3%. Additional devices, such as retrieval baskets, loop snares, coronary guiding catheters and pigtail catheters were also used. A total of 93% of leads were completely extracted (and 5% partially extracted) with a major complication rate of 1.4%, which was statistically significantly higher in women than in men (2.3% vs 0.8%, p <0.01). Only one death was reported (0.04%) and the minor complication rate was also low at 1.7%. The overall complication risk increased significantly with the number of leads removed and less operator experience. The authors concluded that the indication for extraction should be balanced against the risk of complication, and that experienced operators should be conscious of the need to be fully equipped and prepared for every eventuality before undertaking lead extraction.[3]

A newer technique using excimer laser has recently been introduced by Spectranetics (Colorado Springs, CO, USA). Data from the randomised PLEXES (Pacemaker Lead EXtraction with the Excimer laser Sheath) trial indicate that this system is more effective than standard non-laser methods.[4] The Spector laser sheath (SLS) contains optical laser fibres, which allow 308 nm ultraviolet light pulses from a xenon–chloride laser to ablate tissue at the sheath tip allowing it to cut through adherent scar. It is threaded over the pacemaker (or ICD) electrode and advanced towards further fibrous binding sites until the tip of the electrode is reached (Fig. 37.4A, B and C). This system is used in conjunction with the lead

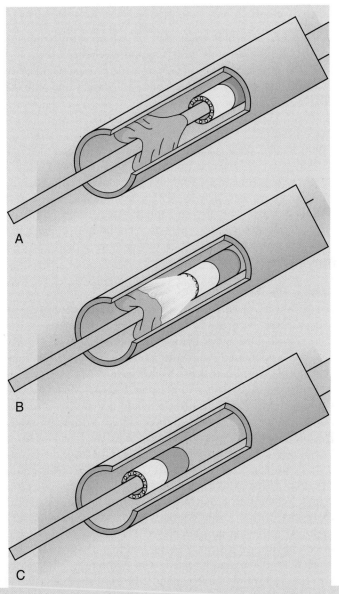

Figure 37.4:
A The laser sheath is advanced over the pacemaker/ICD electrode towards the binding site.
B Controlled bursts of excimer laser energy photo-ablate fibrous tissue. C The laser sheath
is advanced through the binding site to the next site until the lead is released.

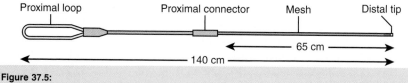

Figure 37.5:
Diagrammatic representation of the lead locking device (LLD).

locking device (LLD) which is comprised of a loop wire handle and a core mandrel that has a stainless steel mesh fixation mechanism (Fig. 37.5). This is inserted down the lumen of the electrode and the proximal end of the mesh is attached to a proximal connector which is used to deploy and lock the device in the electrode.

Left heart

There are only limited data concerning the incidence of retained components within the left heart. However, two series that reviewed 500 and 5400 consecutive elective coronary angioplasty procedures, estimated the risk of retained components to be 0.2%.[5,6] Within this system, the most frequently reported retained fragments are angioplasty guidewires[7] often within the coronary tree. Occlusion devices such as embolisation coils, umbrella duct occluders and detachable balloons are becoming more widely used and may also become misplaced.[8]

Intra-coronary stents

Failure of stent delivery or embolisation has been widely reported and although it is not frequent, may occur in up to 8% of cases.[9] However, delivery success rates have improved with more modern premounted, lower-profile, flexible, slotted-tube stents compared with the previous bare, hand-crimped, rigid Palmaz–Schatz stents. Displaced stents, which have not been fully deployed, can be retrieved using snares, baskets and grasping forceps. Meticulous attention to procedural and peri-procedural details is required if stent loss is to be prevented, although such events are usually unpredictable. Although systemic stent embolisation does not usually result in clinical sequelae, undeployed stents in the coronary arteries should be removed immediately. However, there is surprisingly little literature describing retrieval methods of undeployed stents retained within the coronary tree. Using a technique where a second guidewire was twisted around the first, Veldhuijzen et al. were unsuccessful in removing an undeployed Palmaz–Schatz stent within a right coronary artery in one patient, although they were successful in retrieving an undeployed Wiktor stent, also within a right coronary artery, in another patient.[10] Foster-Smith et al. used a snare to retrieve an undeployed Wiktor stent and a forceps device to retrieve a deployed Wiktor stent from a vein graft, in the same patient.[11] In another patient, an undeployed Gianturco–Roubin stent was removed from the left main coronary artery by inflation of a balloon catheter to 5 atmospheres to trap the stent. It could not, however, be drawn into the guide catheter and was dislodged from the balloon catheter during the attempt. The stent was then retrieved using a multipurpose basket.[11]

More recently, Columbo has described the use of the Amplatz goose neck snare (Fig. 37.2) to retrieve stents both within and outside the coronary tree, and the Cook grasping forceps (Fig. 37.1, top) outside the coronary tree.[12] The goose neck snare may be used in one of two ways (Fig. 37.6). In the proximal grab method, the balloon catheter is removed and the loop of the snare is placed over the proximal end of the guidewire. The snare is advanced until the distal end of the microcatheter is positioned just proximal to the stent. The loop is then opened and advanced around the proximal end of the stent. The loop is then closed to grab the stent and removed into the guide catheter. In the distal wire grab method, the balloon catheter is removed and a second guidewire is positioned adjacent to the stent and distal to the original guidewire. The snare is looped over the

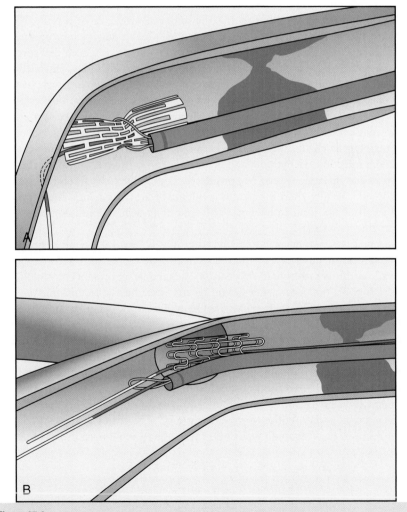

Figure 37.6:
Two methods of stent retrieval using the Amplatz 'Goose neck' microsnare. A The 'proximal grab'; and B the 'distal wire grab' methods.

proximal end of the second guidewire and advanced until the distal end of the microcatheter is positioned distal to the stent and original guidewire. The loop is opened to snare the distal end of the original guidewire. The snare, both guidewires and the stent can then be withdrawn together into the guiding catheter.

MANAGEMENT

The optimal management of intravascular fragment retention has been controversial and remains undefined. It is dependent on the site and situation in which the event occurs and must be tailored to the individual patient's needs and risks. Thus, the retrieval of an undeployed stent within a coronary artery may differ in technique and complexity from that of a pacemaker lead within a great vein.

Although retained components may be removed surgically or percutaneously, they may also be left in situ. There are instances when it may be appropriate and safe to leave a metallic fragment contained within a previously occluded coronary artery, when there is no clear indication for CABG. In their series, Hartzler et al. observed that the intra-coronary retention of equipment fragments were at times well tolerated.[6] However, it is worth noting that in this series only one wire fragment was left in situ in a patent coronary artery. Thus the benign clinical course characteristic of the patients in that series primarily reflected detached wire fragments in chronically occluded arteries. The potential for late perforation, dissection, infection, arrhythmia and proximal propagation of thrombus resulting in myocardial infarction must be considered as possible risks when this strategy is adopted. While there is some evidence that fragments may become endothelialised and remain benign, there is no long-term or pathological data to support this hypothesis.

In some cases, surgery will be required primarily because the initial procedure was unsuccessful and, in these circumstances, the retained fragment can be removed intra-operatively. If myocardial ischaemia is present or threatened, surgical removal of components should be considered early. In unstable patients, attempts at catheter extraction may cause unnecessary delay in mobilising an operating team.

Although transcatheter removal of retained components may be the optimal solution, it may itself result in serious complications. Thrombus deposition on protruding hardware with subsequent systemic embolisation must be considered, although adequate heparinisation should reduce this. Wires and retrieval devices may themselves break and become retained. In addition, fragments may slip free during removal and embolise to other locations.[6] The stiffer devices such as the Dotter retrieval basket should be handled carefully to avoid myocardial or venous perforation.

CONCLUSIONS

The morbidity and mortality associated with retained intravascular fragments are difficult to assess and it is likely that reported cases underestimate the true incidence and early deaths. It is often difficult to conclusively implicate retained fragments as the main cause of death, as this may be ascribed to other causes.

As the applications of conventional angioplasty and intra-coronary stenting expand, the probability of experiencing equipment failure will increase. Therefore, the option of percutaneous extraction of such components in place of invasive surgery will assume increasing importance. Where it can be executed successfully it should substantially diminish clinical risk. In order to achieve this, operators should have a wide selection of retrieval devices and equipment, and be familiar with their use.

REFERENCES

1. Auge JM, Orial A, Serra C, Crexells C. The use of pigtail catheters for retrieval of foreign bodies from the cardiovascular system. Cathet Cardiovasc Diagn 1984; 10:625–8.

2. Krone RJ. Successful percutaneous removal of retained broken coronary angioplasty guidewire. Cathet Cardiovasc Diagn 1986; 12:409–10.

3. Byrd CL, Wilkoff BL, Love CJ et al. Intravascular extraction of problematic or infected permanent pacemaker leads: 1994–1996. PACE 1999; 22:1348–57.

4. Wilkoff BL, Byrd CL, Love CJ et al. Pacemaker lead extraction with the laser sheath: results of the pacing lead extraction with the excimer sheath (PLEXES) trial. J Am Coll Cardiol 1999; 33(6):1671–6.

5. Steffanino G, Meier B, Finci L et al. Acute complications of elective coronary angioplasty: a review of 500 consecutive procedures. Br Heart J 1988; 59:151–8.

6. Hartzler GO, Rutherford BD, McConahay DR. Retained percutaneous transluminal coronary angioplasty equipment components and their management. Am J Cardiol 1987; 60:1260–64.

7. Keltai M, Bartek I, Biro V. Guidewire snap causing left main coronary occlusion during coronary angioplasty. Cathet Cardiovasc Diagn 1986; 12:324–6.

8. Huggon IC, Qureshi SA, Reidy J, Dos Anjos R, Baker EJ, Tynan M. Percutaneous transcatheter retrieval of misplaced therapeutic embolisation devices. Br Heart J 1994; 72:470–5.

9. Cantor WJ, Lazzam C, Cohen EA et al. Failed coronary stent deployment. Am Heart J 1998; 136:1088–95.

10. Veldhuijzen FLMJ, Bonnier HJRM, Michels R, El Gamal MIH, van Gelder BM. Retrieval of undeployed stents from the right coronary artery: Report of two cases. Cathet Cardiovasc Diagn 1993; 30:245–8.

11. Foster-Smith KW, Garratt KN, Higano ST, Holmes DR Jr. Retrieval techniques for managing flexible intra-coronary stent misplacement. Cathet Cardiovasc Diagn 1993; 30:63–8.

12. Colombo A. Stent retrieval. In: Serruys P, Kutryk MJB (eds). Handbook of coronary stents. London: Martin Dunitz 1998:275–81.

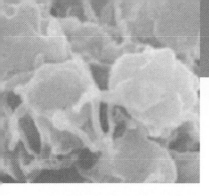

38

Gene therapy and stem cell technology

ANTHONY MATHUR AND MATTHEW LOVELL

KEY POINTS

- Gene and stem cell therapy may well represent the future for the treatment of cardiovascular disease.

- A number of Phase I clinical trials of gene and stem cell therapy for the heart have been published suggesting that these approaches are safe and maybe effective at relieving the symptoms of heart disease.

- Phase II studies have either failed to demonstrate a sustained effect or in the case of stem cell therapy are too few in number to make a definitive conclusion.

- Although few cardiologists will have direct experience of using gene or stem cell therapy to treat their patients most will have faced questions generated by the intense interest these potential treatments have produced in the media.

- The aim of this chapter is to objectively evaluate the current status of both of these exciting fields and to address their current role in the management of patients with cardiovascular disease.

GENE THERAPY

The concept of gene therapy has best been applied to the treatment of diseases where the genetic defect is understood. An example of this is cystic fibrosis where identification of an abnormality in the gene coding for a chloride channel (the cystic fibrosis transmembrane conductance regulator) has lead to the therapeutic approach of transfecting the lung with the normal gene in an effort to correct the abnormality. Unfortunately although successful transfection has occurred, the duration of effect has been short-lived.[1]

Gene therapy in the cardiovascular system has taken a different approach since a single gene defect has not been identified as a sole causative factor in the development of ischemic heart disease. Instead the approach has been taken to identify genes with the potential of correcting the fundamental problem of cardiac ischaemia. Although several different methodologies have been used (reviewed in Table 38.1) the majority of gene therapy studies have targeted genes involved in angiogenesis in an attempt to stimulate a 'repair' process rather than correct a causative factor. However, now more than ten years after the first clinical trials of gene therapy in cardiovascular disease no approach has been shown to be effective in a randomised control trial (major clinical trials summarised in Table 38.2).

In theory, successful gene therapy involves the safe transfer of the gene(s) of interest into the target cell/organ where the gene interacts with the native DNA to produce an effect such as the production of a protein (e.g. vascular endothelial

TABLE 38.1 - POTENTIAL STRATEGIES FOR GENE THERAPY INTERVENTION IN THE CARDIOVASCULAR SYSTEM[4]

DISEASE	THERAPEUTIC TARGET
Ischemic heart disease (prevention or protection)	Antioxidant genes (HO-1, SOD, catalase, GPx)
	Heat Shock Proteins (HSP70,SHP90,HSP27)
	Survival genes (BCL-2, Akt, HGF)
	Inflammatory cytokines, adhesion molecules and TFs (I-CAM,V-CAM,TNF-α,NF-κB)
	Pro-apoptotic genes (Bad, caspase inhibitor p53)
	Coronary vessel tone (eNOS, adenosine receptors)
	Lipid lowering in FHH (LDL receptor)
Rescue coronary artery disease	Proangiogenic factors (VEGF$_{121,165}$, FGF-1,2,4,5, HGF, Ang-1, MCP-1, G-CSF, PDGF-BB, IGF-1,2, HIF-1α/VP16, egr-1, Prox-1)
Heart failure	Contractility or calcium regulation (β-adrenoreceptor, SERCA2A, BARK, phospholamban)
Inherited heart disease	Arrhythmia or channelopathies (SCN5A, I$_k$, HERG, KCNE1, Gαi2, Kir2)
	Cardiomyoplasty (sarcomeric proteins, sarcoglycans)
Congenital heart disease	Heart and Blood Vessels (endoglin, NKx2.5, TBX5, TFAP2B)

Abbreviations: AAV, adeno-associated virus; ACS, acute coronary syndromes; ADV, adenovirus; Ang-1, angiopoietin-1; AS-ODN, antisense oligonucleotide; CAD, coronary artery disease; egr-1, early growth response factor-1; eNOS, endothelial nitric oxide synthase; FGF, fibroblast growth factor; G-CSF, granulocyte colony stimulating factor; GPx, glutathione peroxidase; HF, heart failure; HGF, hepatocyte growth factor; HIF, hypoxia inducible factor; HO-1, heme oxygenase-1; HSP, heat shock protein; IGF; insulin like growth factor; I/R, ischemia and reperfusion, LV, lentivirus; MCP-1 monocyte chemotactic protein-1; MI, myocardial infarction; NF, nuclear factor; PDGF, platelet derived growth factor; RV, retrovirus; SOD, superoxide dismutase; TFs, transcription factors; TNF, tumor necrosis factor; V-CAM, vascular cell adhesion molecule; VEGF, vascular endothelial growth factor.

growth factor (VEGF)). This process requires the completion of several steps before the desired end-point is reached. Transfer of a gene can be performed in a number of ways ranging from the use of a viral vector to infect target cells with the gene to delivery of the 'naked' DNA itself with the aim of incorporation into the target tissue in sufficient amounts. Finding a virus that is safe and can reliably deliver the DNA has been one of the biggest problems confronting this area. Also once delivered the sustained expression of the therapeutic DNA has posed new challenges to scientists. Ultimately deciding which gene to target still remains the key question.

Preclinical trials suggested that the delivery of angiogenic factors to ischemic vascular beds may attenuate the ischaemia and lead to the testing of genes that code for these factors in vivo. The main group of agents were the growth factors VEGF, fibroblast growth factor (FGF) and hepatocyte growth factor (HGF).

In themselves these growth factors consist of groups of proteins containing many isoforms of which only a small proportion have been tested experimentally. The majority of clinical gene transfer experience has accumulated with vectors encoding FGF-1 and FGF-4. Non-viral and viral-based approaches have been used in clinical studies in the belief that a single protein can significantly influence a process such as angiogenesis. A more realistic approach using genes coding for a protein that stimulates a cascade of relevant factors will probably result in more

TABLE 38.2 - CLINICAL TRIALS OF CARDIOVASCULAR GENE TRANSFER[5]

TRANSGENE AND VECTOR	ROUTE AND INDICATION	REFERENCES
VEGF$_{165}$		
Plasmid	Intra-arterial for PAD	Isner et al. (1996) and Makinen et al. (2002)
Plasmid	Intramuscular for PAD	Baumgartner et al. (1998), Baumgartner et al. (2000) and Shyu et al. (2003)
Plasmid	Intra-arterial for CAD	Symes et al. (1999), Vale et al. (2000), Sarkar et al. (2001), Kolsut et al. (2003) and Ueda et al. (1999)
Plasmid	Intra-arterial for TO	Isner et al. (1998)
Plasmid	Intra-arterial for PAD	Makinen et al. (2002)
VEGF$_{121}$		
Adenovirus	Intramuscular for PAD	Rajagopalan et al. (2002) and Rajagopalan et al. (2003)
Adenovirus	Intramyocardial for CAD	Rosengart et al. (1999)
VEGF-2		
Plasmid	Intramyocardial for CAD	Vale et al. (2001) and Losordo et al. (2002)
FGF-1		
Plasmid	Intramuscular for PAD	Comerota et al. (2002)
FGF-4		
Adenovirus	Intra-arterial for CAD	Grines et al. (2002) and Grines et al. (2003)
HGF		
Plasmid	Intramuscular for PAD	Morishita et al. (2004)

Abbreviations: CAD = coronary artery disease; FGF = fibroblast growth factor; HGF = hepatocyte growth factor; PAD = peripheral arterial disease; TO = thromboangiitis obliterans; VEGF = vascular endothelial growth factor.

dramatic results (e.g. hypoxia inducible factor-1α – HIF-1α – coordinates the regulation of multiple angiogenic factors).

The basis for gene delivery to the heart came from the first clinical trials of gene delivery for the treatment of peripheral vascular disease.[2] In a case report from a Phase I study using local delivery of phVEGF$_{165}$, digital subtraction angiography and Doppler flow studies suggested an improvement in the peripheral circulation of an individual with arterial insufficiency. A series of Phase I studies followed (reviewed in[3]) that demonstrated gene delivery of angiogenic factors improved the symptoms of patients with vascular insufficiency. Unfortunately the Phase II studies that followed did not confirm the promising results seen in the Phase I studies although a number of reasons for this (differences in gene delivery and local gene expression) have been put forward.[4,5]

Given the preclinical and clinical experience of gene transfer of phVEGF$_{165}$, it was not surprising that this approach was used in the first clinical studies of cardiac gene transfer.[6] Plasmid coding for VEGF$_{165}$ was injected intramyocardially via a mini-thoracotomy in five patients with angina who were refractory to maximum medical therapy and not amenable to standard revascularization procedures. A reduction in angina and objective evidence of ischaemia (as measured by single photon emission computed tomography – SPECT) was seen in all patients. This approach has been evaluated in small numbers of patients throughout the world with favourable reports of clinical improvement.[7-9] Interpretation of these small studies is limited due to confounding factors such as a lack of control group for the surgical procedure. Indeed the promising results seen in a study in which phVEGF$_{165}$ was injected at the time of elective coronary artery bypass surgery was not found by a larger randomised study due to the small size of the effect seen above that which was achieved by the surgery alone.[10] In order to remove the confounding effects of surgery which in itself leads to an increase in circulating VEGF levels,[11] catheter-based intramyocardial delivery was developed in conjunction with the NOGA electromechanical mapping system (see Fig. 38.1) and tested in a pilot study of

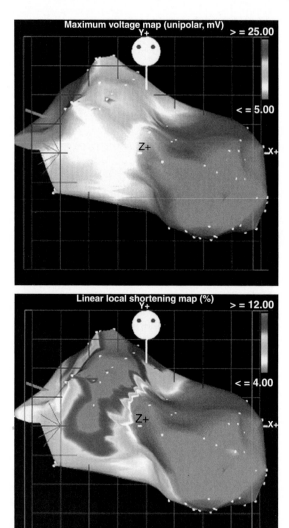

Figure 38.1:
NOGA Evaluation of cardiac function.
Colour contour maps displaying endocardial voltage and local shortening can be produced by the NOGA system that allow the targeting and evaluation of catheter based therapies.

six patients.[12] A steerable, deflectable 8 F catheter incorporating a 27-guage needle was advanced percutaneously to the left ventricular myocardium of six patients with chronic myocardial ischaemia. Patients were randomized (1:1) to receive phVEGF-2 (total dose, 200 μg), which was administered as six injections into ischemic myocardium (total, 6.0mL), or placebo (mock procedure). Patients that received phVEGF-2 experienced reduced angina and reduced nitroglycerin consumption for up to 360 days after gene transfer. Reduced ischaemia by electromechanical mapping and improved myocardial perfusion by SPECT-sestamibi scanning was also seen in the gene transfer group for up to 90 days after treatment when compared with images obtained after control procedures. An initial placebo effect was seen in the control group, which did not persist to the later time points. The larger placebo controlled, double blinded dose escalation study which followed was put on hold by the FDA after the death of a patient in a non-related gene therapy study.[13] Again promising provisional results were seen in the few patients that were recruited.

A different approach using an adenovirus to encode the VEGF protein has also been employed in the hope that the different vector delivery system would lead to long-term protein expression.[14] Again using a mini-thoractomy procedure 21 patients received an adenovirus coding for VEGF121 either as sole therapy or as an adjunct to CABG. An improvement in perfusion was observed using nuclear imaging as seen in previous studies, however, this did not reach statistical significance.

A number of growth factors have been implicated in the biology of angiogenesis and not surprisingly some of these have been used in clinical studies. FGF has been used in a randomised double blind controlled trial of gene transfer for angiogenesis (AGENT).[15] Patients were randomised to adenovirus mediated FGF or placebo injected intracoronary (as distinct from previous studies which had administered the gene product by direct intramuscular injection). Using exercise testing as an outcome measure subgroup analysis demonstrated that those who had exercise treadmill times below ten minutes or those with low baseline titres of neutralising antibodies to adenovirus derived significant benefit from gene transfer. The AGENT 2 study was subsequently designed to assess whether adenovirus mediated FGF gene transfer improves myocardial perfusion using SPECT to assess outcome.[16] Although a reduction in the perfusion defect on SPECT was seen in the gene transfer group compared to controls, no other differences were noted. Expansion of these studied to Phase III unfortunately did not reach a positive conclusion as both the AGENT 3 and 4 studies were stopped in 2004 due to inability to reach the study end-point.

In summary the promising effects on symptoms and myocardial perfusion of angiogenic gene transfer seen in preclinical and Phase I clinical studies has not been demonstrated in larger Phase III studies at least in the case of FGF. Important answers to the question of the role of gene transfer using genes coding for angiogenic proteins needs to be addressed in large scale RCTs. Indeed such studies continue to be designed and in addition the role of other growth factors such a HGF and HIF-1α are being tested.

The future for gene therapy lies not only on the testing of new target proteins and delivery systems but also in identifying mechanisms. New molecular imaging techniques will provide information about local gene expression, protein production and effects that will allow an understanding of the optimisation of these strategies. Cellular therapy may provide a means of delivering candidate genes in an efficient and durable manner thereby improving on current systems. Given that there are still many unanswered questions about the mechanisms of cardiovascular disease gene therapy studies should continue with the emphasis on safety as well as efficacy.

Stem cells

The defining characteristic of a stem cell is the ability to self-renew and if appropriate to form daughter cells of one or more differentiated cell types. The 'ultimate' cell that meets this definition is found in the embryo. Several days after fertilisation the embryo develops into the blastocyst with an outer shield of cells, the trophoblast, and an inner clump of undifferentiated cells known as the inner cell mass. This inner ball of cells contains the pluripotent (definition – see Table 38.3) embryonic stem cells (ESC). These are thought to represent the ultimate stem cell as they have the ability to organise and produce all of the specialised cells and organs needed to form a fully functioning adult, including the heart and blood vessels.[17] ESC gradually disappear and are replaced towards the end of term with adult stem cells (ASC). ASC like ESC have the defining stem cell trait – an endless capacity to self-renew – but have a more limited repertoire of specialised cells that they can produce. The most well known example of an ASC is the haematopoietic stem cell (HSC) that resides in the bone marrow and continuously replaces all the cells of the blood. Thus, each adult organ contains its own reservoir of stem cells that can produce daughter cells appropriate to its location.[18] Hence, adult stem cells are also known as tissue specific or somatic stem cells. It is thought that their purpose is to replace cells lost from adult organs during physiological and pathological cell turnover. As such, ASC are most obvious and consequently best characterised within highly proliferative organs such as the bone, skin and gut. It has taken longer for tissue specific stem cells to be recognised within less proliferative organs such as the heart, but their presence within adult cardiac tissue has now be documented in a variety of species including rats, mice, dogs and humans.[19]

TABLE 38.3 - GLOSSARY OF COMMON STEM CELL TERMINOLOGY

TERM	MEANING	EXAMPLE
Unipotent	Capable of producing only one type of specialised cell	Epidermal stem cell within dermal layer of skin
Multipotent	Can produce a small range of differentiated cell lineages appropriate to their location	HSCs
Pluripotent	Able to differentiate into all cells that arise from the three germ layers	ESCs derived from inner cell mass around five days after fertilisation
Totipotent	Can produce all fully differentiated cells of the body and trophoblastic cells of the placenta	ESCs derived one or two days after fertilisation

Abbreviations: HSCs = Haematopoietic stem cells; ESCs = Embryonic stem cells.

It is hoped that the proliferative and regenerative capacity of both ASC and ESC can be harnessed to produce cardiomyocytes and vascular cells for transplantation into ischaemic and failing hearts. In contrast to current pharmacological therapy such a treatment would directly address the fundamental problems of myocyte loss and lack of an adequate blood supply.

ES cell therapy In 1998, two papers reported that ESC could be isolated from human embryos. This technological advance heralded tremendous interest and excitement in the field of stem cell research leading to claims that stem cell therapy will revolutionise the treatment of chronic conditions such as cardiovascular disease and cancer (see Fig. 38.2).

This claim was initially born from the observation of the potential of human embryonic stem cells (hESC) to spontaneously form functioning cardiomyocytes, smooth muscle cells and endothelial cells in vitro.[20] Furthermore, cardiomyocytes derived in this manner were successfully used to treat myocardial infarction in animal studies, significantly improving cardiac function.[21,22] However,

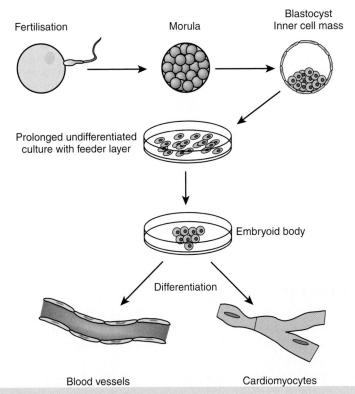

Figure 38.2:
Embryonic stem cells (ESC) can be used to derive cells for transplantation.
Following fertilisation ESC can be obtained from the inner cell mass and maintained in an undifferentiated state with feeder layers until needed. Differentiation into cardiomyocytes, blood vessels and other cells can be started spontaneously by suspending ESC in a hanging drop known as an embryoid body.

considerable development is still needed before these exciting techniques can be trialled in man.

Many technical hurdles remain such as the eradication of animal products currently used in the cell culture of hESC, and the assessment of the tumour potential of transplanted hESC. The last point also reflects the need for techniques of selecting ESC as they start to differentiate towards myocytes; allowing the correct cells to be delivered to the relevant sites. For example, if only cells fated to form ventricular type myocytes were delivered to the left ventricle instead of a heterogonous population of cells, with the potential to become multiple phenotypes, the problems related to subsequent arrythmogenesis induced by non-relevant cell differentiation may be overcome.[21,22] Another question is that of transplant rejection; in theory all recipients of hESC derived cells will need to receive immunomodulatory therapy with the subsequent risk of complications. This may not be the case in future as the promise of successful human therapeutic cloning (Fig. 38.3) nears realisation.

Finally, it should be remembered that the use of any form of embryonic tissue carries with it serious moral and ethical issues that society is struggling to address. For example, many people believe that early human embryos should be accorded the same status as a sentient being and thus their 'harvesting' for stem cells is morally unjustifiable. With this in mind, other sources of stem cells with the potential of ESC are being looked for.

Adult stem cell therapy A large body of evidence now supports the idea that certain adult stem cells, particularly those of bone marrow origin, can engraft alternative locations (e.g. the heart), particularly when the recipient organ is damaged. Furthermore, these cells behave in a contextual manner and transdifferentiate into cell types with functions appropriate to their new location (see Fig. 38.4). For example, mesenchymal stem cells (MSC) taken from bone marrow that are normally capable of producing bone, fat and connective tissue cells, have now been shown to transdifferentiate into cardiomyocytes. Hence, the considerable excitement for using these cells as clinical therapies. This is particularly attractive because bone marrow stem cells are readily obtained from patients by mobilisation into the circulation using a cytokine such as granulocyte-colony stimulating factor (G-CSF). Moreover, if a patient's own stem cells are used in their treatment no immune rejection problems would arise.

Several theories have been proposed as to how transplanted adult stem and progenitor cells improve cardiac function (Fig. 38.5). Firstly it has been suggested that the injected cells are able to form functional myocytes following transplantation. Having done so, these cells would seamlessly integrate into the surrounding myocardium, augmenting cardiac function. Secondly, transplanted cells contribute to new blood vessel formation via vasculogenesis and increase perfusion. The third competing or perhaps complementary mechanism can be thought of as the cytokine hypothesis. Here cardiac function is improved not through direct action and integration but by the release of beneficial cytokines and growth factors. These could reduce necrosis and apoptosis of 'vulnerable' cardiomyocytes as well as facilitating new blood vessel formation. The fourth

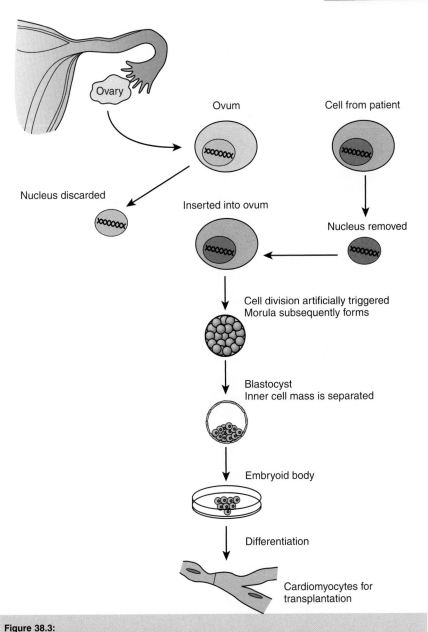

Figure 38.3:
Therapeutic cloning could provide allogenic cells for transplantation in the future.
In somatic cell nuclear transfer or therapeutic cloning the nucleus is removed from surplus ova and
is replaced by a nucleus taken from the patient requiring treatment. Cell division is artificially
triggered and embryonic stem cells can be subsequently isolated from the inner cell mass at the
blastocyst stage embryo.

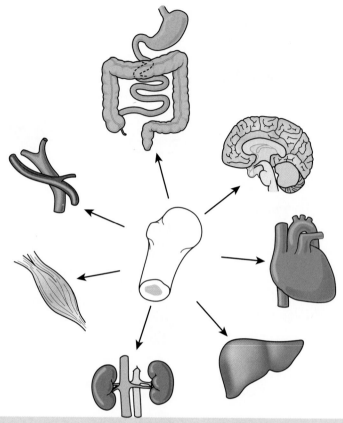

Figure 38.4:
Bone marrow stem and progenitor cells can exhibit plasticity.
It is now felt that these cells can jump lineage boundaries in certain situations and transdifferentiate into functional cells contextual with the need for the damaged organ to heal. In particular this has been seen in the brain, gut, kidney, vasculature, skeletal muscle, liver and heart.

theory is that transplanted cells improve function by fusing with failing local recipient cells.

However, before ASC are seen as the panacea for all ills, it is worth noting that not everyone is convinced of their versatility.[24] The reasons for this include the fact that certain instances of so-called plasticity (the ability to change phenotype) have now been attributed to cell fusion between bone marrow cells and cells of the recipient organ; in addition several remarkable claims in the literature have been difficult to reproduce in other laboratories.[25,26]

In order to circumvent the issues relating to differentiation another approach has been to use cells that already have a muscle phenotype (the skeletal myoblast) to engraft damaged myocardium with the aim of improving cardiac function. Promising preclinical and clinical results have been observed using these cells and the results of large scale clinical trials are awaited.[27,28]

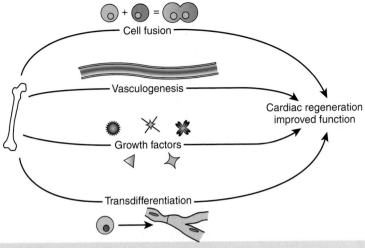

Figure 38.5:
Proposed mechanism of action of bone marrow derived stem and progenitor cells.
How bone marrow derived cells improve cardiac function remains unclear. Currently the main
mechanisms are thought to be vasculogenesis. transdifferentiation, cell fusion and release of
beneficial growth factors which could influence vasculogenesis, apoptosis and necrosis.

Bone marrow Studies using human adult stem cells have shown that they can
ameliorate loss of cardiac function following myocardial infarction in animal
models. Histological examination in these studies demonstrated that the
transplanted cells have in some cases formed new cardiomyocytes and vascular
structures.[22] The positive animal and human studies plus the need for effective
treatments have quickly led to Phase I trials of adult stem and progenitor cells.

Clinical trials of bone marrow derived cells Early clinical trials have used the
mononuclear cell fraction isolated from bone marrow aspirates containing HSC,
MSC and endothelial progenitor cells. So far the studies have involved relatively small
numbers of patients and have demonstrated that adult stem cell therapy
for heart disease appears to be safe and may improve cardiac function (see Tables 38.4
and 38.5). Large randomised control trials are undoubtedly needed before the
true value of this approach can be decided. The trials so far can be divided into
two categories:

1. *Acute studies* – Cells are injected shortly after an acute myocardial infarction
   once the patient has received best medical treatment and primary angioplasty
   to restore flow down the culprit coronary artery (see Fig. 38.6). Bone marrow
   is aspirated from the posterior iliac crest within five days of the infarct.
   Following separation of the mononuclear cellular fraction and sometimes
   following additional culture the cells are injected down the culprit vessel in an
   angioplasty-like procedure. Studies have used between 3–10 injections per
   artery of 2–3 mls of cells through an over-the-wire PTCA balloon inflated for
   up to three minutes at a time. The numbers treated per study ranges from 6 to

TABLE 38.4 - TRIALS OF ADULT STEM CELL AND PROGENITOR THERAPY IN ACUTE MYOCARDIAL INFARCTION

STUDY	INJURY	ROUTE OF DELIVERY	PATIENT NO:	FOLLOW UP	OUTCOME
Strauer et al. 2002	AMI	Intracoronary catheter	10 treated, 10 std Rx	3 months	Significant reduction in hypo/dys/ akinetic segments, improved perfusion, no significant increase in EF
Assmus et al. 2002	AMI	Intracoronary catheter	9 with BM, 11 with EPCs, 11 controls	4 months	EF significantly improved, reduced WMA, improved CFR, improved viability on FDG-PET
Britten et al. 2003	AMI	Intracoronary catheter	14 BMC, 12 CPC	4 months	MRI – significant increase in global EF, decreased LVESV and infarct size.
F-Aviles et al. 2004	AMI	Intracoronary catheter	20 treated, 13 Std treatment	11±5 months	Decrease in LVESV, improved regional & global LV function, increased thickness in infarct wall, re-stenosis rate 15% in cell group
Kang et al. 2004	AMI	Intracoronary catheter & sc G-CSF	10 cells and G-CSF, 10 G-CSF alone, 7 controls	6 months	Increased exercise time, significant increase in EF, CFR and perfusion in cells group
Chen et al. 2004	AMI	Intracoronary catheter	MSCs 34, N-Saline 35	6 months	Significant increase in global EF, decreased perfusion defects, LVEDV, LVESV
Wollert et al. 2004	AMI	Intracoronary catheter	30 Cell and 30 Std Rx	6 months	MRI – EF increased 6.7% in treatment group, 1.1% in controls
Kuethe et al. 2004	AMI	Intracoronary catheter	5 pts, BM-MNCs	3 & 12 months	No improvement in EF or CFR

34 patients and the follow up of the patients has ranged from 3–16 months. Using echocardiography, LV angiography and MRI, the studies have documented an improvement in a range of functional parameters including ejection fraction, wall motion scoring, infarct size, wall thickening and LV dimensions. In addition, thallium and PET results have shown improved perfusion and viability in keeping with results of pressure wire studies

TABLE 38.5 - TRIALS OF ADULT STEM CELL AND PROGENITOR THERAPY IN CHRONIC ISCHAEMIC HEART DISEASE AND CONGESTIVE CARDIAC FAILURE

STUDY	INJURY	ROUTE OF DELIVERY	PATIENT NO.	FOLLOW UP	OUTCOME
Hamano et al. 2001	IHD/CCF	Intramyocardial at CABG	5 treated	1 yr	Stress tests 60% improved
Stamm et al. 2003	IHD/CCF	Intramyocardial at CABG	6 treated	6±3 months	Improved NYHA, EF (minimal) and perfusion.
Tse et al. 2003	IHD/CCF	Percutaneous intramyocardial	8 treated	3 months	Less angina and medication, MRI: improved wall thickening & motion
Perin et al. 2003	IHD/CCF	Percutaneous intramyocardial	14 treated, 7 controls	4 months	One death, NYHA, CCS improved, EF significantly improved, SPECT: less stress defects
Fuchs et al. 2003	IHD/CCF	Percutaneous intramyocardial	10 pts, BM	3 months	Significant increase in CCS, and perfusion on SPECT, trend to increase in ETT
Galinanes et al. 2004	IHD/CCF	Intramyocardial at CABG	14 pts CABG and BM	10 months	Improved NYHA, CCS, LV motion score, in segments revascularised plus cells, no increase in EF

Abbrevations for tables 38.4 and 38.5.

(EF = Ejection fraction; WMA = wall motion abnormality; CFR = coronary flow reserve; FDG-PET = Fluorodeoxyglucose-Positron Emission Tomography, MRI = magnetic resonance imaging; LV = left ventricle, LVEDSV = left ventricular end diastolic volume, LVESV = Left ventricular end systolic volume, G-CSF = Granulocyte colony stimulating factor).

demonstrating improved coronary flow reserve. On a cautionary note, one study was stopped due a trend of in-stent stenosis, but the study was too small for these numbers to reach statistical significance and their findings could well be in the realms of normal outcomes as on average 20% of people will suffer in-stent stenosis following standard PCI.[29]

2. *Chronic studies* – Patients with chronic heart failure secondary to ischaemic heart disease have been treated with cells directly injected into the myocardium or intracoronary either at the time of cardiac bypass surgery or percutaneously (see Fig. 38.6). Both methods of delivery have been used to inject cells overcoming the fact that diseased arteries may not be useful for efficient cell delivery to the target area. Studies have enrolled between 4 and 21 patients with follow up between 3 and 12 months. Some studies have used as many as 16 intramyocardial injections of up to 0.2 ml of cell suspension per injection. The results have shown improved cardiac function and perfusion. Patients at follow up experience fewer symptoms and a reduction in cardiac medications.[30]

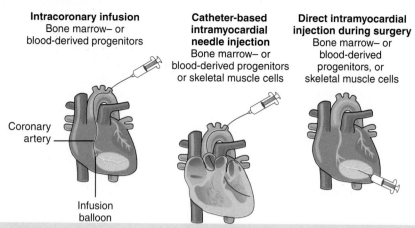

Figure 38.6:
Methods for delivery of stem cells in human trials.

It should be remembered that none of the chronic studies so far have been sufficiently powered to detect significant changes in function and were solely designed to test safety.

Taken together the acute and chronic studies are reassuring and all have confirmed the safety and feasibility of cellular therapy with no significant rise in biochemical markers of myocardial damage, dysrrhythmias or any other adverse event in the treated groups compared to controls. Most have shown functional benefit although only one phase II study was powered to detect this outcome.[31] Many questions remain concerning the use of progenitor cell therapy in the treatment of heart disease: which patients will benefit; what cell types is best; when is the best time to deliver the cells and what delivery technique should be used to do this? We feel that such questions can only be answered by well-designed randomised control trials targeting specific patient groups, carried out using standardised reproducible techniques and adequately powered to detect significant differences in robust outcome measures. Should this approach be bypassed in a haphazard or disjointed fashion the true potential of this revolutionary approach to the treatment of cardiovascular disease may never be realised.

REFERENCES

1. Lee TW, Matthews DA, Blair GE. Novel molecular approaches to cystic fibrosis gene therapy. Biochem J 2005; 387(Pt 1):1–15.

2. Isner JM, Pieczek A, Schainfeld R, Blair R, Haley L, Asahara T, et al. Clinical evidence of angiogenesis after arterial gene transfer of phVEGF165 in patient with ischaemic limb. Lancet 1996; 348(9024):370–4.

3. Yla-Herttuala S, Martin JF. Cardiovascular gene therapy. Lancet 2000; 355(9199):213–22.

4. Melo LG, Pachori AS, Gnecchi M, Dzau VJ. Genetic therapies for cardiovascular diseases. Trends Mol Med 2005; 11(5):240–50.

5. Pisalru S, Simari R. Gene transfer for ischemic cardiovascular disease: is this the end of the beginning or the beginning of the end? Nat Clin Pract Cardiovasc Med 2005; 2(3):138–44.

6. Losordo DW, Vale PR, Symes JF, Dunnington CH, Esakof DD, Maysky M, et al. Gene therapy for myocardial angiogenesis: initial clinical results with direct myocardial injection of phVEGF165 as sole therapy for myocardial ischemia. Circulation 1998; 98(25):2800–4.

7. Kolsut P, Malecki M, Zelazny P, Teresinska A, Firek B, Janik P, et al. Gene therapy of coronary artery disease with phvegf165-early outcome. Kardiol Pol 2003; 59(11): 373–84.

8. Sarkar N, Ruck A, Kallner G, S YH, Blomberg P, Islam KB, et al. Effects of intramyocardial injection of phVEGF-A165 as sole therapy in patients with refractory coronary artery disease-12-month follow up: angiogenic gene therapy. J Intern Med 2001; 250(5):373–81.

9. Vale PR, Losordo DW, Milliken CE, Maysky M, Esakof DD, Symes JF, et al. Left ventricular electromechanical mapping to assess efficacy of phVEGF(165) gene transfer for therapeutic angiogenesis in chronic myocardial ischemia. Circulation 2000; 102(9):965–74.

10. Huwer H, Welter C, Ozbek C, Seifert M, Straub U, Greilach P, et al. Simultaneous surgical revascularization and angiogenic gene therapy in diffuse coronary artery disease. Eur J Cardiothorac Surg 2001; 20(6):1128–34.

11. Cotton JM, Mathur A, Hong Y, Brown AS, Martin JF, Erusalimsky JD. Acute rise of circulating vascular endothelial growth factor-A in patients with coronary artery disease following cardiothoracic surgery. Eur Heart J 2002; 23(12):953–9.

12. Vale PR, Losordo DW, Milliken CE, McDonald MC, Gravelin LM, Curry CM, et al. Randomized, single-blind, placebo-controlled pilot study of catheter-based myocardial gene transfer for therapeutic angiogenesis using left ventricular electromechanical mapping in patients with chronic myocardial ischemia. Circulation 2001; 103(17):2138–43.

13. Losordo DW, Vale PR, Hendel RC, Milliken CE, Fortuin FD, Cummings N, et al. Phase 1/2 placebo-controlled, double-blind, dose-escalating trial of myocardial vascular endothelial growth factor 2 gene transfer by catheter delivery in patients with chronic myocardial ischemia. Circulation 2002; 105(17):2012–18.

14. Rosengart TK, Lee LY, Patel SR, Sanborn TA, Parikh M, Bergman GW, et al. Angiogenesis gene therapy: phase I assessment of direct intramyocardial administration of an adenovirus vector expressing VEGF121 cDNA to individuals with clinically significant severe coronary artery disease. Circulation 1999; 100(5):468–74.

15. Grines CL, Watkins MW, Helmer G, Penny W, Brinker J, Marmur JD, et al. Angiogenic Gene Therapy (AGENT) trial in patients with stable angina pectoris. Circulation 2002; 105(11):1291–7.

16. Grines CL, Watkins MW, Mahmarian JJ, Iskandrian AE, Rade JJ, Marrott P, et al. A randomized, double-blind, placebo-controlled trial of Ad5FGF-4 gene therapy and its effect on myocardial perfusion in patients with stable angina. J Am Coll Cardiol 2003; 42(8):1339–47.

17. Wobus AM, Boheler KR. Embryonic stem cells: prospects for developmental biology and cell therapy. Physiol Rev 2005; 85(2):635–78.

18. Poulsom R, Alison MR, Forbes SJ, Wright NA. Adult stem cell plasticity. J Pathol 2002; 197(4):441–56.

19. Beltrami AP, Barlucchi L, Torella D, Baker M, Limana F, Chimenti S, et al. Adult cardiac stem cells are multipotent and support myocardial regeneration. Cell 2003; 114(6):763–76.

20. Kehat I, Kenyagin-Karsenti D, Snir M, Segev H, Amit M, Gepstein A, et al. Human embryonic stem cells can differentiate into myocytes with structural and functional properties of cardiomyocytes. J Clin Invest 2001; 108(3):407–14.

21. Behfar A, Hodgson DM, Zingman LV, Perez-Terzic C, Yamada S, Kane GC, et al. Administration of allogenic stem cells dosed to secure cardiogenesis and sustained infarct repair. Ann N Y Acad Sci 2005; 1049:189–98.

22. Lovell MJ, Mathur A. The role of stem cells for treatment of cardiovascular disease. Cell Prolif 2004; 37(1):67–87.

23. Hwang WS, Roh SI, Lee BC, Kang SK, Kwon DK, Kim S, et al. Patient-specific embryonic stem cells derived from human SCNT blastocysts. Science 2005; 308(5729):1777–83.

24. Alison MR, Poulsom R, Otto WR, Vig P, Brittan M, Direkze NC, et al. Recipes for adult stem cell plasticity: fusion cuisine or readymade? J Clin Pathol 2004; 57(2):113–20.

25. Balsam LB, Wagers AJ, Christensen JL, Kofidis T, Weissman IL, Robbins RC. Haematopoietic stem cells adopt mature haematopoietic fates in ischaemic myocardium. Nature 2004; 428(6983):668–73. Epub 2004 Mar 21.

26. Murry CE, Soonpaa MH, Reinecke H, Nakajima H, Nakajima HO, Rubart M, et al. Haematopoietic stem cells do not transdifferentiate into cardiac myocytes in myocardial infarcts. Nature 2004; 428(6983):664–8.

27. Menasche P. Skeletal muscle satellite cell transplantation. Cardiovasc Res 2003; 58(2):351–7.

28. Menasche P, Hagege AA, Vilquin JT, Desnos M, Abergel E, Pouzet B, et al. Autologous skeletal myoblast transplantation for severe postinfarction left ventricular dysfunction. J Am Coll Cardiol 2003; 41(7):1078–83.

29. Kang HJ, Kim HS, Zhang SY, Park KW, Cho HJ, Koo BK, et al. Effects of intracoronary infusion of peripheral blood stem-cells mobilised with granulocyte-colony stimulating factor on left ventricular systolic function and restenosis after coronary stenting in myocardial infarction: the MAGIC cell randomised clinical trial. Lancet 2004; 363(9411):751–6.

30. Perin EC, Dohmann HF, Borojevic R, Silva SA, Sousa AL, Mesquita CT, et al. Transendocardial, Autologous Bone Marrow Cell Transplantation for Severe, Chronic Ischemic Heart Failure. Circulation 2003; 21:21.

31. Wollert KC, Meyer GP, Lotz J, Ringes-Lichtenberg S, Lippolt P, Breidenbach C, et al. Intracoronary autologous bone-marrow cell transfer after myocardial infarction: the BOOST randomised controlled clinical trial. Lancet 2004; 364(9429):141–8.

Section Six

Training and Practice Guidelines for Percutaneous Coronary Intervention

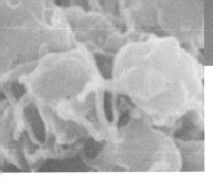

39

Training and practice guidelines for percutaneous coronary intervention

MARTYN THOMAS

KEY POINTS

- There is now a training program that was developed for the practice of PCI.
- It is assumed that prior to specialised training the individual will have performed at least 500 cardiac catheters in the 'core' training.
- In the current system many trainees undergo a period of research before they are appointed as a cardiology trainee.
- An 'exit' exam seems inevitable and is already being planned at a European level.
- All PTCA procedures performed in the UK will be electronically transmitted to a centrally held database.

Training in coronary intervention in the UK has historically been somewhat haphazard. In addition PCI is now regularly performed in the DGH setting without onsite surgical cover. In the 'new world' of clinical governance ad hoc training in this manner in no longer acceptable.

The UK, along with the rest of Europe, is currently trying to develop new methods of training which will allow:

- a systematic curriculum-based training in PCI;
- a methodology which allows selection criteria to enter such a training system;
- a competency-based assessment which will allow certification of a 'fitness to practice';
- a methodology for assessing continuing levels of competency for both performing and training in PCI; and

- recommendations for which centres should perform PCI.

TRAINING IN PCI

Training in PCI in the UK has traditionally been based on an apprenticeship type of model. Emphasis was placed on experience with the number of performed cases being given utmost importance and often there was no formal training scheme or indeed recognition of trainers in PCI.

More recently the British Cardiovascular Intervention Society (BCIS) along with Working Group 10 of the European Society of Cardiology[1] have been developing a more structured competency based training in interventional cardiology.

The modernising medical careers (MMC) programme[2] will result in an abbreviated medical and speciality training, resulting in an early 'core training' in general cardiology. Following this there will be a selection 'process' which will allow selected individuals to enter specialised training; in this instance training in interventional cardiology. The manner by which this selection will take place is still in development but is likely to be in the form of a competitive interview process.

The PCI training programme will consist of a two-year scheme. Learning methods in this two years will consist of multiple facets including:

Apprenticeship learning

Prior to training in PCI a solid grounding in diagnostic angiography is essential. It is assumed that prior to specialised training the individual will have performed at least 500 cardiac catheters in the 'core' training.

The shift towards competency based training with less dependence on numbers of procedure is a welcome change in emphasis but it remains the BCIS view that the number of procedures do still form an important part of training and should remain an integral part of the assessment of a trainee in conjunction with other methods. Defining the minimum number of PCI procedures that constitutes an acceptable training in angioplasty, however, is difficult because individuals learn at different rates and case selection and available facilities will differ between centres. The current recommendation is that trainees perform a minimum of 200 procedures over the last two years of their training programme, with a minimum of 125 procedures as first operator. At least 150 of these procedures should have been undertaken at the tertiary/surgical centre. A number of studies have indicated the link between procedural PCI numbers, for both an individual and an institution, and the recorded outcome of the procedure.[3]

These guidelines (available on the BCIS website[4]) are consistent with other national guidelines such as the ACC/AHA.[5]

Formal learning

A structured formal training timetable should be put in place in training programmes. This will consist of attendance at multidisciplinary meetings (including surgical colleagues) to discuss complex cases and modes of revascularisation in patients with coronary artery disease. Attendance and participation in audit meetings will be expected. Time will be made available to attend local, national and international study days.

In the current system many trainees undergo a period of research before they are appointed as a cardiology trainee. Much of this research is basic science as practical skills have not been acquired to allow clinical research. During the formal PCI training trainees should be exposed to clinical research in interventional cardiology. This may be in the form of local research, recruitment of patients into multi-centre trials or organisation of a clinical audit.

Practical skill learning on simulators

The hardware and software for computer-based simulated PCI is developing rapidly. In the very near future it will be possible to simulate all forms of coronary lesion and also programme 'complication scenarios' in a similar way to flight simulators. This will be a very valuable tool in the learning process. Because of the improved angioplasty technology the learning curve, especially in managing complications, has potentially become quite prolonged. It is now possible that a complication is seen by an individual, for the first time, as a newly appointed consultant in the middle of the night. This is clearly not satisfactory. The possibility to reproduce such complications on a simulator and facilitate actions to successfully resolve these complications will be particularly useful.

Certification of successful training in PCI

One of the potential weaknesses of the current rather ad hoc training schemes is the lack of 'validation' of training in PCI. An individual can 'claim' to be trained in PCI having had very little formal or practical training other than that as a second operator. In the systems currently being designed this will change. Individuals will be allocated training numbers after entry into a formal training scheme following, most likely, a competitive process. They will then appear on a formal 'register' of trainees acknowledged as interventional trainees from that particular scheme. In addition an 'exit' exam seems inevitable and is already being planned at a European level. This exit exam is likely to take the form of a multiple choice written exam and a 'practical' simulator-based case study. Formal certification will follow this process.

Continued competence

Continued competence for individuals once they have become a consultant will generally be assessed within the clinical governance arrangement of any hospital and also in the annual appraisal system. However, the current recommendation is that an individual can be considered an independent operator if he performs a minimum of 75 cases per year. Ideally plans should be in place for the individual to increase this number to 150. In order to be considered a 'trainer' a minimum number of 125 procedures should be performed per year.

INSTITUTIONAL GUIDELINES

Although the numbers of procedures may not be regarded as an important element of quality there is some data which relates institutional numbers to patient outcome. Current BCIS guidelines state that a centre should achieve a minimum of 200 procedures per year but should be aiming to increase to 400 cases per year. Once more this is in line with other (US and European) guidelines. A number of new PCI centres have been set up in the UK. Many of these are based in DGH hospitals and have off-site surgical cover. The process of centre accreditation includes a formal request from the Chief Executive of the institution to BCIS for an institutional review. The site is then visited and a report issued which assesses cardiac network support, the business case, the number of trained operators, arrangements for surgical support and all other infrastructure within the hospital. Importantly the current guidelines state that formal arrangements need to be in place for surgical cover and that it should be possible to institute cardiopulmonary bypass within 90 minutes of any call for emergency bypass surgery.

Institutional and individual operator audit

Audit plays an important part of maintaining and improving both individual and institutional performance in PCI. It should allow identification of factors, whether personal or system based, which lead to adverse outcome for patients. It is vital that any outcome assessment has a link with pre-procedural risk and also has the confidence of the interventional community. Without this element of confidence and the link of outcome to pre-procedural risk the inevitable outcome will be a reluctance of individual operators to 'take on' high risk patients because of the fear of adverse outcomes.

This problem has been highlighted within the surgical community in the UK with the publication of individual operator surgical outcome published in a rather ad hoc non-controlled fashion. Data for this publication was demanded under the Freedom of Information Act (FOI). The interventional community can be protected from these demands by having a plan to produce this type of information and display it in the public domain. If the medical community do this it can be released in a responsible manner with proper risk adjustment to maintain public and physician faith. All of these factors should allow interventional cardiologists to be able to practice in a responsible manner, to keep treatment of individual patients to the foremost and to allow high risk patients to continue to receive high risk interventions despite the potential high complication rates.

To this end BCIS and the Department of Health (DOH) in the UK have established the UKCCAD process. This refers to the system of centrally collected angioplasty data. All PTCA procedures performed in the UK will be electronically transmitted to a centrally held database. This database will be integrated with a myocardial infarction database (MINAP), the surgical (SCTS) database and the Office of National Statistics (ONS, mortality) databases. This will allow true 'tracking' of the patient journey (i.e. diagnosis, treatment modalities and outcome) which will be virtually unique.

Analysis of this data will clearly be sensitive. To this end a 'tripartite group' consisting of BCIS, the Healthcare Commission and the Heart Team (DOH) has been set up. This group will consider requests for data analysis in a scientific manner. Any approved request for data analysis will be passed to an independent unit with statistical expertise which will be charged with data analysis. It is hoped that this process will allow National Audit and quality control within a controlled scientific environment.

CONCLUSIONS

Training in coronary angioplasty has been historically somewhat ad hoc. Given that PCI is now the dominant form of revascularisation worldwide this is no longer acceptable. More formalised European guidelines for training in PCI and continued UK institutional guidelines for standards for hospitals performing PCI should lead to continued high quality delivery of PCI within the UK.

REFERENCES

1. www.escardio.org

2. www.mmc.nhs.uk

3. Moscucci M, Share D, Smith D, O'Donnell MJ, Riba A, McNamara R, Lalonde T, Defranco AC, Patel K, Kline Rogers E, D'Haem C, Karve M, Eagle KA. Relationship between operator volume and adverse outcome in contemporary percutaneous coronary intervention practice: an analysis of a quality-controlled multicenter percutaneous coronary intervention clinical database. J Am Coll Cardiol. 2005 Aug 16; 46(4):625–32.

4. www.bcis.org.uk

5. Smith SC Jr, Dove JT, Jacobs AK, Kennedy JW, Kereiakes D, Kern MJ, Kuntz RE. Popma JJ, Schaff HV, Williams DO. ACC/AHA guidelines of percutaneous coronary interventions (revision of the 1993 PTCA guidelines)-executive summary. A report of the American College of Cardiology/American Heart Association Task Force on Practice Guidelines. J Am Coll Cardiol 2001; 37:2215–38.

Section Seven

Current Major Trials in Interventional Cardiology

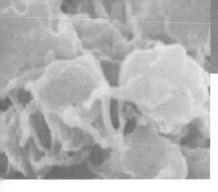

40

Current major trials in interventional cardiology

ANTHONY H. GERSHLICK

KEY POINTS

- Balloon angioplasty is of historic interest only due to the need for excess repeat procedures compared to CABG.

- Bare metal stents made percutaneous intervention safer but patients still require re-intervention more frequently, the difference being 12–15% greater than surgery as a result of in-stent intimal hyperplasia.

- Increased operator skill, newer equipment and the development of new techniques has radically changed the profile of patients undergoing PCI, with those normally receiving surgery (e.g. left main stem disease) now candidates for the percutaneous approach.

- Drug eluting stents have allowed the results of such interventions to be maintained with recurrence rates now <5% for straightforward cases.

- Established DES have been proven to be beneficial in randomised controlled trials versus BMS.

- New stent programmes with new drugs and new platforms are being developed.

- The acute, medium and longer term results of PCI are now robust enough to challenge those of CABG.

- PCI is the dominant therapy for treating patients with coronary artery disease and with the advent of DES may result in CABG becoming a niche therapy.

BACKGROUND

Percutaneous coronary intervention has become the dominant therapy for treating patients with ischaemia due to obstructive coronary artery disease. In 2003, 53 000 UK patients were treated with PCI and 26 000 with surgery. In other European countries the ratio rises to 8 PCIs–1 CABG patient. Such a major change in patient care involving a shift from one therapeutic modality to another over a relatively short time (5–10 years) could only have occurred as a result of a number of reasons. Firstly, there needed to be the drive to perform PCI by enthusiastic operators. Simultaneously techniques and equipment evolved to make the procedure safer and clinically effective and an understanding of the potential and the limitations of the procedure evolved. Finally all of this had to be underpinned by an evidence base consisting of randomised controlled trials (RCT) and registry data. While RCT remain the corner-stone of evidence-based treatment they have the limitations of (over) patient selection and applicability of results to the real world, which often includes patients excluded from the RCT. This review will highlight the key evidence that has led to the opening statement in this article.

PCI (BALLOONS AND BMS) VERSUS CABG

Coronary angioplasty has evolved rapidly. During the early 1990s it was seen as a treatment for predominantly single vessel disease, with coronary surgery for all else. Although studies comparing balloon angioplasty with surgery indicated no difference in myocardial infarction or death, the need for re-vascularisation was about 5% pa with surgery but 30% for balloon angioplasty[1], due to a number of factors including vessel recoil, late remodelling (where the vessel gets smaller after vessel wall injury) and injury-induced scar tissue formation.

Stents arose from the need to reduce *acute* balloon angioplasty induced adverse outcomes (due to intimal dissection). As a bonus stents also reduced recoil and late negative re-modelling with a halving of the need for a repeat procedure to about 15%–20%, but with higher rates in certain sub-groups (diabetics and those with small reference diameters or longer lesions[2,3] Fig. 40.1. The benefit of safer acute outcomes and overall reduction in need for repeat procedures made stenting the standard of care, with >90% PCI patients now receiving stents.

Despite advantages over balloon angioplasty, stenting still resulted in a excess need for repeat intervention compared to multi-vessel stenting with coronary surgery: ARTS 1, SOS and ERACI studies[4-6] indicated a difference in re-intervention between 12%–15% at six months in the stent arm. A meta-analysis comparing PCI and surgery in multi-vessel disease (Mercado *et al.* J Thoracic Cardiovasc. Surg.) suggests no difference in death, AMI, CVA (PCI-8.7% Surgery-9.1 HR=0.95 (95% ci 0.74–1.2). These studies were not trials of simple, single vessel disease-in ARTS-1, for example, there was a mean 2.9 stents/patient and 2.7 grafts/patient- (93% with at least one internal mammary artery).

RESTENOSIS RATES: DVD, LENGTH AND DM

Vessel diameter	Lesion length						
	10 mm	15 mm	20 mm	25 mm	30 mm	35 mm	40 mm
Diabetic patients							
2.5 mm	18%	21%	24%	28%	33%	38%	45%
3.0 mm	12%	14%	16%	18%	21%	25%	29%
3.5 mm	8%	9%	10%	12%	14%	16%	19%
4.0 mm	5%	6%	7%	8%	9%	10%	12%
Non-diabetic patients							
2.5 mm	11%	13%	15%	18%	21%	24%	28%
3.0 mm	7%	8%	10%	11%	13%	15%	18%
3.5 mm	5%	5%	6%	7%	9%	10%	12%
4.0 mm	3%	4%	4%	5%	6%	6%	7%

Figure 40.1:
Factors that influence restenosis rates.

Residual in-stent scar tissue formation remained a clinical limitation of stenting compared to surgery. The concept of delivering drugs from stents at local high concentrations to prevent within tissue in-growth evolved from local balloon drug delivery. Failure to retain drug at the site and inadequate local dose concentration limited the applicability of such balloons. Delivering drugs locally on stents became the goal. A number of drugs to limit the restenotic process have been delivered either by altering the surface of the stent or by utilising a polymer to load the drug.

DRUG ELUTING STENTS VERSUS BARE METAL STENTS

SIROLIMUS-Eluting-STENTS (SES)

Sirolimus (Rapamycin) is the metabolic substrate of the fungus streptomyces hygroscopicus. Loaded onto stents at a dose of 180 µg it inhibits cell proliferation after vessel wall injury by binding to a receptor protein (FKBP12)-the rapamycin/FKB12 complex then binds to mTOR (Mammalian Target Of Rapamycin), preventing its interaction with target proteins, such as regulatory tumour suppressor genes including P27, which are important in signalling pathways leading to cell proliferation.

The first Rapamycin trial (RAVEL[7]) while demonstrating efficacy was criticised for the simple nature of the lesions tested, although inclusion of such patients was appropriate for a 'proof of principle' trial. There were also concerns about 'excess effectiveness' with late loss ('angiographic difference in minimal lumen diameter from immediate post stenting to follow up in mm') approaching 0 mm suggesting complete inhibition of tissue growth with no stent coverage. The US–based SIRIUS trial[8] included more complex lesions and late loss and binary restenosis rate were greater. SIRIUS trial patients with small reference vessel diameters (mean 2.3 mm) had higher target lesion revascularisation (TLR) –7.3% compared to 1.8% in 3.0 mm vessels, and a higher need for revascularisation in diabetics (TLR 7.2%). The TLR rate of 13.9% in insulin-dependant diabetics was particularly worrying although the numbers were small. The NEW-SIRIUS data addressed some of these issues. NEW-SIRIUS represents the pooled results of two trials C-SIRIUS[9] (the Canadian study of 100 patients) and E-SIRIUS[10] (the European study of 352 patients). The trials design was identical. Primary end-point was eight-month angiographic outcome with nine-month clinical follow-up. The late-loss was 0.18 mm in-stent and 0.17 mm outside the stent indicating the so-called 'edge effect' in the SIRIUS trial had been overcome (presumably by a change in technique). The option of direct stenting in NEW-SIRIUS, (30% incidence) also reduced balloon injury. TLR for NEW-SIRIUS was 4% versus control 20.3%. The small-reference vessel subgroups results are better than in SIRIUS with in-stent restenosis rates of 3.8% for vessels with mean size 2.2 mm. TLR rates in diabetics was still around 7%, however. A list of the 'CYPHER Trials' and their outcomes are shown in Table 40.1.

Concerns have been raised that polymer and/or drug could be removed during direct stenting (which accounts for about 30% of all PCI procedures) potentially affecting DES efficacy. In NEW-SIRIUS this was found not to be the case with in-lesion restenosis in the pre-dilatation Sirolimus stenting group 7% versus 2.4% in the direct Sirolimus stent group. Other recently presented data includes longer

STUDY	PTS (N)	DIABETIC PTS (%)	RD (mm)	LESION	% STENOSIS LENGTH (mm)	B2/C LESIONS (%)	100% OCCLS. (%)	TLR % (@ X MONTHS)	MACE
RAVEL	238	19.0	2.62	9.6	63.8	57.0(B2)	0	2.5 (36 mo)	5.8 (36 mo)
SIRIUS	1058	26.0	2.80	14.4	65.3	56	0	6.8 (36 mo)	12.6 (36 mo)
E-SIRIUS	252	23.0	2.55	15.0	65.4	–	0	4.6 (24 mo)	10.3 (24 mo)
C-SIRIUS	100	24.0	2.64	13.5	69.7	59	0	4.0 (9 mo)	4.0 (9 mo)
DIABETES	160	100	2.34	15.0	–	80.1	13.1	7.5 (12 mo)	11.3 (12 mo)
SES-SMART	257	24.9	2.20	11.8	66.8	28.8	0	7.0 (8 mo)	9.3 (8 mo)
SCANDSTENT	322	18.0	2.86	18.0	76.6	–	35.7	2.4 (6 mo)	3.1 (6 mo)

TABLE 40.1 - OUTCOMES FOR CYPHER STENTS RANDOMIZED CYPHER VS. BMS TRIALS TOTAL: 2827 PATIENTS (1420 CYPHER, 1407 BMS)

term follow-up, with the RAVEL results maintained to three years and the FIM (n=45) patients having little loss in any of the measures of initial success out to four years.

Concerning diabetics, Sabaté recently presented the 'DIABETES' study. Angiographic restenosis in the Sirolimus arm was 7.7%, with target lesion revascularisation 7.5% and overall MACE 11.3% – all highly significantly improved (p=0.0001) over the control bare metal stented patients.[11]

PACLITAXEL-ELUTING-STENT (PES)

While it was recognised in the 1960s that the extract of yew-bark killed artificially-preserved leukemia cells and was effective against ovarian tumors, it was only in 1978 that it was shown that it killed cancer cells in a novel way by microtubular stabilization. These properties make it a valuable agent for stent-delivery in the treatment of restenosis.

The agent has been delivered either with or without a polymer carrier. The ELUTES[12] and ASPECT [13]) clinical trials tested paclitaxel applied directly to the stent. Both showed significant reduction in restenosis at dose density of 3 ug/mm^2 of stent. These results led investigators to undertake the pivotal US DELIVER 1 trial, in which paclitaxel was loaded without polymer onto a different stent to that used in either of the other two previous trials. The results were disappointing with no significant benefit in the treated group. The reasons for the differences from ELUTES/ASPECT will probably never be fully understood, but likely due to inability to load the stent with the effective (ELUTES) dose. No further development of a non-polymer stent is likely, which is disappointing now there are concerns about the longer term effect of residual polymer once the any drug has eluted.

The difference in success between the non-polymer and polymer-coated paclitaxel (TAXUS) programmes cannot have been more acute. The success of TAXUS II[14] has been extended to more complex lesions in TAXUS IV.[15] The outcomes for the increasingly complex TAXUS trials are shown in Table 40.2. The end-point of TAXUS IV was clinical with TLR rates of 3% versus 11% in controls (p<0.0001). TLR rates for smaller vessels are similar to the Sirolimus trials (3.4% for TAXUS IV <2.5 mm and 3.6% for mean 2.5 mm in NEW-SIRIUS) but while in the non-direct comparisons outcomes of TAXUS diabetic patients appeared better than Sirolimus (TLR of 4.8% and insulin-dependant diabetics 5.9%), a recently presented direct comparison ISAR-DIABETES[16] gives Sirolimus the edge in these difficult patients. In 250 randomised diabetics showed no difference in death/MI at nine months. However, late lumen loss in the Sirolimus group was 0.43 mm compared 0.67 mm (p=0.002) with TAXUS. The angiographic binary restenosis rates were 6.9% Cypher and 16.5% TAXUS (p=0.03), but the difference in clinical restenosis was not statistically significant (TLR 6.4% versus 12.0%) Fig. 40.2.

Robust efficacy is highlighted in TAXUS VI[17] which included longer lesions (20.6 mm) and multiple stenting. Total stent length of 33.4 mm, and AHA/ACC type C lesions of 55.6%. TLR was 19.4% in the control group and 9.1% in the TAXUS–(53% decrease in TVR, p=0.0027). The difference was independent of classic restenosis risk factors.

TABLE 40.2 - OUTCOME OF THE TAXUS TRIALS RANDOMIZED TAXUS VS. BMS TRIALS TOTAL: 3471 PATIENTS (1732 TAXUS, 1739 BMS)

STUDY	PTS (N)	DIABETIC Pts (%)	RD (mm)	LESION LENGTH (mm)	% STENOSIS	B2/C LESIONS (%)	100% OCCLUS (%)	TLR % (@ X MONTHS)	MACE
TAXUS I	61	18.0	2.97	11.3	56.5	36.0(B)	0	3.0 (24 mo)	3.0 (24 mo)
TAXUS II	536	14.0	2.75	10.4	64.4	–	0	4.7 (12 mo)	10.9 (12 mo)
								5.5 (24 mo)	14.2 (24 mo)
TAXUS IV	1314	24.2	2.75	13.4	66.5	–	0	5.6 (24 mo)	14.7 (24 mo)
TAXUS V	1156	30.8	2.69	7.2	68.3	55.6 (C)	–	8.6 (9 mo)	15 (9 mo)
TAXUS VI	446	19.9	2.79	20.6	65.4	83.4	–	9.7 (9 mo)	21.3 (24 mo)

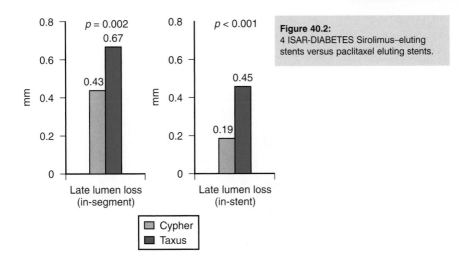

Figure 40.2:
4 ISAR-DIABETES Sirolimus–eluting stents versus paclitaxel eluting stents.

Are all DES equal?

The impact of the two current on clinical outcome DES versus BMS is shown in Fig. 40.3. The recently presented REALITY trial (n=1386)[18] compared SES and TAXUS using eight months angiographic restenosis as primary end point. It show significantly less late loss with SES (0.09 versus 0.31 p<0.001). TLR was no different, however, (5.0% versus 5.4% respectively). Why there was no difference in clinical end point despite a difference in late loss is unclear especially as from the SIRTAX trial[19] less of a difference in LL favouring SES translated into a clinical difference between devices (4.8% TLR Sirolimus versus 8.3% TAXUS p=0.025).

Real world registries

Real world registry data exists for both currently available DES. Such studies, although subject to critism of selection bias, are important since many of the

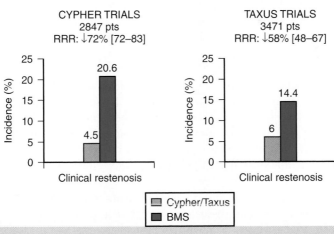

Figure 40.3:
DES versus BMS – clinical outcomes (TLR).

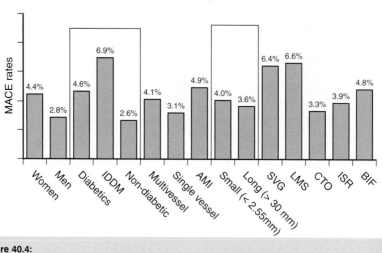

PATIENT SUBSETS: 6 MONTHS MACE
Overall (n = 11159): 3.2% MACE

Figure 40.4:
MACE rates in the real world – e-CYPHER Registry of Sirolimus–eluting stents.

exclusion criteria in the RCT include lesions treated in everyday practice (CTO, in-stent restenosis, bifurcation disease, etc). The e-Cypher registry[20] reached its recruitment target of 15 000 patients in 2004 with 11 159 (87%) evaluated at six months. There are 1.3 stents per lesion and 30% direct stenting. 48.7% of patients were treated 'off-label' (CTO, SVG, etc). Overall MACE was 3.2% with 6.4% in SVG, 6.6% left main stem, non-diabetic 2.6%, diabetic 4.6% and in bifurcation 4.8% (Fig. 40.4) TLR rates are low in all subsets compared to historical data. In a further registry of Cypher stents, clinically driven TLR is 3.7% (n=508) (RESEARCH[21]).

In the WISDOM TAXUS Registry MACE rates of 4.5% and TLR of 1.8% have been reported in 604 patients. The MILESTONE II registry is designed to assess outcome by lesion subsets in 3000 patients. Data collection is ongoing.

Higher risk patient populations
While DES are effective overall (Fig. 40.3) there is no doubt that certain patients are at greater risk of restenosis (see Fig. 40.1). These include those with small vessel disease, long lesions, and those with diabetes and ACS. Additionally we need to know the outcomes for those who have CTO, left main stem and bifurcations. Much of the data is registry or post hoc analyses, but provides some insight into potential outcomes of DES used in such clinical scenarios.

Small vessel disease: Problems occur in patients with small vessel reference diameter because the same tissue response has a greater impact within the confines of a smaller vessel. Even with DES, smaller vessel size is associated with an increased risk of restenosis or repeat revascularisation but the events rates are much reduced compared to BMS (mean late loss value falling from 0.8 to 0.04).

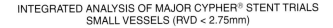

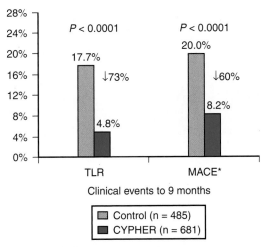

INTEGRATED ANALYSIS OF MAJOR CYPHER® STENT TRIALS
SMALL VESSELS (RVD < 2.75mm)

Figure 40.5:
Randomised trials of SES v BMS in small vessel disease.

Figure 40.5 presents combined data from randomised trials comparing the SES and BMS. Overall binary restenosis is reduced from 42.5% to 9.9% (p <0.0001), with a 73% reduction in TLR from 17.7% to 4.8% (p <0.0001). Similar findings emerge from the randomised TAXUS studies (Fig. 40.6).

Long lesions: Why those with longer lesions should be more prone to restenosis is less clear. However the independent effects of stented lesion length, non-stented lesion length, and excess stent length, on coronary restenosis have been evaluated in 1,181 patients from six BMS trials of de novo lesions in native coronary arteries.[22] Stent length exceeded lesion length in 87% of lesions (mean difference 7.6±7.9 mm). At 6–9 month follow up, mean percent diameter stenosis was 39±20%. In a multivariate model of percent diameter stenosis, each 10 mm of stented lesion length was associated with an absolute increase in percent diameter stenosis of 7.7% (p <0.0001), whereas each 10 mm of excess stent length independently increased percent diameter stenosis by 4.0% (p <0.0001) with increased TLR at nine months (odds ratio 1.12, 95% confidence interval 1.02 to 1.24).

A multiple regression model was used to predict eight-month percent diameter in the angiographic follow-up of the SIRIUS trial (n=699).[23] Stented lesion length and excess stent length were associated with absolute increases in percent diameter stenosis per 10 mm of 9.1% (p<0.0001) and 3.6% (p=0.053) in the bare metal arm but 3.5% (p<0.05) and 2.1% (p<0.05) in the Sirolimus-eluting stent arm Fig. 40.7.

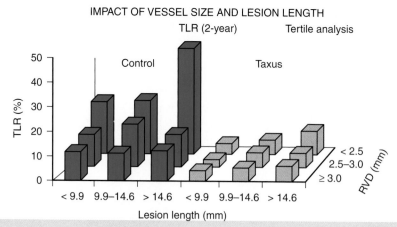

Figure 40.6:
Small vessels and long lesions with the TAXUS stent versus BM controls.

Diabetes This patient group remain a problem. The formation of advanced glycation end products (AGE), in various tissues has been known to enhance immunoinflammatory reactions and local oxidant stresses in long standing diabetes, leading to excessive tissue response.[24] However in diabetic sub-groups randomised to SES or PES versus BMS an important biologically consistent reduction in restenosis (both angiographic and clinical) has been demonstrated with DES (Table 40.3). Data is available that directly compare BMS versus DES in diabetics only (the DIABETES[11] trial see above). At nine months angiographic follow up, the late luminal loss was 0.44 mm in the BMS group and 0.08 mm in the Sirolimus arm (p<0.001).

To test the independent predictor of diabetes for restenosis Dawkins *et al.*[25] have under taken a multivariate logistic regression analysis for TLR with predictors of lesion length (by QCA), RVD (by QCA), treatment (DES/BMS), and

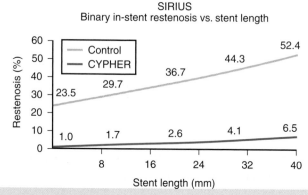

Figure 40.7:
Restenosis does not significantly increase with length of DES compared to BMS.

TABLE 40.3 - OUTCOMES IN DIABETICS IN THE VARIOUS TRIALS

TRIAL (% DIABETICS)	RELATIVE REDUCTION IN BINARY RESTENOSIS (%) IN DIABETICS	TLR RATE IN DIABETICS TREATED WITH DES (%)
RAVEL (18.5%)	100%	0
SIRIUS (26%)	65%	6.9
NEW-SIRIUS	81%	7
TAXUS II (15%)	100%	3.1
TAXUS IV (24%)	82%	5.9
TAXUS VI (19%)	80%	2.6

diabetic status from the pooled database of three randomized TAXUS trials. The diabetic group consisted of 214 patients randomized to the TAXUS stent and 240 patients randomized to BMS control: the non-diabetic group consisted of 919 patients randomized to the TAXUS stent and 903 patients randomized to the BMS. Comparisons of baseline mean lesion length and RVD, as well as the outcome for TLR were made between treatments, and between the diabetic and non-diabetic patient subgroups.

Multivariate logistic regression for patients in the BMS arm indicated no diabetic benefit when controlling for RVD and lesion length. In non-diabetic patients, the 12-month TLR rate was reduced by 69% from 14.0% in Control to 4.3% in TAXUS (p<0.0001). This benefit was maintained in diabetics with a reduction by 63% from 20.2% in Control to 5.6% in TAXUS (p<0.0001). Multivariate logistic regression for patients in the TAXUS arm indicated a diabetic benefit when correcting for RVD and lesion length. Multivariate logistic regression for all patients in both arms indicated that the adjusted odds ratio for TLR for diabetic patients is 1.38 with a 95% confidence interval of (1.004, 1.905).

These results are important since they support the concept that diabetes is an independent risk factor for restenosis that is reduced by DES (in this instance TAXUS) irrespective of other factors that normally influence restenosis.

PCI in AMI The European Society of Cardiology has recently recommended that primary PCI be the preferred treatment for patients suffering acute myocardial infarction.[26] It is thus critical that optimal short, medium and longer term outcomes be achieved in such patients.

BMS implantation has been shown to be better than balloon alone in acute MI.[27,28] However in-stent restenosis and vessel occlusion remained clinical problems. Conversely patients with acute coronary syndromes have increased thrombotic complications after PCI[29,30] and there have been concerns that these will be excessive with DES, with potential vessel re-endothelialisation being delayed by drug elution. The results of various registries of Sirolimus-and Paclitaxel eluting stents in AMI is shown in Table 40.4.[31-33]

Because of the presence of a thrombotic (infarct-precipitating environment) stent thrombosis has received particular attention in this group of patients, however, registry data does not support this concern. DES in AMI appears appropriate.

Drug eluting stents in acute coronary syndromes (NSTEMI): For ACS patients requiring revascularisation the most common form of revascularisation is

TABLE 40.4 - OUTCOMES OF AMI PATIENTS

REGISTRY (N=) FOLLOW UP TIME (MO)	MORTALITY %		TLR %		MACE		STENT THROMBOSIS %	
	BMS	DES	BMS	DES	BMS	DES	BMS	DES
Saia [31] (n=96) (7.2 mo)		7.3		1.1		8.4		0
Lemos [32] (n=186) (10 mo)	8.2	8.3	8.2	1.1	17	9.4	1.6	0
						p=0.02		
Gershlick [33] (n=803) (6 mo)	NA	3.5	NA	1.7	NA	5.3	NA	1.5

PCI and this is usually performed with intra coronary stents (NICE stent submission 2002).

In the RESEARCH registry[34] early outcomes of patients with ACS treated with SES were compared to those treated with BMS. Thirty-day MACE was similar (SES 6.1% vs BMS 6.1% p=0.8), Stent thrombosis was not significantly different between the groups, with even a trend favouring DES (SES 0.5% vs BMS 1.7% p=0.4).

Paclitaxel-eluting Stents have been compared to BMS (n=213) in ACS (35) (n=237). MACE at 30 days were 3.4% PES vs 2.3% BMS p=0.52. One year revascularisation rates were 6.5% PES vs 17.7 % BMS p=0.0003 and MACE 11.1 PES vs 21.7 BMS p=0.003, a reduction in composite MACE of 51%. Stent thrombosis was the same (0.8% PES vs 0.9% BMS). Comparison of unstable vs stable patients all treated with PES had a trend towards a higher rate of stent thrombosis at 30 days in the ACS group (0.8% unstable vs 0% stable p=0.06), but not at one year (0.8% unstable vs 0.5% stable p=0.55).

Both DES have been evaluated in registry[36] containing a high proportion of AMI and unstable angina (55% in each group). There were no differences in death or MI, TVR or MACE at 30 days, six months or one year between the two stent types.

Lesion specific registry data

The registry/RCT outcome data for particular sub-groups is shown in (refs 35–52) (Table 40.5).

Can DES challenge CABG?

Drug eluting stents have been a major advance for interventional cardiology. Target TLR rates have fallen to ~5% (a >70% reduction compared to BMS). Even in complex cases the need for revascularisation is between 5% and 10%.[17] Recently presented data indicated event-free survival between nine months and two years of 92.2% for those in the original TAXUS trials, good considering vein graft attrition rates are between 2.5% and 5% pa, reaching 50% occlusion rate at ten years. The standard of care for PCI is DES even in complex lesions. Recent studies have compared DES in multi-vessel disease to surgery.

TABLE 40.5 - OUTCOME REGISTRY & RCT DATA FOR LESIONS GENERALLY EXCLUDED FROM RANDOMISED TRIALS OF DES

STUDY WITH DATA WHERE AVAILABLE — TRIAL TYPE	FOLLOW-UP MO	TARGET LESION REVASCULARISATION			MACE			LATE LOSS MM / RESTENOSIS %		
		DES	P	BMS	DES	P	BMS	DES	P	BMS
Saphenous vein grafts										
Vermeersch[37] (RCT)	(12)	5%			11%	(NS)	44%	LL 0.49	0.005	1.48
Hoye[38] (Reg)	(12)	NA		NA	26%		NA			
Ge[39] (Reg ~ historical controls)	(6)	3.3%	0.003	19.8%	11.5%	0.02	28.1%			
Bifurcations										
Colombo[40] (RCT~ double versus provisional)	(6)	Overall 8%		(TVF =15 %)				Rest 28%		18.7%
Louvard[41]										
Chronic Total Occlusions										
Simes[42] (RCT bare metal stent trial "SICCO")	(12)	NA		22%	3.6%	<0.05	17.2%	LL 0.13		
Hoye[43](Reg ~ historical controls)	(12)				12.5%	<0.001	47.9%	Rest 8.3%	<0.05	51%
Werner[44] (Reg ~ matched BMS)	(12)									
Left main stem disease										
Silvestri[45] (Reg ~ bare metal stent)	(6)	NA		17.4%	NA					
Tan[46] (Reg ~ bare metal stent)	(19)				6.6%		39.4%			
Gershlick[47] (Reg ~ CYPHER stents)	(6)				10%	<0.0006	35%			
Valgimigli[48](Reg ~ DES versus historical controls)	(12)	6%	<0.0004	23%	2%	<0.0003	18.6	LL 0.05	<0.001	1.27
Park[49] (Reg ~ DES versus historical controls)	(12)				20%	<0.04	35.9%			
Chieffo[50] (Reg ~ DES versus historical controls)	(6)				3.9%					
In-stent restenosis										
Gershlick[51] (Reg ~ CYPHER stents)	(6)	8% (SES)	p<0.02							
Kastrati[52] (RCT ~ SES v PES v balloon)	(6)	19% (PES)						Rest 14.3% (SES) 21.7% (PES)		NA NA

539

The ARTS-2 trial[52] compared SES with the previous ARTS 1 BMS and surgical arms. Freedom from major adverse cardiac and cardiovascular event (MACCE) rate was 89.5% with SES in ARTS 2 (re-vascularisation 7.4% (5.4% re-PCI, 2% CABG), compared to 88.5% MACCE free for ARTS-1 surgery (3% PCI). It would seem that in complex patient subsets DES appear to produce better outcomes than surgery.

Ongoing DES programmes

New programmes in DES are important for a number of reasons.

- Firstly, as we treat more complex lesions, more efficacious agents may be required. Stent delivered agents that are more lipophylic, have greater tissue penetration or greater residency time may have true advantages. We may want agents that are more stable or have different release kinetics or even agents that work in completely different ways. Clinical trials of such new DES will be required by the Regulatory authorities to be tested against currently available DES, not BMS.
- Secondly, we may wish for improved stent platforms. Treating complex lesions and making in-roads into previous surgical cases will be dependant on technology and operator skills, not merely effective DES.
- Thirdly, new DES will result in competition and lower prices for this expensive technology.

SIROLIMUS-DERIVATIVES

Sirolimus has three important chemical regions: the FK binding protein region, the non-protein binding region that influences physical properties and the mTOR binding domain. C-43 sits in the first of these and substitution of the 'HO' produces new agents (Fig. 40.8). The ABT578 53 (substitution at C-43 with 5=N ring formation) has been loaded onto the Medtronic DRIVER stent using a bio-neutral (phosphorylcholine) polymer. The ENDEAVOR programme is based on laboratory and pre-clinical data suggesting ABT578 (10 ug/mm stent) has potent effects on smooth muscle cell growth, inhibiting intimal hyperplasia.

The pivotal ENDEAVOR II trial[54] randomised 1200 patients to ABT578/Biocompatible polymer/Driver stent or BMS. The primary endpoint of target vessel failure (cardiac death, MI, TVR) at nine months occurred in 8.1% ENDEAVOR compared to control 15.4%. TLR rates were 4.7% – competitive with the CYPHER and TAXUS programmes. An interesting aspect of this trial was the 'high' late loss relative to the two other devices: 0.62 mm versus SIRUS-0.17 mm and TAXUS IV–0.39 mm). The relationship between late loss and clinical events is as yet not fully understood, but TLR may only become important only at >0.6 mm.[55] ENDEAVOR III is a US-based 30 centre study of 436 patients randomised 3:1 to ENDEAVOR stent or Cypher. Again primary end point will be angiographic 'in-segment late loss' at eight months because of likely small clinical differences. ENDEAVOR IV is a comparison with the TAXUS stent in 1000 patients.

The Abbott

Everolimus is also a Sirolimus derivative, with reportedly better pharmaco-kinetics, tissue residency and stability than its parent compound[56] but unlike

RAPAMYCIN CHEMICAL MODIFICATIONS

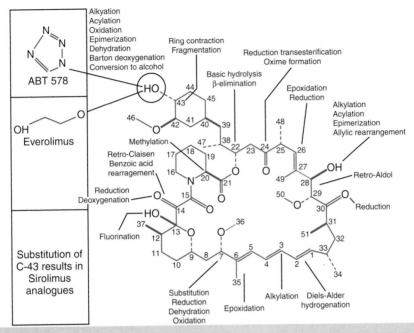

Figure 40.8:
The basic Rapamycin molecule – changes to C-43 produces new anti-restenotic molecules.

ABT578 is currently available, being used in organ transplantation. The Guidant Everolimus programme consists of loading drug onto the Biosensors Champion stent/bio-absorbable polymer (polylactic acid, which breaks down to lactic acid and has a high drug carrying potential) and which is already used in bio-prostheses. Safety and pilot efficacy data with this combination (Future I & II studies (n=42 & 64)) reported MACE rates of 7.7% and 4.8% resp. and low late loss of 0.15 mm. Future III will compare six-month late loss in 800 patients randomised 3:1 to this drug/polymer/stent combination or to bare metal Zeta stent and FUTURE IV will compare this combination with an FDA approved DES control (n=935 randomised 2:1). The future of this drug on the Vision stent will depend on the outcome of merger negotiations between J&J and Guidant.

BiolimusA9 is yet another Sirolimus derivative, claimed to be even more lipophylic with >85% eluting into tissue within eight hours, on a Biosensors stent and is being tested STEALTH trials. It is currently being tested on a conical ('bifurcation') DEVAXX stent.

The CONNOR stent has a unique stent design (Fig. 40.9) with polymer-filled laser cut wells and configurered to release drug toward the vessel wall, toward the lumen or both. Stent deliverability appears good. The PISCES pilot study[57] tested different doses, released over different periods –10 or 30 ug Paclitaxel for between 10 and 30 days. Results suggest an overall 30-day MACE of 4.2%, with

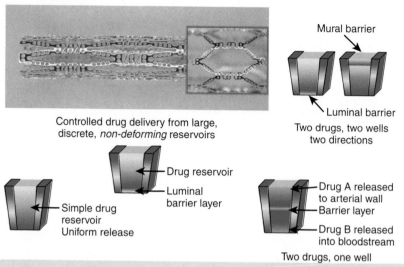

Controlled drug delivery from large,
discrete, *non-deforming* reservoirs

Mural barrier

Luminal barrier

Two drugs, two wells
two directions

Drug reservoir

Luminal
barrier layer

Simple drug
reservoir
Uniform release

Drug A released
to arterial wall

Barrier layer

Drug B released
into bloodstream

Two drugs, one well

Figure 40.9:
The Connor device – a unique stent design.

the best formulations (10 ug/30 day and 30 ug/30 day) being tested on a cobalt chromium Connor stent platform (EuroSTAR trial).

POTENTIAL PROBLEM AREAS

Making PCI safe

Adjunctive therapy

Clopidogrel Since the mid-1990s anti-platelet therapy has been the corner-stone of safe stenting. Recently published data suggests that pre-loading >6 hours with Clopidogrel improves outcome (CREDO[58] (Fig. 40.10)). Some data support the use of 600 mg of Clopidogrel ISAR-REACT[59]. Clopidogrel resistance, its frequency and significance are as yet unresolved.[60,61]

It is clear that with the advent of DES and the potential risk of stent thrombosis (Fig. 40.11) due to the presence of polymer or reduction in rate of re-endothelialisation, dual anti-platelet therapy should be continued, especially in complex cases, for a minimum six months and maybe even for a year with Aspirin being continued forever, although there is no data to support any of these strategies.

GP IIbIIIa The use of GpIIbIIIa during PCI has been well established with Abciximab having been shown to benefit ACS patients, and diabetics undergoing intervention[62–65] Fig. 40.12. Use of Abciximab in patients requiring intervention following an acute event (AMI) has been strengthened by the ADMIRAL[65] trial those receiving ReoPro had a cumulative six-month end-point of 7.4% compared to 15.9% in controls (p=0.02). However, this difference was driven by those patients receiving treatment in a mobile intensive care rather than in the emergency room or pre-procedure.

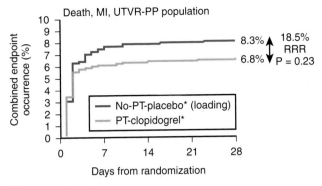

EARLY EFFECTS OF PRETREATMENT
WITH CLOPIDOGREL—28 DAY RESULTS

Figure 40.10:
The CREDO results indicating Clopidogrel given (>6 hours) pre-procedure improve outcome.

Abciximab use increased to >50% as PCI-cases became more complex, but its use has fallen back as stents and operators improve and aim for better acute results. Data suggest it may be cost effective to new anti-thrombins in more routine cases.

Anti-thrombins Anti-thrombins are sophisticated Heparins (consistency of inhibition, lack of need for intermediate anti-thombin and actions independent of

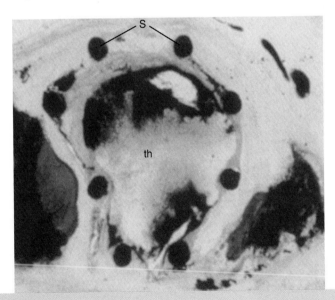

Figure 40.11:
Stent thrombosis.

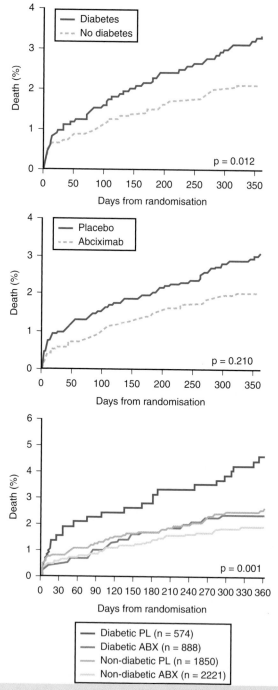

Figure 40.12:
Outcomes from use of Abciximab in diabetic patients.

platelet activity) but are more expensive. In REPLACE-2 trial 6000 patients were randomised to Bivalirudin or Heparin plus Abciximab. The results suggest no difference in 30 days outcome (composite end point reached in about 10% in both groups) and no difference in the longer term although bleeding was less in the Bivalirudin group (major bleed 2.4% versus 4.1% p<0.001).[66] The value of early ambulation, and of cost saving with bivalirudin have also been raised. Concerns have been raised as to whether the patients included are the 'high risk' who would normally have received Abciximab. While 42% included in REPLACE-2 were ACS patients we will need to await the ACUITY study of pure ACS and HORIZONS (STEMI) to have such questions answered. In the mean time bivalirudin has made some inroads into less than straightforward (but not AMI) patients undergoing PCI. They will not be cost effective for straightforward ('Heparin-alone') cases.

Stent thrombosis Stent thrombosis requires special mention although there is little randomised trial data. Late stent thrombosis due to polymer or reduced re-endothelialisation remains the concern with DES, with implications for duration of anti-platelet therapy.

Such concerns were raised through the national reporting service in 2003/4. Review of the NEW SRIUS data, the e-CYPHER registry, world-wide implant data (n=250 000) showed Cypher stent thrombosis rate to be about 0.6% (similar to BMS) and to that seen in the TAXUS IV data.

A number of recent publications have again drawn attention to stent thrombosis.

McFadden reported four cases of stent thrombosis (two Cypher, two TAXUS) all occurring between 300 and 450 days after stent implantation and all soon after both Aspirin and Clopidogrel therapy were stopped.[67]

The database consists of observational and meta-analyses.

Incidence with BMS
- A review 6058 patients with BMS indicates that stent thrombosis was 1.6%. Importantly in the context of worries about DES delayed re-endothelialisation and its impact on late stent thrombosis, 8/24 patients suffered stent thrombosis beyond six months. Overall outcome was poor; six month MACE comprised death (11%), re-infarction (16%), and recurrent stent thrombosis (12%).[68]

BMS v DES
- In a meta-analysis of ten randomised studies, stent thrombosis rate for DES was 0.58% versus 0.54% for bare metal.[69] Stented length was a predictor of thrombosis.
- In a review of 3 cohorts of patients: BMS (n=507) stent thrombosis rate=1.2%, SES (n=1017)=1.0% and PES (989)=1.0%. Mortality was 15% and AMI 60% in those who suffering stent thrombosis.[70]
- A meta-analysis of six CYPHER trials (Sirius, E-Sirius, C-Sirius, Direct, SmVelte, Ravel n=2,074) has been presented[71] stent thrombosis was recorded, as SES 0.6%, control 0.6%.
- Similarly, data from TAXUS II, IV, V, and VI studies (n=3445)[72] showed stent thrombosis from implant to six months was 0.6% for control, 0.7% for

TAXUS (p=0.68). Stent thrombosis to 2 years was 0.7% for control, 1.2% for TAXUS (p = 0.44). However, stent thrombosis between 6 and 24 months was 0.7% control and 1.2% TAXUS which was statistically significant (p=0.014). The data, therefore, do suggest a small increase in late stent thrombosis with TAXUS.

DES v DES

● The REALITY trial[18] which randomised patients to Sirolimus or Paclitaxel eluting stents suggested a non-significant increase in stent thrombosis in the PES group (0.6% versus 1.6% p=0.07)

Higher risk lesions

● Even in the thrombus rich AMI patient the stent thrombosis was not seen in any of the 186 Sirolimus patients compared to 1.6% in those in the bare metal arm (RESEARCH AMI registry).[73]

Precipitating factors

● Certain factors predict stent thrombosis, including stent under-expansion and residual reference diameter,[74] supporting the concept that DES-use is not an excuse for inadequate technique. Most importantly discontinuation of anti-platelet therapy is the most powerful predictor of stent thrombosis (Fig. 40.13).

How long dual anti-platelet therapy should be continued for is unresolved. Further, what to do about the need to stop, versus the risk of stopping, such drugs for non-cardiac procedures and operations is unclear.

In summary we are unsure whether there is an additional problem of stent thrombosis with DES greater than that seen in the BMS era. We are unsure of the incidence of late stent thrombosis and we do not know, therefore, how long to recommend dual anti-platelet therapy for and what to recommend when patients need a non-cardiac surgical procedure. This will require ongoing monitoring.

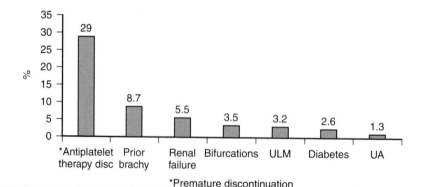

Figure 40.13:
The most common cause of stent thrombosis (thought to be in the order of 2%) is premature discontinuation of anti-platelet therapy.

Trials of diabetes include:

- CARDia (Coronary Revascularisation in Diabetes) is a UK multi-centre trial which will randomise 600 diabetic patients with multi-vessel or complex single-vessel disease to BMS-PCI, DES-PCI or CABG in a 1:1:2 ratio. The primary endpoint is death, MI or CVA at 1 year.
- FREEDOM (Future Revascularization Evaluation in Patients with Diabetes Mellitus: Optimal Management of Multi-vessel Disease) is a NHLBI multi-centre trial that will randomise 2300 patients to DES-PCI or CABG. The primary endpoint is five-year mortality.

Others

- SYNTAX trial. This is an important trial of LMS or three vessel disease randomised to PCI or surgery (n=1500) with separate surgical and PCI registries for patients only considered treatable with one of the procedures.

REFERENCES

1. Pocock SJ, Henderson RA, Rickards AF, *et al*. Meta-analysis of randomised trials comparing coronary angioplasty with bypass surgery. Lancet. 1995 Nov 4; 346(8984):1184–9.

2. Serruys PW, de Jaegere P, Kiemeneij F, *et al*. A comparison of balloon-expandable-stent implantation with balloon angioplasty in patients with coronary artery disease. Benestent Study Group. New England Journal of Medicine. 1994 Aug 25; 331(8):489–95.

3. Mehilli J, Kastrati A, Dirschinger J, *et al*. Comparison of stenting with balloon angioplasty for lesions of small coronary vessels in patients with diabetes mellitus. Am J Med 2002 Jan; 112(1):13–18.

4. Serruys P, Unger F, Sosa J, *et al*. Comparison of CABG and stenting for the treatment of multivessel disease. N Engl J Med 2001; 344:1117–24.

5. SOS authors. Coronary artery bypass surgery versus percutaneous coronary intervention with stent implantation in patients with multivessel coronary artery disease (the Stent or Surgery trial): a randomised controlled trial. Lancet 2002; 360:965–70.

6. Rodriguez A, Bernardi V, Navia J, *et al*. Argentine Randomized Study: Coronary Angioplasty with Stenting versus Coronary Bypass Surgery in patients with Multiple-Vessel Disease (ERACI II): 30-day and one-year follow-up results. ERACI II Investigators. J Am Coll Cardiol 2001; 37:51–8.

7. Morice M, Serruys P, Sousa J, *et al*. A randomised comparison of a sirolimus-eluting stent with a standard stent for coronary revascularisation. N Engl J Med 2002; 346:1773–80.

8. Moses JW, Leon MB, Popma JJ, Fitzgerald PJ, Holmes DR, O'Shaughnessy C, Caputo RP, Kereiakes DJ, Williams DO, Teirstein PS, Jaeger JL, Kuntz RE; SIRIUS Investigators. Sirolimus-eluting stents versus standard stents in patients with stenosis in a native coronary artery. N Engl J Med. 2003; 349:1315–23.

9. Schampaert E, Cohen EA, Schluter M, *et al.* The Canadian study of the sirolimus-eluting stent in the treatment of patients with long de novo lesions in small native coronary arteries (C-SIRIUS). J Am Coll Cardiol 2004; 43:1110–15.

10. Schofer J, Schluter M, Gershlick AH, *et al.* Sirolimus–eluting stents for treatment of patients with long atherosclerotic lesions in small coronary arteries: double-blind, randomised controlled trial (E-SIRIUS). Lancet 2003; 362:1093–9.

11. Sabate M, Jimenez-Quevedo P, Angiovillo D, *et al.* Sirolimus-eluting stent to prevent restenosis after stenting in diabetic patients with de novo coronary stenoses: The DIABETES Trial: 9 month angiographic results. Am J Cardiol 2004; 94(suppl6A):75E.

12. Gershlick A, De Scheerder I, Chevalier B. Inhibition of restenosis with a paclitaxel-eluting, polymer-free coronary stent: the European evaLUation of pacliTaxel Eluting Stent (ELUTES) trial. Circulation. 2004 Feb 3; 109(4):487–93.

13. Hong MK, Mintz GS, Lee CW. Paclitaxel coating reduces in-stent intimal hyperplasia in human coronary arteries: a serial volumetric intravascular ultrasound analysis from the Asian Paclitaxel-Eluting Stent Clinical Trial (ASPECT). Circulation. 2003 Feb 4; 107(4):517–20.

14. Colombo A, Drzewiecki J, Banning A. Randomized study to assess the effectiveness of slow- and moderate-release polymer-based paclitaxel-eluting stents for coronary artery lesions. Circulation. 2003 Aug 19; 108(7):788–94.

15. Stone G, Ellis S, Cox D, *et al.* One year clinical results with the slow-release, polymer-based, paclitaxel-eluting stent: the TAXUS IV trial. Circulation 2004; 109:1942–47.

16. Kastrati A, Dibra A, Mehilli J. ISAR-DIABETES: Paclitaxel-Eluting Stent Versus Sirolimus-Eluting Stent for the Prevention of Restenosis in Diabetic Patients With Coronary Artery Disease Late breaking session ACC 2005.

17. Dawkins K, Grube E, Guagliumi G, *et al.* Clinical efficacy of polymer-based, paclitaxel-eluting stents in the treatment of complex, long coronary artery lesions from a multicentre, randomised trial: support for the use of drug-eluting stents in clinical practice. Circulation 2005 (in press).

18. Morice MC, Serruys P, Colombo A, *et al.* Eight-Month Outcome of the Reality Study: A Prospective Randomized Multi-Center Head-to-Head Comparison of the Sirolimus-Eluting Stent (Cypher) and the Paclitaxel-Eluting Stent (Taxus). Session Number 22: Late-breaking Clinical Trials in Interventional Cardiology, American College of Cardiology Annual Scientific Sessions, Sunday, March 6th, 2005, 9.30 AM–10.30 AM.

19. Windecker S, Remondino A, Erbeli F. Nine-Months results From the SIRTAX Trial A Randomized Comparison of a Sirolimus With a Paclitaxel Stent For Coronary Revascularization. Session number 25: Late breaking Clinical Trials and Trial Updates, American College of Cardiology Annual Scientific Sessions, Sunday, March 6th, 2005, 4.00 PM–5.30 PM.

20. Gershlick A, Guagliumi G, Guyon P, *et al.* Comparison of outcomes for Sirolimus-Eluting stent in the e-CYPHER Registry with those from the randomised controlled trials. JACC (Abst) 45 p 50A 2005.

21. Lemos PA, Serruys PW, van Domburg RT, *et al.* Unrestricted utilization of sirolimus-eluting stents compared with conventional bare stent implantation in the "real world": the

Rapamycin-Eluting Stent Evaluated At Rotterdam Cardiology Hospital (RESEARCH) registry. Circulation 2004; 109:190–5.

22. Mauri L, O'Malley AJ, Cutlip DE, Ho KK, Popma JJ, Chauhan MS, Baim DS, Cohen DJ, Kuntz RE. Effects of stent length and lesion length on coronary restenosis. Am J Cardiol 2004; 93:1340–6.

23. Mauri L, O'Malley AJ, Popma JJ, *et al*. Comparison of thrombosis and restenosis risk from stent length of sirolimus-eluting stents versus bare metal stents. Am J Cardiol. 2005; 95:1140–5.

24. Choi EU, Kwon HM, Chul-Woo. Serum Levels of Advanced Glycation End Products Are Associated with In-Stent Restenosis in Diabetic Patients. Yonsei Med J 2005 February; 46(1):78–85.

25. Dawkins K, Colombo A, Stone G. The Clinical TAXUS Benefit in Diabetic Patients is Independent of Reference Vessel Diameter and Lesion Length Abst Accepted ESC 2005.

26. Silber S, Albertsson P, Avile's FF. Guidelines for Percutaneous Coronary Interventions. The Task Force for Percutaneous Coronary Interventions of the European Society of Cardiology European Heart Journal 2005; 26:804–47.

27. Stone GW, Grines CL, Cox DA, *et al*. Comparison of angioplasty with stenting, with or without abciximab, in acute myocardial infarction. NEJM 2002; 346:957–66.

28. Grines CL, Cox DA, Stone GW, *et al*. Coronary angioplasty with or without stent implantation for acute myocardial infarction. NEJM 1999; 341:1949–56.

29. Schuhlen H, Kastrati A, Dirschinger J, *et al*. Intracoronary stenting and risk for major adverse cardiac events during the first month. Circ 1998; 98:104–11.

30. Thel MC, Califf RM, Tardiff BE, *et al*. Timing of and risk factors for myocardial ischemic events after percutaneous coronary intervention (IMPACT-II). Integrilin to minimize platelet aggrgation and coronary thrombosis. Am J Cardiol 2000; 85:427–34.

31. Saia F, Lemos PA, Lee CH, *et al*. Sirolimus-eluting stent implantation in ST-elevation acute myocardial infarction: a clinical and angiographic study. Circulation. 2003 Oct 21; 108(16):1927–9. Epub 2003.

32. Lemos PA, Saia F, Hofma SH, *et al*. Short- and long-term clinical benefit of sirolimus-eluting stents compared to conventional bare stents for patients with acute myocardial infarction. JACC 2004; 43:704–8.

33. Gershlick AH, Lota C, Urban P, *et al*. treatment of acute myocardial infarction with sirolimus-eluting coronary stents: midterm results from the e-Cypher international registry. Am J Cardiol 2004; 94: 208S abs.

34. Lemos PA, Lee CH, Degertekin M, *et al*. Early outcome after sirolimus-eluting stent implantation in patients with acute coronary syndromes: insights from the Rapamycin-Eluting Stent Evaluated At Rotterdam cardiology Hospital (RESEARCH) registry. JACC 2003; 41:2093–9.

35. Moses JW, Mehran R, Nikolsky E, *et al*. Outcomes with the paclitaxel-eluting stent in patients with acute coronary syndromes. Analysis from the TAXUS-IV trial. JACC 2005; 45:1165–71.

36. Ong ATL, Serruys PW, Aoki J, *et al.* The unrestricted use of paclitaxel- vs sirolimus-eluting stents for coronary artery disease in an unselected population. JACC 2005; 45:1135–41.

37. Vermeersch PH, Van Langenhove G, Verheye S. First Randomized Trial Comparing Sirolimus-Eluting Versus Bare Metal Stents in Severely Diseased Saphenous Vein Graft Treatment: Six-Month Clinical and Angiographic Outcome Presnted at the ACC 2005.

38. Hoye A, Lemos PA, Arampatzis CA, *et al.* Effectiveness of the sirolimus-eluting stent in the treatment of saphenous vein graft disease. J Invasive Cardiol 2004; 16:230–3.

39. Ge L, Iakovou I, Sangiorgi GM, *et al.* Treatment of saphenous vein graft lesions with drug-eluting stents: immediate and midterm outcome. J Am Coll Cardiol 2005; 45:989–94.

40. Colombo A, Moses JW, Morice MC, *et al.* Randomized Study to Evaluate Sirolimus-Eluting Stents Implanted at Coronary Bifurcation Lesions. Circulation 2004; 109:1244–9.

41. Louvard Y, Colombo A, Raghu C, *et al.* Sirolimus-eluting stents in bifurcation lesions:six-month angiographic results according to the implantation technique. J Am Coll Cardiol 2003; 41:53A.

42. Simes PA, Golf S, Myreng Y, *et al.* Stenting in Chronic Coronary Occlusion (SICCO): A randomised, controlled trial of adding stent implantation after successful angioplasty. J Am Coll Cardiol 1996; 28:1444–51.

43. Hoye A, Tanabe K, Lemos PA, Aoki J, Saia F, Arampatzis C, Degertekin M, Hofma SH, Sianos G, McFadden E, van der Giessen WJ, Smits PC, de Feyter PJ, van Domburg RT, Serruys PW. Significant Reduction in Restenosis After the Use of Sirolimus-Eluting Stents in the Treatment of Chronic Total Occlusions. J Am Coll Cardio 2004; 43:1954–8.

44. Werner GS, Krack A, Schwarz G, Prochnau D, Betge S, Figureulla HR. Prevention of Lesion Recurrence in Chronic Total Coronary Occlusions by Paclitaxel-Eluting Stents. J Am Coll Cardiol 2004; 44:2301–6.

45. Silvestri M, Barragan P, Sainsous J. Unprotected left main coronary artery stenting: immediate and medium-term outcomes of 140 elective procedures. J Am Coll Cardiol. 2000 May; 35(6):1543–50.

46. Tan WA, Tamai H, Park SJ. Long-term clinical outcomes after unprotected left main trunk percutaneous revascularization in 279 patients. Circulation. 2001 Oct 2; 104(14):1609–14.

47. Gershlick A, Guagliumi G, Guyon P, *et al.* Comparison of outcomes for Sirolimus-Eluting stent in the e-CYPHER Registry with those from the randomised controlled trials. JACC (Abst) 45 p 50A 2005.

48. Valgimigli M, van Mieghem CA. Ong AT Short- and long-term clinical outcome after drug-eluting stent implantation for the percutaneous treatment of left main coronary artery disease: insights from the Rapamycin-Eluting and Taxus Stent Evaluated At Rotterdam Cardiology Hospital registries (RESEARCH and T-SEARCH).Circulation. 2005 Mar 22; 111(11):1383–9.

49. Park SJ, Kim YH, Lee BK, Lee SW. Sirolimus-eluting stent implantation for unprotected left main coronary artery stenosis: comparison with bare metal stent implantation. J Am Coll Cardiol. 2005 Feb 1; 45(3):351–6.

50. Chieffo A, Stankovic G, Bonizzoni E. Early and mid-term results of drug-eluting stent implantation in unprotected left main. Circulation. 2005 Feb 15; 111(6):791–5.

51. Gershlick A, Guagliumi G, Guyon P, *et al*. Comparison of outcomes for Sirolimus-Eluting stent in the e-CYPHER Registry with those from the randomised controlled trials. JACC (Abst) 45 p 50A 2005.

52. Kastrati A, Mehilli J, von Beckerath N, *et al*. Sirolimus-eluting stent or paclitaxel-eluting stent vs balloon angioplasty for prevention of recurrences in patients with coronary in-stent restenosis: a randomized controlled trial. JAMA. 2005 12; 293(2):165–71.

53. Serruys PW. ARTS II: Arterial Revascularization Therapies Study Part II –Sirolimus-Eluting Stents vs PCI and CABG at 1 Year. American College of Cardiology Annual Scientific Sessions 2005.

54. Buellesfeld L, Grube E ABT–578-Eluting Stents The Promising Successor of Sirolimus- and Paclitaxel-Eluting Stent Concepts? Herz. 2004 Mar; 29(2):167–70.

55. Wijns W, Fajadet JP, *et al*. Results of the ENDEAVOR II trial Late-breaking Clinical Trials in Interventional Cardiology, American College of Cardiology Annual Scientific Sessions, Sunday, March 6th, 2005.

56. Ellis SG, Jeffrey J, Popma JJ, Lasala JM, *et al*. Relationship between angiographic late loss and target lesion revascularization after coronary stent implantation: analysis from the TAXUS-IV Trial J. Am Coll Cardiolo 2005; 45:1193–200.

57. Formica RN Jr, Lorber KM, Friedman AL. The evolving experience using everolimus in clinical transplantation. Transplant Proc. 2004 Mar; 36(2 Suppl):S495–9.

58. Aoki J, Ong ATL, Abizaid A, *et al*. One-year clinical outcome of various doses and pharmacokinetic releaseof paclitaxel eluted from an erodable polymer – insights from thepaclitaxel in-stent controlled elution study (PISCES) JACC Vol. 46, Issue 2, 19 July 2005, Pages 253–60 Posted 7/15/2005.

59. Steinhubl SR, Berger PB, Mann JT 3rd. Early and sustained dual oral antiplatelet therapy following percutaneous coronary intervention: a randomized controlled trial. JAMA. 2002 Nov 20; 288(19):2411–20.

60. Kandzari DE, Berger PB, Kastrati A. Influence of treatment duration with a 600-mg dose of clopidogrel before percutaneous coronary revascularization Journal of the American College of Cardiology 44, 2004, 2133–6.

61. Wenaweser P, Dörffler-Melly J, Imboden K, *et al*. Stent Thrombosis is associated with an impaired response to antiplatelet therapy. J Am Coll Cardiolo 2005, 45:1748–52.

62. Steinhubl SR, Charnigo R, Moliterno DJ. Resistance to antiplatelet resistance is it justified. J Am Coll Cardiol. 2005 Jun 7; 45(11):1757–8.

63. Topol EJ, Moliterno DJ, Herrmann HC, *et al*. Comparison of two platelet glycoprotein IIb/IIIa inhibitors, Tirofiban and abciximab, for the prevention of ischaemic events with percutaneous coronary revascularisation. N Engl J Med 2001; 344:1888–94.

64. Bhatt DL, Marso SP, Lincoff AM. Abciximab reduces mortality in diabetics following percutaneous coronary intervention. J Am Coll Cardiol. 2000 Mar 15; 35(4):922–8.

65. Atwater BD, Roe MT, Mahaffey KW. Platelet glycoprotein IIb/IIIa receptor antagonists in non-ST segment elevation acute coronary syndromes: a review and guide to patient selection. Drugs. 2005; 65(3):313–24.

66. Montalescot G, Barragan P, Wittenberg O. Platelet glycoprotein IIb/IIIa inhibition with coronary stening for acute myocardial infarction The ADMIRAL Trial NEJM 2001; 344: 1895–1903.

67. Lincoff AM, Kleiman NS, Kereiakes DJ. Long-term efficacy of bivalirudin and provisional glycoprotein IIb/IIIa blockade vs heparin and planned glycoprotein IIb/IIIa blockade during percutaneous coronary revascularization: REPLACE-2 randomized trial. JAMA. 2004 Aug 11; 292(6):696–703.

68. McFadden E, Sile E, Regar E, *et al*. Late thrombosis in drug-eluting coronary stents after discontinuation of anti-platelet therapy. The Lancet 2004; 364:1519–21.

69. Wenaweser P, Rey C, Eberli FR, *et al*. Stent thrombosis following bare-metal stent implantation: success of emergency Percutaneous coronary intervention and predictors of adverse outcome. European Heart Journal 2005; 26:1180–7.

70. Moreno R, Fernández C, Hernández R, *et al*. Drug-eluting stent thrombosis: results from a pooled analysis including 10 randomized studies. J Am Coll Cardiol 2005; 45:954–9.

71. Ong AT, Hoye A, Aoki J, *et al*. Thirty-day incidence and six-month clinical outcome of thrombotic stent occlusion after bare-metal, sirolimus, or paclitaxel stent implantation. J Am Coll Cardiol 2005; 45:947–53.

72. Leon MB. Cypher Update. Presented at American College of Cardiology, March 2005. Available at www.tctmd.com

73. Stone GW. Metanalysis of Taxus II, IV, V and VI. Presented at American College of Cardiology, March 2005. Available at www.tctmd.com

74. Saia F, Lemos PA, Lee CH, *et al*. Sirolimus-eluting stent implantation in ST-elevation acute myocardial infarction: a clinical and angiographic study. Circ 2003; 108:1927–9.

75. Fujii K, Carlier SG, Mintz GS, *et al*. Stent underexpansion and residual reference segment stenosis are related to stent thrombosis after sirolimus-eluting stent implantation: an intravascular ultrasound study. J Am Coll Cardiol 2005; 45:995–8.

Index

Index

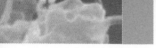

Index